Food–Drug Synergy and Safety

Food–Drug Synergy and Safety

edited by

Lilian U. Thompson
Wendy E. Ward

Taylor & Francis
Taylor & Francis Group

Boca Raton London New York Singapore

A CRC title, part of the Taylor & Francis imprint, a member of the Taylor & Francis Group, the academic division of T&F Informa plc.

Published in 2006 by
CRC Press
Taylor & Francis Group
6000 Broken Sound Parkway NW, Suite 300
Boca Raton, FL 33487-2742

Printed in the United States of America on acid-free paper
10 9 8 7 6 5 4 3 2 1

International Standard Book Number-10: 0-8493-2775-X (Hardcover)
International Standard Book Number-13: 978-0-8493-2775-9 (Hardcover)
Library of Congress Card Number 20050505072

Library of Congress Cataloging-in-Publication Data

Food-drug synergy and safety / edited by Lilian U. Thompson, Wendy E. Ward.
p. cm.
Includes bibliographical references and index.
ISBN 0-8493-2775-X (alk. paper)
1. Drug-nutrient interactions. 2. Drug synergism. 3. Drugs--Safety measures. I. Thompson, Lilian U. II. Ward, Wendy E.

RM302.4.F66 2005
615'.70452--dc22

20050505072

Taylor & Francis Group
is the Academic Division of T&F Informa plc.

Visit the Taylor & Francis Web site at
http://www.taylorandfrancis.com

and the CRC Press Web site at
http://www.crcpress.com

Preface

Elucidating and understanding the potential benefits of food synergy or food–drug synergy are exciting and emerging areas in food, nutrition, and pharmaceutical sciences. Scientific evidence that food synergy and food–drug synergy play an important role in the prevention or management of chronic disease is promising, but the field is in its infancy. In addition to scientific interest in food synergy and food–drug synergy, consumers are increasingly interested in these relationships as they strive to prevent or treat specific diseases by combining a healthful food or diet with pharmacological agents prescribed by their physicians. Results of a follow-up national survey in the United States reported that in 1997, a total of 15 million adults combined drug therapies with alternative therapies, including high-dose vitamins and herbal remedies. Moreover, food companies are marketing a myriad of products that incorporate multiple food components that are known to have healthful effects when consumed individually; however, their combined effect often remains to be determined.

Because of promising scientific data, as well as interest from consumers and the food industry, there is a genuine need to focus attention on the topic of food and food–drug synergy at this time. We have put together this book to both encourage and provide a basis for scientists to design and conduct studies that elucidate food and food–drug synergies. There are few studies that have examined food and food–drug synergy so some topics have a dearth of information available now. Moreover, there are several examples of food and food–drug synergy discussed in the book that are still in the process of publication, emphasizing that this is a cutting-edge area of research.

The book is divided into seven sections with one or more chapters per section. In Section I, the introduction defines and highlights the area of food and food–drug synergy as a significant, emerging area of research focus. Sections II through V are organized to discuss the major chronic diseases and/or diseases of aging such as cardiovascular disease, cancer, osteoporosis, inflammatory diseases, hypertension, and obesity. A chapter on ergogenics, including caffeine, creatine, and ephedrine and/or ephedra, is included in Section 6 because of interest in performance enhancers, and, moreover, there is evidence that these aids may have the potential to influence human health in addition to having ergogenic applications. Within Sections II through VI, the following aspects are discussed in each chapter: food synergy and potential health benefits; food–drug synergy and potential health benefits; and safety aspects that pertain to the food and/or food–drug synergies that are discussed. The final section of the book is devoted to experimental designs for determining not only the health aspects but also the safety aspects of food and food–drug synergy. This is a particularly exciting section as these chapters provide a framework that scientists can use to design experiments to elucidate these synergies.

Most current books on foods and drugs focus on the adverse health effects of foods and drugs. A unique feature of this book is that the focus is on the potential healthful effects of combining foods with drugs, while still considering potential adverse effects, providing a balanced perspective of how foods and drugs can be used in combination to prevent or treat chronic disease. Another unique aspect of this book is that topics are grouped according to disease rather than by a specific food or drug, making it easier for readers to relate both food and drugs to the same specific disease

It is our fervent hope that this book encourages food, nutritional and pharmaceutical scientists, medical and pharmaceutical practitioners, and the food industry to investigate the vast potential to use foods in combination with other foods or with drugs, ultimately leading to improvements in the overall health of our society through the beneficial effects of food and food–drug synergy.

We thank Susan Farmer and Pat Roberson for their support and editorial assistance at CRC Press, and the authors for participating in this endeavor despite their very busy schedules.

We express our sincere thanks to our families for their unconditional support of our academic pursuits.

Lilian U. Thompson and Wendy E. Ward
Department of Nutritional Sciences
Faculty of Medicine
University of Toronto

The Editors

Dr. Lilian U. Thompson obtained her Ph.D. from University of Wisconsin in Madison and is currently a full professor in the Department of Nutritional Sciences, Faculty of Medicine, University of Toronto, Canada. She is internationally recognized for her research on components of plant foods responsible for their health benefits and/or adverse effects, their interactions with drugs, and the mechanisms of their action. She has published numerous papers in refereed journals, book chapters, and books, presented many invited papers in conferences and symposia, and served in several research granting councils and expert committees.

Dr. Wendy E. Ward obtained a Ph.D. in Medical Sciences from McMaster University, Canada, held a National Institute of Nutrition Postdoctoral Fellowship at the University of Toronto, and is currently an assistant professor in the Department of Nutritional Sciences, Faculty of Medicine, University of Toronto, Canada. Her research is focused on the mechanisms by which dietary estrogens and fatty acids regulate bone metabolism, with the long term goal of developing dietary strategies that protect against fragility fracture. Dr. Ward has published many peer-reviewed articles in the area of nutrition and bone health and book chapters on nutrition and women's health issues, particularly osteoporosis. Dr. Ward was an awardee of a Future Leader Award from the International Life Sciences Institute.

Contributors

G. Harvey Anderson
Department of Nutritional Sciences
Faculty of Medicine
University of Toronto
Toronto, Ontario, Canada

Alfred Aziz
Department of Nutritional Sciences
Faculty of Medicine
University of Toronto
Toronto, Ontario, Canada

Angelika de Bree
Unilever Health Institute
Unilever Research
Vlaardingen, The Netherlands

Russell de Souza
Clinical Nutrition & Risk Factor Modification Center
St. Michael's Hospital and Department of Nutritional Sciences
Faculty of Medicine
University of Toronto
Toronto, Ontario, Canada

Hani El-Nezami
Food and Health Research Centre
University of Kuopio
Kuopio, Finland

Azadeh Emam
Clinical Nutrition & Risk Factor Modification Center
St. Michael's Hospital and Department of Nutritional Sciences
Faculty of Medicine
University of Toronto
Toronto, Ontario, Canada

V.J. Feron
TNO — Nutrition and Food Research
Zeist, The Netherlands

Pilar Galan
UMR INSERM U557/INRA/CNAM, ISTNA-CNAM
Paris, France

Terry E. Graham
Department of Human Biology and Nutritional Sciences
University of Guelph
Guelph, Ontario, Canada

J.P. Groten
TNO — Nutrition and Food Research
Zeist, The Netherlands

R.J.J. Hermus
Department of Human Nutrition
Maastricht University
Maastricht, The Netherlands

David J.A. Jenkins
Clinical Nutrition & Risk Factor Modification Center
Department of Medicine, Division of Endocrinology and Metabolism
St. Michael's Hospital
and
Departments of Nutritional Sciences and Medicine
Faculty of Medicine
University of Toronto
Toronto, Ontario, Canada

Peter J.H. Jones
School of Dietetics and Human Nutrition
McGill University
Ste-Anne-de-Bellevue, Québec, Canada

D. Jonker
TNO — Nutrition and Food Research
Zeist, The Netherlands

Cyril W.C. Kendall
Clinical Nutrition & Risk Factor Modification Center
St. Michael's Hospital and Department of Nutritional Sciences
Faculty of Medicine
University of Toronto
Toronto, Ontario, Canada

David D. Kitts
Food, Nutrition and Health
University of British Columbia
Vancouver, British Columbia, Canada

Marlena C. Kruger
Institute of Food, Nutrition and Human Health
Massey University
Palmerston North, New Zealand

Augustine Marchie
Clinical Nutrition & Risk Factor Modification Center
St. Michael's Hospital and Department of Nutritional Sciences, Faculty of Medicine
University of Toronto
Toronto, Ontario, Canada

I. Meijerman
Biomedical Analysis, Drug Toxicology
Faculty of Pharmaceutical Science
Utrecht University
Utrecht, The Netherlands

Louise Mennen
UMR INSERM U557/INRA/CNAM, ISTNA-CNAM
Paris, France

Lesley L. Moisey
Department of Human Biology and Nutritional Sciences
University of Guelph
Guelph, Ontario, Canada

G.J. Mulder
Leiden/Amsterdam Center for Drug Research
Leiden University
Leiden, The Netherlands

Akira Murakami
Division of Food Science and Biotechnology
Graduate School of Agriculture
Kyoto University
Kyoto, Japan

Hannu Mykkänen
Department of Clinical Nutrition
University of Kuopio
Kuopio, Finland

Hajime Ohigashi
Division of Food Science and Biotechnology
Graduate School of Agriculture
Kyoto University
Kyoto, Japan

Raewyn C. Poulsen
Institute of Food, Nutrition and Human Health
Massey University
Palmerston North, New Zealand

Kedar N. Prasad
Premier Micronutrient Corporation
Antioxidant Research Institute
Novato, California

Eeva Salminen
Department of Oncology
University of Turku
Turku, Finland

Seppo Salminen
Functional Foods Forum
University of Turku
Turku, Finland

F. Salmon
TNO — Nutrition and Food Research
Zeist, The Netherlands

E.D. Schoen
TNO TPD
Delft, The Netherlands

Joanne Slavin
Department of Food Science and Nutrition
University of Minnesota
St. Paul, Minnesota

Lyn M. Steffen
Division of Epidemiology and Community Health
School of Public Health
University of Minnesota
Minneapolis, Minnesota

Lilian U. Thompson
Department of Nutritional Sciences
Faculty of Medicine
University of Toronto
Toronto, Ontario, Canada

Rob M. van Dam
Department of Nutrition and Health
Faculty of Earth and Life Sciences
Vrije Universiteit Amsterdam
Amsterdam, The Netherlands

Krista A. Varady
School of Dietetics and Human Nutrition
McGill University
Ste-Anne-de-Bellevue, Québec, Canada

Manuel T. Velasquez
Division of Renal Diseases and Hypertension
Department of Medicine
George Washington University Medical Center
Washington, D.C.

Wendy E. Ward
Department of Nutritional Sciences
Faculty of Medicine
University of Toronto
Toronto, Ontario, Canada

Julia M.W. Wong
Clinical Nutrition & Risk Factor Modification Center
St. Michael's Hospital and Department of Nutritional Sciences
Faculty of Medicine
University of Toronto
Toronto, Ontario, Canada

Jin-Rong Zhou
Nutrition/Metabolism Laboratory
Beth Israel Deaconess Medical
Center
Harvard Medical School
Boston, Massachusetts

Contents

Section VI Ergogenics

Section VII Experimental Designs

Section I

Introduction

1

Understanding Food and Food–Drug Synergy

Wendy E. Ward and Lilian U. Thompson

CONTENTS

1.1 Introduction

Nutrition has a unique and important role in the prevention and treatment of chronic disease. From a prevention perspective, many individuals modify their diet, even subtly, to modify their risk of chronic diseases. Some common reasons for dietary modifications include improving blood lipid profile, controlling blood glucose, maintaining a healthy body weight, and ensuring adequate calcium in the diet to maintain a strong skeleton. While using foods to promote health seems intuitive, delineating the complex interactions within a food and among different foods is challenging and at times perplexing. Moreover, when combining foods with drugs, there are additional interactions, positive or negative, that can influence health outcomes. Using the diet to promote optimal health requires knowledge of the beneficial effects resulting from these interactions among foods, individual food components, and/or drugs.

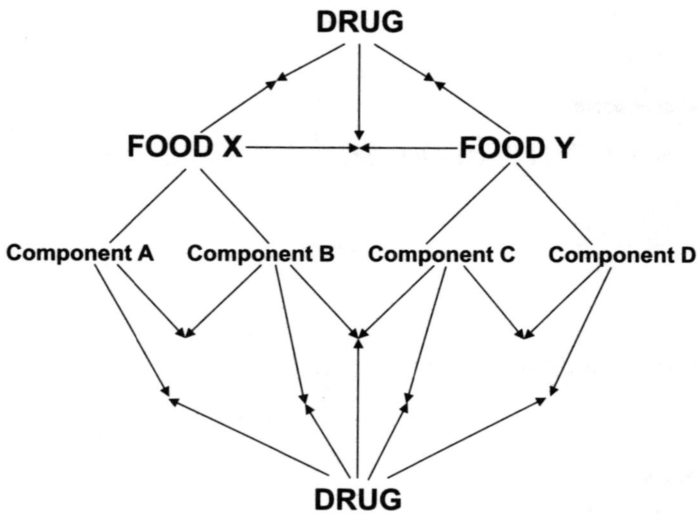

FIGURE 1.1
Potential synergistic interactions of foods and/or drugs.

1.2 Definitions

As shown in Figure 1.1, there are multiple interactions that can occur among foods; components within a food; components from different foods; foods and drugs; or individual food components and drugs. Because of the wide variety of interactions, there is a vast potential for synergistic relationships to be observed.

What is food synergy and food–drug synergy? In the context of this book, food synergy encompasses the following:

- The interaction of two or more components within a food or of two or more foods working together such that the potential health benefit is greater than the effect of the single component or food;
- The additive effects of multiple foods or food components that confer a health benefit;
- The ability of a food or food component to attenuate or negate an unwanted side effect of another food or food component.

Similarly, food–drug synergy includes the following:

- The interaction of a food (or food component) and a specific drug that confers a greater health benefit than either the food (or food component) or drug alone;

- The additive effects of a drug in combination with a food (or food component) that confer a health benefit;
- The ability of a food (or food component) to attenuate or negate a negative side effect of a drug.

1.3 Significance

Why is it important to study food synergy or food–drug synergy? While many individuals alter their diet in an attempt to prevent or delay the development of a chronic disease, many patients also change their diet after the diagnosis of a chronic disease. Since patients are often prescribed a specific drug or multiple drugs to manage a disease, alterations in their diet while taking one or more drugs may prove harmful or helpful. There is the potential for specific foods and/or individual components in a food to interact favorably with a drug such that a lower dose or shorter duration of taking the drug is required, or a decreased adverse reaction is observed. It may also be possible that with the right combination of foods the same effect as the drug alone can be achieved; thus, the need for the drug can be eliminated.

Much of the scientific information about the biological effects of foods is from studies in which the effects of individual foods or food components have been studied in isolation. Although such studies are useful in demonstrating their efficacy, foods are consumed in combination with other foods and sometimes in combination with one or more drugs. Therefore, it is important to consider the interactions of multiple foods and/or foods and drugs with respect to both beneficial and adverse effects.

Most current books focus on the adverse health effects of foods and drugs. A unique feature of this book is that it focuses on the potential healthful effects of combining foods with drugs, while still considering potential adverse effects, thus providing a balanced perspective of how foods and drugs can be used in combination to improve or promote health. Another unique aspect of this book is that topics are grouped according to disease, rather than discussing foods or drugs in isolation. This facilitates the linking of certain foods or food components and drugs to a specific disease.

1.4 Examples of Food Synergy

Throughout this book there are many examples of food synergy but a few are summarized here. While the mechanisms involved with each food synergy are not sometimes known, it is possible that foods or food components may act by similar or complementary mechanisms. They may also have opposing mechanisms, which may negate an undesirable effect of one or more foods or food components.

Examples of food and/or food components working together to achieve an additive or synergistic effect include those in the:

DASH (Dietary Approaches to Stop Hypertension) diet, characterized by high intakes of fruits, vegetables, and low fat dairy products, in combination with a low sodium diet; results in significant lowering of blood pressure;

Portfolio diet, containing plant sterols, viscous fibers, and soy protein; demonstrates reductions in serum low-density lipoprotein (LDL) cholesterol similar to traditional statin drugs;

Mediterranean diet, consisting of a high intake of legumes, grains, fruit, and vegetables, moderate alcohol intake, low to moderate consumption of meats and dairy products, and the use of olive oil for salad dressings and cooking; has been linked to reduced risk of cardiovascular disease.

Other examples abound. The combination of garlic and fish oil has been shown to be beneficial at improving blood lipid profile to a greater extent than garlic or fish oil alone. Garlic attenuates the elevation of LDL cholesterol that occurs with fish oil intervention. With respect to weight loss, consumption of dairy products results in a greater weight reduction than taking calcium alone. This finding suggests that despite the positive effect of calcium on weight loss, additional components in dairy products act synergistically to induce weight loss. Food synergy has been demonstrated with respect to osteoporosis in an animal model. Calcium, in combination with soy isoflavones, preserves bone mineral density to a greater extent than either component alone in ovariectomized rodents. In a murine model of lupus, food restriction in combination with fish oil results in increased life span compared to food restriction or fish oil alone, and in another animal model of inflammation, a diet low in arachidonic acid in combination with fish oil attenuates rheumatoid arthritis.

There are also examples of foods or food components interacting such that a negative effect of a food or food component is attenuated by providing multiple foods, as occurs *in vivo*. Using an athymic mouse model, flaxseed has been shown to attenuate the late-stage mammary tumor–promoting activity of soy. Similarly, lignans derived from flaxseed have been shown to attenuate the late-stage mammary tumor–promoting activity of genistein, which is abundant in soy.

1.5 Examples of Food–Drug Synergy

There are several examples of food–drug synergy. Preliminary results of a randomized clinical trial using high dose multiple antioxidants in combination with chemotherapy provide promising results with respect to survival from non–small cell lung cancer. A commonly used cancer drug, tamoxifen, has been reported to favorably interact with soy protein isolate or flaxseed, resulting in lower tumor size and greater inhibition of chemically induced mammary tumors in rodents or human tumor xenografts in athymic mice. Administration of garlic and omeprazol results in greater inhibition of *Helicobacter pylori*, which is implicated in the etiology of gastric ulcers. Among hypertensives with type II diabetes, a low sodium diet in combination with losartan, an angiotensin II receptor blocker, results in lower blood pressure and proteinuria than the drug alone. Another example includes the synergy of calcium and hormone replacement therapy at preserving bone mineral density, a surrogate measure of risk of fragility fracture, in postmenopausal women.

Other food components attenuate the side effects of drug therapies. Examples include the use of probiotics to lessen the severity of diarrhea and abdominal pain concurrent with many antibiotic regimens and the intake of *n*-3 fatty acids to reduce the adverse side effects of some cancer drugs. The chapters within this book provide details about these and additional examples of food synergy and food–drug synergy.

1.6 Conclusions

The topic of food and food–drug synergy is in its infancy, and the number of studies investigating this area is still limited. Many of the findings discussed in the following chapters are very recent, with some examples being part of ongoing studies.

However, novel findings on beneficial health outcomes of the described food and food–drug synergies provide a solid rationale for continuing to study these types of interactions. Without question, a multitude of studies still need to be conducted on food and food–drug synergies before these interactions can be optimized and exploited in the prevention and management of chronic diseases. Healthful dietary patterns can provide guidance in identifying combinations of foods that can act synergistically. As mechanisms of action of the food, individual food components, and drugs are elucidated, selection of their proper combinations to obtain synergistic effect and optimum health outcome will become more feasible. Conducting the studies with proper experimental design, some of which are described in this book, will make certain that the observed healthful or adverse effects of foods and drugs in combination, not in isolation, are substantive and credible. The challenge is for basic scientists to provide the experimental evidence for the synergy, for the medical and pharmaceutical practitioners to recognize the potential of the marriage between food and drug in the prevention and management of disease, for the food industries to apply the synergies in the formulation of healthful food products, and for the consumers to understand the proper combinations of foods and drugs to help in the maintenance of their optimum health or in the management of their disease. We hope this book will help stimulate and inspire others to do more work in this important scientific endeavor.

Section II

Cardiovascular Disease

2

Lipid Sources and Plant Sterols: Effect of Food and Food–Drug Synergy on Cardiovascular Disease Risk

Krista A. Varady and Peter J.H. Jones

CONTENTS

2.1 Introduction

Though multiple pharmacological treatments for cardiovascular disease exist, it has been shown that certain dietary interventions or supplements may provide similar, yet more cost-effective, benefits. Certain dietary fat constituents, occurring either as natural components of food or as nutritional supplements, have been shown to favorably alter indicators of cardiovascular disease risk when administered to various population groups. Examples of such lipid compounds include fish oils, medium chain triglycerides (MCT), and plant sterols. Though the independent effects of these compounds have been thoroughly studied, their cardioprotective effects when administered in combination have yet to be fully defined. Therefore, the aim of this chapter is to examine whether a synergistic relationship exists between certain dietary fat constituents and whether this synergy alters cardiovascular risk parameters in a way that is more beneficial than that of each intervention alone. Additionally, the potential synergistic relationships between certain dietary lipids and drug therapies used to treat cardiovascular disease are also elucidated. Furthermore, the safety profiles of these foods when administered alone, or in combination, are explored.

2.2 Food Synergy and Cardiovascular Disease

2.2.1 Fish Oil

Polyunsaturated fatty acids, which include n-3 and n-6 fatty acids, are essential for human health and must be consumed as a part of the diet.[1] While the n-3 fatty acid α-linolenic acid (ALA) is available from certain plants, eicosapentanoic acid (EPA) and docosahexanoic acid (DHA) are derived from fish and fish oils. Interest in n-3 fatty acids first arose when it was discovered that the Greenland Inuit experienced low mortality from cardiovascular disease, despite having a diet that was high in fat.[2] Eventually, it was proposed that this decreased risk in mortality could be attributed to the high content of n-3 fatty acids in their diet, which was derived from fish, whale, and seal.[2] Since then several studies have tested the hypothesis that fish oil consumption is associated with a decrease a risk of cardiovascular disease.

Results from numerous recent epidemiological studies have shown an inverse association between fish consumption and the risk of cardiovascular disease.[3,4] In a systematic review of 11 cohort trials,[5] it was concluded that an increased intake of fish markedly decreased cardiovascular disease mortality. In addition to epidemiological and observational evidence, several clinical investigations have tested the cause and effect relationship between fish oil administration and cardiovascular disease risk. In a meta-analysis by Harris,[6] fish oils were shown to consistently lower triglyceride concentrations, while low-density lipoprotein (LDL) cholesterol and high-density lipoprotein (HDL) cholesterol levels were shown to either not change or increase slightly. Similar findings have been noted in other recent clinical intervention trials.[7,8] Thus, although epidemiological studies show that fish oils decrease cardiovascular risk, results from clinical investigations suggest that the cardioprotective effect of fish oils still requires further clarification.

2.2.1.1 Fish Oil Combined with Olive Oil

Since fish oil supplementation alone has been shown repeatedly to decrease the risk of cardiovascular disease, researchers questioned whether there would be an additive or synergistic effect of fish oils when combined with other lipid constituents known for their antiatherogenic effect. One such dietary fat, olive oil, known for its hypocholesterolemic effect,[9,10] soon became a likely candidate for such a combination therapy. In a recent study by Ramirez-Tortosa et al.,[11] the effect of fish oil (16 g/d) combined with olive oil on indicators of cardiovascular disease risk was examined in a randomized, crossover trial. Consumption of olive oil plus fish oil for a period of 3 months significantly decreased plasma triglyceride concentrations when compared with the olive oil and control phases, but had no effect on total, LDL cholesterol, or HDL cholesterol concentrations.[11] Additionally, the susceptibility of LDL to Cu-mediated oxidation was lower in the patients consuming the combination therapy than in the control group.[11] Nestares et al.[12] tested similar objectives in a 15-month crossover trial that included a control diet phase, an olive oil supplement phase, and a fish oil plus olive oil phase. Results from this trial demonstrated that the intake of fish oil combined with olive oil resulted in significantly decreased concentrations of LDL cholesterol when compared with the olive oil, and control phases. However, the combination therapy had no effect on any other lipid parameter measured. Contrary to these findings, when Vognild et al.[13] tested the effect of cod liver oil (15 ml/d) combined with olive oil on cardiovascular disease risk parameters, no significant differences in serum lipid response were found. Therefore, whether the combination of fish oil and olive oil decreases cardiovascular risk more than each constituent alone still needs further clarification. While certain trials demonstrate favorable results with respect to decreasing both LDL cholesterol and triglyceride concentrations, others exhibit no such effect. Thus, more randomized, placebo controlled, clinical trials that test the effect of fish oil combined with olive oil still need to be performed before any definitive conclusions can be made.

2.2.1.2 Fish Oil Combined with γ-Linolenic Acid

The effect of fish oil supplementation in combination with other dietary fats on plasma lipid profiles has also been tested. In a study by Leng et al.,[14] the effect of EPA in combination with γ-linolenic acid on cholesterol concentrations and the number of recurrent cardiovascular disease events was investigated. After 2 years of supplementation, no difference between the treatment and placebo groups was noted with regards to total, LDL cholesterol, HDL cholesterol, or triglyceride concentrations. However, those consuming the combination therapy did experience a slight decrease in cardiovascular disease events when compared with the control group. Thus, these data suggest that although this combination therapy may not affect lipid profiles, the trend toward fewer coronary events in those consuming the combination of EPA and γ-linolenic acid warrants further investigation.

2.2.1.3 Fish Oil Combined with Garlic

In addition to combining fish oil with other dietary fats, the effect of these n-3 fatty acids in combination with nonlipid food constituents has also been examined. In a randomized, placebo controlled clinical trial,[15] the effects of garlic (900 mg/d) and fish oil (12 g/d) supplementation, alone and in combination, on serum lipids in hypercholesterolemic subjects was examined. After 12 weeks, total cholesterol concentrations decreased by 12.2 and 11.5% in the combination and garlic groups, respectively, but showed no difference with fish oil alone. LDL cholesterol concentrations were reduced by 9.5 and 14.2% in the combination and garlic groups, respectively, but were raised by 8.5% with fish oil alone. Conversely, triglyceride concentrations were reduced by 34.3% in the combination group and by 37.3% with fish oil alone. From this, the authors concluded that the combination of garlic and fish oil has the ability to reverse the moderate fish oil–induced rise in LDL cholesterol levels. Additionally, it was concluded that the coadministration of garlic with fish oil favorably alters serum lipid profiles by providing a combined lowering of total, LDL cholesterol, and triglyceride concentrations.

In summary, combining fish oil with certain dietary fats, such as olive oil, may decrease cardiovascular disease risk by decreasing both LDL cholesterol and triglyceride concentrations. Nevertheless, more studies that combine fish oil with other lipid constituents need to be performed before any solid conclusions can be made. Conversely, although only a limited number of studies have been done that examine the effect of fish oil combined with garlic, these results demonstrate that a synergistic effect between these two diet therapies may exist as their combined supplementation results in more favorable lipid alterations than that of each intervention alone.

2.2.2 Oil Containing Medium Chain Triglycerides (MCT Oil)

2.2.2.1 MCT Oil Alone

Medium chain triglycerides contain fatty acid chains that are 6 to 12 carbon atoms in length.[16] Recent evidence suggests that MCT oil is metabolized differently from common fats and oils.[17,18] More specifically, MCT have been shown to be rapidly absorbed through the portal circulation and undergoes oxidation to carbon dioxide or conversion to long chain fatty acids in the liver, thus avoiding deposition in peripheral tissues.[18] Therefore, the supplementation of MCT oil in place of conventional fats has been the subject of much research because this dietary therapy may be beneficial in the prevention and treatment of obesity.

Although the consumption of MCT oil has exhibited beneficial effects with regard to energy expenditure and fat oxidation, the effect of these fats on plasma lipid profiles has not been favorable. Recent human trials,[19,20] examining the effect of MCT oil on plasma lipid concentrations, consistently indicate that MCT oil increases total, LDL cholesterol, and triglyceride concentrations. In a study that compared the lipid effects of a natural food diet supplemented with either MCT oil, palm oil, or high oleic acid sunflower in hypercholesterolemic men, it was shown that the diets containing MCT and palm oil increased both total and LDL cholesterol to the same extent.[19] Similarly, when diets containing MCT versus long chain triglycerides (LCT) were compared, plasma triglycerides were shown to be elevated by the MCT diet but were unchanged by the LCT diet.[20] Therefore, from the standpoint of cardiovascular disease risk, supplementation with MCT oil alone may be unadvisable because this dietary therapy has been shown to unfavorably alter blood lipid concentrations.

2.2.2.2 MCT Oil Combined with n-3 Fatty Acids and Plant Sterols

In contrast, when MCT oil is combined with other dietary fat components, favorable lipid alterations have been observed. As a means of benefiting from the fatty acid oxidation capacity of MCT oil, while offsetting its deleterious effect on lipid profiles, certain functional oils have been created. These functional oils combine MCT oil with other lipids known for their potent hypocholesterolemic effect, i.e., n-3 fatty acids and plant sterols. Recently, Bourque et al.[21] demonstrated that a functional oil containing MCT (50% of fat), plant sterols (45% of fat; 22 mg/kg body weight), and flaxseed derived n-3 fatty acids (5% of fat) improved the overall cardiovascular disease risk profile of obese women when compared with beef tallow. More specifically, the diet containing the functional oil decreased total cholesterol and LDL cholesterol concentrations by 9.1 and 16.0%, respectively, while having no effect on either triglyceride or HDL cholesterol concentrations. Similarly, when St-Onge et al.[22] compared the effect of a diet containing the same functional oil with that of a diet supplemented with olive oil alone, those subjects consuming the functional oil exhibited more favorable lipid alterations. Total cholesterol concentrations were shown to decrease by 12.5 and 4.7% for the functional oil and olive oil diets, respectively. In addition, LDL-cholesterol levels decreased by 13.9% as a result of functional oil administration, while supplementation with the olive oil showed no effect on this lipid parameter.

In sum, these data suggest that a synergistic relationship may exist between these three lipid components and that this synergy not only offsets the deleterious actions of MCT oil when administered alone, but simultaneously alters the lipid profiles in a cardioprotective manner.

2.2.3 Plant Sterols

2.2.3.1 Plant Sterols Alone

Plant sterols are naturally occurring constituents of plant cell membranes and are similar in structure to cholesterol.[23] Although 40 plant sterols exist, the most abundant forms found in nature are β-sitosterol, campesterol, and stigmasterol. Plant sterols exhibit a potent hypocholesterolemic effect by displacing cholesterol from the mixed micelle in the small intestine, thereby reducing the total amount of dietary cholesterol absorbed.[24]

Published data from several randomized control trials repeatedly demonstrate that plant sterols improve plasma lipid profiles by decreasing total and LDL cholesterol concentrations.[25] In contrast, plant sterols generally have little or no effect on HDL cholesterol or triglyceride levels. In a recent review that calculated the placebo-adjusted reduction in LDL cholesterol concentrations across 50 trials, it was shown that plant sterols reduce LDL cholesterol concentrations by approximately 10% on average.[25] The effect appears to be maximal at a dose of 2 g/d, with doses exceeding this amount showing no additional effect.[25]

2.2.3.2 Plant Sterols Combined with Various Food Constituents

Although the effects of foods enriched with plant sterols have been frequently studied, effects of these compounds when placed in combination with other food constituents still require further examination. In one of the few studies that does exist in this area,[26] the effect of a low saturated fat diet containing plant sterols (1.2 g/1000 kcal), soy protein (16.2 g/1000 kcal), viscous fibers (8.3 g/1000 kcal), and almonds (16.6 g/1000 kcal) on lipid profiles was compared to a low saturated fat control diet. Each diet was administered for 4 weeks to hypercholesterolemic, middle aged subjects. LDL cholesterol concentrations were reduced by 35 and 12.1% in the combination and control diets, respectively. In addition, the reduction in the ratio of LDL cholesterol to HDL cholesterol was significantly greater for the combination diet when compared to the control. No post treatment differences were noted with respect to HDL cholesterol, triglycerides, lipoprotein (a), or homocysteine concentrations between the diets. In another study performed by the same group,[27] hypercholesterolemic subjects were randomly assigned to one of three interventions (1) combination diet (same composition as mentioned above), (2) control diet, and (3) control diet plus lovastatin (20 mg/d). Results indicate that LDL cholesterol concentrations were decreased by 28.6, 8.0, and 30.9%, in the combination, control, and levostatin groups, respectively. The reductions in LDL cholesterol concentrations for the combination and statin group were significantly different from the changes in the control group. Interestingly, there were no significant differences in efficacy between the statin and dietary portfolio treatments.

Thus, when plant sterols are combined with other hypocholesterolemic food components, a potentially synergistic relationship may exist between these constituents resulting in a much greater lipid lowering effect than that of plant sterols alone. Moreover, since this combination diet lowers cholesterol concentrations to a similar extent as statins, this diet may potentially be used as an alternative to pharmacological therapy in the prevention and treatment of cardiovascular disease.

2.3 Food–Drug Synergy and Cardiovascular Disease

Nonpharmacological interventions, such as diet and exercise, can help to control weight, blood pressure, and lipid abnormalities, thereby lowering the risk of adverse cardiovascular outcomes.[28] Unfortunately however, patient adherence to such programs is often disappointing.[29] Therefore, managing dyslipidemia effectively, and thus, decreasing the chances of future cardiac events, often requires lipid altering pharmacological therapy. Examples of such agents include statins (3-hydroxy-3-methylglutaryl coenzyme A reductase inhibitors) and fibrates. Treatment with statins has been shown to significantly reduce total and LDL cholesterol, as well as apolipoprotein B concentrations; however, their ability to correct hypertriglyceridemia and low concentrations of HDL cholesterol is limited. Conversely, the use of fibrates has been shown to increase HDL cholesterol, while decreasing triglyceride concentrations; fibrates may, however, deleteriously raise LDL cholesterol and apolipoprotein B concentrations.[30] Thus, combining such pharmacological therapies with certain dietary constituents, and hence favorably altering each lipid parameter, may be the optimal strategy for decreasing cardiovascular disease risk.

2.3.1 Fish Oil Combined with Pharmacological Therapy

2.3.1.1 Fish Oil Combined with Statin Therapy

Recent evidence suggests that combining fish oil with statin therapy may beneficially alter lipid profiles more than each intervention alone. Recently Chan et al.[31] investigated the effects of atorvastatin (40 mg/d) and fish oil (4 g/d), alone and in combination, on indicators of cardiovascular risk in men with hypercholesterolemia. After 6 weeks of supplementation, atorvastatin significantly decreased total and LDL cholesterol concentrations, while fish oil significantly decreased triglyceride and increased HDL cholesterol concentrations. When these two interventions were combined, their effects were shown to be complementary as total and LDL cholesterol, and triglyceride concentrations decreased, while HDL cholesterol concentrations increased. In a study by Durrington et al.,[32] similar results were demonstrated. Patients with coronary heart disease receiving simvastatin (10 to 40 mg/d) were randomized to receive either a fish oil supplement (4 g/d) or placebo for 12 months. Posttreatment lipid results indicated that the fish oil supplement significantly decreased triglyceride concentrations without adversely effecting total, LDL, or HDL cholesterol concentrations. In sum, these data suggest that, when compared with the effects of statins and fish oil alone, this combination therapy may be an optimal therapeutic approach for correcting dyslipidemia.

2.3.1.2 Fish Oil Combined with Other Forms of Pharmacological Therapy

The effect of fish oil supplementation in combination with nifedipine, a calcium channel blocker used to treat hypertension and dyslipidemia, has also been tested. In a double-blind, crossover, placebo-controlled study,[33] the effects of 4 weeks of supplementation with fish oil (4.55 g/d) and nifedipine (40 mg/d), alone or in combination, on blood pressure and serum lipids was assessed in males with hypertension. Four weeks of fish oil treatment alone significantly reduced triglyceride concentrations, yet had no effect on blood pressure values. In contrast, 4 weeks of nifedipine had no effect on lipid concentrations, yet significantly reduced blood pressure. Interestingly, when the fish oil was combined with nifedipine, total and LDL cholesterol concentrations were significantly reduced by 12.0 and 15.0%, when compared with baseline, while the blood pressure decreased to a similar extent as what was noted with the nifedipine therapy alone. Thus, when combined, fish oil and nifedipine may act synergistically to lower lipid and lipoprotein concentrations in a way that cannot be demonstrated when each intervention is administered alone.

2.3.2 Plant Sterols Combined with Pharmacological Therapy

2.3.2.1 Plant Sterols Combined with Statin Therapy

The question of whether there is an additional lowering of LDL cholesterol levels when plant sterols are combined with statins has been tested in several clinical trials. Recently, Simons[34] tested the LDL cholesterol lowering effect of plants sterols (2 g/d) combined with cerivastatin (400 mg/d) compared to each intervention alone. The results indicate that the effect of the combination therapy was additive, producing an overall reduction in LDL cholesterol concentrations of 39% after 4 weeks of treatment. Similarly, when plant sterols (2.5 g/d) were administered to patients with familial hypercholesterolemia treated concurrently with statins, an additional 15% decrease in LDL cholesterol concentrations was noted.[35] In other studies that combined plant stanols (the saturated form of plant sterols) with statin therapy,[36,37] LDL cholesterol levels were shown to decrease by an additional 16 and 20%, respectively. Moreover, other recent trials[38,39] have demonstrated that combining either plant sterols or stanols with statins produces a more sizable LDL cholesterol reduction than what is seen after simply doubling the statin dose. Therefore, although no synergistic relationship between plant sterols and statins has been demonstrated, the results of several clinical trials support the hypothesis that combining sterol therapy with statins has an additive effect in reducing LDL cholesterol concentrations. In conjunction, this combination has been shown to produce more beneficial alterations in LDL cholesterol concentrations than what is seen when the dose of statins is doubled.

2.3.2.2 Plant Sterols Combined with Other Forms of Pharmacological Therapy

The effect of plant sterols in combination with other pharmacological interventions such as fibrates and bile acid sequestrants has also been tested. In a study by Nigon et al.,[40] the objective was to evaluate whether patients receiving fibrates would experience more favorable lipid alterations when this pharmacological therapy was combined with plant sterol (1.6 g/d) supplementation. After 2 months of the combination therapy, total and LDL cholesterol concentrations were reduced by an added 3 and 3.4%, respectively, when compared with the fibrate intervention alone. Adding plant sterols to the fibrate therapy did not have any effect on either HDL cholesterol or triglyceride concentrations. Contrary to these findings, when the bile acid sequestrant, colestipol, was combined with β-sitosterol, total cholesterol concentrations decreased to a lesser extent than with the colestipol alone.[41] Moreover, the combination of colestipol and sterols showed no effect on any of the other lipid parameters measured. Thus overall, plant sterols may be a beneficial adjunctive therapy to fibrates, but should most likely not be used in combination with bile acid sequestrants as they impede on the effectiveness of these pharmacological agents. More data are needed, however, to consolidate these findings as well as to test the effect of plant sterols when combined with ezetimibe and niacin therapy on other cardiovascular disease risk parameters.

2.4 Safety Aspects

2.4.1 Interactions of Fish Oil When Combined with Diet or Drug Therapy

Taking into consideration the potential therapeutic use of fish oils in the treatment and prevention of cardiovascular disease, the determination of any toxic effects that these compounds may exert is essential. Results of several recent trials have demonstrated that the administration of fish oil as a hypocholesterolemic agent is generally safe. At moderate intake levels (approximately 3 to 6 g/d of marine n-3 fatty acids), certain infrequent side effects have been reported, including a fishy aftertaste and gastrointestinal upset.[42] Additionally, concerns have been raised regarding the adverse effects of fish oil supplementation on LDL cholesterol concentrations. Although evidence suggests that small increases in this lipid parameter do occur as a result of fish oil supplementation,[43,44] these effects are unlikely to be harmful as fish oils have been shown time and time again to be cardioprotective.

While no studies to date have examined the adverse interactions between fish oils and lipid altering drug therapies, only one trial has evaluated the interaction between fish oils and other dietary fat constituents on indicators of cardiovascular disease risk. In a study by Haban et al.,[45] the competitive relationship between n-3 fatty acids and oleic acid was examined. The results demonstrated that the supplementation of EPA and DHA lead to the lowering of oleic acid concentrations in serum phospholipids. Since oleic acid has been shown to exert certain favorable effects on the cardiovascular system, the decline of this fatty acid as a result of n-3 fatty acid supplementation can be regarded as a potential problem. Thus, future research should focus on delineating the optimal balance of these two fatty acids when they are administered as a combination therapy for cardiovascular disease.

2.4.2 Interactions of MCT Oil When Combined with Diet or Drug Therapy

Although the safety profile of MCT oil when combined with diet or drug therapies has not yet been clinically evaluated, some trials exist that have documented the toxic effects of MCT oil when supplemented alone. In an earlier study, patients were fed either MCT oil, corn oil, or butter as the sole source of dietary fat for 10 weeks. The only side effect documented for the MCT formula was a transient period of nausea and abdominal fullness during the first 3 to 4 days.[46] In another study,[47] subjects were overfed (150% of estimated energy requirements) two formula diets for 6 days each in a randomized crossover design. The sole source of dietary fat, which accounted for 40% of caloric energy, was either MCT or LCT oil. No significant clinical toxicity was reported; however, a threefold increase in fasting serum triglyceride concentrations was noted for the MCT but not for the LCT diet. Therefore, it is possible that when MCT oil is fed in excess of caloric needs, increased *de novo* fatty acid synthesis and enhanced fatty acid elongation activity in the liver may result.[47] Thus, although MCT oil has been shown to be safe when administered at moderate levels alone, clinical trials should be performed to evaluate the interaction of MCT oil when combined with other lipid altering diet and drug therapies.

2.4.3 Interactions of Plant Sterols When Combined with Diet or Drug Therapy

Oral administration of plant sterols in humans has not been associated with any severe adverse clinical[48] or biochemical[49] effects thus far. In an early study be Lees et al.,[50] supplementation with plant sterols up to 18 g/d for up to 3 years was not associated with any side effects besides mild constipation experienced by only a few subjects. The results from experiments with animal models show similar findings.[51] Plant sterol administration has, however, been associated with decreased absorption of certain vitamins. Since LDL acts as a transporter for certain fat-soluble vitamins and since plant sterols have been shown to lower concentrations of LDL, decreases in the plasma concentrations of β-carotene by 28% and of α-carotene by 9% have been observed after the administration of plant sterols.[25] Although the levels of these vitamins were shown to decline, these decreases did not constitute a health risk. Nevertheless, adding sufficient fruits and vegetables to the diet can prevent these decreases in vitamin concentrations.[52] No studies to date have tested the interaction of plant sterols on the absorption of other lipid or nonlipid food constituents. In contrast, in the several studies that have examined the effect of plant sterols combined with lipid altering drug therapy, no adverse interactions have been reported.[40,41,53]

2.5 Conclusions

In conclusion, it is clear that when combined, certain dietary fats may beneficially alter cardiovascular disease risk parameters more so than that of each lipid constituent alone. More specifically, it has been shown that when fish oils are combined with olive oil or garlic, when MCT oil is combined with certain dietary fats, and when plant sterols are combined with an array of hypocholesterolemic food constituents, positive alterations in cardiovascular risk parameters seem to emerge. Additionally, it has been shown that when fish oils or plant sterols are united with certain lipid altering drug therapies, their combined effect results in more advantageous alterations than that of each intervention alone. Furthermore, although the data are limited, these therapies seem to be well tolerated when administered in combination, as no adverse health outcomes have yet to be documented. In summary, though more evidence is required in certain areas, the administration of these dietary lipids when combined with other food constituents or pharmacological agents may be a simple and safe way to correct certain dyslipidemias, and thus reduce cardiovascular disease risk.

References

1. Kris-Etherton, P.M. et al., Polyunsaturated fatty acids in the food chain in the United States, *Am. J. Clin. Nutr.*, 71, 179, 2000.
2. Din, J.N., Newby, D.E., and Flapan, A.D., Omega 3 fatty acids and cardiovascular disease — fishing for a natural treatment, *Brit. Med. J.*, 328, 30, 2004.
3. Daviglus, M.L. et al., Fish consumption and the 30-year risk of fatal myocardial infarction, *N. Engl. J. Med.*, 336, 1046, 1997.
4. Hu, F.B. et al., Fish and omega-3 fatty acid intake and risk of coronary heart disease in women, *JAMA*, 287, 1815, 2002.
5. Marckmann, P. and Gronbaek, M., Fish consumption and coronary heart disease mortality: a systematic review of prospective cohort studies, *Eur. J. Clin. Nutr.*, 53, 585, 1999.
6. Harris, W.S., Fish oils and plasma lipid and lipoprotein metabolism in humans: a critical review, *J. Lipid. Res.*, 30, 785, 1989.
7. Lovegrove, J.A. et al., Moderate fish-oil supplementation reverses low-platelet, long-chain n-3 polyunsaturated fatty acid status and reduces plasma triacylglycerol concentrations in British Indo-Asians, *Am. J. Clin. Nutr.*, 79, 974, 2004.
8. Piolot, A. et al., Effect of fish oil on LDL oxidation and plasma homocysteine concentrations in health, *J. Lab. Clin. Med.*, 141, 41, 2003.
9. Kris-Etherton, P.M. et al., The role of fatty acid saturation on plasma lipids, lipoproteins, and apolipoproteins: I. Effects of whole food diets high in cocoa butter, olive oil, soybean oil, dairy butter, and milk chocolate on the plasma lipids of young men, *Metabolism*, 42, 121, 1993.
10. Krzeminski, R. et al., Effect of different olive oils on bile excretion in rats fed cholesterol-containing and cholesterol-free diets, *J. Agric. Food. Chem.*, 51, 5774, 2003.
11. Ramirez-Tortosa, C. et al., Olive oil- and fish oil-enriched diets modify plasma lipids and susceptibility of LDL to oxidative modification in free-living male patients with peripheral vascular disease: the Spanish Nutrition Study, *Br. J. Nutr.*, 82, 31, 1999.
12. Nestares, T. et al., Effects of lifestyle modification and lipid intake variations on patients with peripheral vascular disease, *Int. J. Vitam. Nutr. Res.*, 73, 389, 2003.
13. Vognild, E. et al., Effects of dietary marine oils and olive oil on fatty acid composition, platelet membrane fluidity, platelet responses, and serum lipids in healthy humans, *Lipids*, 33, 427, 1998.
14. Leng, G.C. et al., Randomized controlled trial of gamma-linolenic acid and eicosapentaenoic acid in peripheral arterial disease, *Clin. Nutr.*, 17, 265, 1998.
15. Adler, A.J. and Holub, B.J., Effect of garlic and fish-oil supplementation on serum lipid and lipoprotein concentrations in hypercholesterolemic men, *Am. J. Clin. Nutr.*, 65, 445, 1997.
16. Kaunitz, H., Medium chain triglycerides (MCT) in aging and arteriosclerosis, *J Environ. Pathol. Toxicol. Oncol.*, 6, 115, 1986.
17. White, M.D., Papamandjaris, A.A., and Jones, P.J.H., Enhanced postprandial energy expenditure with medium-chain fatty acid feeding is attenuated after 14 d in premenopausal women, *Am. J. Clin. Nutr.*, 69, 883, 1999.

18. DeLany, J.P. et al., Differential oxidation of individual dietary fatty acids in humans, *Am. J. Clin Nutr.*, 72, 905, 2000.
19. Cater, N.B., Heller, H.J., and Denke, M.A., Comparison of the effects of medium-chain triacylglycerols, palm oil, and high oleic acid sunflower oil on plasma triacylglycerol fatty acids and lipid and lipoprotein concentrations in humans, *Am. J. Clin. Nutr.*, 65, 41, 1997.
20. Swift, L.L. et al., Plasma lipids and lipoproteins during 6 d of maintenance feeding with long-chain, medium-chain, and mixed-chain triglycerides, *Am. J. Clin. Nutr.*, 56, 881, 1992.
21. Bourque, C. et al., Consumption of an oil composed of medium chain triacyglycerols, phytosterols, and n-3 fatty acids improves cardiovascular risk profile in overweight women, *Metabolism*, 52, 771, 2003.
22. St-Onge, M.P. et al., Consumption of a functional oil rich in phytosterols and medium-chain triglyceride oil improves plasma lipid profiles in men, *J. Nutr.*, 133, 1815, 2003.
23. de Jong, A., Plat, J., and Mensink, R.P., Metabolic effects of plant sterols and stanols, *J. Nutr. Biochem.*, 14, 362, 2003.
24. Ostlund, R.E., Phytosterols and cholesterol metabolism, *Curr. Opin. Lipidol.*, 15, 37, 2004.
25. Katan, M.B. et al., Efficacy and safety of plant stanols and sterols in the management of blood cholesterol levels, *Mayo Clin. Proc.*, 78, 965, 2003.
26. Jenkins, D.J. et al., The effect of combining plant sterols, soy protein, viscous fibers, and almonds in treating hypercholesterolemia, *Metabolism*, 52, 1478, 2003.
27. Jenkins, D.J. et al., Effects of a dietary portfolio of cholesterol-lowering foods vs lovastatin on serum lipids and C-reactive protein, *JAMA*, 290, 502, 2003.
28. Centers for Disease Control, National Center for Chronic Disease Prevention and Health Promotion. Physical activity and good nutrition: essential elements to prevent chronic diseases and obesity 2003, *Nutr. Clin. Care*, 6, 135, 2003.
29. EUROASPIRE I and II Group, Lifestyle and risk factor management and use of drug therapies in coronary patients from 15 countries: principle results from EUROASPIRE II Euro Heart Survey, *Eur. Heart. J.*, 22, 554, 2001.
30. Watts, G.F. and Dimmitt, S.B., Fibrates, dyslipoproteinaemia and cardiovascular disease, *Curr. Opin. Lipidol.*, 10, 561, 1999.
31. Chan, D.C. et al., Factorial study of the effects of atorvastatin and fish oil on dyslipidaemia in visceral obesity, *Eur. J. Clin. Invest.*, 32, 429, 2002.
32. Durrington, P.N. et al., An omega-3 polyunsaturated fatty acid concentrate administered for one year decreased triglycerides in simvastatin treated patients with coronary heart disease and persisting hypertriglyceridaemia, *Heart*, 85, 544, 2001.
33. Landmark, K. et al., Effects of fish oil, nifedipine and their combination on blood pressure and lipids in primary hypertension, *J. Hum. Hypertens.*, 7, 25, 1993.
34. Simons, L.A., Additive effect of plant sterol-ester margarine and cerivastatin in lowering low-density lipoprotein cholesterol in primary hypercholesterolemia, *Am. J. Cardiol.*, 90, 737, 2002.
35. Neil, H.A., Meijer, G.W., and Roe, L.S., Randomised controlled trial of use by hypercholesterolaemic patients of a vegetable oil sterol-enriched fat spread, *Atherosclerosis*, 156, 329, 2001.

36. Gylling, H., Radhakrishnan, R., and Miettinen, T.A., Reduction of serum cholesterol in postmenopausal women with previous myocardial infarction and cholesterol malabsorption induced by dietary sitostanol ester margarine: women and dietary sitostanol, *Circulation*, 96, 4226, 1997.
37. Vuorio, A.F. et al., Stanol ester margarine alone and with simvastatin lowers serum cholesterol in families with familial hypercholesterolemia caused by the FH-North Karelia mutation, *Arterioscler. Thromb. Vasc. Biol.*, 20, 500, 2000.
38. Blair, S.N. et al., Incremental reduction of serum total cholesterol and low-density lipoprotein cholesterol with the addition of plant stanol ester-containing spread to statin therapy, *Am. J. Cardiol.*, 86, 46, 2000.
39. Bradford, R.H. et al., Expanded clinical evaluation of Lovastatin (EXCEL) study results. I. Efficacy in modifying plasma lipoproteins and adverse event profile in 8245 patients with moderate hypercholesterolemia, *Arch. Intern. Med.*, 151, 43, 1991.
40. Nigon, F. et al., Plant sterol-enriched margarine lowers plasma LDL in hyperlipidemic subjects with low cholesterol intake: effect of fibrate treatment, *Clin. Chem. Lab. Med.*, 39, 634, 2001.
41. Briones, E.R. et al., Primary hypercholesterolemia: effect of treatment on serum lipids, lipoprotein fractions, cholesterol absorption, sterol balance, and platelet aggregation, *Mayo Clin. Proc.*, 59, 251, 1984.
42. Kris-Etherton, P.M., Harris, W.S., and Appeld L.J., AHA scientific statement. Fish consumption, fish oil, omega-3 fatty acids, and cardiovascular disease, *Circulation*, 106, 2747, 2002.
43. Theobald, H.E. et al., LDL cholesterol-raising effect of low-dose docosahexaenoic acid in middle-aged men and women, *Am. J. Clin. Nutr.*, 79, 558, 2004.
44. Rivellese, A.A. et al., Effects of dietary saturated, monounsaturated and n-3 fatty acids on fasting lipoproteins, LDL size and post-prandial lipid metabolism in healthy subjects, *Atherosclerosis*, 167, 149, 2003.
45. Haban, P., Zidekova, E. and Klvanova, J., Supplementation with long-chain n-3 fatty acids in non-insulin-dependent diabetes mellitus (NIDDM) patients leads to the lowering of oleic acid content in serum phospholipids, *Eur. J. Nutr.*, 39, 201, 2000.
46. Hashim, S.A., Arteaga, A., and Van Itallie, T.B., Effect of a saturated medium-chain triglyceride on serum-lipids in man, *Lancet*, 21, 1105, 1960.
47. Hill, J. et al., Thermogenesis in humans during overfeeding with medium-chain triglycerides, *Metabolism*, 38, 641, 1990.
48. Becker, M., Staab, D., and Von Bergmann, K., Treatment of severe familial hypercholesterolemia in childhood with sitosterol and sitostanol, *J. Pediatr.*, 122, 292, 1993.
49. Becker, M., Staab, D., and Von Bergman, K., Long-term treatment of severe familial hypercholesterolemia in children: effect of sitosterol and bezafibrate, *Pediatrics*, 89, 138, 1992.
50. Lees, A.M. et al., Plant sterols as cholesterol-lowering agents: clinical trials in patients with hypercholesterolemia and studies of sterol balance, *Atherosclerosis*, 28, 325, 1977.
51. Malini, T. and Vanithakumari, G., Antifertility effects of beta-sitosterol in male albino rats, *J. Ethnopharmacol.*, 35, 149, 1991.

52. Noakes, M. et al., An increase in dietary carotenoids when consuming plant sterols or stanols is effective in maintaining plasma carotenoid concentrations, *Am. J. Clin. Nutr.*, 75, 79, 2002.
53. Nguyen, T.T. et al., Cholesterol-lowering effect of stanol ester in a US population of mildly hypercholesterolemic men and women: a randomized controlled trial, *Mayo Clin Proc.*, 74, 1198, 1999.

3

Antioxidant Phytochemicals and Potential Synergistic Activities at Reducing Risk of Cardiovascular Disease

David D. Kitts

CONTENTS

3.1 Introduction

Reports from epidemiological studies have linked consumption of fruits and vegetables with lower mortality rates attributed to incidences of coronary heart disease (CHD).[1–4] CHD is a primary cause of death in Western societies and involves a complex number of underlying mechanisms that may be modulated by diet (Table 3.1). Oxidative stress is a well documented etiopathogenic factor of both hypertension and atherosclerosis. Hypertension is a multifactor condition with underlying causes related to overproduction of various reactive oxygen species (ROS), such as the superoxide anion and the hydroxyl radical. The generation of peroxynitrite from these two ROS sources lead to the depletion of nitric oxide and lost relaxation function of smooth muscle and induction of intracellular calcium overload. Peroxynitrite, a powerful oxidant formed *in vivo* from nitric oxide and superoxide, also promotes an endothelial inflammatory response by activating transcriptional factor nFkB, which in turn increases expression of genes encoding proinflammatory cytokines (e.g., TNF-) and enzymes such as inducible nitric oxide synthetase (iNOS) and cyclooxygenase-2 (COX-2). Another mechanism suggests that ROS enhance COX-2 induced activity leading to aggregation of platelets and increased tendency for thrombogenesis. ROS also are involved in depletion of low-density lipoprotein (LDL) antioxidant that results in a propagation chain reaction of low density lipoprotein peroxidation and oxidative modification of LDL cholesterol, a key early step in the pathogenesis of atherosclerosis. Lipid peroxidation during myocardial ischemic-reperfusion[5] and glycooxidation reactions with diabetic conditions,[6] are further examples of the involvement of ROS in different human pathologies that are related to CHD. Specific complications of diabetes include microvascular (e.g., nephropathy) and macrovascular (e.g., arterioscelerotic and cardiac) disorders that are linked to oxidative stress. Dietary antioxidants working through redox properties (e.g., reducing activity, hydrogen donating or transition metal ion chelating activities, inhibitors of lipoxygenase and cycloxygenase enzyme activities, and regulators of signal transduction pathways responsible for combating the effects of ROS) have an important role in reducing the risk of free radical oxidative damage in CHD. Although there is no clearly understood single mechanism underlying these associations, it is important to point out that in the case of fruits and vegetables, a complex milieu of nutrients and phytochemicals exist with established health promoting (e.g., antioxidant, hypolipidemic, antiinflammatory, and antifibrinolytic) activities (Table 3.2). Presently a general consensus exists that a policy of a healthy consumption of fruits and vegetables

TABLE 3.1

Proposed Mechanisms for Etiology of CHD

Causative Factor	Biomarker	Protective Factor
Hypertension Vasoconstriction of efferent and afferent arterioles Smooth muscle efflux of calcium	Diastolic blood pressure	Promote relaxation of cardiovascular smooth muscle (antiarrhythmic effect)
Inflammation Increased cyclooxygenase activity Increased lipooxygenase activity	Cyclooxygenase-derived prostanoids	Inhibit macrophage iNOS, modify eicosanoid biosynthesis (antiprostanoid, antiinflammatory responses)
Clinical outcomes of oxidative stress	Arachidonic acid lipid peroxidation products (i.e., prostaglandin F2α) Antioxidant status of saliva: uric acid products; breath test: pentane assay by GC	Enhanced total serum antioxidant capacity
Decreased balance of antioxidant status	Redox balance; antioxidant/prooxidant molecules; glutathione antioxidant system.	Enhanced antioxidant enzyme status
Increased LDL oxidation	LDL oxidation (e.g., TBARS, conjugated dienes, modified apolipoprotein B-100 and migration on agarose electrophoresis)	Enhanced LDL antioxidant capacity
Increased glycooxidation	Oxidized hemoglobin	Enhanced antioxidant enzyme status
Thrombogenesis	Platelet thromboxane (TXA_2)	
Increased platelet aggregation and lipooxygenase activity	Fibrinolytic effect, vascular cytokines (IL-1) and tumor necrosis factor (TNF-alpha)	Antithrombic effects, improved vascular reactivity.
Dislipidemia Elevated total (T-chol) and LDL cholesterol	Total serum cholesterol concentration; LDL cholesterol; LDL/HDL ratio	Increase bile acid secretion Increase LDL receptor activity Reduce cholesterol absorption
Athrogenesis	Total cholesterol/HDL ratio	

has distinct advantages to the alternative dietary supplement pill method, which supplies individual nutrients in some cases.[7] There is more support concerning a possible synergistic effect from a combination of antioxidant vitamins to prevent cardiovascular disease.[8–10] Epidemiological studies support this philosophy with evidence that substantial benefits to CHD are seen when fruit and vegetable consumption reaches 400 g/d,[11,12] thus suggesting that a critical threshold of multiple nutrients working in an additive or

TABLE 3.2

Some Nutrient and Phytochemical Interactions with Identified Protective Roles against CHD

Nutrient	Proposed Effect	Ref.
Single Nutrient		
Vitamin E	Inversely related to CHD mortality; reduced LDL oxidation and platelet aggregation	174–178
Vitamin C	Inversely related to CHD mortality; protection against ischemia heart disease, improved endothelial function, decreasing LDL induced leukocyte adhesion, stimulating nitric oxide availability	179,180
Carotinoids	Peroxyl and peroxynitrite radical scavengers, reduced plasma LDL oxidation products, reduced carotic artery plaque formation, prevention of carotid intima-media thickness	71–73, 85
n-3 Fatty acids		
Eicosapentaenoic acid (EPA) and doxosahexaenoic acid (DHA)	Lipid (TG, VLDL) lowering; antithrombotic; NO-dependent vasodilation; inhibition COX-2 and PGE_2, inflammatory cytokines	182
Nutrient × Nutrient Interaction		
Ascorbic acid	Regeneration of α-tocopherol	146, 147, 149
Ascorbic acid, glutathione	Regeneration of α-tocopherol (RBC membrane)	150
Ascorbic acid, glutathione	Regeneration of α-tocopherol (platelets)	147
Lycopene	Regeneration of α-tocopherol	80
β-Carotene × vitamin C × vitamin E	Reduced LDL oxidation	10
β-Carotene × vitamin C	Reduced membrane oxidative damage	9
Vitamin E × n-3 fatty acids	Lowered platelet aggregation	183
α-Tocopherol × lycopene	Enhanced endothelial platelet metabolism	86
Multiple vitamin combinations	Optimal antioxidant activity	152
Established Phytochemical × Nutrient Interactions		
Ajoene (garlic) × dipriyirdamole	Enhanced antithrombotic activity	131
EGCg (tea) × α-tocopherol	Enhanced free radical scavenging power	155
Curcumin (spice) × *n*-3 PUFA	Enhanced antiinflammatory response	164
Garlic × *n*-3 PUFA	Enhanced lowering of total cholesterol	165

synergistic mode is required for the effect. In addition, phytochemical-rich beverage consumption, including various teas, has also been related to a reduced risk to mortality caused by CHD.[13] Thus, it stands to reason that additive or synergistic effects between nutrients and bioactive phytochemicals represent important interactions that facilitate promoting protection against CHD. Although patterns of dietary intake of tea and certain herbal preparations (e.g., ginseng) also vary considerably, these products are often consumed either during or in association with exposure to many food systems. Thus the potential interaction between these sources of bioactive phytochemicals and certain food derived nutrients may also exist.

This chapter describes the bioactive nature of specific phytochemicals that have potential for acting to protect against different metabolic etiologies of CHD and the interaction between active plant agent and specific food nutrients in promoting the same.

3.2 Antioxidant Phytochemicals in Food Sources

3.2.1 Tea Polyphenols

Increased plasma antioxidant activity has been reported in humans consuming green and black tea,[14] albeit, there is less evidence to indicate definitively that regular tea drinking results in an increased plasma antioxidant potential.[15] Antioxidant activity of tea flavonoids that protect against LDL oxidation *in vitro*,[16] provide little evidence to indicate more than a marginal effect *in vivo*.[17] However, studies with the consumption of Lung Chen tea have reported delayed atherogenesis and lower risk of CHD, attributed by reduced endothelial cell LDL oxidation and foam cell formation.[18]

The reduced risk to CHD related to ingested tea polyphenols has also been linked, in part, to hypocholesterolemic activities that involve increased fecal excretion of cholesterol and bile acids,[19] as well as a potential probiotic effect of the tea polyphenols that result in stimulated intestinal fermentation and production of volatile fatty acids (VFA).[20] Other workers have reported increased high-density lipoprotein (HDL) cholesterol levels in rats fed green tea and stimulated efflux of accumulated cholesterol.[21] Cell culture work with Hep-G2 cells have shown that green tea has the ability to up-regulate the LDL receptor at the level of gene transcription and to decrease intracellular cholesterol concentration. The up-regulation of LDL receptor and related hypocholesterolemic effect may be mediated by the effect of tea constituents on sterol-regulated element binding protein (SREBP-1) in response to a decrease in the intracellular cholesterol concentration.[22]

3.2.1.1 Phenolic Acids

Simple phenolics (C6), phenolic acids (C6-C1) and cinnamic acids (C6-C3) occur in numerous food products and beverages at concentrations that vary from 1 to 30 mg/100 g for cinnamic acids in plums, cherries, and apples to 250 to 600 mg/100 g for chlorogenic acid in dry tea shoots or a cup of coffee.[23] The phenolic acid caffeic acid (3,4-dihydroxycinnamic acid), is a relatively simple compound with a carboxylic acid group, an aromatic ring

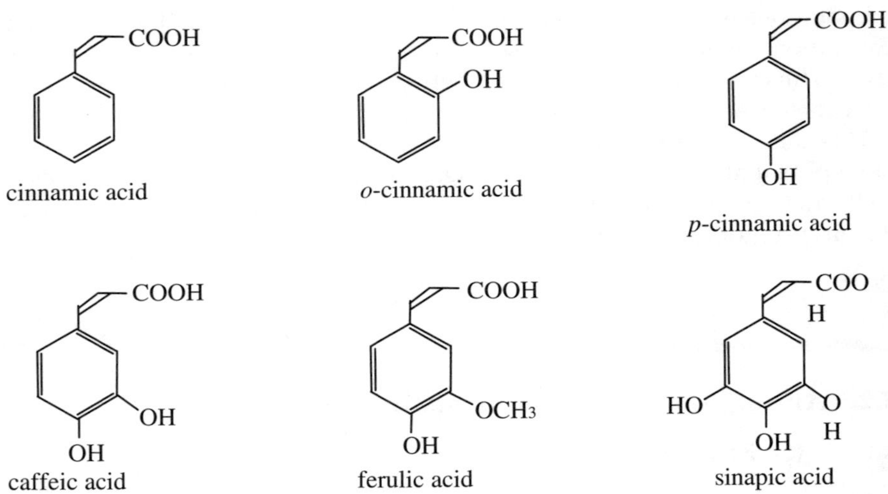

FIGURE 3.1
Some typical simple phenolic acids with noted antioxidant activity.

typical of phenols, and two hydroxyl groups that contribute to the antioxidant activity (Figure 3.1). Caffeic acid contains both antioxidant and reducing activity.[24] Chlorogenic acid (5-caffeoyquinic acid) is another phenolic acid found in green and roasted coffee that exhibits antioxidant activity, with relatively greater activity than both caffeic acid and 3,5-dicaffeolyquinic acid toward H_2O_2-induced hemolysis[25] and peroxyl radical-induced LDL oxidation.[26] Simple phenolics present in barley, notably *p*-coumaric and ferulic acids, have antioxidant activity toward prevention of linoleic acid peroxidation reactions,[27] while apple juice is an excellent source of phenolic antioxidants containing constituents such as chlorogenic, caffeic, and ferulic acids, along with quercetin and rutin. The resulting Trolox equivalent antioxidant capacities toward the scavenging 2,2′-azinobis(3-ethybenzothiazoline-6′-sulfonic acid) ($ABTS^{\cdot+}$) radical exceed those of ascorbic acid.[28]

3.2.1.2 Flavonoids

Flavonoids represent a wide range of distinct polycyclic compounds that are derived from a confluence of the acetate-malonate and shikimate pathways, ubiquitous in foods of plant origin (e.g., fruits, vegetables, soybeans, cocoa, herbs). This family of compounds have been described as having a stability that exceeds the presence of ascorbate[29]; thus they represent important sources of dietary antioxidants. Sustained circulating levels reaching 1 to 10 μ*M* can be obtained in subjects fed a normally high flavonoid containing diet. Flavonoids are categorized into six groups and contain two aromatic rings (e.g., rings A and B) that are linked to a heterocyclic ring (e.g., ring C) structure and sugar molecules (catechins being the only exception), which accounts for their lipophilic and hydrophilic characters (Figure 3.2). A variety

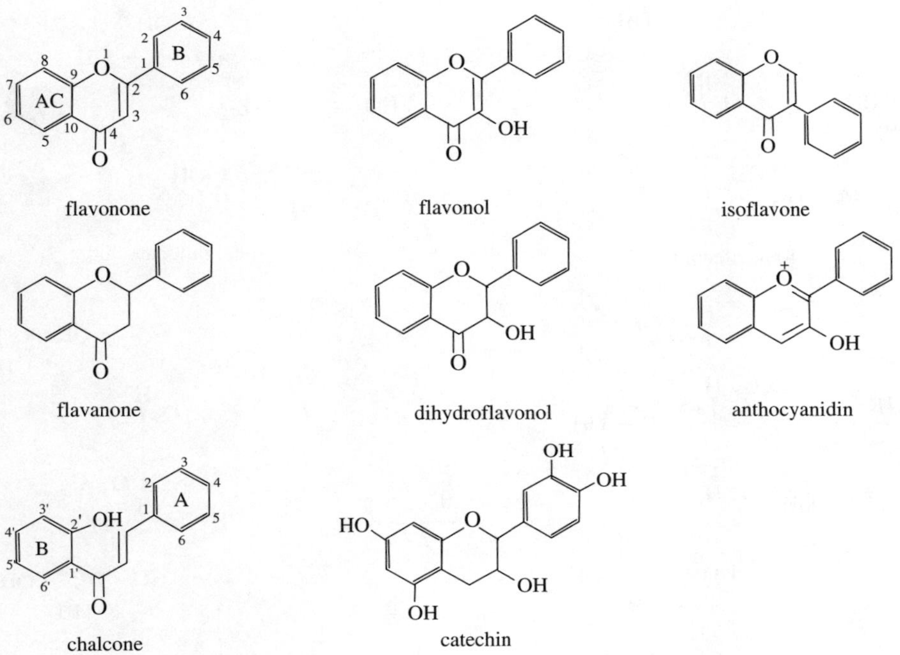

FIGURE 3.2
Chemical structures of common flavonoids.

of bioactive mechanisms that potentially reduce the risk of cardiovascular disease (CVD) associated with flavonoids have been proposed.[30–34] This includes reducing hypertension through vasodilatation of afferent and efferent arterioles and inhibiting calcium flux, thereby blocking excitation coupling of smooth muscle. Artichoke derived flavonoids (e.g., luteolin) induce endothelial NO synthase (eNOS) gene expression and nitric oxide production in vascular endothelial cells, which contributes to enhanced endothelial-dependent vasodilatation.[35] Flavonoids also potentially contribute to strengthening antioxidant defense systems and interacting with intracellular signaling mechanisms. The free radical scavenging activity of flavonoids to protect against oxidation of LDL is inversely related to the concentration of flavonoids in macrophages.[36]

3.2.1.3 Catechins

Catechins belong to the flavan-3-ol category of flavonoids and have a series of bioactivities that range from antioxidant and antiinflammatory activity to immune stimulant and weight loss actions. Catechins (e.g., a mixture of catechin, epicatechin, epigallocatechin, epicatechin gallate, epigallocatechin gallate) consist of 80 to 90% of the total flavonoid content in tea (Figure 3.3). Epigallocatechin gallate (EGCg) accounts for 50 to 60% of the total catechin

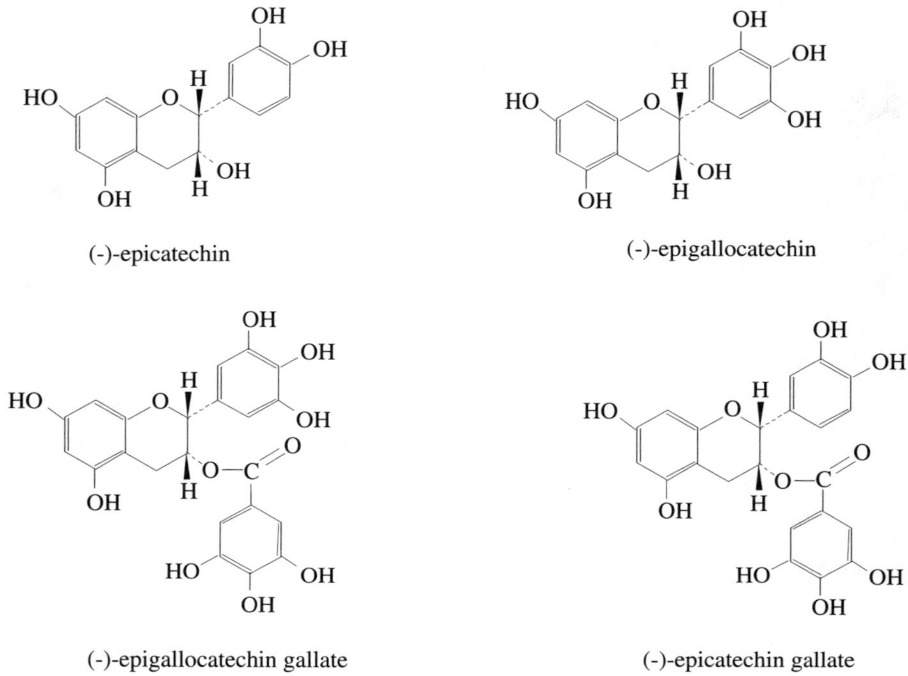

FIGURE 3.3
General structure of bioactive tea catechins.

in tea and represents the greatest antioxidant activity. The beneficial effect of daily tea catechin intake in reducing the risk of cardiovascular disease has in part been attributed to the protection of oxidative modification of plasma lipoproteins.[37] In particular, tea catechins inhibit lipoxygenase activity and act as scavengers for radicals and chain-breaking antioxidants that suppress endothelial cell induced–LDL oxidation through these mechanisms.[38] Moreover, the significant bioavailabity of catechins[39] facilitates potential protection of LDL from direct oxidation from attack by free radicals, or indirectly, by maintaining and regenerating α-tocopherol.

The number and arrangement of phenolic hydroxyl groups specific to the structure of the individual tea flavonoids influences the affinity to which they scavenge free radicals and sequester potential prooxidant transition metal ions.[38,40] For the catechin gallates (EGC and EGCg), the presence of 3′4′5′-OH groups in the B ring and a gallate moiety located in the C ring have been associated with increased antioxidant activity.[41] The *ortho*-dihydroxyl group (*o*-3′4′-OH) in the B ring also participates in electron delocalization and stabilizes the radical form.[40] The process of fermenting tea to produce black tea results in the generation of bioactive large polyphenol polymers, referred to as theaflavins and thearubigins.

3.2.1.4 Tannins

In addition to catechins, green tea contains tannins, which inhibit peroxynitrite (ONOO) formation by direct scavenging, or by removal of precursors nitric oxide (NO) and superoxide (O_2^-).[42] The removal of NO^- and O_2^- by tannins explains the protective effects of green tea tannin against LLC-PK1 cell injury that is linked to ischemia-reperfusion. Moreover, EGCg is effective at inhibiting mitogen-stimulated nitrite production by mouse macrophages,[43] and thus may have a role in reducing an inflammatory response that could contribute to endothelial dysfunction and development of atherosclerosis. Tannins also scavenge hydroxyl radicals, a known decomposition product of ONOO. In doing so, tannins inhibit lipid peroxidation chain reactions that are induced by the hydroxyl radical. This could have an impact on another mechanism of action whereby the prevention of endothelial cell-mediated LDL lipid peroxidation by tea catechins results in down-regulation of hemoxygenase activity.[44] Hemoxygenase activity is linked to macrophage-generated ROS.

3.2.2 Fruits and Vegetables

Flavonoids are also widely distributed in various fruits, vegetables, and grains, and contribute to antioxidant activity that is also associated with vitamins C and E, and β-carotene.[45,46] Antioxidant activity of many different fruits has been characterized using the ORAC (oxygen radical absorbance capacity) method to give relative estimates of total antioxidant capacity.[47] Simple phenolics and flavonoids account for a majority of antioxidant activity found in apples,[48] with the phenolic content in apple peel accounting for majority of antioxidant and antiproliferating activity.[49] In contrast, only 0.4% of total antioxidant activity was estimated to come from vitamin C in apple skin.[50] Taken together, important potential additive or synergistic antioxidant activity exist with flavonoids and vitamins C or E interactions in fruits and vegetables.

3.2.2.1 Flavonols

Flavonols have a characteristic double-bonded oxygen atom attached to position 4 and a hydroxyl group at position 3, and are further identified by the number and placement of hydroxyl groups on the three-ring structure (Figure 3.4). The most common flavonols are quercetin, mycertin, and kaempferol. Relatively strong antioxidant activity of quercetin, in particular, has been attributed to the 2-3 double bond and 4-oxo structure, which scavenge free radicals such as superoxide anions and lipid peroxyl radicals, and interrupts free radical chain reactions. In addition, quercetin has been shown to modify eicosanoid biosynthesis and exhibit antithrombotic and antihypertensive activities. These activities are relevant to potential anti-inflammatory responses, protection against LDL oxidation, and prevention of platelet

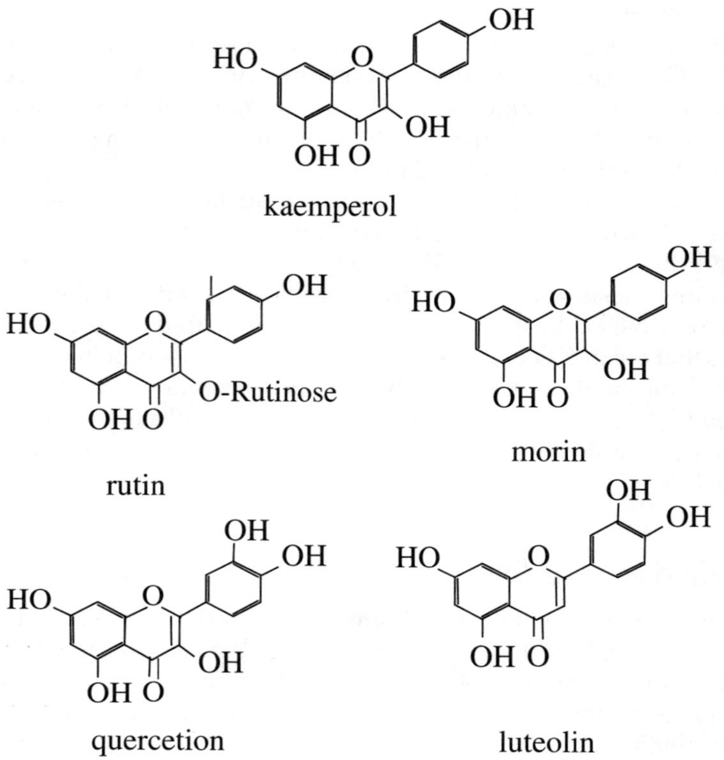

FIGURE 3.4
Structural differences between bioactive flavonols, kaemperol, quercetin, rutin, morin, and flavone luteolin (note the absence of hydroxyl group on C-3 in luteolin).

aggregation. Moreover, the bioflavonol rutin (querecetin-3-*O*-β-rhamnosyl-glucose) can suppress the production of advanced glycation end products (AGEs), known to accumulate in various tissues of diabetic subjects, in part due to an oxidative stress, and linked to health complications that include vascular disease.[51] The presence of kaempferol, quercetin, isorhamnetin, and associated glycoside derivatives have also been identified as antioxidant components in the *Ginko biloba* therapeutic herb standardized extract, Egb761 with effective scavenging of both superoxide and hydroxyl radicals.[52] Bioavailability of flavonols, such as quercetin has been estimated from rat studies that reported circulating plasma concentrations of both quercetin (e.g.,19 μ*M*) and isorhamnetin (101 μ*M*) after 2 weeks feeding on diets containing 0.25% w/w quercetin.[53]

3.2.2.2 Flavones

Typical flavone compounds, including tangeritin, luteolin, nobilitin, and apigenin, are present in both free and glycosylated forms. Interactions between flavones and flavonols can occur with luteolin and quercetin, both of which have double bond between carbons 2 and 3 in the C-ring and hydroxyl groups on the 3 and 4 carbons in the B-ring. This similar structure provides access to protein kinase substrate binding sites required for regulating cell proliferation.[54] Both luteolin and quercetin greatly reduced protein phosphorylation at 20 μ*M*, and cell proliferation after 24-h exposure. Moreover, the two adjacent polar hydroxyl groups located on carbons 3 and 4 on B-ring are required for suppressing kinase activity. Decreased cellular protein phosphorylation occurs with both luteolin (49%) and quercetin (27%) at 50 μ*M* and roughly to the same extent when added together at 20 μ*M* concentrations. Total flavones extracted from sea buckthorn (*Hippophae rhamnoides* L) prevent thrombogenesis *in vivo* and platelet aggregation *in vitro* through a mechanism that may involve suppression of arachidonic acid synthesis.[55] Recent studies have shown that luteolin-rich extracts derived from dandelion flower possess affinities that can reduce hydroxyl radical–induced DNA scission and scavenge peroxyl radicals in chemical model systems.[56] Luteolin prooxidant activity enhances Cu^{2+}-catalyzed LDL oxidation only at low concentrations, while antioxidant protection against transition metal ion–induced LDL oxidation occurs at higher concentrations. In addition to exhibiting antioxidant activity, luteolin and luteolin-*O*-glucoside can scavenge reactive nitrogen species and suppress iNOS and COX-2 activity in cultured macrophage cells.[57]

3.2.2.3 Flavonones

Flavonones are commonly found in citrus fruits, such as orange, grapefruit and lemon. Naringin is a water soluble glycone and is hydrolyzed by intestinal enzymes to yield the bioactive aglycone naringenin. Naringin and hesperidin exhibit antioxidant, antiinflammatory, antithrombotic, and antiatherogenic activities.[58] The presence of naringenin in atherogenic diets fed to rats was also found to lower hepatic triacylglycerides and inhibit the rate limiting cholesterol synthesis enzyme, HMG-CoA (3-hydroxy-3-methylglutaryl-Coenzyme A) reductase.[59] A similar synergistic effect was obtained with the lowering of acyl coenzyme A:cholesterol acyltransferase (ACAT) enzyme, important for the conversion of free cholesterol to cholesterol ester. Reduction of ACAT leads to lower plasma very low density lipoprotein (VLDL) and LDL apo-B concentrations by reducing hepatic VLDL–apo-B secretion. The suppression of ACAT activity paralleled a reduction in aortic fatty streak areas.[60]

3.2.2.4 Anthocyanidins

Anthocyanidins represent an important group of flavonoids with polyphenolic structures that provide color and antioxidant activity to many fruits and vegetables,[61,62] as well as pigmented cereals[63, 64] and sorghums.[65] More common individual anthocyanidins include peonidin, cyanidin, delphinidin,

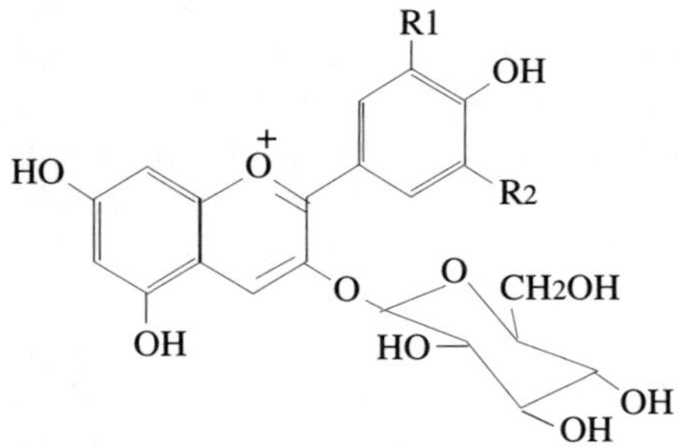

R1=OH, R2=H,	cyanidin 3-O-B-glucoside
R1=H, R2=H,	pelargonidin 3-O-B-glucoside
R1=OH, R2=OH,	delphinidin 3-O-B-glucoside

FIGURE 3.5
Chemical structure of anthocyanidin.

peunidin, and malvidin; all of which vary in structural aspects by the number of hydroxyl groups attached, the type and position of sugar attachments, and the degree of methylation of hydroxyl groups (Figure 3.5). The water soluble β-D-glucoside conjugate form of cyanidin and delphinidin have both been identified as antioxidant pigments derived from red and black beans, respectively.[65] Moreover, anthocyanidin pigment has been shown to reduce the extent of atherosclerosis as a result of potential antioxidant and antiinflammatory activity[66] (Figure 3.5). A diverse combination of cardioprotection pathways have also been attributed to antioxidant activities of proanthocyanindins found in grape seed. Free radical scavenging activity resulting in reduced formation of reactive oxygen species,[67,68] and possibly regenerating other oxidized antioxidants[69] have been linked to activities related to reduced ischemic-reperfusion mediated injury[67] and have improved the recovery of coronary and aortic flow.

3.2.2.5 Carotenoids

Carotenoids are lipophilic pigments found within cell membranes of fruits and vegetables, and microorganisms, but are not synthesized in animals (Figure 3.6). Once absorbed, carotenoids appear unchanged in the circulation and peripheral tissue where they are transported in lipoprotein particles. Antioxidant activity from a hydrophobic chain of polyene units quenches singlet oxygen and stabilizes peroxyl radicals at characteristically low oxygen tensions, demonstrating the properties of chain-breaking antioxidants in radical-initiated reactions including lipid peroxidation.[70] Carotenoids react with radicals via electron transfer, which produces a carotenoid radical cation. The efficiency of the electron transfer depends on the carotenoid structure; the greater the number of coplanar conjugated double bands, the higher the reaction rate. The presence of hydroxyl- and keto groups will lower the reaction rate with electron transfer.

Carotenoids also directly quench peroxynitrite, an oxidant produced from nitric oxide and superoxide. This particular ROS destroys protein-lipid complexes, a hallmark of the atherosclerosis event, by reacting discriminatively

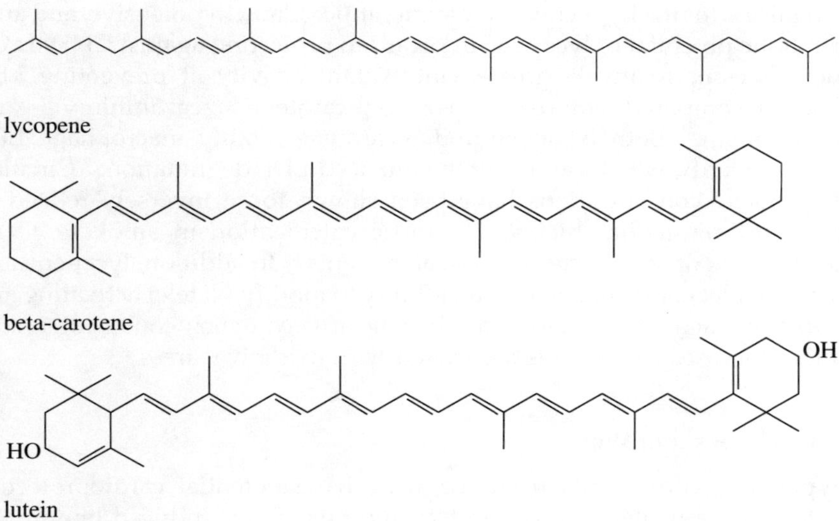

FIGURE 3.6
Structures of antioxidant carotenoids, lycopene, β-carotene, and lutein.

with lipids and amino acid residues.[71] Moreover, *in vitro* enrichment of LDL with β-carotene protects against endothelial cell–mediated oxidation.[72] Carotenoids thus appear to have a role in the prevention of arterial plaque formation, as shown by studies that indicated a lower prevalence of carotid arterial plaque in subjects with higher carotenoid intake.[73] Functional modulation of the atherogenic processes involving the vascular endothelium includes reduced adhesion, or binding, between monocytes and aortic endothelial cells by different carotenoids that produce structure-specific membrane changes that alter the expression of adhesion molecules.[74] Although β-carotene has been shown to protect LDL from endothelial cell–mediated oxidation both *in vitro* and *in vivo*,[75] some clinical studies have not indicated a positive effect of β-carotene on CHD.[76] This is surprising since the level of β-carotene in body fluids or tissues is linked with a reduced risk of CVD.[77,78]

3.2.2.5.1 Lycopene

Lycopene is a linear open-chain lipophilic (possessing 11 conjugated and 2 nonconjugated double bonds) carotenoid antioxidant that has no provitamin A activity and is located within cell membranes and in close contact with other lipid components[78] (Figure 3.6). This molecule has nonoxidative effects, including inhibition of HMG-CoA reductase activity,[79] thus protecting against elevated LDL. Related to this is the antioxidant potential that lowers LDL oxidation,[80] which protects against oxidized LDL-induced inhibition of the endothelial L-arginine–nitric oxide pathway,[81] key components required for prevention of platelet aggregation, aterial vasodilation, and blood pressure control. Collectively, therefore, these activities are important underlying mechanisms for the hypocholesterolemic, antioxidant, hypotensive, and antithrombotic potential of lycopene in regard to protecting against CHD. Lycopene possesses relatively greater antioxidant activity at preventing LDL oxidation, compared with α-tocopherol > β-carotene > zeazanthin = β-carotene > lutelin.[82] Both lycopene and β-carotene modify macrophage LDL receptor activity, which can result in enhanced LDL degradation.[79] Circulating lycopene concentrations have been shown to be inversely related to carotid intima-media thickness,[83] aortic calcification in smokers,[84] and increased risk of atherosclerotic vascular events.[85] In addition, lycopene and tomato extract constituents have an affinity to modify platelet activating and acyl-platelet activating factors in a beneficial way, which could potentially reduce atherosclerotic events associated with oxidative stress.[86]

3.2.3 Grapes and Wine

Polyphenolic compounds from red wine have potential cardioprotective effects that are related to reduced transition metal ion–induced lipoprotein oxidation,[87] inhibition of LDL cholesterol oxidation and endothelium dysfunction and vasospasm,[88] and inhibition of platelet aggregation.[89] Consumption of polyphenols from wine can enhance the serum antioxidant capacity,[90] and there is evidence that wine consumption will also increase plasma cytokine (e.g., IL-6) concentrations in men; however, it is not certain if this effect is partly related to the coingestion of alcohol.[91] On the other hand, red wine constituents can inhibit platelet thrombosis and vasoconstriction through a single mechanism related to prostacyclin release, which is dependent on protein kinase C activity.[92] Moreover, strong evidence exists that wine polyphenols increase endothelial nitric oxide and cyclooxygenase-2 (COX-2) activities, which are related to increased endothelium-dependent relaxation.[93] The various bioactive properties associated with wine polyphenols helps explain the well recognized French Paradox with regard to prevention of cardiovascular disease.[94]

3.2.3.1 Resveratrol

This relatively simple polyphenol found in grapes has a myriad of biological activities, including antioxidant, anticancer, and antiinflammatory activities. The presence of a 4-hydroxy in ring B and the *meta*-hydroxy structure in ring A are essential for the antioxidant activity of resveratrol[95] (Figure 3.7). Resveratrol also has a role in reducing oxidative stress, which is a relevant factor for cardioprotection, as shown by findings of a resveratrol-induced up-regulation of nitric oxide production[96] and peroxyl radical scavenging activity with reduced malonaldehyde (MDA) formation in effluents of isolated hearts.[95] Pretreatment with resveratrol will reduce ischemia-reperfusion injury and improved postischemic ventricular function and greater postischemic functional recovery,[97] but no effect on ischemic-reperfusion-induced arrhythmias and mortality has been reported.[98]

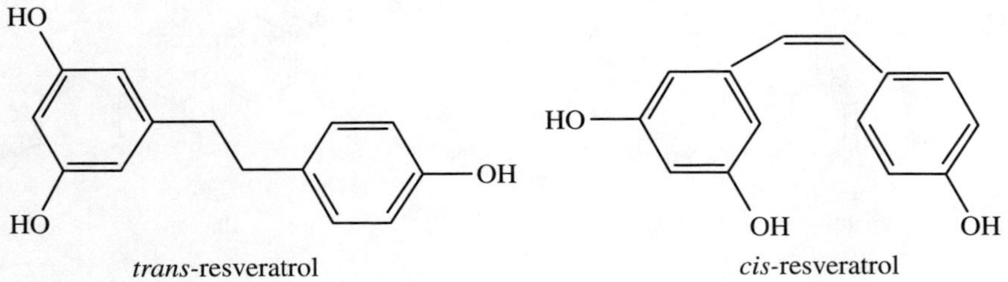

FIGURE 3.7
Structures of bioactive *trans*-resveratrol and *cis*-resveratrol.

Other indications of resveratrol antioxidant activity include the inhibitory effect on AGE-stimulated proliferation, DNA synthesis, and collagen synthesis activity in stroke prone, spontaneously hypertensive rats.[99] AGEs accumulate in plasma proteins and slower turnover tissue proteins, and have been linked to diabetic complications, including vascular diseases.[100]

3.2.4 Soybeans

Soybean and soya-based products contain many beneficial bioactive phytochemical constituents, which include isoflavones, lignans, and phenolic acids, all of which have in common a potential antioxidant activity.[101,102]

3.2.4.1 Isoflavones

Isoflavones are naturally occurring flavonoids with a multitude of potential bioactive activities, including antioxidant, antiestrogenic, and antiosteoporotic effects. Soybeans contain a large amount of isoflavones with genistin, daidzin, and their respective aglycones, genistein and daidzein, representing the primary isoflavones. Unlike flavones, which have their B-ring attached to position 2 of the C-ring, isoflavones have the B-ring attached to position 3. The number and position of hydroxyl groups attached at positions 5, 7 and 4 distinguish the individual isoflavones (Figure 3.8). Isoflavones have moderate cardioprotective, antiinflammatory, and antioxidant activity. In particular, the antioxidative effect of genistein is related to structural features that include positioning of hydroxyl groups at the C5, 7, and 4 position. For example, both genistsein and daidzein inhibit peroxynitrite-mediated LDL oxidation and reduce formation of 3-nitrotyrosine,[103] whereas related glucoside conjugates have lower activity.[103] The isoflavone metabolites dihydrodaidzein and dehydroequol improved endothelial nitric oxide function in apoE0/HF mice through antioxidant activity that protects endothelial cells against the cytotoxicity of oxidized LDL.[104] Genistein, has also been shown to inhibit NFkB-induced TNF-α activation in human lymphocytes, thereby indicating genistein plays a role in gene regulatory activity and signal transduction pathways.[105]

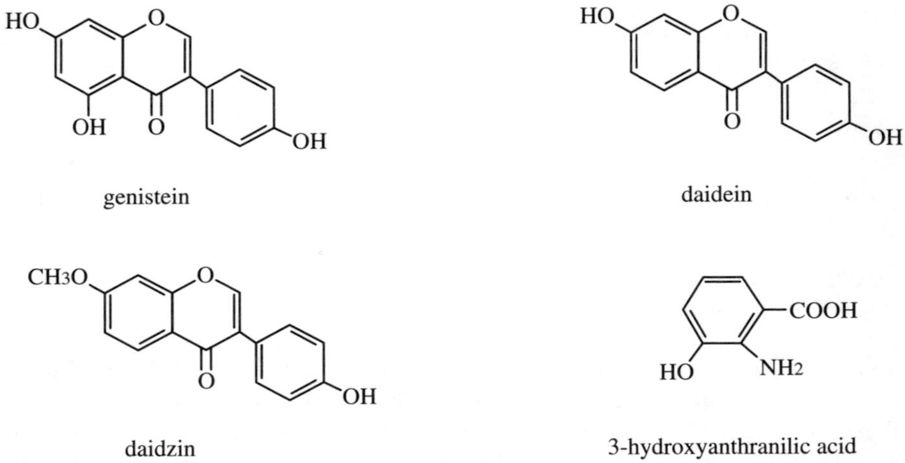

FIGURE 3.8
Structures of isoflavones and 3-hydroxyanthranilic acid isolated from soybean.

In addition, soy polyphenols can lower cholesterol.[106] Increased plasma isoflavone concentrations are associated with diets high in isoflavones; increased plasma HDL cholesterol and apolipoprotein A-1 concentrations are also seen in healthy normolipidemic subjects.[107] There is no effect on transforming growth factor $_1$ or fibrinogen concentrations, factor VII coagulant activity, or plasminogen activator inhibitor type 1 activity. The underlying mechanism for the reduction in plasma cholesterol attributed to isoflavones is the loss of bile acids and the up-regulation of the LDL receptor.[108]

Protective antiatherosclerotic properties of isoflavones are a result of many diverse biological activities, including beneficial effects on plasma lipids, prevention of lipid peroxidation, antiproliferative effects on vascular smooth muscle cells, inhibition of platelet aggregation, and facilitated endothelium-dependent vasodilation. Vasodilatory effects of isoflavones may also be related to a structural similarity with estradiol and preferential binding to estrogen receptor β.[108] Genistein also inhibits protein-tyrosine kinase topoisomerase II enzymes, which are critical for cell proliferation. The inhibitory potential of genistein toward tyrosine kinase reduces the depressed postischemic myocardial function in isolated papillary muscle by increasing Ca^{2+} sensitivity of the myofilaments.[109] This effect has a beneficial role on the ischemia-reperfusion cycle. The affinity of genistein to inhibit both *in vivo* thrombogenesis, and *in vitro* platelet aggregation induced by collagen, involves inhibition of tyrosine kinase activation.[110] A similar observation has been made with the soybean isoflavones, genistein, daidzein, and glycitein, which inhibit *in vitro* platelet aggregation and DNA synthesis of aortic smooth muscle cells (SMC) in stroke-prone, spontaneously hypertensive rats.[111] In addition, genistein is an inhibitor of angiogenesis and steroid metabolizing enzymes such as aromatase and 5-α-reductase. The finding that isoflavonoids can also suppress platelet-endothelial adhesion by inhibiting deposition of platelets on damaged vessel walls[112] is a further indication of the numerous mechanisms whereby isoflavones prevent thrombogenesis.

3.2.5 Garlic and Onion

Chronic garlic consumption has been shown to prevent myocardial ischemia-reperfusion injury associated with oxidative stress and ultrastructural changes.[113] Aged garlic extracts inhibit the activation of the oxidant-induced transcription factor, nuclear factor NFkB, which has clinical significance in human atherogenesis.[114] Other studies have confirmed that aged garlic extract, but not raw garlic, increases the resistance of LDL to oxidation.[115] The antioxidant activity of aged garlic extract may be useful in preventing atherosclerotic disease through separate mechanisms that involve enhancement of cellular antioxidant enzyme systems, such as superoxide dismutase, catalase, and glutathione peroxidase, or by direct scavenging of ROS; the combination of these two mechanisms results in increased cellular glutathione content.[116] Other evidence of aged garlic extract antioxidant activity involves protection of DNA against free radical–mediated damage and inhibition of carcinogenesis as well as protection against some forms of UV-induced immunosuppression.[117] Aged garlic extract lowers ischemia-reperfusion damage of endothelial cells by reducing lipid peroxidation–induced oxidative modification of LDL. In other studies, an aged garlic extract–related suppression of iNOS mRNA and protein expression in both LPS- and IFNg-induced murine macrophage cell line RAW264.7 correspond to similar activity with rat aortic smooth muscle cells that were stimulated with LPS plus cytokines.[114] This result corresponds to other findings of a significantly increased cGMP production by eNOS without changes in activity, protein levels, and cellular distribution of eNOS. Therefore, components of garlic extract differentially regulate NO production by inhibiting macrophage expression of iNOS, but at the same time enhancing NO synthesis in endothelial cells. This selective regulation may contribute to the anti-inflammatory effect of garlic that works toward prevention of atherosclerosis.

The selective inhibitions of platelet function, which include platelet aggregation and adhesion, have further importance for the development of cardiovascular events such as myocardial infarction and ischemic stroke. Underlying mechanism(s) of garlic-induced antiplatelet activity include its ability to reduce thromboxane formation from arachidonic acid, and to inhibit the required products of platelet phospholipase and lipoxygenase activities.[118] Both the synthesis and the incorporation of arachidonic acid in platelet phospholipids are inhibited by water soluble garlic extracts. Constituents present in garlic oil have also been shown to inhibit platelet aggregation induced by several platelet agonists, and also platelet thromboxane formation *in vitro*.[119] It is of interest that similar constituents present in onion oil also inhibit both platelet cyclooxygenase and 12-lipoxygenase activities, as well as reducing platelet aggregation–induced by epinephrine and ADP.[120] Reduced deacylation of platelet phospholipids upon stimulation with the calcium ionophore-A23187 occurred in the presence of garlic extracts, thereby reducing eicosanoid synthesis. Aged garlic extract will reduce platelet aggregation in response to collagen and epinephrine, but not to von Willebrand factor.[116] Additional garlic related effects concerning inhibition of platelet aggregation involve modifying platelet membrane composition, which results in reduced calcium mobilization and impaired platelet metabolism of arachidonic acid.[121] The inhibition by garlic of thrombin-induced synthesis of platelet TXB2 during clotting of rabbit blood *in vitro* indicates that garlic contains many constituents that have an inhibitory effect at different stages of platelet aggregation and thromboxane synthesis.

Another viable mechanism for the cardioprotective effects of garlic includes the dose-dependent cholesterol lowering capacity in hypercholesterolemic experimental animals fed garlic extracts.[122] This observation involves the underlying inhibitory activity of cholesterol synthesis by decreasing such enzymes as 3-hydroxyl-3 methylglutaryl (HMG)-CoA reductase and acetyl-CoA synthetase activities.[123] Similarly, the antiatherogenic effect of the aged garlic extract product Kyolic is associated with the lowering of plasma cholesterol levels and reduced fatty streak formation, as well as inhibiting smooth muscle cell proliferation of aortic vessels in hyperlipidemic rabbits.[124] Diets supplemented with garlic resulted in marked reductions in total serum cholesterol and triglycerides, and significantly increased HDL cholesterol levels as well as fibrinolytic activity in patients with coronary artery disease. Plasma cholesteryl ester transfer protein (CETP) activity is lowered with garlic feeding, thus reducing the concentration of total cholesterol and triglycerides, LDL-C, and VLDL-C.[125] These changes have been attributed to delayed progression of atherosclerosis in aortic tissues.

3.2.5.1 Organosulfur Compounds

Organosulfur compounds (OSC) are primary bioactive phytochemicals present in garlic and onion. The four prominent OSCs, diallyl sulfide (DAS) and diallyl disulfide (DADS), which represent two lipophilic constituents, and *S*-ethylcysteine (SEC) and *N*-acetylcysteine (NAC), the hydrophilic compounds, are linked to cardioprotective activity through both antioxidant and antiglycation properties.[126] DADS has been shown to possess the strongest antioxidant activity to prevent LDL oxidation, and SEC has the relatively greatest antiglycation activity. *S*-Allyl cysteine (SAC) suppresses production of hydroxyl radicals, confirming antioxidant activity for this particular OSC.[114]

Allium derivatives have also been shown to reduce serum lipid and cholesterol levels.[127] SAC, DADS, and allicine and its derivative ajoene contribute to a hypocholesterolemic effect by decreasing several enzymes (e.g.,

HMG-CoA reductase, squalene monooxygenase, and squalene synthase) involved in cholesterol biosynthesis.[128] HMG-CoA reductase is susceptible to inactivation by phosphorylation and sulfhydryl oxidation. Garlic containing *S*-alkyl cysteines (e.g., SAC, SEC, and *S*-propyl cysteine [SPC], can depress HMG-CoA reductase activity. In addition, the reported deactivation of HMG-CoA reductase with DADS and SAC has been attributed to the formation of intramolecular disulfide bonding and increasing sulfhydryl oxidation.[129] In addition, squalene epoxidase activity, an enzyme in the downstream pathway of cholesterol synthesis involving catalysis of squalene epoxide (e.g., 2,3-oxidosqualene), is reduced by OSC. Four OSC (e.g., SAC, allicin, DADS, and DATS) have the ability to inhibit squalene monoxygenase, which in turn represents another potential mechanism for reduced cholesterol biosynthesis.[128]

Ajoene represents another OSC derived from allicin in garlic, which contains noted antithrombotic action. Ajoene is found in processed garlic products, such as garlic oil, and acts to prevent thrombosis by inhibiting platelet binding to fibrinogen, thus reducing platelet aggregation.[130] Ajoene reduces platelet membrane receptor binding to respective proaggregatory ligands, thus interfering with a cascade of metabolic events that influences conversion of arachidonic acid to potent proinflammatory agents and inducers of platelet aggregation and platelet granule release. Since ajoene inhibits receptor-ligand interactions at later stages of whole platelet activation, a synergistic effect between ajoene and the antithrombotic agent dipriyirdamole would be expected because dipriyirdamole reduces platelet aggregation differently.[131] Moreover, the alkenyl thiosulfates derived from onion and garlic, notably sodium *n*-propyl thiosulfate (NPTS) and sodium 2-propenyl thiosulfate (2PTS), also reduced the reaction time for PMA-induced O_2^- generation in canine polymorphonuclear leukocytes (PMNs). These compounds also inhibit ADP-induced platelet aggregation in both canine and human platelets. Taken together, these findings indicate that NPTS and 2PTS are potential promoters of immune functions that act to prevent cardiovascular diseases.[132]

3.2.6 Ginseng

Ginseng has a history of use dating back 2000 years as a herbal medicine with pharmacological and therapeutic use for treatment and prevention of many different stress related conditions, such as impaired memory and immune activity, and has protective effects against diabetes, cardiovascular disease and cancer.[133] The antioxidant activity of crude ginseng extracts has been reported in both Asian (Panax ginseng, C.A. Meyer)[134] and North American (*Panax quinquefolium*).[135] Extracts of Panax ginseng (0.5% w/v) reduced the loss of arachidonic acid following forced peroxidation with nitrolotriacetate and hydrogen peroxide.[134] Electron spin resonance (ESR) analysis confirmed that 0.25% ginseng extract was the minimal concentration required to scavenge free radicals generated in an aqueous reaction system. North American ginseng root extracts exhibit inhibition against Fenton reaction–induced hydroxyl radical scavenging activity.[135] Studies confirmed that ginseng root extracts were effective at inhibiting peroxyl radical–induced lipid oxidation in bilayer lamella suspensions and incubated human LDL oxidation models.[136] Moreover, protection against peroxyl radical–induced DNA damage was reported at 30 mg/mL concentration. These results help to explain the observations made with human subjects that smoked for 4 weeks while supplemented with vitamin E, β-carotene, and red ginseng. Smokers receiving 1.9 g red ginseng exhibited significantly higher concentrations of plasma antioxidants and reduced plasma malonaldehyde concentrations.[137]

3.2.6.1 Ginsenosides

Ginsenosides represent a primary group of bioactive phytochemicals unique to ginseng plants (e.g., Panax ginseng, C.A. Meyer and North American ginseng; *Panax quinquefolium*) that are categorized as terpenoid saponins (Figure 3.9). Model antioxidant studies have shown notable protection against Cu^{2+}-induced LDL oxidation from ginsenoside, Rb1 and a relatively lower peroxidation propagation rate of North American ginseng compared to Asian ginseng at preventing supercoiled DNA oxidation.[136] North American ginseng contains a greater Rb1/Rb2 concentration ratio than Asian

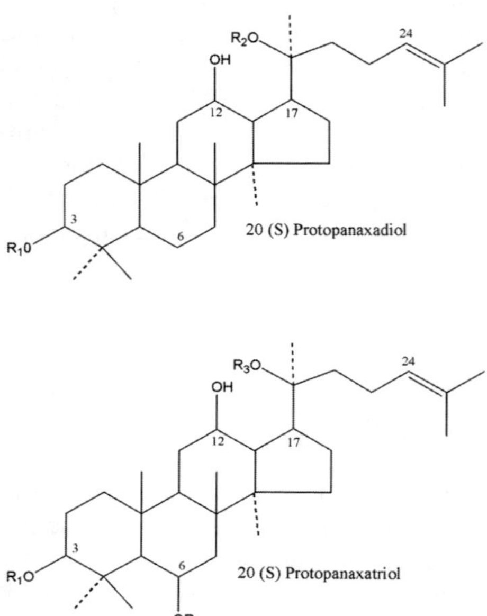

20 (S)-Protopanaxadiol

	R1	R2
Rb1	O-G-G	O-G-G
Rb2	O-G-G	O-G-Ap
Rb3	O-G-G	O-G-X
Rc	O-G-G	O-G-Af
Rd	O-G-G	O-G
Rg3	O-G-G	O-H
Rh2	O-G	O-H
Aglycone (PD)	O-H	O-H

20 (S)-Protopanaxatriol

	R1	R2	R3
Re	O-H	O-G-R	O-G
Rf	O-H	O-G-G	O-H
Rg1	O-H	O-G	O-G
Rg2	O-H	O-G-R	O-H
Rh1	O-H	O-G	O-H
Aglycone (PT)	O-H	O-H	O-H

FIGURE 3.9
Structures of specific ginsenosides identified by R1, R2, and R3 residue (Ap-arabinopyranose, Af-arabinofuranose, G-glucopyranose, R-rhamnopyranose, X-xylopyranose) components.

ginseng. Other studies using forced peroxidation of human erythrocytes have reported similar findings of antioxidant activity from Rb1 and Rc.[138]

Predominate ginsenosides Rb1 and Rb2 undergo metabolism to 20-β-*O*-glucopyranosyl-20(S)-prootopanaxadiol (e.g., Compound K) by intestinal microflora.[139] The acidic conditions of the stomach are likely involved in the hydrolysis of Rb1 to Rb3, which can then be further metabolized by colonic bacteria to ginsenoside Rh2. Moreover, the thermal processing of North American ginseng leaf also yields significant concentrations of both Rg3 and Rh2.[140] Rh2 has cytotoxic activity against many different cell lines,[141,142] as well as antiinflammatory activity in cultured macrophage cells.[143] In the latter example, Compound K was shown to reduce LPS-induced iNOS and COX-2 expression in cultured RAW 264.7 macrophages[143] and to reduce inflammatory responses to induced brain injury in rats.[144] Similarly, overexpression of proinflammatory enzyme COX-2 was significantly reduced by topical application of Rg3 in mice.[145]

3.3 Positive Interactions and Synergies

3.3.1 Nutrient-Nutrient Antioxidant Interactions

A well identified example of synergistic activity derived from established nutrients can be made with the enhanced antioxidant activity resulting from different vitamin interactions (Table 3.2). The interaction between ascorbic acid and α-tocopherol,[146–148] β-carotene and ascorbic acid,[9] and glutathione and α-tocopherol [149,150] are typical examples of enhanced antioxidant activity related to recycling of oxidized lipophilic antioxidant vitamin E and extended half-life of antioxidant activity. For example, the reducing activity of ascorbic acid regenerates α-tocopherol from α-tocopheryl radical, thus extending the free radical quenching power of α-tocopherol. There are, however, some examples with vitamin mixtures, such as retinol and β-carotene, where the combination had no effect on primary prevention of CHD.[151] On the other hand, multiple vitamin mixtures in normal subjects[152] and vitamin and zinc mixtures in smokers [153] have produced positive antioxidant results with significant increases in LDL oxidation lag times.

3.3.2 Polyphenol-Nutrient Antioxidant Interactions

Model studies have shown a similar synergistic mode of action for numerous polyphenols derived from various food systems that enhance the antioxidant activity of vitamin C and α-tocopherol (Table 3.2). Caffeic acid has been shown to act synergistically with α-tocopherol in regard to providing greater antioxidant activity.[24] The regeneration of the vitamin E radical to a reduced state by caffeic acid extends the antioxidant capacity. In addition, caffeic acid

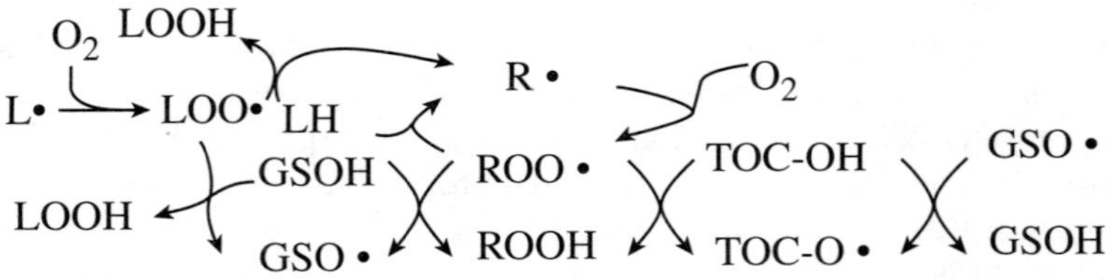

FIGURE 3.10
Scheme of antioxidant mechanism of green tea phenols (GSOH) involving lipid oxidation resulting in initiation and propagation of the peroxyl radical (R·) by lipid hydroperoxide (LOOH), trapping the peroxyl radical with α-tocopherol (TOC-OH), reducing the α-tocopheroxyl radical (TOC-O·) to recycle α-tocopherol (TOC-OH).

is an efficient quencher of hydroxyl, superoxide, and peroxyl radicals,[102] by both donating hydrogen atoms and stabilizing phenoyl radicals formed by reducing activity. When LDL containing α-tocopherol is exposed to ferrylmyoglobin, α-tocopherol is depleted as a function of myoglobin concentration. The presence of caffeic acid prevents the oxidation of α-tocopherol by acting through a one electron transfer reaction mechanism between ferrylmyoglobin and caffeic acid, which reduces the ferrylmyoglobin to a ferric state. The addition of caffeic acid prior to oxidation delays α-tocopherol consumption; however, when added simultaneously with the oxidation reaction, the α-tocopherol is restored.

Examples of green tea catechins regenerating α-tocopherol have been reported with *in vitro* linoleic peroxidation,[154] direct *in vitro* scavenging of DPPH free radical,[155] depletion of antioxidant status in plasma,[156] and LDL particles.[157] The antioxidant activity of catechins, sparing α-tocopherol, can occur by either chelating prooxidant metal ions with its redox properties, by scavenging free radicals, or, alternatively, by recycling oxidized α-tocopherol to active form (Figure 3.10). Similar antioxidant synergy activities between caffeic or *p*-coumaric acids with ascorbate have been reported in this regard.[158] Feeding rats dietary tea catechins produced significant increases in plasma α-tocopherol[159] and maintaining and regenerating antioxidant activity in human LDL.[157]

In human studies, intake of green tea did not change plasma ascorbate concentrations *ex vivo*; however, both α-tocopherol and β-carotene concentrations were enhanced.[160] These results suggest that the presence of tea polyphenols in plasma spares the *in vivo* consumption of lipid soluble antioxidants and that a daily consumption of green tea could protect against oxidative modification of LDL, either directly or indirectly by reducing the depletion of LDL-containing antioxidative vitamins. Evidence exists that the recycling of α-tocopherol by water-soluble antioxidants, including ascorbate, thiols, and also green tea epicatechin derivatives, is potentially important for the enhanced antioxidant protection of LDL and the reduced risk of cardiovascular disease.[10] Similar results have been observed with polyphenolic compounds in red wine, which act to prevent the α-tocopherol depletion and cholesterol oxidation in LDL and protect against vascular endothelium dysfunction.[161] Moreover, the fact that lycopene and other phytochemicals, such as garlic and rosemarinic acid, accumulate in serum VLDL and LDL fractions also suggests an additive antioxidant effect with vitamin E to reduce LDL oxidation.[162] In the case of ginseng, a synergistic, or antagonistic (e.g., prooxidant), activity exists in relation to the activity of individual antioxidant on vitamin E activity. For example, a synergistic activity between α-tocopherol and ginsenosides Rc, Rb1, Rg2, Rh1, and Re has been noted, whereas the presence of Rg3, Rh2, and Rd actually decreased the antioxidant activity of α-tocopherol.[138]

The synergistic effects between phytochemical and nutrient vitamin actions are not confined to antioxidant activities. For example, the inhibitory effect of naringin on HMG-CoA reductase activity is enhanced in the presence of vitamin E,[59] and the combination of ascorbic acid with citrus extracts decreases lipids and susceptibility of lipoprotein oxidation in hypercholesterolemic animals.[163] Bioactive components found in spices, such as curcumin and eugenol, perform in a similar fashion with vitamin E to reduce liver peroxidation susceptibility in rats fed dietary n-3 fatty acids[164] by stimulating specific antioxidant enzyme activities. Notwithstanding this, the combination of garlic constituents and very long chain n-3 fatty acids (EPA and DHA) has been shown to produce synergistic effects on lowering total cholesterol, LDL cholesterol, triacylglycerides, and atherogenic indexes such as LDL-HDL, and total cholesterol-HDL ratios,[165] which could indirectly have an impact on reducing lipoprotein oxidation. In the case of lycopene, the direct protective effect of lycopene and potential synergy with vitamin E toward reducing LDL oxidation goes beyond quenching of ROS, as evidenced by the interactive effect of lycopene and α-tocopherol in modifying platelet-activating factors in endothelial cells.[86]

Other evidence of potential synergies between plant derived antioxidant constituents involves polyphenol-phytochemical interactions. For example, the flavonoids quercetin and catechin act in a synergistic manner to reduce intracellular hydrogen peroxide production and platelet dysfunction.[166] The suggestion has also been made that mixtures of carotenoids are more effective than single compounds for exhibiting antioxidant activity, as evidenced by the synergistic action of lycopene and lutein on protecting against oxidation of multilamella liposomes.[167]

3.4 Adverse Reactions

3.4.1 Redox-Active Metals and Reducing Agents

Interactions between polyphenols and mineral ions can lead to the creation of stable complexes and reduced mineral bioavailability, a well known and characterized antinutritional event.[168] In addition, several natural phytochemicals have been shown to autoxidize and generate ROS, such as hydrogen peroxide (H_2O_2). Phytochemicals with reducing activity can transform ferric (Fe^{3+}) to ferrous (Fe^{2+}) ion, with the subsequent reaction between Fe^{2+} and H_2O_2, resulting in the generation of hydroxyl radicals via the Fenton reaction. Reducing agents, such as ascorbic acid and various polyphenols, including many flavonoids, have the capacity to exhibit prooxidant activity when in the presence of free transition metal ions. For example, both vitamin C[169] and flavonoids[170,171] have the capacity to accelerate lipid peroxidation and LDL oxidation when in the presence of free transition metal ions, such as $CuCl_2$. In general, compounds with a catechol moiety have the potential for prooxidant activity under specific conditions.[172] Similar prooxidant activity of α-tocopherol has also been reported in situations where tocopheroxyl radicals generated from the interaction of high concentrations of α-tocopherol with peroxyl radicals, derived from oxidized polyunsaturated fatty acids, will in fact enhance tocopherol-mediated peroxidation. Tocopherol-mediated peroxidation reaction, following exposure to transition metal ions or free radical peroxinitrite, has also been shown to generate prooxidant activity that results in oxidation of human LDL, especially in the absence of ascorbic acid.[173] The specific conditions that involve interaction of vitamins with transition metal ions, reducing agents, and presence of free radicals will therefore dictate the oxidative-antioxidative balance. Although this is an important consideration for food systems, the significance of the potential prooxidant activity of phytochemical-nutrient interactions *in vivo* is likely small and remains to be determined.

3.5 Conclusions

A number of epidemiological studies have showed a negative correlation between the incidence of CHD and dietary intake of fruits and vegetables. In addition, biochemical research has identified oxidative stress as a common underlying factor in the development of many chronic disease conditions that contribute to CHD. Oxidative stress refers to the imbalance between antioxidant and oxidizing agents that will lead to cellular injury. Many studies have shown phytochemicals that possess antioxidant activity, may also potentially modulate the degree of oxidative stress that underscores the development of CHD. In addition to providing antioxidant activity, many of these compounds need also to be evaluated for bioactivity that is related to regulatory functions triggered through signal transduction and enzyme pathways, and that work beyond a pure chemical antioxidant property. In addition, both synergistic, or inhibitory, roles of phytochemicals with other important nutrients linked to cardioprotection makes the field especially challenging and susceptible to misinterpretation. This chapter reviewed the protective role of a number of phytochemicals that are associated with reducing the risk of CHD and the potential interaction with relevant nutrients in both a positive (e.g., synergistic activity) and adverse (e.g., prooxidant activity) manner.

References

1. Ness, A.R. and Powels, J.W., Fruit and vegetables and cardiovascular disease: a review, *Int. J. Epidemiol.*, 26, 1, 1997.
2. Aldercreutz, H. and Mazur W., Phytoestrogens and western disease, *Ann. Med.*, 29, 95, 1995.
3. Liu, S., Lee, I.M., Ajani, U., Cole, S.R., Buring, J.E., and Manson, J.E., Intake of vegetables rich in carotenoids and risk of cardiovascular disease in men: The Physicians' Health Study, *Int. J. Epidemiol.*, 30, 130, 2001.
4. Truswell, A.S., Cereal grains and coronary heart disease, *Eur. J. Clin. Nutr.*, 56, 1, 2002.
5. Iqbal, K., Rauoff, M.A., Mir, M.M., Tramboo, N.A., Malik, J.A., Naikoo, B.C., Dar, M.A., Masoodi, S.R., and Khan, A.R., Lipid peroxidation during acute coronary syndromes and its intensification at the time of myocardial ischemia reperfusion, *Am. J. Cardiol.*, 89, 334, 2002.
6. Uesugi, N., Sakata, N., Horiuchi, S., Nagai, R., Takeya, M., Meng, J., Saito, T., and Takebayashi, S., Glycoxidation modified macrophages and lipid peroxidation products are associated with the progression of human diabetic nephropathy, *Am. J. Kidney Dis.*, 38, 1016, 2001.
7. Trichopoulou, A., Naska, A., Antoniou, A., Friel, S., Trygg, K., and Turrini, A., Vegetable and fruit: the evidence in their favour and the public health perspective, *Inter. J. Vitamin Nutr. Res.*, 73, 63, 2003.
8. Marchioli, R., Antioxidant vitamins and prevention of cardiovascular disease: laboratory, epidemiological and clinical trial data, *Pharmacol.Res.*, 40, 227, 1999.
9. Wieseman, H., Dietary influence on membrane function: Importance in protection against oxidative damage and disease. *J. Nutr. Biochem.*, 7, 2, 1996.
10. Mosca, L., Rubenfire, M., Mandel, C., Rock, C., Tarshis, T., Tsai, A. and Pearson, T., Antioxidant nutrient supplementation reduces the susceptibility of low density lipoprotein to oxidation in patients with coronary artery disease, *J. Am. Coll Cardiol.*, 30, 392, 1997.
11. Van't Veer, P., Jansen, M.C.J., Klerk, M., and Kok, F., Fruits and vegetables in the prevention of cancer and cardiovascular disease. *Public Health Nutr.*, 3, 103, 2000.
12. Brandt, K., Christenen, L.P., Hansen-Moller, H., Hansen, S.L., Haralsdottir, H., Jespersen, L., Purup, S., Kharazmi, A., Barkholt, V., Froliaer, H., and Kobaek-Larsen, M., Health promoting compounds in vegetables and fruits: A systematic approach for identifying plant components with impact on human health, *Trends Food Sci. Technol.*, 15, 384, 2004.
13. Sesso, H.D., Gaziano, J.M., Buring, J.E., and Hennekens, C.H., Coffee and tea intake and risk of myocardial infarction, *Am. J. Epidemiol* 149, 162, 1999.
14. Serafini, M., Ghiselli, A., and Ferro-Luzzi, A., *In vivo* antioxidant effect of green and black tea in man, *Eur. J. Clin. Nutr.* 50, 79, 1996.

15. Cherubini, A., Beal, M.F., and Frei, B., Black tea increases the resistance of human plasma to lipid peroxidation *in vitro*, but not ex vivo, *Free Rad. Biol. Med.*, 27, 381, 1999.
16. Ishikawa, T., Suzukawa, M., Toshimitsu, I.,Yoshida, H., Ayori, M., Nishikawa, M., Ishikawa, M., Yonermura, A., Hara, Y., and Nakamura, H., Effect of tea flavonoids supplementation on the susceptibility of low-density lipoprotein to oxidative modification, *Am. J. Clin. Nutr.*, 66, 261, 1997.
17. Hodgson, J.M., Odgson, J.M., Puddey, I.B., Burke, V., Beilin, L.J., and Jordan, N., Effects on blood pressure of drinking green and black tea, *J. Hypertension,* 17, 457, 2000.
18. Yang, T.T. and Koo, M.W., Inhibitory effect of Chinese green tea on endothelial cell-induced LDL oxidation, *Atherosclerosis*, 148, 67, 2000.
19. Matsumoto, N., Okushio, K., and Hara, Y., Effect of black tea polyphenols on plasma lipids in cholesterol-fed rats, *J. Nutr. Sci. Vitaminol.*, 44, 337, 1998.
20. De Vos, S., and DeSchrijver, R., Lipid metabolism, intestinal fermentation and mineral absorption in rats consuming black tea, *Nutr. Res.*, 23, 527, 2003.
21. Yokozawa, T., Nakagawa, T., and Kitani, K., Antioxidant activity of green tea polyphenols in cholesterol-fed rats, *J. Agric. Food Chem.*, 50, 3549, 2000.
22. Bursill, C., Roach, P.D, Bottema, C.D. and Pal, S., Green tea up-regulates the low-density lipoprotein receptor through the sterol-regulated element binding protein in HepG2 liver cells, *J. Agric. Food Chem.*, 49, 5639, 2001.
23. Stich, H F. and Powrie, WD., Plant phenolics as genotoxic agents and as modulators for the mutagenicity of other food components, in *Carcinogens and Mutagens in the Environment*, Vol. 1, Stich, H.F. (ed). CRC Press, Boca Raton, FL, 1982, pp. 136–145.
24. Laranjinha, J., Vieira, O., Madeira, V., and Almeida, L., Two related phenolic antioxidants with opposite effects on vitamin E content in low density lipoproteins oxidized by ferrylmyoglobin: consumption vs regeneration, *Arch. Biochem. Biophys.*, 323, 373, 1995.
25. Ohnishi, M., Morishita, H., Iwahashi, H., Toda, S., Shirataka, Y., Kimura, M., and Kido, R., Inhibitory effects of chlorogenic acids on linoleic acid peroxidation and haemolysis, *Phytochemistry*, 36, 579, 1994.
26. Laranjinha, J.A.N., Almeida, L.M., and Madieire, V.M.C., Reactivity of dietary phenolic acids with peroxyl radicals: antioxidant activity upon low density lipoprotein peroxidation, *Biochem. Pharmacol.*, 48, 487, 1994.
27. Millard, M.N. and Berset, C., Evalution of antioxidant activity during kilning. Role of insoluble bound phenolic acids of barley and malt, *J. Agric. Food Chem.*, 43, 1789, 1994.
28. Miller, N.A., Diplock, A.T., and Rice-Evans, C.A., Evaluation of the total antioxidant activity as a marker of the deterioration of apple juice on storage, *J. Agric. Food Chem.*, 43, 1794, 1994.
29. Miller, N.A. and Rice–Evans, C.A., The relative contributions of ascorbic acid and phenolic antioxidants to the total antioxidant activity of orange and apple fruit juices and black-current drink, *Food Chem.*, 60, 331, 1997.
30. Joudad, D., Lacaille-Dubois, M.A., Lyoussi, B., and Eddouks, M., Effects of flavonoids extracted from *Spergularia purpurea* Pers on arterial blood pressure and renal function in normal and hypertensive rats, *J. Enthopharmacol.*, 76, 159, 2002.
31. Steinberg, F., Bearden, M.M., and Keen, C.L., Cocoa and chocolate flavonoids: implications for cardiovascular health, *J. Am. Dietetic Assoc.*, 103, 215, 2003.

32. Aviram, M. and Fuhrman, B., Polyphenolic flavonoids inhibit macrophage-mediated oxidation of LDL and attenuate atherogenesis, *Atherosclerosis*, 137, S45, 1998.
33. Safari, M.R. and Sheikn, N., Effects of flavonoids on the susceptibility of low-density lipoprotein to oxidative modification, *Prostaglandins Leukot. Essen. Fatty Acids*, 69, 73, 2003.
34. Karaim, M., McCormick, K., and Kappogoda, C.T., Effects of cocoa extracts on endothelium-dependent relaxation, *J. Nutr.*, 130, 2105S, 2000.
35. Li, I.H., Xia, N., Brausch, I., Yao, Y., and Forstermanu, U., Flavonoids from artichoke (*Cynara scolymus L.*) upregulate eNOS gene expression in human endothelial cells, *J. Pharmacol. Exp. Ther.*, 310, 926, 2004.
36. Aviram, M. and Fuhrman, B., Polyphenolic flavonoids inhibit macrophage-mediated oxidation of LDL and attenuate atherogenesis, *Atherosclerosis* 137, S45, 1998.
37. Miyazawa, T., Absorption, metabolism and antioxidant effects of tea catechins in humans, *Biofactors*, 13, 55, 2000.
38. Salah, N., Miller, N.J., Paganga, G., Tijburg, L., Bolwell, G. P., and Rice Evans, C., Polyphenolic flavonols as scavengers of aqueouos phase radicals and as chain-breaking antioxidants, *Arch. Biochem. Biophys.*, 322, 339, 1995.
39. Van Het Hof, K.H., Kivitis, G.A.A., Weststrate, J.A., and Tijburg, L.B.M., Bioavailability of catechins from tea: the effect of milk, *Eur. J. Clin. Nutr.*, 52, 356, 1998.
40. Rice-Evans, C.A., Miller, N.J., and Pagana, G., Structure-antioxidant activity relationships of flavonoids and phenolic acids, *Free Rad. Biol. Med.*, 20, 933, 1996.
41. Nanjo, F., Mor, M., Goto, K., and Hara, Y., Radical scavenging activity of tea catechins and their related compounds. *Biosci. Biotechnol. Biochem.*, 63, 1621, 1999.
42. Nakagawa, A., Beal, M.F., and Frei, B., Direct scavenging of nitric oxide and superoxide by green tea, *Food Chem. Toxicol.* 40, 1745, 2002.
43. Chan, M. M-Y., Ho, C.T., and Huang, H.I., Effects of three dietary phytochemicals from tea, rosemary, and tumeric on inflammation-induced nitrite production, *Cancer Letts.*, 96:, 23, 1995.
44. Soriani, M., Rice-Evans, C.A., and Tyrell, R.M., Modulation of the UV activation of haem oxygenase, collagenase and cyclooxygenase expression by epigallocatechin in human skin cells, *FEBS Letts*. 439, 253, 1995.
45. Sun, J., Chu, Y.F., Wu, X., and Liu, R.I., Antioxidant and antiproliferative activities of common fruits, *J. Agric. Food Chem*. 50, 7449, 2002.
46. Miller, H.E., Pigelhof, F., Marquart, L., Prakash, A., and Kanter, M., Antioxidant content of whole grain breakfast cereals, fruits and vegetables, *J. Am. Coll. Nutr.*, 19, 312S, 2000.
47. Wang, H., Cao, G., and Prior, R.L., Total antioxidant capacity of fruits, *J. Agric. Food Chem*. 44, 701, 1996.
48. Lee, K.W., Kim, Y.J., Kim, D.O., and Lee, C.Y., Major phenolics in apple and their contribution to the total antioxidant capacity. *J. Agric. Food Chem.*, 51, 6516, 2003.
49. Wolfe, K., Liu, X., and Liu, R.H., Antioxidant activity of apple peels, *J. Agric. Food Chem*. 51, 609, 2003.
50. Liu, R.H., Health benefits of fruit and vegetables are from additive and synergistic combinations of phytochemicals, *Am. J. Clin. Nutr.*, 78, 517S, 2003.

51. Nagasawa, T., Tabata, N., Ito,Y., Aiba,Y., Nishizawa, N., and Kitts, D.D., Dietary G-rutin suppresses glycation in tissue proteins of streptozotocin-induced diabetic rats, *Mol. Cell Biochem.*, 252, 141, 2003.
52. Marcocci, L., Packer, L., Droy-Lefaix, M-T., Sekaki, A., and Gardes-Albert, M., Antioxidant action in ginkgo biloba extract Egb761, in *Methods of Enzymology — Oxygen Radicals in Biological Systems*, Vol 234, Packer, L., Ed., Academic Press, San Diego, 1994, p. 462.
53. Manach, C., Morand, C., Texiert, O., Favier, M. L., Agullo, G., Demigne, C., Regerat, F., and Remesy, C., Quercetin metabolites in plasma of rats fed diets containing rutin or quercetin, *J. Nutr.*, 125, 1911, 1995.
54. Huang, Y.T., Hwang, J.J., Lee, P.P., Ke, F. C., Huang, C. J., Kandaswami, C., Middleton, E., and Lee, M.T., Effect of luteolin and quercetin inhibitors of tyrosine kinase on cell growth and metastasis-associated properties in A431 cells over expressing epidermal growth factor receptor, *Br J. Pharmacol.*, 128, 999, 1999.
55. Cheng, J., Kondo, K., Suzuki, Y., Ikeda, Y., Meng, X., and Umemura, K., Inhibitory effects of total flavones of *Hippophae Rhammoides L* on thrombosis in mouse femoral artery and *in vitro* platelet aggregation, *Life Sci.*, 72, 2263, 2003.
56. Hu, C. and Kitts, D., Antioxidant, prooxidant and cytotoxic activities of solvent-fractionated dandelion (*Taraxacum officinale*) flower extracts *in vitro, J. Agric. Food Chem.*, 51, 301 2003.
57. Hu, C. and Kitts, D.D., Luteolin and luteolin-7-O-glucoside from dandelion flower suppress iNOS and COX-2 in RAW264.7 cells, *Mol. Cell Biochem.*, 265, 107, 2004.
58. Wilcox, L.J., Borradaile, N.M., and Huff, M.W., Antiatherogenic properties of naringenin, a citrus flavonoid, *Cardiovasc. Drug Rev.*, 17, 160, 1999.
59. Choi, M-S., Do, K-M, Park, Y-B., Jeon, S-M., Jeong, T-S., Lee, Y-K., Lee, M-K., and Bok, S-H., Effect of naringin supplementation on cholesterol metabolism and antioxidant status in rats fed high cholesterol with different levels of vitamin E, *Ann. Nutr. Metab.*, 45, 193, 2001.
60. Chen, C.H., Jeong, T.S., Choi, Y.K., Hyun, B.H., Oh, G.T., Kim, E.H., Kim, J.R., Han, J.I., and Bok, S.H., Anti-atherogenic effect of citrus flavonoids, naringin and naringenin, associated with hepatic ACAT and aortic VCAM-1 and MCP-1 in high cholesterol-fed rabbits, *Biochem. Biophys. Res. Commun.*, 284, 681, 2001.
61. Kalt, W., Forney, C., Marin, A., and Prior, R.L., Antioxidant capacity of vitamin C, phenolics and anthocyanins after fresh storage of small fruits, *J. Agric. Food Chem.*, 47, 4638, 1999.
62. Wang, H., Nair, M.G., Strasburg, G., Chang, Y.C., Booren, A M., Gray, J.I., and DeWitt, D.L., Antioxidant and antinflammatory activities of anthocyanins and their aglycon, cyaniding form tart cherries, *J. Nat. Prod.*, 62, 294, 1999.
63. Hu, C., Zawistowski, J., Ling, W., and Kitts, D.D., Black rice (*Oryza sativa* L. indica) pigmented fraction suppresses both reactive oxygen species and nitric oxide in chemical and biological model systems, *J. Agric. Food Chem.*, 51, 5271, 2003.
64. Awika, J., Rooney, L.W., and Waniska, R.D., Properties of 3-deoxyanthocyanins from sorghum, *J. Agric. Food. Chem.*,52, 4388, 2004.
65. Tsuda, T., Ohshima, K., Kawakishi, S. and Osawa, T., Antioxidant pigments insolated from the seed of *Phaseolus vulgaris* L., *J. Agric. Food Chem.*, 42 248, 1994.

66. Xia, M., Ling, W., Ma, J., Kitts, D.D., and Zawistowski, J., Supplementation of diets with black rice pigment fraction attenuates atherosclerotic plaque formation in apolipoprotein E deficient mice, *J. Nutr.*, 133, 744, 2003.
67. Sato, M., Bagchi, D., Toskai, A., and Das, D.K., Grape seed proanthocyanidin reduces cardiomyocyte apoptosis by inhibiting ischemia/reperfusion-induced activation of JNK-1 and C-JUN, *Free Rad. Biol. Med.*, 31,729, 2001.
68. Bagchi, S., Sen, C.K., Ray, S.D., Das, D.K., Bagchi, M., Preuss, H.G., and Vinson, J.A., Molecular mechanisms of cardioprotection by a novel grape seed proanthocyanidin extract, *Mutat. Res.*, 523–524, 87, 2003.
69. Patraki, T., Bak, I., Kovacs, P., Bagchi, D., Das, D.K., and Tosaski, A., Grape seed proanthocyanidins improved cardiac recovery during reperfusion after ischemia in isolated rat hearts, *Am. J. Clin. Nutr.*, 75, 894, 2002.
70. Paiva, S.A. and Russell, R. M., Beta-carotene and other carotenoids as antioxidants, *J. Am. Coll Nutr.*, 18, 426, 1999.
71. Panasenko, O.M., Sharov, V.S., Briviba, K., and Sies, H., Interaction of peroxynitrite with carotenoids in human low density lipoproteins, *Arch. Biochem. Biophys.*, 373, 302, 2003.
72. Dugas, T.R., Morel, D.W., and Harrison, E.H., Dietary supplementation with β-carotene, but not with lycopene, inhibits endothelial cell-mediated oxidation of low density lipoproteins, *Free Rad. Biol. Med.*, 26, 1238, 1999.
73. Kritshevsky, S.B., Tell, G. S., Shimakawa, T., Dennis, B., Li, R., Kohlmeier, L., Steere, E., and Heiss, G., Provitamn A carotenoid intake and carotid artery plaques: the atherosclerosis risk in communities study, *Am. J. Clin. Nutr.*, 68, 726, 1998.
74. Martin, K.R., Wu, D., and Meydani, M., The effects of carotenoids on the expression of cell surface adhesion molecules and binding of monocytes to human aortic endothelial cells, *Atherosclerosis*, 150, 265, 2000.
75. Tavani, A. and La Vecchia, C., Beta-carotene and risk of coronary heart disease, A review of observational and intervention studies, *Biomed. Pharmacoltherapy*, 53, 409, 1999.
76. Van Poppel, G., Epidemiological evidence for beta-carotene in prevention of cancer and cardiovascular disease, *Eur J. Clin. Nutr.*, 50, S57, 1996.
77. Greenberg, R.E., Baron, J.A., Karagas, M.R., Stukel, T.A., Nierenberg, D.W., Stevens, M M., Mandel, J. S., and Haile, R.W., Mortality associated with low plasma concentration of beta-carotene and the effect of oral supplementation, *JAMA*, 275, 699, 1996.
78. Rao, A.V., Lycopene, tomatoes and the prevention of heart disease, *Exp. Biol. Med.*, 227, 908, 2002.
79. Fuhrman, B., Elis, A., and Aviram, M., Hypocholesterolemic effect of lycopene and beta-carotene is related to suppression of cholesterol synthesis and augmentation of LDL receptor activity in macrophages, *Biochem. Biophys. Res. Commun.*, 233, 658, 1997.
80. Fuhrman, B., Volkova, N., Rosenblat, M., and Aviram, M., Lycopene synergistically inhibits LDL oxidation in combination with vitamin E, glabridin, rosemarinic acid, carnosic acid or garlic. *Antioxid. Redox Signal*, 2, 491, 2000.
81. Moncada, S. and Higgs, A., The L-arginine-nitric oxide pathway. *New Eng. J. Med.*, 329, 2002, 1993.
82. Esterbauer, H., Gebicki, J., Puhl, H., and Jurgens, G., The role of lipid peroxidation and antioxidants in oxidative modification of LDL. *Free Rad. Biol. Med.*, 13, 341, 1992.

83. Gianetti, J., Pedrinelli, R., Petrucci, R., Lazzerini, G., De Caterina, M., Bellomo, G., and De Caterina, R., Inverse association between carotid-media thickness and the antioxidant lycopene in atherosclerosis. *Am. Heart J.* 143, 467, 2002.
84. Klipstein-Grobusch, K., Launer, L. J., Geleijnse, J. M., Boeing, H., Hofman, A., and Witteman, J. C., Serum carotenoids and atherosclerosis, the Rottendam study, *Atherosclerosis,* 148, 49, 2000.
85. Rissanen, T.H., Voutilainen, S., Nyyssonen, K., Lakka, T.A., Sivenius, J., Salonen, R., Kaplan, G.A., and Salonen, J.T., Low serum lycopene concentration is associated with an excess incidence of acute coronary events and stroke: the Kuopio Ischaemic Heart Disease Risk Factor Study, *Br J. Nutr.,* 85, 749, 2000.
86. Balestrieri, M.L., De Prisco, R., Nicolaus, B., Pari, P., Schiano Moriello, V., Strazzullo, G., Iorio, E.L., Servillo, L., and Balestrieri, C., Lycopene in association with alpha-tocopherol or tomato lipophilic extracts enhances acyl-platelet-activating factor biosynthesis in endothelial cells during oxidative stress, *Free Rad. Biol. Med.,* 36, 1058, 2004.
87. Ivanov, V., Carr, A.C., and Frei, B., Red wine antioxidants bind to human lipoproteins and protect them from metal ion-dependent and -independent oxidation. *J. Agric. Food Chem.,* 49, 4442, 2001.
88. Deckert, V., Desrumaux, C., Athias, A., Duverneuil, L., Palleau, V., Gambert, P., Masson, D., and Lagrost, L., Prevention of LDL alpha-tocopherol consumption, cholesterol oxidation, and vascular endothelium dysfunction by polyphenolic compounds from red wine, *Atherosclerosis,* 165, 41, 2002.
89. De Lange, D.W., Van Golde, P.H., Scholman, W.L.G., Kraaijenhagen, R.J., Akkerman, J.W.N., and Van De Wiel, A., Red wine and red wine polyphenolic compounds but not alcohol inhibit ADP-induced platelet aggregation, *Eur. J. Intern. Med.,* 14, 361, 2003.
90. Whitehead, T.P., Robinson, D., Sallaawaay, S., Syms, J., and Hale, A., Effect of red wine on the antioxidant capacity of serum, *Clin. Chem.,* 41, 32, 1995.
91. Williams, M.J., Sutherland, W.H., Whelan, A.P., McCormick, M.P., and De Jong, S.A., Acute effect of drinking red and white wines on circulating levels of inflammation-sensitive molecules in men with coronary artery disease, *Metabolism,* 53, 318, 2004.
92. Schramm, D.D., Pearson, D.A., and German, J.B., Endothelial cell basal PGI_2 release is stimulated by wine *in vitro*: One mechanism that may mediate the vasoprotective effects of wine, *J. Nutr. Biochem.,* 8, 647, 1997.
93. Diebolt, M., Bucher, B., and Andrianstisohaina, R., Wine polyphenols decrease blood pressure, improve NO vasodilation and induce gene expression, *Hypertension,* 38, 159, 2001.
94. Landrault, N., Poucheret, P., Ravel, P., Gasc, F., Cros,G., and Teissedre, P.L., Antioxidant capacities and phenolic levels of French wines from different varieties and vintages. *J. Agric. Food Chem.,* 49, 3341, 2001.
95. Ray, P.S., Maulik, G., Cordis, G.A., Bertelli, A.A., Bertelli, A., and Das, D.K. The red wine antioxidant resveratrol protects isolated rat hearts from ischemia reperfusion injury, *Free Rad. Biol. Med.,* 27, 160, 1999.
96. Hung. L.M., Chen, J.K., Huang. S.S., Lee, R. S., and Su, M.J., Cardioprotective effect of resveratrol, a natural antioxidant derived from grapes, *Cardiovasc Res.,* 47, 549, 2000.

97. Bradamante, S., Barenghi, L., Piccinini, F., Bertelli, A. A., De Jong, R., Beemster, P., and De Jong, J.W., Resveratrol provides late-phase cardioprotection by means of a nitric oxide- and adenosine-mediated mechanism, *Eur. J. Pharmacol.,*, 465, 115, 2003.
98. Fremont, L., Biological effects of resveratrol, *Life Sci.*, 66, 663, 2000.
99. Mizutani, K., Ikeda, K., and Yamori, Y., Resveratrol inhibits AGE-s induced proliferataion and collagen synthesis activity in vascular smooth muscle cells from stroke-prone spontaneously hypertensive rats, *Biochem. Biophys. Res. Comm.*, 274, 61, 2000.
100. Chappey, O., Dosquet, C., Wautier, M-P., and Wautier, J.L., Advanced glycation end-products, oxidative stress and vascular lesions, *Eur J. Clin. Invest.*, 27, 97, 1997.
101. Kitts, D.D., Yuan, Y.V., Wijewickreme, A.N., and Thompson, L.U., Antioxidant activity of flaxseed lignan secoisolariciresinol diglycoside and its mammalian lignan metabolites enterodiol and enterolactone, *Mol. Cell Biochem.*, 202, 545, 1999.
102. Sroka, Z. and Cisowski, W., Hydrogen peroxide scavenging, antioxidant and anti-radical activity of some phenolic acids. *Food Chem. Toxicol.*, 41, 753, 2003.
103. Lai, H.H. and Yen G.C., Inhibitory effect of isoflavones on peroxynitrite-mediated low-density lipoprotein oxidation, *Biosci. Biotechnol. Biochem.*, 66, 22, 2002.
104. Jiang, F., Jones, G.T., Husband, A.J., and Dusting, G.J., Cardiovascular protective effects of synthetic isoflavone derivatives in apolipoprotein E-deficient mice, *J. Vasc. Res.*, 40, 276, 2003.
105. Davis, J.N., Kucuk, O., Djuric, Z., and Sarkar, F.H., Soy isoflavone supplementation in healthy men prevents NF-kappa B activation by TNF-alpha in blood lymphocytes, *Free Rad. Biol. Med.*, 30, 1293, 2001.
106. Jenkins, D. J., Kendell, C.W., Jackson, C. J., Connelly, P.W., Parker, T., Faulkner, D., Vidgene, E., Cunnane, S.C., Leiter, L.A., and Josse, R.G., Effects of high- and low-isoflavone soyfoods on blood lipids, oxidized LDL, homocysteine, and blood pressure in hyperlipidemic men and women, *Am. J. Clin. Nutr.*, 76, 365, 2002.
107. Sanders, T.A., Dean, T.S., Grainger, D., Miller, G.J., and Wiseman, H., Moderate intakes of intact soy protein rich in isoflavones compared with ethanol-extracted soy protein increase HDL but do not influence transforming growth factor beta(1) concentrations and hemostatic risk factors for coronary heart disease in healthy subjects, *Am. J. Clin. Nutr.*, 76, 373, 2002.
108. Nestel, P., Isoflavones: their effects on cardiovascular risk and functions, *Curr. Opin. Lipidol.*, 14, 3, 2003.
109. Min, J.Y., Liao, H., Wang, J.F., Sullivan, M.F., Ito, T., and Morgan, J.P., Genistein attenuates post-ischemic depressed myocardial function by increasing myofilament Ca^{2+} sensitivity in rat myocardium, *Exp. Biol. Med.*, 227, 632, 2002.
110. Kondo, K., Suzuki, Y., Ikeda, Y. and Umemura, K. Genistein, an isoflavone included in soy, inhibits thrombotic vessel occlusion in the mouse femoral artery and *in vitro* platelet aggregation. *Eur. J. Pharmacol.*, 455, 53, 2002.
111. Pan, W., Ikeda, K., Takebe, M., and Yamori, Y., Genistein, daidzein and glycitein inhibit growth and DNA synthesis of aortic smooth muscle cells from stroke-prone spontaneously hypertensive rats, *J. Nutr.*, 131, 1154, 2001.

112. Mruk, J.S., Webster, M.W., Heras, M., Reid, J.M., Grill, D.E, and Chesebro, J.H., Flavone-8-acetic acid (flavonoid) profoundly reduces platelet-dependent thrombosis and vasoconstriction after deep arterial injury *in vivo*, *Circulation,* 101, 324, 2000.
113. Sahu, S.C., Dual role of organosulfur compounds in foods: a review, *J. Environ. Sci. Health,* 20, 61, 2002.
114. Ali, M., Al-Qattan, K.K., Al-Enezi, F., Khanafer, R.M., Mustafa, T., Effect of allicin from garlic powder on serum lipids and blood pressure in rats fed with a high cholesterol diet, *Prostaglandins Leukot. Essent. Fatty Acids,* 62, 253, 2000.
115. Chernyad'eva, I.F., Shil'nikova, S.V., Rogoza, A.N., and Kukharchuk, V.V., Dynamics of interrelationships between the content of lipoprotein particles, fibrinogen, and leukocyte count in the plasma from patients with coronary heart disease treated with Kwai, *Bull. Exp. Biol. Med.,* 135, 436, 2003.
116. Borek, C., Antioxidant health effects of aged garlic extract, *J. Nutr.,* 131, 1010S, 2001.
117. Banerjee, S.K., Dinda, A.K., Manchanda, S.C., and Maulik, S.K., Chronic garlic administration protects rat heart against oxidative stress induced by ischemic reperfusion injury, *BMC Pharmacol.,* 2, 16, 2002.
118. Ackermann, R.T., Mulrow, C.D., Ramirez, G., Gardner, C.D., Morbidoni, L., and Lawrence, V.A., Garlic shows promise for improving some cardiovascular risk factors, *Arch. Intern. Med.,* 161, 813, 2001.
119. Ali, M., Thomson, M., and Afzal, M., Garlic and onions: their effect on eicosanoid metabolism and its clinical relevance, *Prostaglandins Leukot. Essen. Fatty Acids,* 62, 55, 2000.
120. Tapiero, H., Townsend, D.M., and Tew, K., Organosulfur compounds from alliaceae in the prevention of human pathologies, *BioMed. Pharmacother.,* 58, 183, 2004.
121. Thomson, M., Mustafa, T., and Ali, M., Thromboxane-B2 levels in serum of rabbits receiving a single intravenous dose of aqueous extract of garlic and onion, *Prostaglandins Leukot. Essen. Fatty Acids,* 63, 217, 2000.
122. Slowing, K., Ganado, P., Sanz, M., Ruiz, E., and Tejerina, T., Study of garlic extracts and fractions on cholesterol plasma levels and vascular reactivity in cholesterol-fed rabbits, *J. Nutr.* 131, 994S, 2001.
123. Focke, M., Feld, A., and Lichtenthaler, K., Allicin, a naturally occurring antibiotic from garlic, specifically inhibits acetyl-CoA synthetase, *FEBS Lett* 26, 106, 1990.
124. Efendy, J.L, Simmons, D.L., Campbell, G.R., and Campbell, J.H., The effect of the aged garlic extract "Kyolic," on the development of experimental atherosclerosis, *Atherosclerosis,* 132, 37, 1997.
125. Kwon, M.-J., Song, Y.-S., Choi, M.-S., Park, S.-J., Jeong, K.-S., and Song,Y.-O., Cholesteryl ester transfer protein activity and atherogenic parameters in rabbits supplemented with cholesterol and garlic powder, *Life Sci.,* 72, 2953, 2003.
126. Yin, M.C., Tsao, S.M., and Lin, M.C., Protective action on human LDL against oxidation and glycation by four organosulfur compounds derived from garlic, *Lipids,* 38, 219, 2003.
127. Loy, M. and Rovlin, R., Garlic and cardiovascular disease, *Nutr. Clin. Care,* 3, 145, 2000.
128. Gupa, N. and Porter, T.D., Garlic and garlic-derived compounds inhibit human squalene monooxygenase, *J. Nutr.,* 131, 1662, 2003.

129. Liu, L. and Yeh, Y., S-Alk(en)yl cysteines of garlic inhibit cholesterol synthesis by deactivating HMG-CoA reductase in cultured rat hepatocytes, *J. Nutr.*, 132, 1129, 2002.
130. Teranishi, K., Apitz-Castro, R., Robson, S.C., Romano, E., and Cooper, D.K., Inhibition of baboon platelet aggregation *in vitro* and *in vivo* by the garlic derivative, ajoene, *Xenotransplant*, 10, 374, 2003.
131. Apitz-Castro, R., Escalanate, J., Vargas, R., and Jain, M.K., Ajoene, the antiplatelet principle of garlic, synergistically potentiates the anti-aggregatory action of prostacyclin, forskolin, indomethacin and dypridamole on human subjects, *Thromb Res.*, 42, 303, 1986.
132. Change, H.S., Yamato, O., Sakai, Y., Yamasaki, M., and Maede, Y., Acceleration of superoxide generation in polymorphonuclear leukocytes and inhibition of platelet aggregation by alk(en)yl thiosulfates derived from onion and garlic in dogs and humans, *Prostaglandins Leukot. Essent. Fatty Acids*, 70, 77, 2004.
133. Kitts, D.D. and Popovich, D.G., Ginseng, in *Performance Functional Foods*, Watson D.H. (ed), Woodhead Publishing Ltd. Cambridge England, 2003, p. 78.
134. Zhang, D., Ysuda, T., Yu, Y., Zheng, P., Kawabata, T., Ma, Y., and Okada, S., Ginseng extract scavenges hydroxyl radical and protects unsaturated fatty acids from decomposition caused by iron-mediated lipid peroxidation, *Free Rad. Biol. Med.*, 20, 145, 1996.
135. Kitts, D.D., Wijewickreme, A.N., and Hu, C., Antioxidant properties of a North American ginseng extract, *Mol. Cell Biochem.*, 203, 1, 2000.
136. Hu, C. and Kitts, D.D., Free radical scavenging capacity as related to antioxidant activity and ginsenoside composition of Asian and North American ginseng extracts. *J. Am. Chem. Soc.*, 78, 249, 2001.
137. Kim, H.S. and Lee, B.M., Protective effects of antioxidant supplementation on plasma lipid peroxidation in smokers, *J. Toxicol. Environ. Health*, 63, 583–589, 2001.
138. Liu, Z., Luo, X., Sun, Y., Chen, Y., and Wang, Z., Can ginsenosides protect human erthrocytes against free-radical induced hemolysis? *Biochim. Biophys. Acta* 1572, 58, 2002.
139. Bae, E.A., Han, M.J., Choo, M.K., Park, S.Y., and Kim, D.H., Metabolism of 20(S)- and 20(R)-ginsenoside Rg3 by human intestinal bacteria and its relation to *in vitro* biological activities, *Biol. Pharmacol.Bull.*, 25, 58, 2001.
140. Popovich, D.G. and Kitts, D.D., Generation of ginsenosides Rg3 and Rh2 from North American ginseng. *Phytochemistry* 65, 337, 2004.
141. Popovich, D.G. and Kitts D.D., Ginsenosides 20(S)-protopanaxadiol and Rh2 reduce cell proliferation and increase sub-G1 cells in two cultured intestinal cell lines, Int-407 and Caco-2, *Can. J. Physiol. Pharmacol.*, 82,183, 2004.
142. Bae, E.A., Choo, M.K., Park, E.K., Park, S.Y, Shin, H.Y., and Kim, D.H., Metabolism of ginsenoside Rc by human intestina bacteria and its related antiallergic activity, *Biol. Pharmaceut. Bull.* 25, 743, 2002.
143. Oh, G.S., Pae, H.O., and Cho, B.M., 20(S)-Protopanaxatriol, one of ginsenoside metabolites inhibits inducible nitric oxide synthase and cyclooxygenase-2 expressions through inactivation of nuclear factor-*k*B in RAW 264.7 macrophages stimulated with lipopolysaccharides, *Cancer Lett.*, 205, 23, 2004.
144. Park, E.K., Choo, M.K., Oh, J.K., Ryu, J.H., and Kim, D.H., Ginsenoside Rh2 reduces ischemic brain injury in rats, *Biol. Pharmacol. Bull.*, 27, 433, 2003.

145. Keum, Y.S., Han, S.S., Chun, K.S., Park, K.K., Park, J.H., Lee, S.K., and Surh, Y.J., Inhibitory effects of ginsenoside Rg3 on phorbol-ester-induced cyclooxygenase-2 expression, NFKB activation and tumor promotion, *Mutat Res.*, 523, 75, 2003.
146. Packer, J.E., Slater, T.F., and Wilson, R.L., Direct observation of a free radical interaction between vitamin E and vitamin C., *Nature*, 278, 737, 1979.
147. Kagan V.E., Serbinova, E.A., Forte, T., Scita, G., and Packer, L., Recycling of vitamin E in human low-density lipoproteins, *J. Lipid Res.*, 33, 385, 1992.
148. Packer, J.E., Weber, S., and Rimbach, G., Molecular aspects of alpha tocotrienol antioxidant action and cellular signaling, *J. Nutr.*, 131, 369S, 2001.
149. Chan, A.C., Tran, K., Raynor, T., Ganz, P.R., and Chow, C.K., Regeneration of vitamin E in human platelet, *J. Biol. Chem.*, 266, 17290, 1990.
150. Constantinescu, A., Han, D., and Packer, L., Vitamin E recycling in human erythrocyte membranes, *J. Biol. Chem.*, 268, 10906, 1993.
151. Omenn, G.S., Goodman, G.E., Thornquist, M.D. et al., Effects of a combination of beta-carotene and vitamin A on lung cancer and cardiovascular disease, *New Engl. J. Med.*, 334, 1150, 1996.
152. Chen, H. and Tappel. A., Protection by multiple antioxidants against lipid peroxidation in rat liver homogenates, *Lipids*, 31, 47, 1996.
153. Abbey, M., Nestell, P.J., and Baghurst, P.A., Antioxidant vitamins and low density lipoprotein oxidation, *Am. J. Clin. Nutr.*, 58, 525, 1993.
154. Jia, Z.S., Zhou, B., Yang, L, Wu, L.M., and Liu, Z.L., Antioxidant synergism of tea polyphenols and alpha-tocopherol against free radical induced peroxidation of linoleic acid in solution, *J. Chem. Soc. Perkin-Transaction.*, 4, 911, 1998.
155. Hu, C and Kitts, D.D., Evaluation of antioxidant activity of epigallocatechin gallate in biphasic model systems *in vitro*, *Mol. Cell Biochem.*, 218, 147, 2001.
156. Lotito, S.B and Fraga, C G., Catechins delay lipid oxidation and alpha tocopherol and beta-carotene depletion following ascorbate depletion in human plasma, *Proc. Soc. Exp. Biol. Med.*, 225, 32, 2000.
157. Zhu, Q.Y., Huang, Y., Tsang, D., and Chen, Z.-Y., Regeneration of alpha tocopherol in human low-density lipoprotein by green tea catechin, *J. Agric. Food Chem.*, 47, 2020, 1999.
158. Vieira, O., Laranginka, J., Madeira, V., and Almeida, L., Cholesterol ester hydroperoxide formation in myoglobin-catalyzed low-density lipoprotein oxidation: concerted antioxidant activity of caffeic and *p*-coumaric acids with ascorbate, *Biochem. Pharmacol.*, 55, 333, 1998.
159. Nanjo, F., Honda, M., Okushio, K., Matsumoto, N., Ishigaki, F., Ishigami, Y., and Hara, Y., Effects of dietary tea catechins on alpha-tocopherol levels, lipid peroxidation, and erythrocyte deformability in rats fed on high palm oil and peril oil diets, *Biol. Pharm. Bull.*, 16, 1156, 1993.
160. Miura, Y., Chiba T., Miura S., Tomita, I., Umegaki, K., Ikeda M., and Tomita, T., Green tea polyphenols (flavan-3-ols) prevent oxidative modification of low density lipoproteins: and ex vivo study in humans, *J. Nutr. Biochem.*, 11, 216, 2000.
161. Deckert, V., Desrumauz, C., Athias, A., Durerneuil, L., Palleau, V., Gambert, P., Masson, D., and Lagrost, L., Prevention of LDL alpha-tocopherol consumption, cholesterol oxidation and vascular endothelium dysfunction by polyphenolic compounds from red wine, *Atherosclerosis*, 165, 41, 2002.

162. Fuhrman, B., Volkova, N., Rosenblat, M., and Aviram, M., Lycopene synergistically inhibits LDL oxidation in combination with vitamin E, glabridin, rosemarinic acid, carnosic acid or garlic, *Antioxid. Redox. Signal*, 2, 491, 2000.
163. Vinson, J.A., Hu, S.J., Jung, S., and Stanski, A., A citrus extract plus ascorbic acid decreases lipids, lipid peroxides and lipoprotein oxidative susceptibility and atherosclerosis in hypercholesterolemic hamster. *J. Agric. Food Chem.*, 46, 1453, 1998.
164. Reddy, A.C.P. and Lokesh, B.R., Alterations in lipid peroxidation in rat liver by dietary n-3 fatty acids: modulation of anti-oxidant enzymes by curcumin, eugenol and vitamin E, *J. Nutr. Biochem.*, 5, 181, 1994.
165. Alder, A.J. and Holub, B.J., Effect of garlic and fish oil supplementation on serum lipid and lipoprotein concentrations in hypercholesterolemic men, *Am. J. Clin. Nutr.*, 65, 445, 1997.
166. Pignatelli, P., Pulcenelli, F.M., Celestine, A., Lenti, L., Ghisellin A., Gazzanega, P.P., and Violi, F., The flavonoids quercetin and catechin synergistically inhibit platelet function by antagonizing the intracellular production of hydrogen peroxide, *Am. J. Clin. Nutr.*, 72, 1150, 2000.
167. Stahl, W., Junghans, A., deBoer, B., Driomina, E.S., Briviba, K., and Sies, H., Carotenoid mixtures protect multimamellar liposomes against oxidative damage: synergistic effects of lycopene and luein, *FEBS Lett.*, 427, 305, 1998.
168. Hurell, R.F., Reddy, M., and Cook, J.D., Inhibition of non-haem iron absorption in man by polyphenolic containing beverages, *Br. J. Nutr.*, 81, 289, 1999.
169. Laudicina, D.C. and Marnett, L.J., Enhancement of hydroperoxide-dependent lipid peroxidation in rat microsomes by ascorbic acid, *Arch. Biochem. Biophys.*, 278, 73, 1990.
170. Laughton, M.J., Halliwell, B., Evans, P.J., and Hoult, J.R.S., Antioxidant and prooxidant actions of plant phenolics, quercetin, gossypol and myricetin, *Biochem. Pharmacol.*, 38, 859, 1989.
171. Hu, C. and Kitts, D.D., Studies on the antioxidant activity of Echinacea root extract, *J. Agric. Food Chem.*, 48, 1466, 2000.
172. Cao, G., Sofic, E., and Prior, R.L., Antioxidant and prooxidant behavior of flavonoids: structure-activity relationships, *Free Rad. Biol. Med.*, 22, 749, 1997.
173. Bowry, V.W. and Ingold, K.U., The unexpected role of vitamin E in the peroxidation of human low-density lipoprotein, *Acc. Chem. Res.*, 32, 27, 1998.
174. Gey, K.F., Puska, P., Jorden, P.K, and Moser, U., Inverse correlation between plasma plasma vitamin E and mortality from ischemic heart disease in a cross-cultural epidemiology, *Am. J. Clin. Nutr.*, 53, 326, 1992.
175. Knipping. G., Rothneder, M., Strriegly, G., and Esterbauder, H., Antioxidants and resisitance against oxidation of procine LDL subfractions, *J. Lipid Res.*, 31, 1965, 1990.
176. Hodis, H.N., Mack, W.J., La Bree, L., Cashin-Hemphill, L., Sevanian, A., Johnson, R., and Azen, S.P., Serial coronary angiographic evidence that antioxidant vitamin intake reduces progression of coronary artery atherosclerosis, *J. Am. Med. Assoc.*, 273, 1849, 1995.
177. Reaven, P.D., Khou, A., Beltz, W.F., Parthasarathy, S., and Witztum, J.L., Effect of dietary antioxidant combinations in humans. Protection of LDL by vitamin E but not beta carotene, *Arteriosclerosis Thrombosis*, 13, 590, 1993.
178. Krichevsky, S.B., Shimakawa, T., Tell, G.S., Dennis, B., Carpenter, M., Echfeldt, J.H., Peacher-Ryan, H., and Heiss, G., Dietary antioxidants and carotid artery wall thickness: The ARIC study, *Circulation*, 92, 2142, 1995.

179. Gey, K.F., Brubacker, G.B., and Stahelin, H.B., Plasma levels of antioxidant vitamins in relation to ischemic heart disease and cancer, *Am. J. Clin. Nutr.*, 45, 1368, 1987.
180. Tousoulis, D., Davies, G., and Toutouzas, P., Vitamin C increase nitric oxide availability in coronary heart atherosclerosis, *Ann. Intern. Med.*, 131, 156, 1999.
181. Osganian, S.K., Stampfer, M.J., Rimm, E., Spiegelman, D., Hu, F.B., Mauson, J.E., and, Willett, W.C., Vitamin C and risk of heart disease in women, *J. Am. Coll. Cardio.*, 42, 246, 2003.
182. Holub, B.J., Omega-3 fatty acids in cardiovascular care, *Can. Med. Assoc. J.*, 166, 608, 2002.
183. Schoene, H.W., Vitamin E and omega-3 fatty acids: effecting platelet responsiveness. *Nutrition*, 17, 793, 2001.

4

Synergy of Portfolio Diet Components and Drugs in Coronary Heart Disease

David J.A. Jenkins, Augustine Marchie, Julia M.W. Wong, Russell de Souza, Azadeh Emam, and Cyril W.C. Kendall

CONTENTS

4.1 Introduction

Coronary heart disease (CHD) is one of the major causes of mortality in Western communities. This disease has strong and long established links to lifestyle. It is therefore not surprising, since diet is an integral part of lifestyle, that dietary approaches to prevent and treat CHD are analogous and complementary to the drug approaches that have been developed.

Regrettably, there are few regimens where diet and drugs are used to complement each other. The reasons are likely to relate to the difficulty of sustaining dietary change and the comparative ease of complying with drug treatment in tablet form together with the financial advantage to industry of drugs over diet through patent protection. This chapter therefore focuses largely on the potential for complementary or synergistic effects of drugs and food components in the portfolio diet (soy protein, viscous fibers, plant sterols and stanols, and nuts) especially in relation to CHD risk reduction (through reduction in blood pressure, blood lipids, and inflammation) and diabetes, including glycemic control and insulin resistance.

4.2 CHD Risk Reduction

4.2.1 Blood Lipids

The desired lipid profile would include a low LDL-C concentration[1] ideally with a large LDL particle size (>260 Å)[2,3] together with high HDL-C[1] and low triglyceride levels[1] and a corresponding low apolipoprotein B (apo B) and high apo A1 concentration.[4]

The current dietary advice of the Adult Treatment Panel III (ATP III)[1] of the National Cholesterol Education Program (NCEP) includes a saturated fatty acid (SFA) intake of less than 7% of calories and no more than 200 mg cholesterol daily. This diet is similar to the previous step 2 diet, whereas the original step 1 diet (less than 10% SFA calories and less than 300 mg dietary cholesterol)[5] has now been eliminated. Compared to a typical North American diet (14% SFA, 147 mg cholesterol/1000 kcal), the ATP III diet may reduce LDL cholesterol by as much as 18%.[6] Decreased intake of commonly used carbohydrates (presumably higher glycemic index) will tend to increase LDL particle size, while low glycemic index diets appear to raise HDL cholesterol[7,8] and lower serum triglyceride.[9]

However the U.S. Food and Drug (FDA) health claims for dietary components that may reduce the risk of CHD are new. These components include soy protein (25 g/d)[10], the viscous fibers psyllium (6.8 g/d) and oat β-glucan (3 g/d),[11,12] plant sterols (1.3 g/d) and stanols (3.4 g/d),[13] and most recently nuts (42 g/d).[14] Further support has been gained from the ATP recommendation to add 10 to 25 g/d of viscous fiber along with 2 g/d of plant sterols to the diet.[1] The American Heart Association (AHA) has also supported the use of soy protein and nuts.[15] As mentioned, the portfolio diet is made up of these food components.[16]

4.2.2 Food Components and Drugs with Similar Mechanisms of Action

4.2.2.1 Viscous Fibers and Anion Exchange Resins

The earliest effective drugs in common use to lower serum cholesterol were the anion exchange resins (e.g., cholestyramine), which bound bile acids and resulted in their increased elimination in the feces.[17] By causing a reduction in the bile acid pool, bile acids would be replenished after synthesis from circulating cholesterol and thus reducing LDL-C levels.

Viscous fibers, although they do not "bind" bile acids, prevent bile acid reabsorption in the terminal ileum, presumably because the fibers develop viscosity as they pass along the small intestine. Bulk diffusion of bile acids is also reduced as the thickness of the unstirred water layer is increased. The uptake of bile acids by the enterocyte in the terminal ileum is therefore reduced, and the increased bile acid losses in the feces is associated with a reduction in LDL-C,[18] an outcome similar in effect although not in magnitude to the anion exchange resins (about one-quarter of the bile acid loss and LDL reduction for acceptable amounts of viscous fiber [10 g/d] compared with cholestyramine [20 g/d]). Thus for psyllium, 12 g/d reduces LDL-C by about 9[19] or 6.7%,[20] while 20 g of cholestyramine will reduce LDL-C by approximately 20%.[17] Fiber consumption has been associated with reduced CHD risk.[21] The majority of associations have been with cereal fiber for which mechanistic explanations are not obvious. However a study by Pereira and colleagues[21] found that fruit fiber, which is high in the soluble fiber pectin, was associated with a decreased risk of CHD. Some epidemiological studies[22,23] support the protective effects of soluble fibers in CHD risk while others[24,25] have failed to find an association, possibly because of the relative lack of data on soluble fiber and the absence of tables for viscous fiber contents of foods.

Fiber and bile acid sequestrants, such as cholestyramine, have, in general, not been used in combination although there would be good reason. Cholestyramine is constipating while the viscous fiber, psyllium, is a laxative. This combination could potentially achieve increased cholesterol lowering together with the absence of the side effect, constipation.[26]

4.2.2.2 Soy, Vegetable Proteins, and Statins

Currently the world's most used class of drug, the statins, have taken on the role as the primary cholesterol lowering medication. Their mechanism is through hydroxymethylglutaryl-coenzyme A (HMG-CoA) reductase inhibition, a key stage in cholesterol biosynthesis. These drugs have pleiotrophic effects, including triglyceride reduction, HDL-C elevation, anticancer properties, possibly by reducing angiogenesis, osteoporosis prevention, and Alzheimer's disease amelioration.[27–30]

Soy proteins appear to reduce serum cholesterol by decreasing the stimulus for cholesterol synthesis, in common with other vegetable proteins, possibly related to soy proteins and peptides.[31] For some time now these components, or the lack of excess essential amino acids, have been considered to be responsible for the lower serum cholesterol levels.[32] Increased LDL receptor activity has also been reported after soy feeding.[33] Originally the isoflavone component of soy was considered to be responsible for the cholesterol lowering activity.[34] Although there remains some evidence for this suggestion,[35,36] the data are not consistent and the effect, though present, may not be great.[37,38]

In the original 1995 meta analysis of 38 soy trials with a total of 743 individuals, a 13% reduction in LDL-C was seen for a mean intake of 47 g/d soy protein.[34] A more recent meta-analysis suggested a more modest effect (4%),[38] and it is possible that at low levels of saturated fat intake (8 to 9 g/d) the hypocholesterolemic effect of soy may be attenuated.[37] Nevertheless one of the advantages of plant proteins, and foods made from them, is that they may be made cholesterol free and with very low saturated fat levels. This compositional change in diet alone may be responsible for a proportion of the reduction in serum cholesterol observed with soy foods.

The combination of soy and statins has not been reported on specifically, but soy studies where some subjects have also been taking a statin have not reported differences between statin users and nonusers in the cholesterol lowering effect of soy.[39,40] Soy has not been shown to reduce the risk of heart diseases in North American or European cohort studies since the low level of soy intake has not made such assessments possible. However the epidemiology of soy consumption globally strongly suggests that such a relationship would be seen because of the very low CHD rates in countries where soy consumption is high.[41] However, such a conclusion might be criticized because of the many other differences in diet and lifestyle also seen in the parts of the world where soy is eaten. Nevertheless in the absence of more definitive data, those that are available support a benefit for soy.

4.2.2.3 Plant Sterols and Ezetimibe

Ezetimibe acts by reducing absorption of cholesterol from the small intestine. It reduces not only cholesterol but sterol absorption in general.[42] Plant sterols and stanols (hydrogenated sterols) reduce cholesterol uptake by reducing cholesterol incorporation into the micelle and hence its absorption by the enterocyte. Both drug and food component thus increase fecal elimination of cholesterol (both endogenous or synthesized, and exogenous or dietary).

In situations where there are abnormalities in the ABC G5 or G8 genes, there may be increased sterol absorption; in the rare homozygotes, there is severe CHD with tendonous xanthomata and plaque formation in the coronary arteries.[43] The composition of the plaque appears to relate to the mix of cholesterol and plant sterols in the serum. It is of interest that the stanols do not appear to be absorbed either in health or disease.[44,45] Although heterozygotes do not appear to be greatly influenced by increases in dietary sterol intake,[43] it has been reported that relatively small elevations of plant sterols in the serum considerably increase the risk of CHD.[46,47] The implications of these observations are not clear since vegetarians have considerably higher plant sterol blood levels[48] due to consumption of vegetable oils, nuts, seeds, and leafy vegetables, which are the dietary sources of plant sterols. Furthermore, both plant foods and vegetarian diets have more generally been seen as reducing the risk for CHD.[49] This issue needs further work to establish a cause and effect relation between plant sterol consumption, serum levels, and atheroma formation, rather than simply an association.

There are no data on plant sterol intakes and reduction of CHD risk. However the occurrence of plant sterols in plant foods and oils recommended for CHD risk reduction together with the superior CHD health of vegetarians, who routinely consume high levels of plant sterols, suggests that plant sterols also may have beneficial effects for CHD risk.

The sterols, stanols, and ezetimibe do not appear to have been given together to determine their combined effects. A recent meta-analysis[50] indicated that 2 g of plant sterols gave a maximum reduction in LDL-C of 10 to 15%. As with soy, and possibly fiber, this effect may be attenuated at low SFA intakes.[51] Ezetimibe may also result in an 18% reduction in LDL-C.[52] Interestingly its effects appear to be restricted to those subjects who, presumably due in part to their ABC G5 or G8 status, are hyperabsorbers. In those for whom synthesis is the main determinant of serum cholesterol, statins work well and ezetimibe may have little effect.[53]

Although no data are available for the sterol or stanol plus ezetimibe combination, there are definite implications for combination therapy employing synthesis inhibitors with agents with a different spectrum of activity such as cholesterol absorption blockers.

4.2.2.4 *Nuts*

Nuts contain a combination of many of the hypocholesterolemic plant food components already discussed. Therefore their effect on CHD may relate to the additive or synergistic action of all these components. Almonds and most of the nuts contain large amounts of oleic acid, which may raise HDL cholesterol and possibly lower LDL-C.[54] If they are substituted for high glycemic index carbohydrates, they may lower serum VLDL-TG.[55] They contain a vegetable protein that may also lower LDL-C, by analogy with soy protein, and they contain fiber and other phytochemicals such as flavonoids and resveratrol, which may have additional actions.[56] For almonds and other nuts, 1 oz of nuts results in approximately a 4% reduction in LDL-C[57,58]; in some cases the effect is greater[59,60] and in other situations less.[61,62] Nut consumption has been found to be associated with reduction in CHD risk in virtually all studies in which this has been examined. Significant studies have included the 7th Day Adventist Cohort, the Nurses Health Study, the Physicians' Health Study, and the Iowa Women's Health Study.[63–67] The reduction in risk has been considerable (18 to 48%) for comparatively modest increments of nut consumption (8 to 20 g/d).[63–67]

4.2.2.5 *Food Combination or Portfolio Effects with Drugs*

Fibrates (fibric acid drugs) that lower triglycerides have been used with cholestyramine to address the concern of raised triglycerides, which may

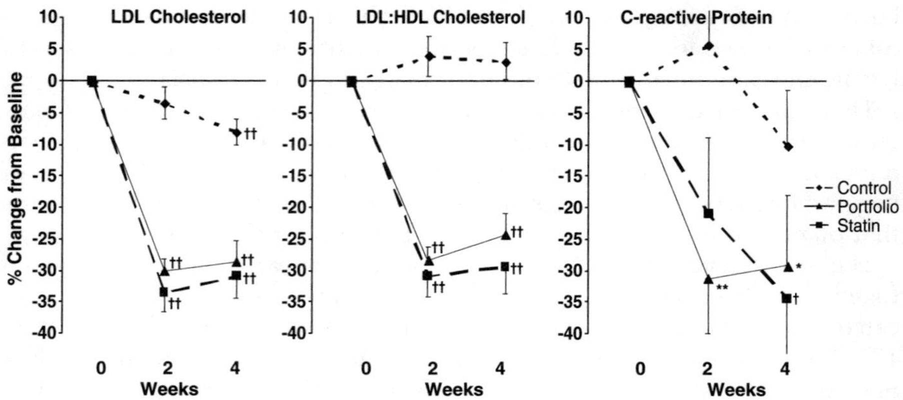

Figure 4.1
Percent change from baseline in LDL-cholesterol, the ratio of LDL:HDL-cholesterol and C-reactive protein on the Portfolio (n = 16) (▲), Control (n = 16) (◆), and Statin (n = 14) (■) diets. Values are mans ± SE since, with the number of subjects involved, approximately twice the SE represents a significance difference. Significantly different from baseline: $^*P < 0.02$; $^{**}P < 0.003$; $\dagger P < 0.002$; $\dagger\dagger P \leq 0.001$.

accompany use of bile acid sequestrants.[68] Now ezetimibe and statins may be used together to maximize the cholesterol lowering potential of drug therapy.[69] Despite the lack of studies with food–drug combinations, this approach is now being used with cholesterol lowering food combinations or dietary portfolios. The aim of the dietary portfolio was to provide on a daily basis about 1.0 g plant sterols per 1000 kcal of diet in a plant sterol ester–enriched margarine; about 10 g of viscous fibers per 1000 kcal of diet from oats, barley, and psyllium; about 20 g of soy protein per 1000 kcal as soy milk and soy meat analogs; and about 14 g of whole almonds per 1000 kcal of diet.[16,70,71]

Recent studies have demonstrated that 28 to 35% reductions in LDL-C can be achieved with such a diet in hyperlipidemic individuals, even in those who are already following a step 2 diet.[16,70,71] These effects are in the same range as seen with the starting dose of the earlier statins, which have reduced CHD rates by 25 to 35% in large clinical trials (Figure 4.1).[72,73] Furthermore, C-reactive protein (CRP), the inflammatory biomarker, seen as an important emerging nonlipid risk factor for CHD, has also been reduced in two portfolio studies.[70,71]

In addition studies of a combination of medium chain fatty acids, long chain fatty alcohols, and plant sterols have been undertaken recently with spectacular falls in serum cholesterol and triglyceride and with a rise in HDL cholesterol, and associated weight loss.[74] To these and other portfolio approaches may also be added policosanols derived from Cuban sugar cane.[75] Policosanols are a mixture of aliphatic alcohols that appear to lower LDL-C concentrations and raise HDL-C levels, possibly by reducing hepatic cholesterol biosynthesis while enhancing LDL clearance. Similar materials have also been identified in beeswax and may be found in other plant materials.

The recent interest in the role of inflammatory processes in CHD will continue with the focus on the biomarker CRP. CRP reduction is a feature of statins, may occur on the current portfolio diet possibly in association with low glycemic index diets,[73,76,77] and may be enhanced by vegetable n-3 fats from such vegetable sources such as alpha-lindenic acid from walnuts, flaxseed, and soy and canola oils.[78] Portfolio diets, which were developed to reduce the lipid risk factors for CHD, are likely to be expanded to cover other risk factors for heart disease and will likely become an important prerequisite for initial treatments before drug therapy is initiated. Such diets will continue to be the background therapy even after drug therapy has commenced.

4.2.3 Blood Pressure

Raised blood pressure is a major risk factor for both stroke and CHD.[1] In turn it is associated with renal damage, diabetes, and vascular disease. It is also one of the metabolic or insulin resistance syndrome associated disorders.[1] Pharmacological approaches to its control include diuretics, especially thiazide diuretics, β blockers, ACE inhibitors, angiotensin II receptor blockers and calcium channel blockers. Drug combination therapy is routinely practiced, effective, and recommended to achieve blood pressure control.[79]

As with blood lipids, recommendations on the acceptable blood pressure values have become increasingly stringent with the original upper levels for hypertension control reduced from 140/90 to 130/85 mm Hg.[79] As a result a major attempt has been made to make diet more effective in an age of powerful medications and combinations of medications. Indeed it has been the development of effective pharmacological control of hypertension that has reduced interest in effective diets such as the fruit and rice diet of Kempner, a diet which was high in potassium and low in sodium.[80] More recently this diet in reengineered form has been reintroduced as the Dietary Approaches to Stop Hypertension (DASH) diet. In its purest form, this diet is a largely lactovegetarian, low saturated fat diet that has shown itself to be as effective as the initial dose of some antihypertensive medications.[81] Part of its success may be the increased intake of potassium and also calcium[81] and the low level of sodium intake that can be achieved.

The DASH diet is highly effective and should be the basis on which pharmacological therapy is initiated, if required. However, only now are there official trials to assess the initiation of this diet with combinations or single components of pharmacological therapy, including studies examining elements of the DASH diet in combination with drugs (e.g., raised calcium intake with, for example, calcium channel blockers) which have shown considerable success.[82]

If hyperinsulinism is likely to be part of the reason for hypertension through the action of insulin on the kidney in enhancing sodium retention, then weight loss, exercise, and perhaps low glycemic index diets should be encouraged with the DASH diet. As yet reports of studies of these combinations are only beginning to emerge.[83] However the creation of low glycemic index diets by the use of acarbose, the α glycoside inhibitor in the STOP NIDDM trial, has demonstrated that new cases of hypertension can be reduced by 50%.[84] This approach now opens the way for diet and possibly diet-acarbose combinations to achieve blood pressure reduction. Hypertension is therefore a further fruitful area in which to explore diet-pharmacological combinations and synergy in the control of major pathophysiological disorders.

4.3 Type 2 Diabetes

Type 2 diabetes is another lifestyle disease where diet and medication play important roles. Overall goals have been to preserve β-cell function for insulin secretion and to reduce peripheral insulin resistance and hepatic glucose output. The drugs used are many, including sulfonylureas to enhance insulin secretion, biguanides to reduce peripheral insulin resistance, thiazolidinediones (glitazones) as PPAR agonists, and acarbose to slow carbohydrate absorption and create low glycemic index diets. Again drugs are used in combination, although care should be taken with glitazones as negative cardiovascular side effects have been reported.[85]

Although considered the cornerstone of prevention and management, there is yet to be a consensus on the optimal diet for diabetes management; however, it is agreed that less is best and weight loss is the goal. The trials of diet, weight loss, and exercise have shown impressive results in prevention of diabetes in high risk groups.[86–88] Currently there is much interest in high protein and low carbohydrate diets, with protein acting as a stimulus to insulin secretion and the low carbohydrate reducing postprandial insulin demand. However these diets have not been used in planned studies in combination with sulfonylureas. Nor have the combination of acarbose and low glycemic index diets been assessed, nor in fact have there been reports of the effect of acarbose combined with diets where carbohydrate intakes have been reduced. The drug–diet interactions in the treatment of diabetes therefore remain largely to be explored.

4.4 Conclusions

There are few studies where the interaction and potential synergy of pharmacological and "nutraceutical" or functional food approaches to disease prevention or treatment have been examined. However, there are a number of drug and nutrient treatment options in the area of chronic disease prevention that may be complementary or synergistic. For the most part, the dietary strategies lack side effects and could reduce the dose of medications required to achieve a therapeutic effect. In view of more stringent guidelines for the control of risk factors and the inevitability of the request for more people to be treated with medications and with increased dosages of drugs, there is an urgent need to develop dietary approaches that can be used with drugs to maximize effects. This approach provides a potentially valuable option to reduce side effects while ensuring therapeutic goals are met.

References

1. Expert Panel on Detection, Evaluation, and Treatment of High Blood Cholesterol in Adults, Executive summary of the third report of the National Cholesterol Education Program (NCEP) Expert Panel on Detection, Evaluation, and Treatment of High Blood Cholesterol in Adults (Adult Treatment Panel III), *JAMA*, 285, 2486, 2001.
2. Gardner, C.D., Fortmann, S.P., and Krauss, R.M., Association of small low-density lipoprotein particles with the incidence of coronary artery disease in men and women, *JAMA*, 276, 875, 1996.
3. Lamarche, B. et al., Small, dense low-density lipoprotein particles as a predictor of the risk of ischemic heart disease in men. Prospective results from the Quebec Cardiovascular Study, *Circulation*, 95, 69, 1997.
4. Walldius, G. and Jungner, I., Apolipoprotein B and apolipoprotein A-I: risk indicators of coronary heart disease and targets for lipid-modifying therapy, *J. Intern. Med.*, 255, 188, 2004.
5. Report of the National Cholesterol Education Program Expert Panel on Detection, Evaluation, and Treatment of High Blood Cholesterol in Adults. The Expert Panel, *Arch. Intern. Med.*, 148, 36, 1988.
6. Schaefer, E.J. et al., Efficacy of a National Cholesterol Education Program step 2 diet in normolipidemic and hypercholesterolemic middle-aged and elderly men and women, *Arterioscler. Thromb. Vasc. Biol.*, 15, 1079, 1995.
7. Jenkins, D.J. et al., Low glycemic index carbohydrate foods in the management of hyperlipidemia, *Am. J. Clin. Nutr.*, 42, 604, 1985.
8. Frost, G. et al., Glycaemic index as a determinant of serum HDL-cholesterol concentration, *Lancet*, 353, 1045, 1999.
9. Liu, S. et al., Dietary glycemic load assessed by food-frequency questionnaire in relation to plasma high-density-lipoprotein cholesterol and fasting plasma triacylglycerols in postmenopausal women, *Am. J. Clin. Nutr.*, 73, 560, 2001.
10. U.S. Food and Drug Administration, FDA final rule for food labeling: health claims: soy protein and coronary heart disease, *Fed. Regist.*, 64, 57699-733, 9-26, 1999.
11. U.S. Food and Drug Administration, Food labeling: health claims; soluble fiber from whole oats and risk of coronary heart disease [Docket No. 95P-0197], 15343, 2001.

12. U.S. Food and Drug Administration, Food Labeling: Health Claims; Soluble fiber from certain foods and coronary heart disease [Docket No. 96P-0338], 1998.
13. U.S. Food and Drug Administration, FDA authorizes new coronary heart disease health claim for plant sterol and plant stanol esters, Washington, DC, U.S. FDA, Docket Nos. 001-1275, OOP-1276, 2000.
14. U.S. Food and Drug Administration, Food labeling: health claims: nuts & heart disease, *Fed. Regist.*, [Docket No. 02P-0505], 2003.
15. Krauss, R.M. et al., AHA dietary guidelines revision 2000: a statement for healthcare professionals from the Nutrition Committee of the American Heart Association, *Circulation*, 102, 2284, 2000.
16. Jenkins, D.J. et al., A dietary portfolio approach to cholesterol reduction: combined effects of plant sterols, vegetable proteins, and viscous fibers in hypercholesterolemia, *Metabolism*, 51, 1596, 2002.
17. The Lipid Research Clinics Coronary Primary Prevention Trial results. I. Reduction in incidence of coronary heart disease, *JAMA*, 251, 351, 1984.
18. Jenkins, D.J. et al., Effect on blood lipids of very high intakes of fiber in diets low in saturated fat and cholesterol, *N. Engl. J. Med.*, 329, 21, 1993.
19. Olson, B.H. et al., Psyllium-enriched cereals lower blood total cholesterol and LDL cholesterol, but not HDL cholesterol, in hypercholesterolemic adults: results of a meta-analysis, *J. Nutr.*, 127, 1973, 1997.
20. Anderson, J.W. et al., Cholesterol-lowering effects of psyllium intake adjunctive to diet therapy in men and women with hypercholesterolemia: meta-analysis of 8 controlled trials, *Am. J. Clin. Nutr.*, 71, 472, 2000.
21. Pereira, M.A. et al., Dietary fiber and risk of coronary heart disease: a pooled analysis of cohort studies, *Arch. Intern. Med.*, 164, 370, 2004.
22. Pietinen, P. et al., Intake of dietary fiber and risk of coronary heart disease in a cohort of Finnish men. The Alpha-Tocopherol, Beta-Carotene Cancer Prevention Study, *Circulation*, 94, 2720, 1996.
23. Bazzano, L.A. et al., Dietary fiber intake and reduced risk of coronary heart disease in US men and women: the National Health and Nutrition Examination Survey I epidemiologic follow-up study, *Arch. Intern. Med.*, 163, 1897, 2003.
24. Liu, S. et al., A prospective study of dietary fiber intake and risk of cardiovascular disease among women, *J. Am. Coll. Cardiol.*, 39, 49, 2002.
25. Wolk, A. et al., Long-term intake of dietary fiber and decreased risk of coronary heart disease among women, *JAMA*, 281, 1998, 1999.
26. Maciejko, J.J. et al., Psyllium for the reduction of cholestyramine-associated gastrointestinal symptoms in the treatment of primary hypercholesterolemia, *Arch. Fam. Med.*, 3, 955, 1994.
27. Bauer, D.C. et al., Use of statins and fracture: results of 4 prospective studies and cumulative meta-analysis of observational studies and controlled trials, *Arch. Intern. Med.*, 164, 146, 2004.
28. Buxbaum, J.D., Cullen, E.I., and Friedhoff, L.T., Pharmacological concentrations of the HMG-CoA reductase inhibitor lovastatin decrease the formation of the Alzheimer beta-amyloid peptide in vitro and in patients, *Front. Biosci.*, 7, a50–a59, 2002.
29. Kawata, S. et al., Effect of pravastatin on survival in patients with advanced hepatocellular carcinoma. A randomized controlled trial, *Br. J. Cancer.*, 84, 886, 2001.

30. Schaefer, E.J. et al., Comparisons of effects of statins (atorvastatin, fluvastatin, lovastatin, pravastatin, and simvastatin) on fasting and postprandial lipoproteins in patients with coronary heart disease versus control subjects, *Am. J. Cardiol.*, 93, 31, 2004.
31. Bosisio, E. et al., Effects of dietary soy protein on liver catabolism and plasma transport of cholesterol in hypercholesterolemic rats, *J. Steroid. Biochem.*, 14, 1201, 1981.
32. Kurowska, E.M. and Carroll, K.K., Effect of high levels of selected dietary essential amino acids on hypercholesterolemia and down-regulation of hepatic LDL receptors in rabbits, *Biochim. Biophys. Acta.*, 1126, 185, 1992.
33. Baum, J.A., Long-term intake of soy protein improves blood lipid profiles and increases mononuclear cell low-density-lipoprotein receptor messenger RNA in hypercholesterolemic, postmenopausal women, *Am. J. Clin. Nutr.*, 68, 545, 1998.
34. Anderson, J.W., Johnstone, B.M., and Cook-Newell, M.E., Meta-analysis of the effects of soy protein intake on serum lipids, *N. Engl. J. Med.*, 333, 276, 1995.
35. Crouse, J.R., 3rd., A randomized trial comparing the effect of casein with that of soy protein containing varying amounts of isoflavones on plasma concentrations of lipids and lipoproteins, *Arch. Intern. Med.*, 159, 2070, 1999.
36. Gardner, C.D. et al., The effect of soy protein with or without isoflavones relative to milk protein on plasma lipids in hypercholesterolemic postmenopausal women, *Am. J. Clin. Nutr.*, 73, 728, 2001.
37. Jenkins, D.J. et al., Effects of high- and low-isoflavone soyfoods on blood lipids, oxidized LDL, homocysteine, and blood pressure in hyperlipidemic men and women, *Am. J. Clin. Nutr.*, 76, 365, 2002.
38. Weggemans, R.M. and Trautwein, E.A., Relation between soy-associated isoflavones and LDL and HDL cholesterol concentrations in humans: a meta-analysis, *Eur. J. Clin. Nutr.*, 57, 940, 2003.
39. Jenkins, D.J. et al., Combined effect of vegetable protein (soy) and soluble fiber added to a standard cholesterol-lowering diet, *Metabolism*, 48, 809, 1999.
40. Jenkins, D.J., et al., The effect on serum lipids and oxidized low-density lipoprotein of supplementing self-selected low-fat diets with soluble-fiber, soy, and vegetable protein foods, *Metabolism*, 49, 67, 2000.
41. Menotti, A. et al., Food intake patterns and 25-year mortality from coronary heart disease: cross-cultural correlations in the Seven Countries Study. The Seven Countries Study Research Group, *Eur. J. Epidemiol.*, 15, 507, 1999.
42. Salen, G., Ezetimibe effectively reduces plasma plant sterols in patients with sitosterolemia, *Circulation*, 109, 966, 2004.
43. Kwiterovich, P.O. Jr. et al., Response of obligate heterozygotes for phytosterolemia to a low-fat diet and to a plant sterol ester dietary challenge, *J. Lipid. Res.*, 44, 1143, 2003.
44. de Jong, A., Plat, J., and Mensink, R.P., Metabolic effects of plant sterols and stanols, *J. Nutr. Biochem.*, 14, 362, 2003.
45. Ostlund, R.E. Jr. et al., Gastrointestinal absorption and plasma kinetics of soy Delta(5)-phytosterols and phytostanols in humans, *Am. J. Physiol. Endocrinol. Metab.*, 282, E911, 2002.
46. Sudhop, T., Gottwald, B.M., and von Bergmann, K., Serum plant sterols as a potential risk factor for coronary heart disease, *Metabolism*, 51, 1519, 2002.
47. Assmann, G. et al., Elevation in plasma sitosterol concentration is associated with an increased risk for coronary events in the PROCAM study. American Heart Association Scientific Sessions, Orlando, 2003.

48. Vuoristo, M. and Miettinen, T.A., Absorption, metabolism, and serum concentrations of cholesterol in vegetarians: effects of cholesterol feeding, *Am. J. Clin. Nutr.*, 59, 1325, 1994.
49. Key, T.J. et al., Mortality in vegetarians and nonvegetarians: detailed findings from a collaborative analysis of 5 prospective studies, *Am. J. Clin. Nutr.*, 70, 516s, 1999.
50. Law, M., Plant sterol and stanol margarines and health, *Br. Med. J.*, 320, 861, 2000.
51. Mussner, M.J. et al., Effects of phytosterol ester-enriched margarine on plasma lipoproteins in mild to moderate hypercholesterolemia are related to basal cholesterol and fat intake, *Metabolism*, 51, 189, 2002.
52. Knopp, R.H. et al., Evaluation of the efficacy, safety, and tolerability of ezetimibe in primary hypercholesterolaemia: a pooled analysis from two controlled phase III clinical studies, *Int. J. Clin. Pract.*, 57, 363, 2003.
53. Ballantyne, C.M. et al., Effect of ezetimibe coadministered with atorvastatin in 628 patients with primary hypercholesterolemia: a prospective, randomized, double-blind trial, *Circulation.*, 107, 2409, 2003.
54. Mensink, R.P. and Katan, M.B., Effect of dietary fatty acids on serum lipids and lipoproteins. A meta-analysis of 27 trials, *Arterioscler. Thromb.*, 12, 911, 1992.
55. Grundy, S.M., Comparison of monounsaturated fatty acids and carbohydrates for lowering plasma cholesterol, *N. Engl. J. Med.*, 314, 745, 1986.
56. Kris-Etherton, P.M. et al., The effects of nuts on coronary heart disease risk, *Nutr. Rev.*, 59, 103, 2001.
57. Jenkins, D.J. et al., Dose response of almonds on coronary heart disease risk factors: blood lipids, oxidized low-density lipoproteins, lipoprotein(a), homocysteine, and pulmonary nitric oxide: a randomized, controlled, crossover trial, *Circulation.*, 106, 1327, 2002.
58. Sabate, J. et al., Serum lipid response to the graduated enrichment of a step I diet with almonds: a randomized feeding trial, *Am. J. Clin. Nutr.*, 77, 1379, 2003.
59. Sabate, J. et al., Effects of walnuts on serum lipid levels and blood pressure in normal men, *N. Engl. J. Med.*, 328, 603, 1993.
60. Kris-Etherton, P.M. et al., High-monounsaturated fatty acid diets lower both plasma cholesterol and triacylglycerol concentrations, *Am. J. Clin. Nutr.*, 70, 1009, 1999.
61. Morgan, W.A. and Clayshulte, B.J., Pecans lower low-density lipoprotein cholesterol in people with normal lipid levels, *J. Am. Diet. Assoc.*, 100, 312, 2000.
62. Curb, J.D. et al., Serum lipid effects of a high-monounsaturated fat diet based on macadamia nuts, *Arch. Intern. Med.*, 160, 1154, 2000.
63. Fraser, G.E. et al., A possible protective effect of nut consumption on risk of coronary heart disease. The Adventist Health Study, *Arch. Intern. Med.*, 152, 1416, 1992.
64. Fraser, G.E. and Shavlik, D.J., Risk factors for all-cause and coronary heart disease mortality in the oldest-old. The Adventist Health Study, *Arch. Intern. Med.*, 157, 2249, 1997.
65. Hu, F.B. et al., Frequent nut consumption and risk of coronary heart disease in women: prospective cohort study, *Br. Med. J.*, 317, 1341, 1998.
66. Albert, C.M. et al., Nut consumption and decreased risk of sudden cardiac death in the Physicians' Health Study, *Arch. Intern. Med.*, 162, 1382, 2002.

67. Ellsworth J.L., Kushi, L.H., and Folsom, A.R., Frequent nut intake and risk of death from coronary heart disease and all causes in postmenopausal women: the Iowa Women's Health Study, *Nutr. Metab. Cardiovasc. Dis.*, 11, 372, 2001.
68. Leitersdorf, E. et al., Efficacy and safety of triple therapy (fluvastatin-bezafibrate-cholestyramine) for severe familial hypercholesterolemia, *Am. J. Cardiol.*, 76, 84A, 1995.
69. Goldberg, A.C. et al., Ezetimibe Study Group. Efficacy and safety of ezetimibe coadministered with simvastatin in patients with primary hypercholesterolemia: a randomized, double-blind, placebo-controlled trial, *Mayo Clin. Proc.*, 79, 620, 2004.
70. Jenkins, D.J. et al., Effects of a dietary portfolio of cholesterol-lowering foods vs lovastatin on serum lipids and C-reactive protein, *JAMA*, 290, 502, 2003.
71. Jenkins, D.J. et al., The effect of combining plant sterols, soy protein, viscous fibers, and almonds in treating hypercholesterolemia, *Metabolism*, 52, 1478, 2003.
72. Scandinavian Simvastatin Survival Study Group, Randomized trial of cholesterol lowering in 4444 patients with coronary heart disease: the Scandinavian Simvastatin Survival Study (4S), *Lancet*, 344, 1383, 1994.
73. Downs, J.R. et al., Primary prevention of acute coronary events with lovastatin in men and women with average cholesterol levels: results of AFCAPS/TexCAPS. Air Force/Texas Coronary Atherosclerosis Prevention Study, *JAMA*, 279, 1615, 1998.
74. Bourque, C. et al., Consumption of an oil composed of medium chain triacyglycerols, phytosterols, and N-3 fatty acids improves cardiovascular risk profile in overweight women, *Metabolism*, 52, 771, 2003.
75. Varady, K.A., Wang, Y., and Jones, P.J., Role of policosanols in the prevention and treatment of cardiovascular disease, *Nutr. Rev.*, 61, 376, 2003.
76. Liu, S. et al., Relation between a diet with a high glycemic load and plasma concentrations of high-sensitivity C-reactive protein in middle-aged women, *Am. J. Clin. Nutr.*, 75, 492, 2002.
77. Nissen, S.E. et al., Effect of intensive compared with moderate lipid-lowering therapy on progression of coronary atherosclerosis: a randomized controlled trial, *JAMA*, 291, 1071, 2004.
78. Kris-Etherton, P.M. et al., Omega-3 fatty acids and cardiovascular disease: new recommendations from the American Heart Association, *Arterioscler. Thromb. Vasc. Biol.*, 23, 151, 2003.
79. Chobanian, A.V. et al., Seventh report of the Joint National Committee on Prevention, Detection, Evaluation, and Treatment of High Blood Pressure, *Hypertension*, 42, 1206, 2003.
80. Bloch, J., [Rice-fruit diet in hypertension (Kempner rice diet); metabolic and clinical aspects], *Wien. Med. Wochenschr.*, 100, 672, 1950.
81. Appel, L.J., A clinical trial of the effects of dietary patterns on blood pressure. DASH Collaborative Research Group, *N. Engl. J. Med*, 336, 1117, 1997.
82. Conlin, P.R. et al., The DASH diet enhances the blood pressure response to losartan in hypertensive patients, *Am. J. Hypertens.*,16, 337, 2003.
83. Appel, L.J., Lifestyle modification as a means to prevent and treat high blood pressure, *J. Am. Soc. Nephrol.*, 14, S99, 2003.
84. Chiasson, J.L. et al., Acarbose treatment and the risk of cardiovascular disease and hypertension in patients with impaired glucose tolerance: the STOP-NIDDM trial, *JAMA*, 290, 486, 2003.

85. Cheng, A.Y. and Fantus, I.G., Thiazolidinedione-induced congestive heart failure, *Ann. Pharmacother.*, 38, 817, 2004.
86. Knowler, W.C. et al., Reduction in the incidence of type 2 diabetes with lifestyle intervention or metformin, *N. Engl. J. Med.*, 346, 393, 2002.
87. Tuomilehto, J. et al., Prevention of type 2 diabetes mellitus by changes in lifestyle among subjects with impaired glucose tolerance, *N. Engl. J. Med.*, 344, 1343, 2001.
88. Pan, X.R. et al., Effects of diet and exercise in preventing NIDDM in people with impaired glucose tolerance. The Da Qing IGT and Diabetes Study, *Diabetes Care*, 20, 537, 1997.

5

The Role of Complementary Vitamins, Folate, Vitamin B_6, and Vitamin B_{12}, in Cardiovascular Disease

Louise Mennen, Pilar Galan, and Angelika de Bree

CONTENTS

5.1 Introduction

This chapter describes the role of three important B vitamins, folate, vitamin B_6, and vitamin B_{12}, on the development of cardiovascular diseases (CVD). These three vitamins are all involved in the metabolism of homocysteine, which in turn is related to CVD. These vitamins may have also an effect on CVD that is independent of the total homocysteine concentration (tHcy) in plasma, but the exact mechanisms still need to be clarified.

The three different vitamins and their basic role in the body are described briefly in the introduction, after which homocysteine metabolism is described in detail. The synergistic effect of the B vitamins and other components on the metabolism of homocysteine and their role in CVD are then covered. Finally, possible interactions with drugs and some safety aspects are discussed.

5.1.1 Folate

Folate was first isolated from spinach in 1941, and its chemical structure and synthesis was finally determined in 1946.[1] Folate is the generic name for all derivatives of the B vitamin that have the biological activity of pteroylmonoglutamic acid (PGA). Folic acid is the most stable synthetic form and does not occur in significant amounts in natural products, but it is used in supplements and food fortification. The richest source of folates is liver, but otherwise they are mainly present in green leafy vegetables (the Latin word for "leaf" is *folium*), citrus fruits, broccoli, and also some fermented cheeses.[2] The bioavailability of food folates varies between 50 and 75% relative to folic acid delivered by supplements.[3,4]

The physiological role of folate is to act as a one-carbon donor for DNA and protein methylation, and for methionine biosynthesis. In addition, when not used for methylation reactions, it is used for purine and pyrimidine nucleotide biosynthesis.[5]

A severe folate deficiency, which may originate from a reduced intake and/or absorption or an increased demand, results in megaloblastic anemia.[1]

A suboptimal folate status is associated with several disease conditions, such as CVD, described in this chapter, congenital malformations such as neural tube defects,[6] neurocognitive dysfunction,[7] certain types of cancer,[8] and recently it has also been linked to osteoporosis.[9,10]

The recommended daily intake for folate in France is 300 and 330 μg/d for adult women and men, respectively,[11] whereas it is 400 μg/d for men and women in the United States.[12] With respect to the prevention of neural tube defects, women who wish to become pregnant are recommended to take a daily supplement with 400 μg folic acid in many countries, while a few countries have preferred to implement obligatory fortification of flour with folic acid.[13]

Folate status can be evaluated by measuring the plasma folate or red blood cell folate concentration. Both measures are used depending on the study question; red blood cell folate reflects the folate intake over the last 3 months because red blood cells only live for that long. The plasma folate concentration reflects the more recent folate intake and may be more relevant in relation to plasma tHcy concentrations.[14]

5.1.2 Vitamin B_6

Vitamin B_6 (pyridoxine) was first isolated by Birch and György in 1936.[15] It is present in foods in several forms, which are readily interconverted in the tissues and are of equal biological value. Vitamin B_6 provides the coenzyme for over 60 different decarboxylation and transamination reactions involving amino acids and has therefore an important role in protein metabolism in the human body. Deficiency of vitamin B_6 is rare because it is found in a large variety of foods; cereals, meat, fruits, and vegetables all contain moderate amounts of vitamin B_6.[1] It is highly bioavailable (between 70 and 80%), and the recommended daily intake is 1.5 and 1.8 mg/d for adult women and men, respectively, in France[11] and 1.3 mg/d for men and women in the United States.[12] The plasma concentration of pyridoxal-5'-phosphate (PLP) is considered to be the best measure of vitamin B_6 status.

5.1.3 Vitamin B_{12}

Vitamin B_{12} (cobalmin) was isolated almost simultaneously for the first time in 1948 by British and American scientists.[16,17] It plays a role together with folate in the synthesis of thymine, the characteristic base of DNA, from deoxyuridine. Furthermore, it plays a separate biochemical role, unrelated to folate, in the maintenance of myelin in the nervous system. Deficiency of vitamin B_{12} may lead to megaloblastic anemia or more commonly to neurological disorders.[1] Because vitamin B_{12} is only present in products of animal origin (liver is a very rich source) and not in plant foods, vegans are at high risk of vitamin B_{12} deficiency. Bioavailability of vitamin B_{12} from animal products is estimated to be around 50%, but data on specific foods are scanty.[18] With respect to vitamin B_{12} deficiency, serum vitamin B_{12} does not seem to be an appropriate tool for the evaluation of vitamin B_{12} status. It has been suggested that plasma tHcy concentration, methylmalonic acid, or holotranscobalamin II be used as indicators for vitamin B_{12} status,[19] whereas in epidemiological studies, plasma vitamin B_{12} is often used.[20] The recommended dietary intake for vitamin B_{12} is 2.4 μg/d for an adult in France[11] and in the United States.[12]

5.2 Homocysteine Metabolism

5.2.1 Homocysteine Metabolizing Pathways

Foods rich in proteins from animal origin, especially meat, contain the essential amino acid methionine. After absorption of methionine in the body, cells metabolize methionine and form it into homocysteine, a sulfur-containing amino acid.[21] Homocysteine is not used for the synthesis of proteins, and foods only contain traces of homocysteine. The intracellular homocysteine concentration is precisely regulated, and any excess is transported to the plasma. In plasma approximately 99% is oxidized to disulfides. The vast majority of these disulfides is bound to proteins; only about 1% is reduced "free" homocysteine, unbound to proteins. The tHcy concentration comprises all these forms of homocysteine in the plasma.[22] No clear cutoff points have been established yet, but roughly, moderate elevations in the tHcy concentration refer to fasting plasma concentrations greater than 15 to 30 μmol/L, intermediate hyperhomocysteinemia refers to concentrations between 30 to100 μmol/L, and severe hyperhomocysteinemia refers to concentrations greater than 100 μmol/L.[23]

In case of an excess in methionine, intracellular homocysteine is irreversibly degraded to cysteine through the transsulfuration pathway, which is mainly limited to cells of the liver and kidneys. The enzymes needed in this pathway are cystathionine β-synthase and γ-cystath]ionase. They are both dependent on the cofactor pyridoxal-5′-phosphate, a biologically active form of vitamin B_6. Under conditions of negative methionine balance, homocysteine is primarily remethylated to methionine through the remethylation pathway. This pathway needs the enzyme methionine synthase, which uses methyl-cobalamin (a biologically active form of vitamin B_{12}) as a cofactor. The methyl group for the latter reaction is donated by 5-methyltetrahydrofolate. This form of folate is produced by the enzyme 5,10-methylene-tetrahydrofolate reductase (MTHFR). MTHFR in turn uses a biologically active form of vitamin B_2 (flavin adenine dinucleotide) as a cofactor.[24,25] In an alternative remethylation route, which is also mainly restricted to the liver and kidney, betaine is used as the methyl donor by the enzyme betaine-homocysteine methyltransferase to remethylate

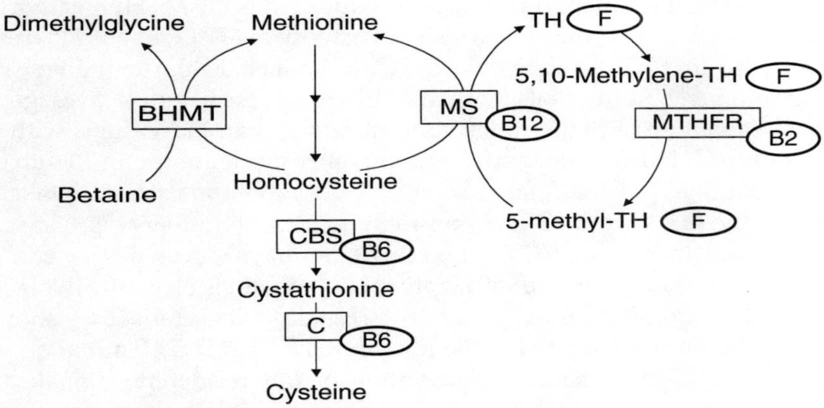

FIGURE 5.1
Simplified intracellular homocysteine metabolism. BHMT, betaine-homocysteine methyltransferase; CBS, cystathionine β-synthase; γ-C, γ-cystathinase; MS, methionine synthase, MTHFR, 5,10-methylene-tetrahydrofolate reductase; F, folate.

homocysteine into methionine.[24] An overview of homocysteine metabolism is presented in Figure 5.1.

5.2.2 Genetic Determinants of Homocysteine

Disturbances in intracellular homocysteine metabolism lead in most cases to elevated tHcy levels. Genetically determined functional deficiencies of enzymes in the homocysteine metabolism, like deficiency of cystathionine β-synthase, can have an extremely large effect on the tHcy concentration. Subjects with this defect not only have elevated tHcy concentrations in plasma (severe hyperhomocysteinemia) but also excrete large amounts with urine.[26] Other examples of inborn errors leading to extreme tHcy elevation are defects in vitamin B_{12} metabolism and deficiency of MTHFR.[27] On the population level, these inborn errors of homocysteine metabolism are not important causes of elevations in tHcy concentrations because they are rare; homozygous cystathionine β-synthase deficiency is the most common inborn error and has a prevalence of about 1:335,000.[28,29]

In addition, there are genetic variants (polymorphisms) that have a less pronounced effect on the activity of the enzyme they encode for. The only polymorphism that has been consistently linked to elevated tHcy concentrations is the 677 C>T mutation (an alanine to valine change) in the gene encoding for MTHFR.[30] The homozygous mutant from (677TT) is relatively prevalent in the general population depending on its origin; the prevalence of the 677TT genotype varies between 5 and 15% in most Caucasian populations.[31,32] MTHFR catalyzes the formation of 5-methyl-tetrahydrofolate from 5,10-methylene-tetrahydrofolate; the former folate derivative is necessary for the remethylation of homocysteine to methionine (see also Figure

5.1). The 677 C>T mutation results in a reduced specific MTHFR activity in isolated lymphocytes (about 34% residual activity in 677TT, about 71% residual activity in 677CT relative to 677CC),[33] which leads to higher tHcy concentrations[30]; individuals with the TT genotype have on average 2.5 μmol/L (about 25%) higher tHcy concentrations than individuals with the CC genotype.[32] Higher tHcy concentrations are especially seen in TT subjects with a marginal plasma folate status[34–37] or a suboptimal folate intake.[38,39] This was the first identified gene–nutrient interaction influencing tHcy concentrations. The fact that 677TT subjects do not have elevated tHcy concentrations when their folate status is optimal (adequate) is elegantly explained by a recent study of Guenther et al.[25] In *Escherichia coli* bacteria, they showed that a mutation homologous to the human MTHFR 677 C>T mutation was associated with an enhanced dissociation of flavin adenine dinucleotide (FAD, the cofactor form of vitamin B_2). An optimal folate supply prevented the loss of FAD binding and in this way suppressed the inactivation of the enzyme. Finally, the MTHFR 677 C>T polymorphism influences the relation between vitamin B_{12} status and tHcy; vitamin B_{12} status is only related to tHcy in subjects carrying the 677 T allele.[40]

A second polymorphism in the same MTHFR gene is an A to C substitution (a glutamate to alanine change) at basepair 1298. There are no data thus far to suggest that the 1298A>C polymorphism alone influences the tHcy concentration, but combined heterozygosity for the 1298A>C and 677C>T polymorphism is associated with increased tHcy concentrations.[41,42] Furthermore, in individuals carrying the wild type of this polymorphism, vitamin B_{12} status is not related to tHcy, whereas it is in individuals carrying the C allele.[40] Other polymorphisms are described either in the genes coding for methionine synthase, methionine synthase reductase, and cystathionine β-synthase, and in genes involved in vitamin B_{12} metabolism. The prevalence of these variants is generally low, and in most cases, it is not clear whether it concerns a functional polymorphism.[43,44] It is not known whether these variants result in important changes in enzymatic activity or in tHcy concentrations.[43–45]

5.2.3 Environmental Determinants of Homocysteine

Because of the role of folate and vitamins B_6 and B_{12} in the metabolism of homocysteine, the intake of these vitamins is one of the most important environmental determinants of the tHcy concentration. Their effect on the tHcy concentration is described in Section 5.4. Other important determinants are age, sex, smoking, and coffee and alcohol consumption.

Increasing age and male sex are associated with a higher tHcy concentration.[46–48] The difference between the sexes could be due to the larger muscle mass in men because the formation of muscles is associated with the simultaneous formation of homocysteine in connection with creatine and creatinine synthesis.[49] It could also be due to the influence of sex hormones,[48] as was confirmed in a study with transsexual males and females.[50] Part of the relation with age in women might be explained by the menopause because tHcy concentration was found to be higher in postmenopausal women compared with premenopausal women.[48,51]

Smoking is positively associated with the tHcy concentration,[52–54] but smokers generally consume a less healthy diet,[55] thus residual confounding of, for example, B vitamin intake cannot be fully excluded. The exact mechanism behind the increase in the tHcy concentration is unidentified; smoking may induce local effects in cells exposed to cigarette smoke,[56] may influence the tHcy concentration by changing the plasma thiol redox status,[57–59] or may inhibit enzymes such as methionine synthase.[60]

Coffee consumption is positively associated with the tHcy concentration in both men and women,[52–54] a relationship that has been recently confirmed to be causal in several intervention trials.[61–63] Caffeine might be the factor that elevates the tHcy concentration,[53,62,64] because it may inhibit the conversion of homocysteine to cysteine by acting as a vitamin B_6 antagonist.[62] Additionally, recent evidence showed that chlorogenic acid, a polyphenol that is present in coffee in the same amount as caffeine, may also partly be responsible for the increase in the tHcy concentration. When polyphenols are metabolized, methyl groups from methionine are necessary, which results in a higher production of homocysteine.[65] Both caffeine and chlorogenic acid are also present in tea, although in smaller doses, which explains the absence of a clear association between tHcy and tea consumption.

The relation between alcohol consumption and the tHcy concentration is complex. It is clear that alcoholics have highly elevated tHcy concentrations.[66] In the general population positive, inverse, J-shaped, and sometimes no relations have been observed.[46,52–54,67–71] These differences are probably due to the type of alcoholic beverage. Wine and spirit consumption have been shown to increase the tHcy concentration, whereas beer consumption had no effect.[72] It has been hypothesized that consumption of beer, because of its B vitamin (B_2, B_6, and folate) content, may to some extent counteract the tHcy increasing effect of alcohol, whereas the betaine content in wine[73] is too low to counteract the negative effects of alcohol on tHcy.[67]

5.3 Homocysteine and Cardiovascular Diseases

5.3.1 History

The process of identifying homocysteine as a possible risk factor for vascular disease had already started in 1964. By that time, Mudd and coworkers[26] showed that the accumulation of homocysteine in blood, and consequently in urine leading to homocystinuria, was due to deficiency of the enzyme cystathionine β-synthase (CBS). After this discovery, McCully[74] observed that a patient with CBS deficiency had comparable arterial damage as another patient with a different enzymatic abnormality that also led to homocystinuria. Since both abnormalities only shared the accumulation of homocysteine, McCully postulated that homocysteine itself, or one of its derivatives, was responsible for the arterial damage.[74] This formed the basis for the hypothesis that moderate elevations in tHcy in blood may be a risk factor for atherosclerosis in the general population.[75] This hypothesis was first tested in 1967 by Wilcken and Wilcken,[76] who showed that patients with coronary artery disease suffered more often from an abnormal homocysteine metabolism than controls.

5.3.2 Meta-Analyses of Observational Studies

The first meta-analysis[77] summarized 11 retrospective and cross-sectional studies that all showed a significantly increased risk of coronary heart disease (CHD) for each 5 μmol/L increase in the tHcy concentration. This meta-analysis was updated by Refsum et al.[78] Of the additional 16 retrospective and cross-sectional studies only 3 did not find a positive association between the tHcy concentration and the risk of CHD. In 1998, another meta-analysis was performed that calculated the relative risk for prospective and retrospective studies separately.[79] The summary relative risk of CHD for the retrospective studies was 1.6 (95% confidence interval: 1.4 to 1.7) and for the prospective studies 1.3 (1.1 to 1.5). The reason that prospective studies show a weaker relation than retrospective studies is that in retrospective studies the tHcy concentration is measured after the event (in prospective studies the blood is collected before the onset of disease) and so the event may thus have influenced the tHcy concentration. When prospective studies include subjects at risk for CHD (subjects with preexisting disease), stronger associations between the tHcy concentration and CHD are found.[80] Therefore, two more recent meta-analyses were based on studies for which (except one) subjects were not selected for their increased risk of CHD. They showed that each 5 μmol/L increase in the tHcy concentration was associated with a 20% increase in risk of CHD.[81,82] Finally, in 2002 the Homocysteine Studies Collaboration published a meta-analysis including data from 30 prospective or retrospective studies involving a total of 5,073 ischemic heart disease and 1,113 stroke events. After adjustment for known cardiovascular risk factors and regression dilution bias in the prospective studies, a 25% lower tHcy concentration (about 3 μmol/L) was associated with a 11% lower ischemic heart disease and a 19% lower stroke risk.[83] This latter estimation is lower than those resulting from the earlier meta-analyses, probably because of a more appropriate adjustment for cardiovascular risk factors and regression dilution bias. If these modest associations are causal, then the implications for public health of decreasing the population mean tHcy concentration could still be substantial.

One way to investigate whether this relation is causal is to evaluate the relation between genotypes related to the tHcy concentration and CVD. The genotype is present at birth; it cannot be influenced by disease onset or lifestyle, so bias due to confounding is therefore much less. The number of cases required for such an evaluation is calculated to be between 7,800 to 16,300, with an equal number of controls. This calculation is based on the average difference in tHcy concentration between 677TT and 677CC subjects, which is about equal to 2.6 μmol/L.[32] This difference in tHcy concentration might produce a relative risk of 1.1 to 1.2.[81] The small relative risk explains the larger number of subjects necessary to identify a statistically significant relative risk of this size with a statistical power of 80%.[81] Wald et al.[84] and Klerk et al.,[85] respectively, evaluated 48 studies (12,193 cases and 11,945 controls) and 34 published and 6 unpublished studies (11,162 cases and 12,758 controls) on the relation between the MTHFR 677C>T genotype and ischemic heart disease. In addition, Wald et al.[84] also evaluated 7 studies (1217 cases) on stroke. The calculated increased risk for ischemic heart disease for subjects carrying the TT genotype compared to those with the CC genotype was almost similar in both studies: 21%[84] and 16%.[85] This increase was 31% for stroke, but this was not statistically significant, probably because of the lack of power. In addition, in the study of Klerk et al.[85] there was significant heterogeneity between the results obtained in European populations compared with North American populations: the risk was only statistically significant in Europe. This may largely be explained by the interaction between this polymorphism and the folate status because folate status in North America is higher as a result of the implementation of food fortification with folic acid.[13] It thus seems that individuals with the MTHFR 677 TT genotype have a significantly higher risk of CHD, particularly in the setting of low folate status. This supports the hypothesis that high tHcy concentrations are causally related to increased risk of this disease. However, only well designed (randomized double-blind placebo-controlled) intervention trials may give final proof for this hypothesis. Several of these trials are currently ongoing and are discussed in Section 5.5.

5.4 Folate, Vitamin B_6, and B_{12} Synergy in Lowering Homocysteine

5.4.1 Effect of Folate, Vitamin B_6, and B_{12} on Homocysteine Concentration

A higher dietary folate intake is associated with a lower tHcy level in adults and is independent of other dietary and lifestyle factors.[53,86–88] These results complement those found in observational studies on dietary folate intake and the tHcy concentration in middle aged[89–91] and elderly subjects.[54,91–93] The observed inverse relations between vitamin B_6 and tHcy concentrations as observed in many studies could well be due to inadequate corrections for the intake of other dietary components like methionine and alcohol.[53,54,87,89–93] A lower tHcy concentration at higher B_{12} intakes was only observed in study samples with elderly and middle aged subjects.[89–91] This is not surprising because the intake level of vitamin B_{12} is generally higher than the recommended level in developed countries. Furthermore, in the elderly, malabsorption of vitamin B_{12} from the diet is more common as a result of atrophic gastritis.[94]

Folate is the most important dietary determinant of tHcy concentrations, which is in line with its metabolic role. Folate is used as a substrate: it donates the methyl group for the conversion of homocysteine to methionine (Figure 5.1). On the contrary, vitamin B_6 and B_{12} are not utilized when homocysteine is metabolized; they function as cofactors of enzymes involved in homocysteine metabolism.

Several intervention studies have provided evidence for the importance of the interaction of B vitamins in homocysteine metabolism.[95] Not only folic acid supplements (synthetic form of folate) but also combinations of folic acid, vitamin B_6 and B_{12} effectively reduced the tHcy concentration in subjects with normal[96,97] and elevated baseline levels.[98–102] A meta-analyses of 12 randomized trials showed that folic acid supplementation reduced tHcy concentrations by 25% with similar effects in a daily dosage of 500 to 5,000 μg. This reduction in tHcy concentration was based on an average pretreatment level of 12 μmol/L; however, higher pretreatment concentrations result in even a larger reduction of tHcy in response to folic acid treatment.[103] Vitamin B_{12} in an average dose of 500 μg produced an additional reduction in tHcy of 7%. Vitamin B_6 did not appear to have a significant effect on the tHcy concentration when in combination with other B vitamins. However, the summarized trials in this meta-analyses did not assess the effects on the tHcy concentration after a methionine load, which is influenced by vitamin B_6.[104] A recent dose-finding study in older adults showed that a daily supplementation with 400 μg folic acid is the minimum dose required for adequate tHcy reduction, which is at 90% of the maximal decrease.[105] However, one study showed that elderly people who already consume a diet fortified with folic acid (mean daily intake probably around 400 μg/d) still may benefit from a multivitamin supplement containing among other vitamins about 100% of the daily recommended value for folic acid, vitamin B_6, and B_{12}.[106]

It has to be noted that this tHcy-lowering effect is dependent on the MTHFR 677 C>T genotype; the effect of supplementation is larger in individuals carrying the TT genotype, but they require higher folate intakes to achieve similar low tHcy concentrations as those carrying only one or no T allele.[107–109]

There seems to be no synergy between the B vitamins in lowering tHcy concentration. Each individual vitamin lowers the tHcy concentration, but when folic acid is given, further supplementation with vitamin B_{12} has only an additive effect[110,111] and B_6 has no additive effect, at least not on the fasting tHcy concentration.[112] On the other hand, there is a metabolic interaction between vitamin B_{12} and folic acid. Folic acid supplements can correct the anemia associated with vitamin B_{12} deficiency. Unfortunately, folic acid will not correct changes in the nervous system that result from vitamin B_{12} deficiency. Permanent nerve damage can occur if vitamin B_{12} deficiency is not treated.[113,114] Therefore, the Institute of Medicine recommends that the intake of supplemental folic acid should not exceed 1000 μg/d to prevent folic acid from masking symptoms of vitamin B_{12} deficiency.[12] It is very important for the elderly to be aware of the relationship between folic acid and vitamin B_{12} because they are at greater risk of having a vitamin B_{12} deficiency.[94,115]

5.4.2 The Effect of [6S]-5-Methyltetrahydrofolate

For a long time only folic acid was available in the form of a supplement and has been tested in previously mentioned trials. Recently a reduced form of folate, [6S]-5-methyltetrahydrofolate (5-MTHF), the major circulating form of folate in the body, also exists as a supplement. The potential advantage of 5-MTHF over folic acid is that it is unlikely to mask a vitamin B_{12} deficiency.[116]

Several intervention trials showed that 5-MTHF and folic acid supplementation increase blood folate indices to a similar extent; furthermore, the effect on the tHcy concentration is also similar. Bostom et al.[117] were first to compare folic acid (15 mg/d) with 5-MTHF supplementation (equimolar dose of 17 mg/d) on tHcy lowering in hemodialysis patients with hyperhomocysteinemia. The percentage decrease in the tHcy concentration was similar for both supplements (15 vs. 17%). Venn et al.[118] showed in a randomized double-blind placebo-controlled intervention study that, although the increases in plasma and red blood cell folate did not differ between supplementation with equimolar amounts of folic acid or 5-MTHF, the latter was slightly more effective in lowering tHcy. However, in a more recent study this was not confirmed, and a similar tHcy lowering effect was observed after supplementation with either 400 μg folic acid or an equimolar dose of 416 μg 5-MTHF. Furthermore, this study showed that a dose of 416 μg 5-MTHF had no greater effect on the tHcy concentration than a dose of 208 μg 5-MTHF (equivalent to 200 μg of folic acid) when given for 6 months.[119] This seems to contradict the results of van Oort et al.,[105] described in Section 5.4.1; however, the latter dose-finding study took place over a period of only 3 months. Thus, a maximum decrease in tHcy concentration within 3 months can be obtained with a dose of 400 μg of folic acid; for a longer-term optimal low tHcy concentration about 200 μg may be sufficient.

Finally, like folic acid and dietary folate (see Section 5.4.1), the effect of 5-MTHF on the tHcy concentration is larger in individuals carrying the 677 TT genotype compared with those carrying the 677 C allele.[116] It is thus clear that 5-MTHF supplementation has at least the same tHcy-lowering effect as folic acid supplementation and may therefore be equally effective, if proven, to reduce risk of CVD.

5.4.3 Folate Fortification

It has been shown that an increase in folate intake and status is more easily achieved by increasing the consumption of folic acid fortified foods than by increasing the consumption of foods naturally rich in folate.[120,121] Consumption of foods, such as bread, cereals, and mineral water fortified with folic acid, vitamin B_6, and B_{12} effectively improve the B vitamin status and lower tHcy concentrations.[122,123] Furthermore, campaigns to make women of childbearing age aware of the importance of taking a folic acid supplement at least 4 weeks before and 10 weeks after conception to prevent neural tube defects have not been very effective.[124–126] An additional problem in this respect is that a large number of pregnancies are unplanned.[127] Therefore the U.S. Food and Drug Administration made fortification of flour with folic acid mandatory from 1998 onward.[128] Thus far Canada and Chile are the only other countries who have implemented mandatory folate fortification. Quinlivan and Gregory[13] have recently evaluated the folic acid intake as a result of fortification in the United States; typical intakes of folic acid after fortification are more than twice the level originally predicted, as has also been seen in other evaluations.[129–131] As a result, the folate status has significantly improved upon fortification in the countries where this is allowed.[132–136] Consequently, the mean tHcy concentration in these different populations has also decreased.[132,134,137,138]

Fortification with folic acid also seems to have an effect on its primary aim: prevention of neural tube defects. In Canada, the prevalence of neural tube defects decreased from 1.89 per 1000 total births to 1.28 per 1000, a decrease of 32%,[139] and in the United States a reduction of 19% was reported.[140,141] Fortification might also offer a secondary benefit: the reduced tHcy concentrations may lead to a decline in death rates due to CVD and stroke. One study with 2481 consecutive patients with CHD was not able to indicate a difference in mortality from CHD in patients followed during the prefortification period and patients followed in the fortification period. This null finding was observed despite a moderate decrease in median tHcy concentrations.[137] Data released by the Centers for Disease Control[142] show a more positive picture: CDC researchers compared the annual mortality rates for stroke and CHD in individuals aged 40 and above for the periods 1994 to 1996 (prefortification) and 1998 to 2000 (fortification). These rates were based on analysis of death certificates. On average, stroke mortality was 10% to 15% lower in the latter study period across nearly all age and racial groups. The stroke mortality rate declined by about 1% per year during the earlier period, compared with 4.5% per year after 1997. The researchers took into account other changes in major cardiovascular risk factors, such as smoking, obesity, cholesterol, high blood pressure, and obesity. Most of these did not change or get worse and could account for no more than a third of the total decline in recent years.[142]

In conclusion, fortification with folic acid seems to have its intended effect. In addition to the prevention of NTDs it may also have other favorable health effects such as a reduction in CVD risk. The risk of masking a vitamin B_{12} deficiency may be decreased if 5-MTHF is used instead of folic acid. However, this form of folate in expensive and less stable. Another option would be to add vitamin B_{12} as well.[135,143] However, the amount would have to be very high to correct deficiencies due to absorption problems like pernicious anemia (about 2% of all cases)[144]; in those cases only about 1% is absorbed via passive absorption.

Dietary counseling to increase natural folate intake seems like an interesting option because altered food consumption patterns lead to beneficial increased intakes of several other vitamins and minerals and decreased intakes of saturated fat.[145] Yet, it has to be noted that on a population level, dietary counseling is very costly, and its long term effectiveness is unclear.

5.5 Folate, Vitamin B_6, and Vitamin B_{12} Synergy and Cardiovascular Disease

5.5.1 Prospective Cohort Studies

The relations between plasma or serum folate, vitamin B_6, and vitamin B_{12}, and CVD have been evaluated in a number of case control and prospective cohort studies. We only review the results from prospective studies because this type of study design is more appropriate for determining causal relations.

Most of the prospective studies evaluating the relation between folate status and CVD observed an inverse association in women only,[146,147] in men as well as in women,[148] or in men only.[149] Two studies did not find statistically significant associations,[150,151] although the risk estimate was compatible with the hypothesis that high folate levels might contribute to protection against CHD. In addition, prospective studies that investigated the relation between folate status and all CVD[152–154] or stroke[155] as endpoints showed a beneficial effect of higher folate levels. Seven studies estimated the folate intake and related it to the incidence of CHD,[150,156,157] stroke[158–160] and peripheral arterial disease.[161] Only, two of these studies[150,160] did not find a protective effect of higher folate intake.

The results of prospective studies evaluating the relation between the vitamin B_6 status and CVD are not entirely consistent. Some studies suggest that the vitamin B_6 concentration is inversely associated with the risk of CHD,[150] although the results were not always statistically significant[151] another found no association.[147] Two studies indicate a protective effect of a higher vitamin B_6 intake on the prevalence of CHD,[150,156] but another study did not find a protective effect against stroke.[159] The plasma vitamin B_{12} concentration was not related to the risk of CHD.[147,150] However, the intake of vitamin B_{12} was inversely associated with CHD,[149] peripheral arterial disease,[161] and stroke.[159]

Taking the above information together, a beneficial effect of a higher folate intake on CVD seems likely, however, it is not clear whether vitamin B_6 or B_{12} have any additive effect.

5.5.2 Intervention Trials

Because of the tHcy-lowering effect of folic acid, several studies investigated the effect of folic acid supplementation on intermediate endpoints of vascular damage. Brown and Hu[162] recently reviewed trials that considered the effect of folic acid supplementation on endothelial function. The general picture that emerges from these studies is that folic acid (5 to 10 mg/d) improves or restores endothelium dependent vasodilation and may decrease the chance of thrombosis by reducing levels of coagulation factors in healthy subjects and in patients with high tHcy concentrations.[162] The observed benefit is probably largely explained by the lowering of tHcy concentrations. There are several short term intervention trials on the effect of folic acid supplementation, in combination with vitamin B_{12} and B_6, on other intermediary endpoints of CVD. Two Dutch trials showed that supplementation with folic acid (5 mg) and vitamin B_6 (250 mg) reduces the risk of cardiovascular events (coronary, peripheral, and cerebral) in patients with high tHcy concentrations and existing CVD, to the level of patients with existing CVD, but with normal tHcy concentration.[163,164] Another trial investigated the effect of folic acid (2.5 mg), vitamin B_6 (25 mg), and vitamin B_{12} (250 μg) on the regression of carotid plaques. Vitamin supplementation resulted in a decreased rate of progression of the plaque growth in 101 patients with vascular disease with normal and elevated tHcy concentrations.[165]

Besides these noncontrolled trials, the results of three double-blind, randomized, placebo-controlled trials are also available.[166–168] All trials used intermediate endpoints. Vermeulen et al.[167] observed fewer abnormal exercise electrocardiography tests after 2 years of supplementation with 5 mg folate and 250 mg vitamin B_6 (n=78) compared to the placebo group (n=80). However, the internal validity of the exercise electrocardiography tests is questioned.[169] Moreover, an effect of treatment on other surrogate endpoint measures (ankle-brachial pressure index and duplex-scanning of the carotid and peripheral arteries) was not observed.[167] The intervention study of Schnyder et al.[168] was double-blind and investigated the effect of a daily combination (1 mg) of folic acid, vitamin B_{12} (400 μg), and pyridoxine (10 mg) on the rate of the restenosis after angioplasty. After 6 months of supplementation, the intervention group (n=105) showed a significant reduction of the rate of restenosis compared with the placebo group (n=100) as assessed by quantitative coronary angiography. More recently, Lange et al.[166] published a study with a similar design that showed an opposite effect. Differences between the studies were that Lange et al. used only patients that received a stent after angioplasty; started the trials with an intravenous injection with 1 mg of folic acid, 5 mg of vitamin B_6 and 1 mg vitamin B_{12};

and supplemented the subjects with a lower dose of vitamin B_{12} (60 μg) and a higher dose of vitamin B_6 (48 mg). That this study showed an adverse effect of B vitamin supplementation is surprising, and more research is necessary to indicate whether B vitamins may be harmful in certain patients, such as those that receive a stent.

In conclusion, the results of most of these studies favor the hypothesis that lower tHcy concentrations are causally associated with a decreased risk of vascular disease in patients with CVD and in healthy subjects. Yet, in all intervention trials folic acid was used. Because this vitamin may have a favorable effect on, for example, endothelial function[170,171] independent of the tHcy concentration, it is not clear whether the observed effect is due to a direct folic acid effect or to a decrease in tHcy concentration. Furthermore, nothing can be said about the individual or possible synergistic effects of the vitamins, as each trial used a combination of the B vitamins.

Several secondary prevention trials will be able to answer the question whether a lower tHcy concentration through vitamin supplementation (folic acid, vitamins B_6 and B_{12}) has an effect on "hard" endpoints like CHD and stroke.[172,173] Almost all of these trials use pharmacological doses of the B vitamins, which, in case of a positive outcome, precludes lowering the tHcy concentration in high-risk subjects by means of low doses of supplemental folic acid, fortification, or dietary measures. This is unfortunate because the effects of long-term supplementation with folic acid are unknown.[174] Only one trial uses nutritional doses, and this trial also uses 5-MTHF instead of folic acid, which is the form of folate that is predominantly present in plasma and may not induce side effects.[175] Furthermore, all studies except one use a combination of B vitamins supplementation without separating the effects of a single vitamin, and no conclusions can be drawn on possible additive or synergistic effects. Some of these trials are performed in countries with mandatory folic acid fortification (Table 5.1) and some in countries without (Table 5.2). Results have become available for two trials so far. The Vitamin Intervention for Stroke Prevention (VISP) trial showed a moderate reduction of the tHcy concentration after daily supplementation with a combination of 25 mg vitamin B_6, 0.4 mg vitamin B_{12}, and 2.5 mg folic acid compared

TABLE 5.1

Trials in "Folic Acid-Fortified" Populations

Trial	Prior disease	No. to be randomised	Scheduled duration (years)	Vitamin Regimen (mg/d) Folic acid	Vitamin B_{12}	Vitamin B_6
HOPE-2	CHD	5522	5.5	2.5	1.0	50
WACS	CHD	5500	7	2.5	1.0	50
VISP	Stroke	3680	2[a]	2.5	0.4	25
FAVORIT	Renal	4000	5	2.5	0.4	20
VA Trial	Renal	2000	5	40.0	0.5	100

[a] This trial has terminated prematurely after 2 years of follow-up.

TABLE 5.2
Trials in "Nonfortified" Populations

Trial	Prior disease	No. to be randomised	Scheduled duration (years)	Vitamin Regimen (mg/d) Folic acid	Vitamin B_{12}	Vitamin B_6
CHAOS-2	CHD	1,880	2[a]	5.0	—	—
SU.FOL.OM3	CHD/stroke	3,000	5	0.5[b]	0.02	3
WENBIT	CHD	3,000	3	0.8	0.4	40
NORVIT	CHD	3,750	3	0.8	0.4	40
SEARCH	CHD	12,064	5	2.0	1.0	—
VITATOPS	Stroke	8,000	3	2.0	0.5	25

[a] This trial has terminated prematurely after 1.7 years of follow-up.
[b] 5-Methyltetrahydrofolate is used instead of folic acid.

with a low-dose supplementation using a combination of 200 μg vitamin B_6, 6 μg vitamin B_{12}, and 20 μg of folic acid, but there were no effects on vascular outcomes during the 2 years of follow-up.[176] The trial was terminated prematurely due to the lack of power to address the hypothesis, because the effect of supplementation may have been lower then expected because of the introduction of mandatory folic acid fortification. The Second Cambridge Heart Antioxidant Study (CHAOS-2) was also prematurely terminated (after a median treatment period of 1.7 years) because of perceived lack of power. It was reported that folic acid supplementation (5 mg/d) had no effect on any vascular outcome, even though tHcy concentration decreased by 13%.[177]

Especially for the trials performed in the "fortified countries," it is questionable whether they are able to show a reduction in CVD because they will likely suffer from a lack of power as a result of the mandatory folic acid fortification[178] and the duration of the trials may be too short. Therefore, a collaboration (Homocysteine Lowering Treatment Trialists' Collaboration) has been set up to perform a prospective meta-analysis once all the data of these trials have become available. Analyses of the combined data (the 12 trials involve 52,000 participants) should have adequate power to show (or not) a preventive effect of these B vitamins.

Finally, almost all trials include a combination of folic acid and vitamins B_6 and B_{12} and will, therefore, not be able to show which of them has the main effect on CVD, whether there is an additive effect of a combination, or whether there is synergy between these three vitamins. Because the effect on the tHcy concentration is additive for folic acid and vitamin B_{12}, no synergy is expected for the effect on CVD. B vitamins may also have an effect on CVD independent of the tHcy concentration as results from several prospective studies suggest for vitamin B_6 and folic acid.[150,151,170,171,179,180] If this is indeed true, a synergistic effect of these vitamins may be possible. This latter question cannot be answered by the ongoing trials. If trials would include other tHcy-lowering compounds such as betaine,[181] they may be able to show whether a lower tHcy concentration or a higher B vitamin intake (or both) are causes of a reduction in CVD. However, it is not inconceivable that extra betaine will affect the availability of folates by influencing methyl group metabolism, and therefore it may still not be possible to indicate which is the causal component.

5.6 B Vitamins and Other Food Components Synergy and Cardiovascular Disease

5.6.1 B Vitamins and n-3 Fatty Acids

Already in 1963, Mueller and Iacono[182] postulated that vitamin B_6 deficiency inhibits the conversion of α-linolenic acid (n-3) and linoleic acid (n-6) into longer chain polyunsaturated fatty acids. Further animal studies showed that supplementation with fish oil rich in n-3 fatty acids in vitamin B_6–deficient rats counteracts the decrease in n-3 fatty acids.[182] The same has been shown for folate; animal studies clearly illustrate that folate metabolism is linked with that of long-chain n-3 fatty acids.[182] Human studies on this research topic are scarce. One study indicated synergistic effects of folic acid (10 mg/d) and vitamin B_6 (80 mg/d) together with fish oil (30 ml/d) on the atherogenic index and fibrinogen concentration in a cross-over study with intervention periods of 4 weeks.[184] The atherogenic index (i.e., [total cholesterol – HDL cholesterol]/HDL cholesterol) decreased by 12% during supplementation with only fish oil, whereas it decreased with 24% during supplementation with a combination of fish oil, folic acid, and vitamin B_6. Furthermore, a 9% greater decrease in plasma fibrinogen concentration (6% with the fish oil only supplementation, 15% with the fish oil with folic acid and vitamin B_6) was observed. Finally, the effect on the concentration of triglycerides, high density lipoprotein (HDL) cholesterol, glucose, and on fibrinolysis was also more beneficial, although not statistically significant in comparison with the fish oil–only supplement.[183] Although these results are promising, they were produced in a very small selective (12 males who were healthy or had slightly increased blood lipid levels) study population. Thus, confirmation in large well-designed intervention trials is warranted. The SU.FOL.OM3 trial may clarify this issue because the study contains a group supplemented with n-3 fatty acids, a group receiving a placebo, and a group that receives both treatments as well as a group receiving a combination of the B vitamins.[175]

5.6.2 B Vitamins and Antioxidant Vitamins

A possible interaction between B vitamins and antioxidant vitamins has been evaluated in one well designed placebo-controlled, double-blind, randomized intervention trial. In this study, using a factorial design including 101 men, subjects received either a combination of 1 mg of folic acid, 7.2 mg of vitamin B_6, and 0.02 mg of vitamin B_{12}, or a combination of 150 mg vitamin C, 67 mg vitamin E, and 9 mg β-carotene, both the vitamin B and antioxidant treatment, or a placebo for 8 weeks. Homocysteine concentrations decreased significantly in both groups receiving B vitamins either with or without antioxidants. There was no evidence of any interaction between the two groups of vitamins on the tHcy concentration.[185]

These results were confirmed in a more recent trial with a similar design, but with only vitamin C as the antioxidant vitamin; no interaction between folic acid (5 mg/d) and vitamin C (500 mg/d) on the tHcy concentration was observed in the group that received both supplements.[186]

5.6.3 B Vitamins and Iron

Biochemical evidence collected from both clinical and noninstitutionalized populations indicate that iron and folate deficiencies frequently occur simultaneously.[187] Controlled animal trials in which dietary iron and folate content have been systematically manipulated reveal that iron deficiency can cause altered folate utilization and that the impact of iron deficiency on folate metabolism is most dramatic during the reproductive and neonatal states of the life cycle.[187] Further *in vitro* studies using cells of animal origin have shown that iron can scavenge non–protein-bound folates and thereby increase folate catabolism.[188] It is not clear yet whether the simultaneous consumption of iron and folate in low or high doses has any effect.

5.6.4 B Vitamins and Alcohol

Alcohol interferes with normal folate transport and metabolism by disrupting intestinal absorption, reducing uptake and storage in the liver, increasing urinary loss, inhibiting methionine synthase activity, and activating oxidative catabolism of folate.[189] Rimm et al.[156] were the first to show an interaction between folate, vitamin B_6 intake, and alcohol consumption in the Nurses' Health Study; the inverse association between folate and vitamin B_6, and CVD was stronger in women who drank alcohol regularly than in nondrinkers. This interaction was confirmed by Jiang et al.[190] who showed that heavy drinkers (more than 30 g alcohol/d) with a low folate intake had the highest risk for chronic disease (CVD and cancer). Interactions with alcohol consumption have also been observed for the relation between folate intake and the plasma tHcy concentration: at a low folate intake nondrinkers had a higher tHcy concentration than drinkers, whereas at a high folate intake no difference was present between nondrinkers and drinkers.[54,88] Adequate folate intake may therefore be especially important in individuals who do not drink or who drink more alcohol than average.[191]

5.7 Food–Drug Synergy and Cardiovascular Disease

5.7.1 Lipid-Lowering Drugs and B Vitamins

Basu and Mann[192] showed that in rats high pharmacological doses of niacin interferes with the metabolism of methionine, leading to hyperhomocysteinemia and hypocysteinemia, through a lower vitamin B_6 status. The tHcy and cysteine levels in plasma were normalized when vitamin B_6 was added to the diet, without any effect on the hypolipidemic action of the drug. Subsequent studies in humans by Dierkes et al. and Westphal et al.[193,194] showed that lipid-lowering drugs have an elevating effect on the tHcy concentration; homocysteine increased by 44% after administration of fenofibrate (200 mg/d) and 17.5% after bezafibrate (400 mg/d), which was not explained by changes in vitamin concentrations.[193] This increase in homocysteine in response to fenofibrate may counteract the cardioprotective effect of lipid lowering. Addition of 650 μg folic acid, 50 μg vitamin B_{12}, and 5 mg vitamin B_6 per day for 6 weeks reduced the fenofibrate induced tHcy increase from 44 to 13%.[195] This was confirmed in another study among 22 patients who received fenofibrate with or without 10 mg of folic acid every other day.[196] It seems thus clear that fibrate therapy and especially fenofibrate therapy should be accompanied by B vitamin supplementation.[197]

Finally, a pilot study of the SEARCH trial investigated a potential interaction between simvastatin and folic acid–vitamin B_{12} treatment in a 2×2 factorial design in 141 patients who received daily (1) 80 mg simvastatin, (2) a combination of 2 mg folic acid and 0.8 mg vitamin B_{12}, (3) both the simvastatin and B vitamin treatment, or (4) a placebo. The combination group and the vitamins alone group experienced similar homocysteine lowering, which means that no interaction or synergy between simvastatins and B vitamins was observed.[198]

5.7.2 Other Drugs and B Vitamins

Several oral and transdermal hormone replacement regimens containing estrogen alone or combined estrogen and progestogen have been shown to reduce fasting tHcy concentrations.[199–201] The majority of randomized placebo controlled trials showed a decrease in tHcy after oral as well as transdermal hormone replacement therapy, although the reduction was larger after oral estrogen administration than after transdermal estrogen or oral estrogen plus gestodene therapy.[202] Related to this, it has been shown that tamoxifen, a nonsteroidal estrogen agonist and antagonist that is used for the treatment of advanced breast cancer, lowered plasma tHcy with 15 to 30% in postmenopausal women with breast cancer as well as in healthy women.[203,204] This may be due to a tamoxifen induced increase in folate status.[204] Furthermore, raloxifene, a novel nonsteroidal compound has also been shown to significantly reduce plasma tHcy concentrations (8% after 6 months and 16% after 12 months) in postmenopausal women.[205,206] With respect to risk of CVD, which is increased in postmenopausal women, it would be interesting to know whether a combination of these drugs with B vitamins has any synergistic effect, but so far nothing is known on this topic.

Finally, drugs with a free thiol group, such as *N*-acetylcysteine, D-penicillamine, or cysteamine can react with the disulfide forms of homocysteine (99% of plasma tHcy). When this reaction takes places, free homocysteine remains, which is available for cellular uptake, metabolic conversion, and (possibly) excretion. Administration of these types of drugs may decrease tHcy concentrations in patients with renal failure who are not responding to B vitamin or betaine therapy. It is possible that combined intake of B vitamins with these drugs may have an even greater effect, but so far no study has been undertaken to evaluate this.

5.8 Safety Aspects of Folate, Vitamin B_6, and Vitamin B_{12}

5.8.1 B Vitamins

With respect to the safety of folic acid intake, most experts would consider an intake of 1 mg/d to be safe to avoid masking of vitamin B_{12} deficiency.[207] Our knowledge of how frequently masking occurs and of the lowest dose of folic acid that produces masking is limited, and the long term effect of free folic acid in serum is unknown.[174,208] Although the U.S. Department of Agriculture chose a fortification level (140 μg/100 flour) that they believed would limit exposure to less than 1 mg folic acid/d in almost everybody, the actual fortification level in foods is considerably higher[13,130] and an increase of undiagnosed vitamin B_{12} deficiency would be expected. However, no evidence of an increase in low vitamin B_{12} concentrations without anemia has been observed in a population of patients at the Veterans Affairs Medical Center in Washington DC, where the vitamin B_{12} concentration was measured.[208] This suggests that masking of vitamin B_{12} deficiency does probably not occur at levels obtained by dietary intake of fortified foods and that the safe level of intake is probably higher than 1 mg/d.

Excessive amounts of vitamin B_6 (greater than 200 mg/d) can cause peripheral neuropathy in persons with normal renal function.[209,210] On the other hand, studies involving large patient groups who receive 100 to 150 mg/d have shown minimal or no toxicity in 5- to 10-year studies.[211] Women self-medicating for premenstrual syndrome taking 500 to 5000 mg/d have shown peripheral neuropathy within 1 to 3 years. It would appear that vitamin B_6 is safe at doses of 100 mg/d or less in adults.[211]

Although intravenous injection of vitamin B_{12} may have unwanted side effects such as reddish discoloration of the skin, mucous membranes, and urine, oral intake of vitamin B_{12} does not seem to induce any negative effects, at least up to 1 mg/d.[212,213]

5.8.2 Interactions of B Vitamins with Other Drugs

Several drugs interfere with folate absorption and metabolism.[80] Antiepileptic drugs are suspected to inhibit enzymes involved in folate metabolism,[214] and methotrexate inhibits the conversion of dihydrofolates to tetrahydrofolates, thereby depleting cells of reduced folates.[215] Other antifolates are sufasalazine, raltritrexed, trimetrexate, and trimethoprim.[216]

Furthermore, metformin, a drug used in diabetes, decreases B vitamin concentrations,[216] and several other vitamin B_6 antagonists exist.[199] Also drugs that need methylation before they are activated or detoxified (for example, the Parkinson's disease drug L-dopa and the anticancer drug 6-mercaptopurine) and immunosuppressive drugs like cyclosporine may increase tHcy concentration.[199,218,219] Thus, all these drugs diminish the beneficial effects of B vitamins on CVD. Thus folic acid supplementation may be warranted for patients at high risk for CVD, such as those with hyperlipemia or diabetes.[196,198] This is certainly true for patients who receive phenytoin therapy, which should be combined with folic acid supplementation.[220,221]

5.9 Conclusions

In conclusion, the combination of folate, vitamin B_6, and vitamin B_{12} has a potential beneficial effect on cardiovascular disease. Intervention trials provide evidence that supplementation with these three vitamins results in favorable effects on cardiovascular outcomes, including a regression of carotid plaques and a reduced rate of restenosis. Studies aimed at determining potential synergy of folate, vitamin B_6, and vitamin B_{12} with respect to cardiovascular outcomes are ongoing. Further studies are required to elucidate the potential synergy of folate, vitamin B_6, and/or vitamin B_{12} with drugs used for prevention and/or management of cardiovascular disease.

References

1. Passmore, R., and Eastwood, M.A., *Human Nutrition and Dietetics*, Churchill Livingstone, New York, 1986.
2. Holland, B., Welch, A.A., Unwin, I.D., Buss, D.H., and Southgate, P.A.A., *McCance and Widdowson's The Composition of Foods*, The Royal Society of Chemistry, London, 1991.

3. Melse-Boonstra, A. et al., Bioavailability of heptaglutamyl relative to monoglutamyl folic acid in healthy adults, *Am. J. Clin. Nutr.*, 79, 424–429, 2004.
4. Sauberlich, H.E. et al., Folate requirement and metabolism in nonpregnant women, *Am. J. Clin. Nutr.*, 46, 1016–1028, 1987.
5. Blakley, R.L. and Benkovic, S.J., *Folates and Pterins. Chemistry and Biochemistry of Folates*, John Wiley& Sons, New York, 1984.
6. Medical Research Council Vitamin Study Research Group, Prevention of neural tube defects: results of the Medical Research Council Vitamin Study, *Lancet*, 338, 131–137, 1991.
7. Selhub J. et al., B vitamins, homocysteine, and neurocognitive function in the elderly, *Am. J. Clin. Nutr.*, 71, 614S–620S, 2000.
8. Choi, S.W. and Mason, J.B., Folate and carcinogenesis: an integrated scheme, *J. Nutr.*, 130, 129–132, 2000.
9. van Meurs, J.B.J. et al., Homocysteine levels and the risk of osteoporotic fracture, *N. Engl. J. Med.*, 350, 2033–2041, 2004.
10. McLean R.R. et al., Homocysteine as a predictive factor for hip fracture in older persons. *N. Engl. J Med.*, 350, 2042–9, 2004.
11. Martin A., *Apports Nutritionnels Conseillés pour la Population Française*, Technique & documentation, Paris: 2001.
12. Institute of Medicine and Food and Nutrition Board, Dietary reference intakes: thiamin, riboflavin, niacin, vitamin B_6, folate, vitamin B_{12}, pantothenic acid, biotin, and choline, National Academy Press, Washington DC, 1998, pp. 1–567
13. Quinlivan, E.P. and Gregory, J.F.I., Effect of food fortification on folic acid intake in the United States, *Am. J. Clin. Nutr.*, 77, 221–225, 2003.
14. Shane, B., Folate chemistry and metabolism, in *Folate in Health and Disease*, Bailey LB, Ed., Marcel Dekker, New York, 1995, 1–22.
15. Birch, T.W. and György, P., A study of the chemical nature of vitamin B_6 and methods for its preparation in a concentrated state. *Biochem. J.*, 30, 304–315, 1936.
16. Smith, E.L. and Parke. L.F.J., Purification of the antipernicious anemia factor, *Biochem. J.*, 43, viii, 1948.
17. Rickes, E.L. et al., Crystalline vitamin B_{12}, *Science*, 107, 396–397, 1948.
18. Heyssel R.M. et al., Vitamin B_{12} turnover in man, The assimilation of vitamin B_{12} from natural foodstuff by man and estimates of minimal daily dietary requirements, *Am. J. Clin. Nutr.*, 18, 176–184, 1966.
19. Hvas, A.M. and Nexo, E., Holotranscobalamin as a predictor of vitamin B_{12} status, *Clin. Chem. Lab. Med.*, 41, 1489–1492, 2003.
20. Herrmann, W. and Geisel, J., Vegetarian lifestyle and monitoring of vitamin B_{12} status, *Clin. Chim. Acta*, 326, 47–59, 2002.
21. Finkelstein, J.D., The metabolism of homocysteine: pathways and regulation, *Eur. J. Pediat.r*, 157 (Suppl 2), S40–S44, 1998.
22. Ueland, P.M. and Refsum, H., Plasma homocysteine, a risk factor for vascular disease: plasma levels in health, disease, and drug therapy, *J. Lab. Clin. Med.*, 114, 473–501, 1989.
23. Kang, S.S., Wong, P.W., and Malinow, M.R., Hyperhomocyst(e)inemia as a risk factor for occlusive vascular disease, *Annu. Rev. Nutr.*, 12, 279–298, 1992.
24. Finkelstein, J.D., Methionine metabolism in mammals, *J. Nutr. Biochem.*, 1, 228–237, 1990.
25. Guenther, B.D. et al., The structure and properties of methylenetetrahydrofolate reductase from Escherichia coli suggest how folate ameliorates human hyperhomoycsteinemia, *Nat. Struc. Biol.*, 6, 359–365, 1999.

26. Mudd, S.H. et al., Homocysteinuria: an enzymatic defect, *Science,* 143, 1443–1445, 1964.
27. Rosenblatt, D.S., Inborn errors of folate and cobalamin metabolism, in *Homocysteine in Health and Disease,* Carmel, R. and Jacobsen D.W., Eds. Cambridge University Press, London, 2001, pp. 244–258.
28. Rosenblatt, D.S., Inherited disorders of folate transport and metabolism, in *The Metabolic Basis of Inherited Disease,* Scriver, C.R., Beaudet, A.L., Sly, W.S, and Valle, D., Eds. McGraw-Hill, New York,1989, 2049–2064.
29. Mudd, S.H., Levy, H.L., and Skovby, F., Disorders of transsulfuration, in *The Metabolic Basis of Inherited Disease,* Scriver, C.R., Beaudet, A.L., Sly, W.S, and Valle, D., Eds. McGraw-Hill, New York,1989, pp. 693–734.
30. Frosst, P. et al., A candidate genetic risk factor for vascular disease: a common mutation in methylenetetrahydrofolate reductase, *Nat Genet.,* 10, 111–113, 1995.
31. Meleady, R. et al., Thermolabile methylenetetrahydrofolate reductase, homocysteine, and cardiovascular disease risk: the European Concerted Action Project, *Am. J. Clin. Nutr.,* 77, 63–70, 2003.
32. Brattstrom, L. et al., Common methylenetetrahydrofolate reductase gene mutation leads to hyperhomocysteinemia but not to vascular disease: the result of a meta-analysis, *Circulation,* 98, 2520–2526, 1998.
33. van der Put, N.M. et al., Decreased methylene tetrahydrofolate reductase activity due to the 677C>T mutation in families with spina bifida offspring, *J. Mol. Med.,* 74, 691–694, 1996.
34. Jacques, P.F. et al., Relation between folate status, a common mutation in methylenetetrahydrofolate reductase, and plasma homocysteine concentrations, *Circulation,* 93, 9, 1996.
35. Kauwell, G.P. et al., Methylenetetrahydrofolate reductase mutation (677C>T) negatively influences plasma homocysteine response to marginal folate intake in elderly women, *Metabolism,* 49, 1440–1443, 2000.
36. de Bree, A. et al., Effect of the methylenetetrahydrofolate reductase 677C>T mutation on the relations among folate intake and plasma folate and homocysteine concentrations in a general population sample, *Am. J. Clin. Nutr.,* 77, 687–693, 2003.
37. Shelnutt, K.P. et al., Folate status response to controlled folate intake is affected by the methylenetetrahydrofolate reducatse 677C>T polymorphism in young women, *J. Nutr.,* 133, 4107–4111, 2003.
38. McQuillan, B.M. et al., Hyperhomocsyteinemia but not the C677T mutation of methylenetetrahydrofolate reductase is an independent risk determinant of carotid wall thickening — The Perth carotid Ultrasound Disease Assessment Study (CUDAS), *Circulation,* 99, 2383–2388, 1999.
39. Alfthan, G. et al., Folate intake, plasma folate and homocysteine status in a random Finnish population, *Eur. J. Clin. Nutr.,* 57, 81–88, 2003.
40. Bailey, L.B. et al., Vitamin B-12 status is inversely associated with plasma homocysteine in young women with C677T and/or 1298C methylenetetrahydrofolate reductase polymorphisms, *J. Nutr.,* 132, 1878, 2002.
41. Meisel, C. et al., Identification of six methylenetetrahydrofolate reductase (MTHFR) gentoypes resulting from common polymorphisms: impact on plasma homocysteine levels and development of coronary artery disease. *Atherosclerosis,* 154, 651–658, 2001.
42. Lievers, K.J.A. et al., A second common variant in the methylenetetrahydrofolate reductase (MTHFR) gene and its relationship to MTHFR enzyme activity, homocysteine, and cardiovascular disease risk, *J. Mol. Med.,* 79, 522–528, 2001.

43. Rozen, R., Polymorphisms of folate and cobalamin metabolism, in *Homocysteine in Health and Disease*, Carmel, R, and Jacobsen, D.W., Eds., Cambridge University Press, London, 2001, pp. 259–270.
44. Winkelmayer, W.C. et al., Effects of TCN2 776C>G on vitamin B, folate, and total homocysteine levels in kidney transplant patients, *Kidney Int.*, 65, 1877–1881, 2004.
45. Kluijtmans, L.A.J. et al., Genetic and nutritional factors contributing to hyperhomocysteinemia in young adults, *Blood*, 101, 2483–2488, 2003.
46. Lussier-Cacan, S. et al., Plasma total homocysteine in healthy subjects: sex-specific relation with biological traits, *Am. J. Clin. Nutr.*, 64, 587–593, 1996.
47. de Bree, A. et al., The homocysteine distribution: (Mis)judging the burden, *J. Clin. Epidemiol.*, 54, 462–469, 2001.
48. Andersson, A. et al., Plasma homocysteine before and after methionine loading with regard to age, gender and menopausal status, *Eur. J. Clin. Invest.*, 22, 79–87, 1992.
49. Norlund, L. et al., The increase of plasma homocysteine concentrations with age is partly due to the deterioration of renal function as determined by plasma cystatin C. *Clin. Chem. Lab. Med.*, 36, 175–178, 1998.
50. Giltay, E.J. et al., Effects of sex steroids on plasma total homocysteine levels: a study in transsexual males and females. *J. Clin. Endocrinol. Metab.*, 83, 550–553, 1998.
51. Wouters, M.G.A.J. et al., Plasma homocysteine and menopausal status, *Eur. J. Clin. Invest.*, 25, 801–805, 1995.
52. de Bree, A. et al., Lifestyle factors and plasma homocysteine concentrations in a general population sample, *Am. J. Epidemiol.*, 154, 150–154, 2001.
53. Jacques, P.F. et al., Determinants of plasma total homocysteine concentration in the Framingham Offspring cohort, *Am. J. Clin. Nutr.*, 73, 613–621, 2001.
54. Koehler, K.M. et al., Association of folate intake and serum homocysteine in elderly persons according to vitamin supplementation and alcohol use. *Am. J. Clin. Nutr.*, 73, 628–37, 2001.
55. Dallongeville, J. et al., Cigarette smoking is associated with unhealthy patterns of nutrient intake: a meta-analyses, *J. Nutr.*, 128, 1450–1457, 1998.
56. Piyathilake, C.J. et al., Effect of smoking on folate levels in buccal mucosal cells, *Int. J. Cancer*, 52, 566–569, 1992.
57. Pryor, W.A. and Stone, K., Oxidants in cigarette smoke. Radicals hydrogen peroxide, peroxynitrate and peroxynitrite, *Ann. N.Y. Acad. Sci.*, 686, 12–27, 1993.
58. Mansoor, M.A. et al., Redox status and protein binding of plasma homocysteine and other aminothiols in patients with early-onset peripheral vascular disease. Homocysteine and peripheral vascular disease, *Arterioscler. Thromb. Vasc. Biol.*, 15, 232–240, 1995.
59. Bergmark, C. et al., Redox status of plasma homocysteine and related aminothiols in smoking and nonsmoking young adults, *Clin Chem,*, 43, 1997–1999, 1997.
60. Blom, H.J., Determinants of plasma homocysteine, *Am. J. Clin. Nutr.*, 67, 188–189, 1998.
61. Urgert, R. et al., Heavy coffee consumption and plasma homocysteine: a randomized controlled trial in healthy volunteers, *Am. J. Clin. Nutr.*, 72, 1107–1110, 2000.
62. Grubben, M.J. et al., Unfiltered coffee increases plasma homocysteine concentrations in healthy volunteers: a randomizd trial, *Am. J. Clin. Nutr.*, 71, 480–484, 2000.

63. Christensen, B. et al., Abstention from filtered coffee reduced the concentration of plasma homocysteine and serum cholesterol — a randomized controlled trial, *Am. J. Clin. Nutr.*, 74, 307, 2001.
64. Nygard, O. et al., Coffee consumption and plasma total homocysteine: the Hordaland Homocysteine Study, *Am. J. Clin. Nutr.*, 65, 136–43, 1997.
65. Olthof, M.R. et al., Consumption of high doses of chlorogenic acid, present in coffee, or of black tea increases plasma total homocysteine concentrations in humans, *Am. J. Clin. Nutr.*, 73, 532–538, 2001.
66. Cravo, M.L. et al., Hyperhomocysteinemia in chronic alcoholism: correlation with folate, vitamin B-12, and vitamin B-6 status, *Am. J. Clin. Nutr.*, 63, 220–224, 1996.
67. Mennen, L.I. et al., Relation between homocysteine concentrations and the consumption of different types of alcoholic beverages: the French Supplementation with Antioxidant Vitamins and Minerals Study, *Am. J. Clin. Nutr.*, 78, 334–338, 2003.
68. Halsted, C.H., Lifestyle effects on homocysteine and an alcohol paradox, *Am. J. Clin. Nutr.*, 73, 501–502, 2001.
69. de Bree, A. et al., Alcohol consumption and plasma homocysteine: What's brewing? *Int. J. Epidemiol.*, 30, 626–627, 2001.
70. Mayer, O., Jr., Simon, J., and Rosolova, H., A population study of the influence of beer consumption on folate and homocysteine concentrations, *Eur. J. Clin. Nutr.*, 55, 605–609, 2001.
71. Burger, M. et al., Alcohol consumption and its relation to cardiovascular risk factors in Germany, *Eur. J Clin. Nutr*, 58, 605–614, 2004.
72. van der Gaag, M.S. et al., Effect of consumption of red wine, spirits, and beer on serum homocysteine, *Lancet*, 335, 1522, 2000.
73. Mar, M.H. and Zeisel, S.H., Betaine in wine: answer to the French paradox? *Med. Hypoth.*, 53, 383–385, 1999.
74. McCully, K.S., Vascular pathology of homocysteinemia: implications for the pathogenesis of arteriosclerosis, *Am. J. Pathol.*, 56, 111–128, 1969.
75. McCully, K.S. and Wilson, R.B., Homocysteine theory of arteriosclerosis, *Atherosclerosis*, 22, 215–227, 1975.
76. Wilcken, D.E. and Wilcken, B., The pathogenesis of coronary artery disease. A possible role for methionine metabolism, *J. Clin. Invest.*, 57, 1079–1082, 1967.
77. Boushey, C.J. et al., A quantitative assessment of plasma homocysteine as a risk factor for vascular disease, *JAMA*, 274, 1049–1057, 1995.
78. Refsum, H. et al., Homocysteine and cardiovascular disease, *Annu. Rev. Med.*, 49, 31–62, 1998.
79. Danesh, J. and Lewington, S., Plasma homocysteine and coronary heart disease, *J. Cardiovasc. Res.*, 5, 229–32, 1998.
80. de Bree, A. et al., Homocysteine determinants and the evidence to what extent homocysteine determines the risk of coronary heart disease, *Pharm. Rev.*, 54, 599–618, 2002.
81. Ueland, P.M. et al., The controversy over homocysteine and cardiovascular risk, *Am. J. Clin. Nutr.*, 72, 324–32, 2000.
82. Ford, E.S. et al., Homocyst(e)ine and cardiovascular disease: a systematic review of the evidence with special emphasis on case-control studies and nested case-control studies, *Int. J. Epidemiol.*, 31, 59–70, 2002.
83. The Homocysteine Studies Collaboration, Homocysteine and risk of ischemic heart disease and stroke, *JAMA*, 288, 2015–2022, 2002.

84. Wald, D.S., Law, M., and Morris, J.K., Homocysteine and cardiovascular disease: evidence on causality from a meta-analysis, *Br. Med. J.*, 325, 1202–1206, 2002.
85. Klerk, M. et al., MTHFR 677C>T polymorphism and risk of coronary heart disease, A meta-analysis, *JAMA*, 288, 2023–2031, 2002.
86. Mennen, L.I. et al., Homocysteine, cardiovascular disease risk factors, and habitual diet in the French Supplementation with Antioxidant Vitamins and Minerals Study, *Am. J. Clin. Nutr.*, 76, 1279–1289, 2002.
87. Rasmussen L.B. et al., Folate intake, lifestyle factors, and homocysteine concentrations in younger and older women, *Am. J. Clin. Nutr.*, 72, 1156–1163, 2000.
88. de Bree, A. et al., Association between B vitamin intake and plasma homocysteine concentration in the general Dutch population aged 20–65 y, *Am. J. Clin. Nutr.*, 73, 1033, 2001.
89. Shimakawa, T. et al., Vitamin intake: a possible determinant of plasma homocyst(e)ine among middle aged adults, *Ann. Epidemiol.*, 7, 285–293, 1997.
90. Ubbink, J.B. et al., Homocysteine and ischaemic heart disease in the Caerphilly cohort, *Atherosclerosis*, 140, 349–356, 1998.
91. Saw S.M. et al., Genetic, dietary, and other lifestyle determinants of plasma homocysteine concentrations in middle-aged and older Chinese men and women in Singapore, *Am. J. Clin. Nutr.*, 73, 232–239, 2001.
92. Selhub, J. et al., Vitamin status and intake as primary determinants of homocysteinemia in an elderly population, *JAMA*, 270, 2693–2698, 1993.
93. Bates, C.J. et al., Plasma total homocysteine in a representative sample of 972 British men and women aged 65 and over, *Eur. J. Clin. Nutr.*, 51, 691–697, 1997.
94. van Asselt, D.Z.B. et al., Role of cobalamin intake and atrophic gastritis in mild cobalamin deficiency in older Dutch subjects, *Am. J. Clin. Nutr.*, 68, 328–334, 1998.
95. Bailey L.B., Rampersaud, G.C., and Kauwel, G.P.A., Folic acid supplements and fortification affect the risk for neural tube defects, vascular disease and cancer: evolving science, *J. Nutr.*, 133, 1961S–1968S, 2003.
96. Ward, M. et al., Plasma homocysteine, a risk factor for cardiovascular disease, is lowered by physiological doses of folic acid, *Quart. J. Med.*, 90, 519–524, 1997.
97. Brouwer, I.A. et al., Low-dose folic acid supplementation decreases plasma homocysteine: a randomized trial, *Am. J. Clin. Nutr.*, 69, 99–104, 1999.
98. Brattstrom, L. et al., Folic acid — an innocuous means to reduce plasma homocysteine, *Scan. J. Clin. Lab. Invest.*, 48, 215–221, 1988.
99. Olszewski, A.J. et al., Reduction of plasma lipid and homocysteine levels by pyridoxine, folate, cobalamin, choline, riboflavin and troxerutin in atherosclerosis, *Atherosclerosis*, 75, 1–6, 1989.
100. Ubbink, J.B. et al., Hyperhomocysteinemia and the response to vitamin supplementation, *Clin. Invest.*, 97, 993–998, 1993.
101. Ubbink, J.B. et al., Vitamin requirements for the treatment of hyperhomocysteinemia in humans, *J. Nutr.*, 124, 1927–1933, 1994.
102. Wald, D.S. et al., Randomized trial of folic acid supplementation and serum homocysteine levels, *Arch. Int. Med.*, 161, 695–700, 2001.
103. Homocysteine Lowering Trialists' Collaboration, Lowering blood homocysteine with folic acid based supplements: meta-analysis of randomised trials, *Br. Med. J.*, 316, 894–898, 1998.
104. Bostom, A.G. et al., Post-methionine load hyperhomocysteinemia in persons with normal fasting total plasma homocysteine: initial results from the NHLBI Family Heart Study, *Atherosclerosis*, 116, 147–151, 1995.

105. van Oort, F.V.A. et al., Folic acid and reduction of plasma homocysteine concentrations in older adults: a dose-response study, *Am. J. Clin. Nutr.*, 77, 1318–1323, 2003.
106. McKay, D.L. et al., Multivitamin/mineral supplementation improves plama B-vitamin status and homocysteine concentration in healthy older adults consuming a folate-fortified diet, *J. Nutr.*, 130, 3090–3096, 2000.
107. Ashfield-Watt, P.A.L. et al., Methylenetetrahydrofolate reductase 677C>T genotype modulates homocysteine responses to a folate-rich diet or a low-dose folic acid supplement: a randomized controlled trial, *Am. J. Clin. Nutr.*, 76, 180–186, 2002.
108. Nelen, W.L. et al., Methylenetetrahydrofolate reductase polymorphism affects the change in homocysteine and folate concentrations resulting from low dose folic acid supplementation in women with unexplained recurrent miscarriages, *J. Nutr.*, 128, 1336–1341, 1998.
109. Malinow, M.R. et al., The effects of folic acid supplementation on plasma total homocysteine are modulated by mutivitamin use and methylenetetrahydrofolate reductase genotypes, *Arterioscler. Thromb. Vasc. Biol.*, 17, 1157–1162, 1997.
110. Brönstrup, A. et al., Effects of folic acid and combinations of folic acid and vitamin B-12 on plasma homocysteine concentrations in healthy, young women, *Am. J. Clin. Nutr.*, 68, 1104–1110, 1998.
111. Sato, Y. et al., Hyperhomocysteinemia in Japanese patients with convalescent stage ischemic stroke: effect of combined therapy with folic acid and mecobalamine, *J. Neurol. Sci.*, 202, 65–68, 2002.
112. Dierkes J., Kroesen M., and Pietrzik, K., Folic acid and vitamin B_6 supplementation and plasma homocysteine concentrations in healthy young women, *Int. J. Vitam. Nutr. Res.*, 68, 98–103, 1998.
113. Scott, J.M. and Weir, D.G., The methyl folate trap. A physiological response in man to prevent methyl group deficiency in kwashiorkor (methionine deficiency) and an explanation for folic acid-induced exacerbation of sub-acute combined degeneration in pernicious anaemia, *Lancet*, 2, 337–340, 1981.
114. Weir, D.G. and Scott, J.M., Brain function in the elderly: role of vitamin B-12 and folate, *Br. Med. Bull.*, 55, 669–682, 1999.
115. Pennypacker, L.C. et al., High prevalence of cobalamin deficiency in elderly patients, *J. Am. Geriatr. Soc.*, 40, 1197–1204, 1992.
116. Fohr, I.P. et al., 5,10-Methylenetetrahydrofolate reductase genotype determines the plasma homocysteine-lowering effect of supplementation with 5-methyltetrahydrofolate or folic acid in healthy young women, *Am. J. Clin. Nutr.*, 75, 275–282, 2002.
117. Bostom, A.G. et al., Controlled comparison of l-5-methyltetrahydrofolate versus folic acid for the treatment of hyperhomocysteinemia in hemodialysis patients, *Circulation*, 101, 2829–2832, 2000.
118. Venn, B.J. et al., Comparison of the effect of low-dose supplementation with l-5-methyltetrahydrofolate or folic acid on plasma homocysteine: a randomized placebo-controlled study, *Am. J. Clin. Nutr.*, 77, 658–662, 2003.
119. Lamers, Y. et al., Supplementation with [6S]-5-mehtyltetrahydrofolate or folic acid equally reduces plasma total homocysteine concentrations in healthy women, *Am. J. Clin. Nutr.*, 79, 473–478, 2004.
120. Cuskelly, G.J., McNulty H., and Scott, J.M., Effect of increasing dietary folate on red-cell folate: implications for prevention of neural tube defects, *Lancet*, 347, 657–659, 1996.

121. Ashfield-Watt, P.A.L. et al., A comparison of the effect of advice to eat either '5-a-day' fruit and vegetables or folic acid-fortified foods on plasma folate and homocysteine, *Eur. J. Clin. Nutr.*, 57, 316–323, 2003.
122. Tucker, K.L. et al., Breakfast cereal fortified with folic acid, vitamin B-6, and vitamin B-12 increases vitamin concentrations and reduces homocysteine concentrations: a randomized trial, *Am. J. Clin. Nutr.*, 79, 805–811, 2004.
123. Tapola, N.S. et al., Mineral water fortified with folic acid, vitamins B_6, B_{12}, D and calcium improves folate status and decreases plasma homocysteine concentration in men and women, *Eur. J. Clin. Nutr.*, 58, 376–385, 2004.
124. Clark, N.A. and Fisk, N.M., Minimal compliance with the Department of Health recommendation for routine folate prophylaxis to prevent fetal neural tube defects, *Br. J. Obstetr. Gynaecol.*, 101, 709–710, 1994.
125. McDonnell, R. et al., Folic acid knowledge and use among expectant mothers in 1997: a comparison with 1996, *Ir. Med. J.*, 92, 296–299, 1999.
126. de Walle, H.E. et al., Effect of mass media campaign to reduce socioeconomic differences in women's awareness and behaviour concerning use of folic acid: cross sectional study. *Br. Med. J.*, 319, 291–292, 1999.
127. Smith, J.B., Potts, D.M., and Fortney, J.A., Political constraints on contraceptive development in the United States, *N. C. Med. J.*, 52, 484–488, 1991.
128. Food and Drug Administration, Food standards: amendment of standards of identity for enriched grain products to require addition of folic acid, *Fed. Regist.*, 61, 8781–8797, 1996.
129. Lewis, C.J. et al., Estimated folate intakes: data updated to reflect food fortification, increased bioavailabitliy, and dietary supplement use, *Am. J. Clin. Nutr.*, 70, 198–207, 1999.
130. Rader, J.I., Weaver, C.M., and Angyal, G., Total folate in enriched cereal-grain products in the United States following fortification, *Food Chem.*, 70, 275–289, 2000.
131. Choumenkovitch, S.F. et al., Folic acid intake from fortification in United States exceeds predictions, *J. Nutr.*, 132, 2792–2798, 2002.
132. Jacques, P.F. et al., The effect of folic acid fortification on plasma folate and total homocysteine concentrations, *N. Engl. J. Med.*, 340, 1449–1454, 1999.
133. Choumenkovitch, S.F. et al., Folic acid fortification increases red blood cell folate concentrations in the Framingham Study, *J. Nutr.*, 131, 3277–3780, 2001.
134. Miriuka, S.G. et al., Effects of folic acid fortification and multivitamin therapy on homocysteine and vitamin B_{12} status in cardiac transplant recipients, *J. Heart Lung Transplant*, 23, 405–412, 2004.
135. Ray, J.G. et al., Persistence of vitamin B_{12} insufficiency among elderly women after folic acid food fortification, *Clin. Biochem.*, 36, 387–391, 2003.
136. Hertrampf, E. et al., Consumption of folic acid-fortified bread improves folate status in women of reproductive age in Chile, *J. Nutr.*, 133, 3166–3169, 2003.
137. Anderson, J.L. et al., Effect of folic acid fortification of food on homocysteine-related mortality, *Am. J. Med.*, 116, 158–164, 2004.
138. Selhub, J. et al., Relationship between plasma homocysteine and vitamin status in the Framingham study population. Impact of folic acid fortification, *Public Health Rev.*, 28, 117–145, 2000.
139. De Wals, P. et al., Trend in prevalence of neural tube defects in Quebec, *Birth Defects Res.*, 67, 919–923, 2003.
140. Honein, M.A. et al., Impact of folic acid fortification of the US food supply on the occurrence of neural tube defects, *JAMA*, 285, 2981–2986, 2001.

141. Williams, L.J. et al., Prevalence of spina bifida and anencephaly during the transition to mandatory folic acid fortification in the United States, *Teratology,* 66, 33–39, 2002.
142. Yang, Q., Presentation, American Heart Association 44th annual Conference on Cardiovascular Disease Epidemiology and Prevention, San Francisco, March 5, 2004 (Abstract LB27).
143. Tucker, K.L. et al., Folic acid fortification of the food supply. Potential benefits and risks for the elderly population, *JAMA,* 276, 1879–1885, 1996.
144. Carmel, R., Prevalence of undiagnosed pernicious anemia in the elderly, *Arch. Intern. Med.,* 156, 1097–1100, 1996.
145. Venn, B.J. et al., Dietary counselling to increase natural folate intake: a randomized, placebo-controlled trial in free-living subjects to assess effects on serum folate and plasma total homocysteine, *Am. J. Clin. Nutr.,* 76, 765, 2002.
146. Morrison, H.I. et al., Serum folate and risk of fatal coronary heart disease, *JAMA,* 275, 1893–1896, 1996.
147. de Bree, A. et al., Coronary heart disease mortality, plasma homocysteine, and B-vitamins: a prospective study, *Atherosclerosis,* 166, 369–377, 2003.
148. Giles, W.H. et al., Serum folate and risk for coronary heart disease: results from a cohort of US adults, *Ann. Epidemiol.,* 8, 490–496, 1998.
149. Voutilainen, S. et al., Low serum folate concentrations are associated with an excess incidence of acute coronary events: the Kuopio Ischaemic Heart Disease Risk Factor Study, *Eur. J. Clin. Nutr.,* 54, 424–428, 2000.
150. Folsom, A.R. et al., Prospective study of coronary heart disease incidence in relation to fasting total homocysteine, related genetic polymorphisms, and B vitamins, *Circulation,* 98, 204–210, 1998.
151. Chasan-Taber, L. et al., A prospective study of folate and vitamin B_6 and risk of myocardial infarction in US physicians, *J. Am. Coll. Nutr.,* 15, 136–143, 1996.
152. Ford, E.S., Byers, T.E., and Giles, W.H., Serum folate and chronic disease risk: findings from a cohort of United States adults, *Int. J. Epidemiol.,* 27, 592–598, 1998.
153. Loria, C.M. et al., Serum folate and cardiovascular disease mortality among US men and women, *Arch. Intern. Med.,* 160, 3258–3262, 2000.
154. Zeitlin, A., Frishman, W.H., and Chang, C.J., The association of vitamin B_{12} and folate blood levels with mortality and cardiovascular morbidity incidence in the old old: the Bronx aging study, *Am. J. Ther.,* 4, 275–281, 1997.
155. Giles, W.H. et al., Serum folate and risk for ischemic stroke, *Stroke,* 26, 1166–1170, 1995.
156. Rimm, E.B. et al., Folate and vitamin B_6 from diet and supplements in relation to risk of coronary heart disease among women, *JAMA,* 279, 359–364, 1998.
157. Voutilainen, S. et al., Low dietary folate intake is associated with an excess incidence of acute coronary events, *Circulation,* 103, 2674–2680, 2001.
158. Bazzano, L.A. et al., Dietary intake of folate and risk of stroke in US men and women, *Stroke,* 33, 1183–1189, 2002.
159. He, K. et al., Folate, vitamin B_6, and B_{12} intakes in relation to risk of stroke among men, *Stroke,* 35, 169–174, 2004.
160. Al Delaimy, W.K. et al., Folate intake and risk of stroke among women.,*Stroke,* 35, 1259–1263, 2004.
161. Merchant, A.T. et al., The use of B vitamin supplements and peripheral arterial disease risk in men are inversely related, *J. Nutr.,* 133, 2863–2867, 2003.

162. Brown, A.A. and Hu, F.B., Dietary modulation of endothelial function: implications for cardiovascular disease, *Am. J. Clin. Nutr.*, 73, 673–686, 2001.
163. de Jong, S.C. et al., Normohomocysteinaemia and vitamin-treated hyperhomocysteinaemia are associated with similar risks of cardiovascular events in patients with premature peripheral arterial occlusive disease. A prospective cohort study. *J Intern Med*, 246, 87–96, 1999.
164. Vermeulen, E.G.J. et al., Normohomocysteinaemia and vitamin-treated hyperhomocysteinaemia are associated with similar risk of cardiovascular events in patients with premature atherothrombotic cerebrovascular disease. A prospective cohort study, *Neth. J. Med.*, 56, 146, 2000.
165. Hackam, D.G., Peterson, J.C., and Spence, J.D., What level of plasma hmocyst(e)ine should be treated? Effects of vitamin therapy on progression of carotid atherosclerosis in patients with homocyst(e)ine levels above and below 14 μmol/L, *Am. J. Hyperten.*, 13, 105–110, 2000.
166. Lange, H. et al., Folate therapy and in-stent restenosis after coronary stenting, *N. Engl. J. Med.*, 350, 2673–2681, 2004.
167. Vermeulen, E.G.J. et al., Effect of homocysteine-lowering treatment with folic acid plus vitamin B_6 on progression of subclinical atherosclerosis: a randomised, placebo-controlled trial, *Lancet*, 355, 517–522, 2000.
168. Schnyder, G. et al., Effect of homocysteine-lowering therapy with folic acid, vitamin B_{12}, and vitamin B_6 on clinical outcome after percutaneous coronary intervention. The Swiss Heart Study: a randomized controlled trial, *JAMA*, 288, 973–979, 2002.
169. Bostom, A.G. and Garber, C., Endpoints for homocysteine-lowering trials, *Lancet*, 355, 511–512, 2000.
170. Verhaar, M.C. et al., 5-methyltetrahydrofolate, the active form of folic acid, restores endothelial function in familial hypercholesterolemia,. *Circulation*, 97, 237–241, 1998.
171. Stroes, E.S. et al., Folic acid reverts dysfunction of endothelial nitric oxide synthase, *Circ. Res.*, 86, 1129–1134, 2000.
172. Clarke, R. and Collins, R., Can dietary supplements with folic acid or vitamin B_6 reduce cardiovascular risk? Design of clinical trials to test the homocysteine hypothesis of vascular disease, *J. Cardiovasc. Risk*, 5, 249–255, 1998.
173. Clarke, R. and Armitage, J., Vitamin supplements and cardiovascular risk: review of the randomized trials of homocysteine-lowering vitamin supplements, *Semin. Thromb. Haemost.*, 26, 341–348, 2000.
174. Kelly, P. et al., Unmetabolized folic acid in serum: acute studies in subjects consuming fortified food and supplements, *Am. J. Clin. Nutr.*, 65, 1790–1795, 1997.
175. Galan, P. et al., Background and rationale of the SU.FOL.OM3 study: double-blind randomized placebo-controlled secondary prevention trial to test the impact of supplementation with folate, vitamin B_6 and B_{12} and/or omega-3 fatty acids on the prevention of recurrent ischemic events in subjects with atherosclerosis in the coronary or cerebral arteries, *J. Nutr. Health Aging*, 7, 428–35, 2003.
176. Toole, J.F. et al., Lowering homocysteine in patients with ischemic stroke to prevent recurrent stroke, myocardial infarction, and death, *JAMA*, 291, 565–575, 2004.
177. Baker, F., Picton, D., and Blackwood, S., Blinded comparison of folic acid and placebo in patients with ischemic heart disease: an outcome trial, *Circulation*, 106, A3642, 2002.

178. Bostom, A.G. et al., Power shortage: clinical trials testing the "homocysteine hypothesis" against a background of folic acid-fortified cereal grain flour, *Ann. Intern. Med.*, 135, 133–137, 2001.
179. Robinson, K. et al., Low circulating folate and vitamin B_6 concentrations. Risk factors for stroke, peripheral vascular disease, and coronary artery disease, *Circulation*, 97, 437–443, 1998.
180. Brattstrom, L. et al., Impaired homocysteine metabolism in early-onset cerebral and peripheral occlusive arterial disease. Effects of pyridoxine and folic acid treatment, *Atherosclerosis*, 81, 51–60, 1990.
181. Brouwer, I.A., Verhoef, P., and Urgert, R., Betaine supplementation and plasma homocysteine in healthy volunteers, *Arch. Intern. Med.*, 160, 2546–2547, 2000.
182. Mueller, J.F. and Iacono, J.M., Effect of desoxypyridoxine-induced vitamin B_6 deficiency on polyunsaturated fatty acid metabolism in human beings, *Am. J. Clin. Nutr.*, 12, 358–367, 1963.
183. de Bree A. et al., Evidence for a protective (synergistic?) effect of B-vitamins and omega-3 fatty acids on cardiovacular diseases, *Eur. J. Clin. Nutr.*, 58, 732–744, 2004.
184. Haglund, O. et al., Effects of fish oil supplemented with pyridoxine and folic acid on triglycerides, glucose, homocysteine and fibrinolysis in man, *Nutr. Res.*, 13, 1351–1365, 1993.
185. Woodside, J.V. et al., Effect of B-group vitamins and antioxidant vitamins on hyperhomocysteinemia: a double-blind, randomized, factorial-design, controlled trial, *Am. J. Clin. Nutr.*, 67, 858–866, 1998.
186. Cafolla, A. et al., Effect of folic acid and vitamin C supplementation on folate status and homocysteine level: a randomised controlled trial in Italian smoker-blood donors, *Atherosclerosis*, 163, 105–111, 2002.
187. O'Connor, D.L., Interaction of iron and folate during reproduction, *Prog. Food Nutr. Sci.*, 15, 231–254, 1991.
188. Suh, J.R., Herbig, A.K., and Stover, P.J., New perspectives on folate catabolism, *Annu. Rev. Nutr.*, 21, 255–282, 2001.
189. Halsted, C.H., Alcohol and folate interaction: clinical implication, in *Folate in Health and Disease*, Bailey, L.B, Ed., New York, NY: Marcel Dekker, New York, 1995, pp. 313–328.
190. Jiang, R. et al., Joint association of alcohol and folate intake with risk of major chronic disease in women, *Am. J. Epidemiol.*, 158, 760–771, 2003.
191. Mennen, L., High alcohol and low folate intake increases risk of major chronic disease in women, *Evidence-based Healthcare*, 8, 71–73, 2004.
192. Basu, T.K. and Mann, S., Vitamin B-6 normalizes the altered sulfur amino acid status of rats fed diets containing pharmacological levels of niacin without reducing niacin's hypolipidemic effects, *J. Nutr.*, 127, 117–121, 1997.
193. Dierkes, J., Westphal, S., and Luley, C., Serum homocysteine increases after therapy with fenofibrate or bezafibrate, *Lancet*, 354, 219–220, 1999.
194. Westphal, S., Dierkes, J., and Luley, C., Effects of fenofibrate and gemfibrozil on plasma homocysteine, *Lancet*, 358, 39–40, 2001.
195. Dierkes, J. et al., Vitamin supplementation can markedly reduce the homocysteine elevation induced by fenofibrate, *Atherosclerosis*, 158, 161–164, 2001.
196. Stulc, T. et al., Folate supplementation prevents plasma homocysteine increase after fenofibrate therapy, *Nutrition*, 17, 721–723, 2001.

197. Dierkes, J., Westphal, S., and Luley, C., The effect of fibrates and other lipid-lowering drugs on plasma homocysteine levels, *Expert. Opin. Drug Safety,* 3, 101–111, 2004.
198. MacMahon, M. et al., A pilot study with simvastatin and folic acid/vitamin B_{12} in preparation for the Study of the Effectiveness of Additional Reductions in Cholesterol and Homocysteine (SEARCH), *Nutr. Metab. Cardiovasc. Dis.,* 10, 195–203, 2000.
199. Blom, H.J., Diseases and drugs associated with hyperhomocysteinemia, in *Homocysteine in Health and Disease,* Carmel, R. and Jacobsen, D.W., Eds., Cambridge University Press, London, 2001, pp. 331–340.
200. Mijatovic, V. and van der Mooren, M.J., Homocysteine in postmenopausal women and the importance of hormone replacement therapy, *Clin. Chem. Lab. Med.,* 39, 764–767, 2001.
201. Whitmer, R.A. et al., Hormone replacement therapy and cognitive performance: the role of homocysteine, *J. Gerontol. A Biol. Sci. Med. Sci.,* 58, 324–330, 2003.
202. Smolders, R.G. et al., A randomized placebo-controlled study of the effect of transdermal vs. oral estradiol with or without gestodene on homocysteine levels. *Fertil. Steril.,* 79, 261–267, 2003.
203. Cattaneo, M. et al., Tamoxifen reduces plasma homocysteine levels in healthy women, *Br. J. Cancer,* 77, 2264–2266, 1998.
204. Anker, G. et al., Plasma levels of the atherogenic amino acid homocysteine in post-menopausal women with breast cancer treated with tamoxifen, *Int. J. Cancer,* 60, 365–368, 1995.
205. Walsh, B.W. et al., The effects of hormone replacement therapy and raloxifene on C-reactive protein and homocysteine in healthy postmenopausal women: a randomized, controlled trial, *J. Clin. Endocrinol. Metab.,* 85, 214–218, 2000.
206. Mijatovic, V. et al., Randomized, double-blind, placebo-controlled study of the effects of raloxifene and conjugated equine estrogen on plasma homocysteine levels in healthy postmenopausal women, *Fertil. Steril.,* 70, 1085–1089, 1998.
207. Savage, D.G. and Lindenbaum, J., Folate-cobalamin interactions, in *Folate in Health and Disease,* Bailey, L.B., Ed., Marcel Dekker, New York, 1995, pp. 237–285.
208. Mills, J.L. et al., Low vitamin B-12 concentrations in patients without anemia: the effect of folic acid fortification of grain, *Am. J. Clin. Nutr.,* 77, 1474–1477, 2003.
209. Parry, G.J. and Bredesen, D.E., Sensory neuropathy with low-dose pyridoxine, *Neurology,* 35, 1466–1468, 1985.
210. Albin, R.L. et al., Acute sensory neuropathy-neuronopathy from pyridoxine overdose, *Neurology,* 37, 1729–1732, 1987.
211. Bernstein, A.L., Vitamin B_6 in clinical neurology, *Ann. N. Y. Acad. Sci.,* 585, 250–260, 1990.
212. Forsyth, J.C. et al., Hydroxocobalamin as a cyanide antidote: safety, efficacy and pharmacokinetics in heavily smoking normal volunteers, *J. Toxicol. Clin. Toxicol.,* 31, 277–294, 1993.
213. Nyholm, E. et al., Oral vitamin B_{12} can change our practice. *Postgrad Med J,* 79, 218–20, 2003.
214. Lambie, D.G. and Johnson, R.H., Drugs and folate metabolism, *Drugs,* 30, 145–155, 1985.
215. Refsum, H., and Ueland, P.M., Clinical significance of pharmacological modulation of homocysteine metabolism, *Trends Pharmacol. Sci.,* 11, 411–416, 1990.

216. Haagsma, C.J. et al., Influence of sulphasalazine, methotrexate and the combination of both on plasma homocsyteine concentrations in patients with rheumatoid arthritis, *Ann. Rheum. Dis.*, 58, 79–84, 1999.
217. Yeromenko, Y., Lavie, L., and Levy, Y., Homocysteine and cardiovascular risk in patients with diabetes mellitus, *Nutr. Metab. Cardiovasc. Dis.*, 11, 108–116, 2001.
218. Blandini, F. et al., Plasma homocysteine and l-dopa metabolism in patients with Parkinson disease, *Clin. Chem.*, 47, 1102–1104, 2001.
219. Schneede, J., Refsum, H., and Ueland, P.M., Biological and environmental determinants of plasma homocysteine, *Semin. Thromb. Haemost.*, 26, 263–279, 2000.
220. Seligmann, H. et al., Phenytoin-folic acid interaction: a lesson to be learned, *Clin. Neuropharmacol.*, 22, 268–272, 1999.
221. Lewis, D.P. et al., Phenytoin-folic acid interaction, *Ann. Pharmacother.*, 29, 726–735, 1995.

6

Food Synergy in Dietary Patterns and Risk for Chronic Diseases

Rob M. van Dam

CONTENTS

6.1 Introduction

6.1.1 Why Are Dietary Patterns of Interest?

Until recently, studies that examined the relation between diet and risk for chronic diseases have predominantly focused on individual nutrients. However, it is unlikely that the effect of diet on health is fully represented by this approach. Additives, contaminants, and unknown compounds, as well as the physical properties of foods may also play a role. Moreover, synergy or antagonism between food components can be highly relevant when determining the effects of diet on chronic disease risk. For example, the high vitamin E content of vegetable oils may modify the effect of the polyunsaturated fatty acids in these oils on arteriosclerosis.[1] High intake of polyunsaturated fatty acids increases the susceptibility of low density lipoprotein (LDL) particles to oxidation. Oxidized LDL may contribute to arteriosclerosis. However, the intake of polyunsaturated fatty acids has been shown to decrease risk for coronary heart disease. Possibly, the high vitamin E content of vegetable oils can prevent oxidation of the fatty acids. In addition to different components of a food, synergy or antagonism may also exist for components of different foods and drinks that are included in the dietary pattern of an individual. For example, alcohol from alcoholic beverages may affect the health effects of folate from vegetables or grain products. Alcohol can reduce intestinal folate uptake, interfere with folate metabolism, and increase urinary folate loss.[2] In a study among U.S. women, low folate intake was associated with a substantially increased risk for major chronic disease among women with high alcohol intake but not among alcohol abstainers.[2] Synergy and antagonism is likely to exist for multiple known and unknown food components from different foods and drinks consumed by an individual. As a result, health effects of overall dietary patterns may be different than predicted from the study of individual food components. Hence, the study of overall dietary patterns in relation to chronic disease risk can be an important complementary approach to the study of individual food components.

6.1.2 How Can Dietary Patterns Be Studied?

Different methodologies have been used to study dietary patterns. Two main approaches can be distinguished.[3] First, an exploratory approach that identifies combinations of foods and drinks as they are consumed in reality in a particular population. Second, a hypothesis-oriented, *a priori* approach that uses predefined criteria for dietary patterns based on prior knowledge of health effects.

6.1.2.1 Exploratory Approach

For the exploratory approach, principal components analysis (commonly referred to as "factor analysis") has frequently been used to identify dietary patterns. This data reduction technique constructs a limited number of new variables ("factors") based on the correlation matrix of the original variables. The factors are linear combinations of the original variables, explaining as much of the variation in the original variables as possible. For the analysis of dietary patterns, factor analysis is applied to a set of food variables. Factor analysis can then derive factors that reflect combinations of the original food variables, maximally explaining the variation in the original food variables. Based on the factor loadings of the food variables, dietary pattern scores can be calculated that reflect the degree to which a person's diet conforms to a dietary pattern. The use of factor analysis to derive dietary pattern scores requires several arbitrary choices such as the original variables to include and the number of dietary patterns to identify.[4] However, the obtained dietary patterns seem to be robust for different options.[5] In a study in U.S. men, reproducibility,[6] tracking over a period of 8 years,[5] and validity for dietary patterns based on information from food frequency questionnaires as compared with diet records were satisfactory.[6] Cluster analysis is a similar data reduction technique that has also been used to identify dietary patterns.[7] A difference with factor analysis is that cluster analysis does not result in scores for different patterns for each person, but categorizes persons into one dietary pattern cluster.

The explanatory approach is based on the combinations of foods as they are consumed in reality in a particular population. This can have both advantages and disadvantages. A potential disadvantage is that the dietary patterns that are identified are not necessarily relevant for disease risk because they are based on dietary behavior and not on known health effects. In addition, the derived dietary patterns are specific for a study population, which may limit possibilities to replicate findings. However, one could use the same pattern score calculation in other populations, instead of generating a new population-specific pattern variable. An advantage of the study of existing food combinations is that it may provide insight into possibilities for dietary changes and can be used for setting priorities for changing dietary patterns in a population by public health action.

6.1.2.2 Hypothesis-Oriented Approach

For the hypothesis-orientated approach, a dietary score can be constructed to reflect the degree to which a person's diet conforms with a dietary pattern that was defined *a priori* based on presumed health effects. For example, scores based on dietary recommendations and characteristics of the traditional Mediterranean diet have been used. Deciding the weight of different components of an *a priori* score still requires arbitrary choices. This approach does not have the advantages of studying existing dietary behavior but can capture the greater effects of the overall diet as compared with individual components, and it can be used to test the validity of dietary recommendations.

In observational studies of individual dietary components, confounding by other dietary variables and the inability to disentangle effects of highly correlated dietary variables can complicate the interpretation of the findings. An advantage of both exploratory and hypothesis-oriented dietary patterns is that potential dietary confounders are largely incorporated in the dietary pattern score.

6.2 Evidence for Health Benefits of Various Dietary Patterns

6.2.1 Mediterranean Dietary Pattern

The first studies on the health effects of the "Mediterranean diet" were based on the traditional dietary pattern found in olive-growing areas of Crete,

Greece, and southern Italy in the late 1950s and early 1960s.[8] This diet was characterized by a high consumption of legumes, grains, fruit, and vegetables, a moderate alcohol intake, a low to moderate consumption of meats and dairy products, and the use of olive oil for salad dressings and for cooking.[8] Interest in this Mediterranean diet has been stimulated by the observation that incidence of coronary heart disease was low in Mediterranean countries as compared with northern European countries and the United States.[8] The association between adherence to a traditional Mediterranean diet and mortality was examined in a population-based cohort study in Greece.[9] A 10-point Mediterranean diet score was used, with higher scores indicating greater adherence to a traditional Mediterranean diet. The components that comprised this diet score are shown in Table 6.1. For presumably beneficial components, those whose consumption was at or above the median (or within a predefined range for alcohol) were assigned a value of 1, the others were assigned a value of 0. For components presumed to be detrimental, persons with consumption below the median were assigned the value 1 and others the value of 0. The used Mediterranean diet score was the sum of the values for these components. Greater adherence to the Mediterranean diet was associated with lower all-cause mortality (adjusted rate ratio for a 2-point increment in the diet score, 0.75, 95% confidence interval 0.67 to 0.87) during a median of 44 months of follow-up. The Mediterranean diet score was also inversely associated with coronary heart disease and cancer mortality. Associations for the individual components included in the score were weaker, suggesting that synergy of different aspects of the Mediterranean diet may contribute to reduced premature mortality. Data from prospective studies of the Mediterranean diet and incidence of coronary heart disease (not only mortality) have not been published.

Two randomized intervention studies have examined the effect of diets with "Mediterranean" characteristics on cardiovascular disease. The Lyon Diet Heart Study was a randomized intervention study testing the effect of a Mediterranean diet on the recurrence of cardiovascular disease after a first myocardial infarction.[10] The experimental diet was rich in fruit, vegetables, bread, and fish, and low in red meat. In addition, it included a margarine high in α-linolenic acid. The recurrence of cardiovascular disease was substantially lower for the group that followed the experimental diet as compared with those that followed a prudent Western type diet after a mean of 46 months of follow-up. In the second trial, effects of an "Indo-Mediterranean diet" on progression of coronary heart disease was tested in Indian patients with angina pectoris, myocardial infarction, or other biological risk factors for coronary heart disease.[11] The experimental diet included more fruits, vegetables, legumes, walnuts, almonds, whole grains, and mustard or soybean oil (oils high in α-linolenic acid) than the control diet. The experimental diet was associated with substantially fewer cases of myocardial infarction or sudden cardiac death (rate ratio 0.50, 95% confidence interval 0.34 to 0.73), as compared with a prudent control diet over 2 years of follow-up. Although the experimental diets of the two intervention studies had several charac-

TABLE 6.1

Characteristics of Dietary Patterns That Have Been Studied in Relation to Risk for Chronic Diseases

Mediterranean[a]	Prudent[b]	DASH[c]	Healthy Diet Indicator[d]	Healthy Eating Index[e]	Alternate Healthy Eating Index[f]
Vegetables (high)	Vegetables(high)	Vegetables(high)	Fruit and vegetables (> 400 g/d)	Vegetables (high)	Vegetables (high)
Legumes (high)	Fruit (high)	Fruit (high)	Nuts, seeds, legumes (> 30 g)	Fruit (high)	Fruit (high)
Fruit and nuts (high)	Fish (high)	Low-fat dairy (high)	Saturated fat (0–10 en%)	Grains (high)	Nuts, soy products (high)
Cereal(high)	Poultry (high)	Whole grains (high)	Polyunsaturated fat (3–7 en%)	Milk (high)	Ratio of white to red meat (high)
Fish (high)	Whole grains (high)	Poultry (high)	Cholesterol (0–300 mg/d)	Meat (high)	Cereal fiber (high)
Red meat (low)		Fish (high)	Protein (10–15 en%)	Total fat (30 en%)	*trans*-fat (low)
Poultry (low)		Nuts, seeds, legumes (high)	Complex carbohydrates (50–70 en%)	Saturated fat (<10 en%)	P:S ratio (high)
Dairy products (low)		Red meat (low)	Mono-and disaccharides (0–10 en%)	Cholesterol (<300 mg/d)	Multivitamin use (≥ 5 yr)
Alcohol (men 10–50 g, women 5–25 g)		Sweets (low)	Fiber (27–40 g/d)	Sodium (<2400 mg/d)	Alcohol(men 1.5–2.5, women 0.5–1.5 units/d)
M:S ratio (high)		High sugar beverages (low)		Variety (high no. different foods)	

En% denotes percentage of total energy intake, M:S ratio denotes the ratio of monounsaturated fatty acids to saturated fatty acids, P:S ratio denotes the ratio of polyunsaturated fatty acids to saturated fatty acids

[a]Trichopoulou, A. et al., *N. Engl. J. Med.*, 348, 2599–2608, 2003.
[b]Hu, F.B. et al., *Am. J. Clin. Nutr.*, 72, 912–921, 2000.
[c]Sacks, F.M. et al., *N. Engl. J. Med.*, 344, 3–10, 2001.
[d]Huijbregts, P. et al., *Brit. Med. J.*, 315, 13–17, 1997.
[e]McCullough, M.L. et al., *Am. J. Clin. Nutr.*, 72, 1214-1222, 2000.
[f]McCullough, M.L. et al., *Am. J. Clin. Nutr.*, 76, 1261-1271, 2002.

teristics of the traditional Mediterranean diet, they were also high in α-linolenic acid and had a lower content of olive oil and monounsaturated fat. These intervention studies indicate that changes of overall dietary patterns can have major effects on the secondary prevention of coronary heart disease.

In addition to the traditional Mediterranean diet, traditional Asian, South American, and vegetarian dietary patterns may also have desirable aspects with regard to prevention of chronic disease.

6.2.2 Major Dietary Patterns in Western Countries

Factor analysis has been used successfully to identify interpretable dietary patterns in Western populations. As described previously, this method yields dietary pattern scores that reflect the combinations of foods as they are consumed in reality. In U.S. studies, a "Western" and a "prudent" dietary pattern were identified in diverse populations.[6,12,13] The prudent pattern was characterized by higher consumption of vegetables, fruit, fish, poultry, and whole grains. The Western pattern was characterized by a higher consumption of red meat, processed meat, french fries, high-fat dairy, refined grains, and sweets and desserts. Higher scores for the prudent dietary pattern were associated with a lower risk for coronary heart disease.[14,15] Higher scores for the Western dietary pattern were associated with a substantially higher risk for coronary heart disease,[14,15] colon cancer,[12,13] and type 2 diabetes.[5] These associations were independent of body mass index, physical activity, cigarette smoking, and other potential confounders. In the study of type 2 diabetes, associations with foods that characterized the Western dietary pattern (red meat, processed meat, refined grains, high-fat dairy) were also examined in relation to type 2 diabetes.[5] Associations for the Western dietary pattern score were stronger than for these individual food groups. In a subsample of a study in male U.S. health professionals, a higher Western pattern score was associated with higher blood concentrations of insulin, C-peptide, and homocysteine, and lower concentrations of folate.[16] A higher prudent pattern score was associated with higher folate concentrations, and lower insulin and homocysteine concentrations. In other populations, the identified dietary patterns were different. In a Dutch[17] and United Kingdom (U.K.) study,[18] four types of dietary patterns were observed: traditional, convenience, refined foods, and cosmopolitan. The traditional and convenience dietary patterns had characteristics of the Western dietary pattern observed in the U.S. studies, and the cosmopolitan dietary pattern had characteristics of the prudent dietary pattern. In the Dutch study, the cosmopolitan pattern was characterized by higher intakes of fried vegetables, salad, rice, chicken, fish, and wine, the traditional pattern by higher intakes of red meat and potatoes, and lower intakes of low-fat dairy and fruit, and the refined foods pattern by higher intakes of french fries, high-sugar beverages, and white bread, and lower intakes of whole grain bread and boiled vegetables.[17] Independent of other lifestyle factors and body mass index, the cosmopolitan pattern score was significantly associated with lower blood pressure and higher high density lipoprotein (HDL) cholesterol, and the traditional pattern score with higher blood pressure and higher HDL cholesterol, total cholesterol, and glucose concentrations. The refined foods pattern score was associated with a higher total cholesterol concentration. Thus, findings on dietary patterns and biological risk factors were consistent with the associations observed with risk for type 2 diabetes and coronary heart disease.

6.2.3 Dietary Approaches to Stop Hypertension

Vegetarians tend to have a lower blood pressure than nonvegetarians, and a vegetarian diet lowered blood pressure in trials.[19] It has been suggested that the blood pressure lowering effect of these vegetarian diets may have been due to the higher level of fiber, potassium, or magnesium, or the lower fat content. However, in trials that tested the effect of these dietary components individually, effects on blood pressure have generally been small and inconsistent.[19] A possible explanation is that the blood pressure lowering effects of vegetarian diets were due to other components. Alternatively, the effect of individual components of diet may have been too small to detect in these trials, whereas the cumulative effect may be sufficient for detection. In addition, synergy between different dietary components may result in stronger effect on blood pressure. The Dietary Approaches to Stop Hypertension (DASH) trial was an 8-week randomized feeding study in 459 adults that tested the effects of changing the overall dietary pattern on blood pressure.[19] The DASH diet was characterized by high intakes of fruits, vegetables, and low fat dairy products. It further includes whole grains, poultry, fish, and nuts, and only small amounts of red meat, sweets, and sugar-containing beverages. The diet on average included more than nine servings of fruits and vegetables per day. In persons with hypertension, the DASH diet reduced systolic and diastolic blood pressure by 11.4 and 5.5 mm Hg, respectively, more than the control diet. In persons without hypertension, the corresponding reductions were 3.5 mm Hg and 2.1 mm Hg.[19] The blood pressure reduction in participants with hypertension is similar in magnitude to that observed in trials of drug monotherapy for mild hypertension. The effect of a combination of the DASH diet and a reduced sodium intake has also been tested, and effects were greater than for either intervention alone.[20] The combined effect was not as great as would be estimated on the basis of additivity, perhaps because the effects of high potassium or magnesium intake in the DASH diet attenuated the effects of low sodium intakes. With regard to blood lipids, the DASH diet lowered the total and LDL cholesterol concentration, but also lowered HDL cholesterol.[21] Effects on the total to HDL cholesterol ratio were neutral. In summary, these studies showed that in addition to weight loss, increased physical activity and reducing sodium intake, changing the dietary pattern, i.e., adopting the DASH diet, can lower blood pressure substantially. However, long-term adherence to the DASH diet may be difficult because it is so different from the current eating patterns in most Western populations.

6.2.4 Dietary Recommendations

Several studies have used dietary pattern scores to examine the relation between adherence to dietary recommendations and risk for chronic diseases[22–24] or premature mortality.[25,26] The World Health Organization's guidelines for the prevention of chronic diseases were used to calculate a healthy diet indicator in five cohorts of men aged 50 to 70 years at baseline in Finland, the Netherlands, and Italy.[26] The criteria for the components of the healthy diet indicator are shown in Table 6.1. For each intake in the recommended range, a person received 1 point, resulting in a sum score of 0 to 9 points. The relative risk for mortality over 20 years of follow up was 0.87 (95%, CI 0.77 to 0.98) for the highest tertile of the healthy diet indicator as compared with the lowest tertile after adjustment for age, smoking, and alcohol consumption.

Kant et al. examined the association between diet quality and mortality in U.S. women with a mean age of 61 years.[25] Diet quality was quantified by a Recommended Food Score (RFS): the sum of the number of foods that are generally recommended by guidelines (fruits, vegetables, whole grains, low-fat dairy, and lean meats and poultry). The relative risk of mortality during 5.6 years of follow-up was 0.69 (95% CI 0.61 to 0.78) for the highest as compared with the lowest quintile after adjustment for potential confounders. A significant reduction in risk was also observed for mortality due to cancer, coronary heart disease, and stroke.

The association between three indicators of adherence to dietary guidelines and risk for major chronic disease during 8 to 12 years of follow-up was examined in U.S. cohorts of female nurses and male health professionals.[22–24] Major chronic disease was defined as stroke, myocardial infarction, or non-traumatic death. The examined indicators were the RFS (see above), the healthy eating index (HEI), and the Alternate Healthy Eating Index (AHEI). The HEI measures adherence to the major recommendations of the Dietary Guidelines for Americans and the food guide pyramid (see Table 6.1).[24] The AHEI is an index developed by Harvard researchers (see Table 6.1).[22] In women, the multivariate-adjusted relative risk for major chronic disease for the highest as compared with the lowest quartile was 0.98 (95% CI 0.90 to 1.06) for the RFS, 0.97 (95% CI 0.89 to 1.06) for the HEI, and 0.89 (0.82 to 0.96) for the AHEI. In men, the multivariate-adjusted relative risk for major chronic disease for the highest as compared with the lowest quartile was 0.93 (95% CI 0.83 to 1.04) for the RFS, 0.89 (95% CI 0.79 to 1.00) for the HEI, and 0.80 (0.71 to 0.91) for the AHEI.[23] Inverse associations with risk for major cardiovascular disease were stronger (relative risk of 0.61 for women and 0.72 for men for the highest versus the lowest AHEI quintile), but none of the scores was substantially associated with risk for cancer. Some of the components of the AHEI were already known to predict chronic disease in these cohorts. Therefore, the observation of a stronger association for the AHEI as compared with the other indices should be confirmed in other populations. With regard to the RFS, the authors noted that it was heavily weighted toward fruit and vegetable consumption (75% of the recommended foods in their studies, 65% in the study by Kant et al.).[22] A larger weight for other aspects of the dietary pattern may result in better prediction of chronic diseases. In general, the inclusion of more specific dietary recommendations (for example, on specific vegetables instead of total vegetable consumption) may be necessary to better reflect the potential effect of dietary patterns on cancer incidence.

6.2.5 Other Approaches to Study Dietary Patterns

In addition to the type of foods and drinks consumed, meal frequency may also affect risk for chronic diseases. In a clinical trial, a diet consisting of 17 snacks per day significantly reduced LDL cholesterol and the mean insulin concentration as compared with an otherwise identical diet consisting of three meals per day.[27] Unfortunately, increasing meal frequency may increase caloric intake and induce weight gain if the size of the meals is not reduced sufficiently. The meal pattern is an aspect of dietary patterns that has not been considered in the discussed studies and may be worthwhile to include in future studies.

Another approach to dietary patterns is the use of indices that quantify specific metabolic effects of dietary patterns. The glycemic index of the diet reflects the effect of a person's diet on postprandial hyperglycemia. The glycemic index of a food is the glycemic response to ingestion of a fixed amount of available carbohydrate of that food as compared with the response to the same amount of available carbohydrate from a standard food consumed by the same subject.[28] To calculate the glycemic index of the total diet, one can multiply the proportion contribution of each individual food to carbohydrate intake by its glycemic index, and sum these values. It has been suggested that a lower glycemic index and the resulting attenuation of postprandial glycemic responses can have various beneficial health benefits, particularly improvement of glycemic control in persons with diabetes mellitus.[28] Although concerns have been raised about the methodology of the study of the dietary glycemic index in relation to risk for chronic diseases,[29] the approach of quantifying a specific metabolic effect of a dietary pattern is of interest.

6.3 Conclusions

Evidence from the studies discussed in this chapter indicates that changing dietary patterns can have substantial effects on risk for major chronic diseases. This evidence includes results from secondary prevention trials of cardiovascular diseases, intervention studies with blood pressure as an endpoint, cross-sectional studies of biomarkers of disease, and cohort studies of incidence of chronic diseases and mortality. For observational studies, the possibility that residual confounding or measurement error affected the strength of the observed associations should be considered. On the one hand, incomplete adjustment for confounders associated with dietary behavior and risk for chronic diseases may have resulted in stronger observed associations. On the other hand, nondifferential misclassification as a result of inevitable errors in the measurement of diet is likely to have attenuated the observed associations. For effects on cardiovascular diseases, however, the consistency between observational and experimental studies is reassuring. Generally, studies showed stronger effects for dietary patterns than for individual foods and nutrients. This may indicate that synergy between food components may indeed play an important role in the prevention of chronic diseases.

Although different approaches have been used to define dietary patterns, similarities are apparent. As shown in Table 6.1, dietary patterns that were considered beneficial were characterized by a high consumption of minimally processed plant foods such as vegetables, fruit, legumes, nuts, and whole grains. This is consistent with the hypothesis that balanced consumption of a wide array of plant components, including vitamins, nonvitamin antioxidants, minerals, phytoestrogens, plant enzymes and plant hormones may confer health benefits in humans.[30] The studied "beneficial" dietary patterns were also characterized by foods that contribute to appropriate intakes of fatty acids, for example low red meat consumption and regular fish consumption, providing long-chain n-3 fatty acids. In the secondary cardiovascular prevention trials,[10,11] sources of the n-3 fatty acid α-linolenic acid were also included in the experimental diet.

A dietary pattern approach can also be useful for health education and public health action. Data on the association between exploratory dietary patterns (which reflect the combinations of foods as they are used in reality) and disease risk in a population may help in prioritizing public health efforts. Furthermore, insight into patterns of food use may contribute to successful interventions because dietary changes may be more readily achieved if recommendations are compatible with existing patterns. Food based messages may be preferable for dietary advice to the public because people choose foods rather than nutrients. Traditional dietary patterns such as the traditional Mediterranean diet can be used as a model in these food based messages.[31] Adherence to dietary advice based on traditional dietary patterns may be better, because they combine health benefits with culinary attractiveness.

References

1. Zock, P.L. and Katan, M.B., Diet, LDL oxidation, and coronary artery disease, *Am. J. Clin. Nutr.*, 68, 759-60, 1998.
2. Jiang, R. et al., Joint association of alcohol and folate intake with risk of major chronic disease in women, *Am. J. Epidemiol.*, 158, 760-71, 2003.
3. Schulze, M.B. et al., Risk of hypertension among women in the EPIC-Potsdam Study: comparison of relative risk estimates for exploratory and hypothesis-oriented dietary patterns, *Am. J. Epidemiol.* 158, 365-73, 2003.
4. Martinez, M.E., Marshall, J.R., and Sechrest, L., Invited commentary: Factor analysis and the search for objectivity, *Am. J. Epidemiol.*, 148, 17-9, 1998.
5. van Dam, R.M. et al., Dietary patterns and risk for type 2 diabetes mellitus in U.S. men, *Ann. Intern. Med.*, 136, 201-9, 2002.
6. Hu, F.B. et al., Reproducibility and validity of dietary patterns assessed with a food- frequency questionnaire, *Am. J. Clin. Nutr.*, 69, 243-9, 1999.
7. Wirfalt, E. et al., Food patterns and components of the metabolic syndrome in men and women: a cross-sectional study within the Malmö Diet and Cancer cohort, *Am. J. Epidemiol.*, 154, 1150-9, 2001.
8. Martinez-Gonzalez, M.A. et al., The emerging role of Mediterranean diets in cardiovascular epidemiology: monounsaturated fats, olive oil, red wine or the whole pattern?, *Eur. J. Epidemiol.*, 19, 9-13, 2004.
9. Trichopoulou, A. et al., Adherence to a Mediterranean diet and survival in a Greek population, *N. Engl. J. Med.*, 348, 2599-608, 2003.
10. de Lorgeril, M. et al., Mediterranean diet, traditional risk factors, and the rate of cardiovascular complications after myocardial infarction: final report of the Lyon Diet Heart Study, *Circulation*, 99, 779-85, 1999.
11. Singh, R.B. et al., Effect of an Indo-Mediterranean diet on progression of coronary artery disease in high risk patients (Indo-Mediterranean Diet Heart Study): a randomised single-blind trial, *Lancet*, 360, 1455-61, 2002.
12. Fung, T. et al., Major dietary patterns and the risk of colorectal cancer in women. *Arch. Intern. Med.*, 163, 309-14, 2003.
13. Slattery, M.L. et al., Eating patterns and risk of colon cancer, *Am. J. Epidemiol.*, 148, 4-16, 1998.
14. Hu, F.B. et al., Prospective study of major dietary patterns and risk of coronary heart disease in men, *Am. J. Clin. Nutr.*, 72, 912-21, 2000.
15. Fung, T.T. et al., Dietary patterns and the risk of coronary heart disease in women, *Arch. Intern. Med.*, 161,1857-62, 2001.
16. Fung, T.T. et al., Association between dietary patterns and plasma biomarkers of obesity and cardiovascular disease risk, *Am. J. Clin. Nutr.*, 73, 61-7, 2001.
17. van Dam, R.M. et al., Patterns of food consumption and risk factors for cardiovascular disease in the general Dutch population, *Am. J. Clin. Nutr.*, 77, 1156-63, 2003.
18. Barker, M.E. et al., Dietary behaviour and health in Northern Ireland: an exploration of biochemical and haematological associations, *J. Epidemiol. Community Health*, 46, 151-6, 1992.
19. Appel, L.J. et al., A clinical trial of the effects of dietary patterns on blood pressure, DASH Collaborative Research Group, *N. Engl. J. Med.*, 336, 1117-24, 1997.

20. Sacks, F.M. et al., Effects on blood pressure of reduced dietary sodium and the Dietary Approaches to Stop Hypertension (DASH) diet, DASH-Sodium Collaborative Research Group, *N. Engl. J. Med.*, 344, 3-10, 2001.
21. Obarzanek, E. et al., Effects on blood lipids of a blood pressure-lowering diet: the Dietary Approaches to Stop Hypertension (DASH) Trial, *Am. J. Clin. Nutr.*, 74, 80-9, 2001.
22. McCullough, M.L. et al., Diet quality and major chronic disease risk in men and women: moving toward improved dietary guidance, *Am. J. Clin. Nutr.*, 76, 1261-71, 2002.
23. McCullough, M.L. et al., Adherence to the Dietary Guidelines for Americans and risk of major chronic disease in men, *Am. J. Clin. Nutr.*, 72, 1223-31, 2000.
24. McCullough, M.L. et al., Adherence to the Dietary Guidelines for Americans and risk of major chronic disease in women, *Am. J. Clin. Nutr.*, 72, 1214-22, 2000.
25. Kant, A.K. et al., A prospective study of diet quality and mortality in women, *JAMA*, 283, 2109-15, 2000.
26. Huijbregts, P. et al., Dietary pattern and 20 year mortality in elderly men in Finland, Italy, and The Netherlands: longitudinal cohort study, *BMJ*, 315, 13-7, 1997.
27. Jenkins, D.J. et al., Nibbling versus gorging: metabolic advantages of increased meal frequency, *N. Engl. J. Med.*, 321, 929-34, 1989.
28. Jenkins, D.J. et al., Glycemic index: overview of implications in health and disease, *Am. J. Clin. Nutr.*, 76, 266S-73S, 2002.
29. Pi-Sunyer, F.X., Glycemic index and disease, *Am. J. Clin. Nutr.*, 76, 290S-8S, 2002.
30. Jacobs, D.R. Jr. and Murtaugh, M.A., It's more than an apple a day: an appropriately processed, plant-centered dietary pattern may be good for your health, *Am. J. Clin. Nutr.*, 72, 899-900, 2000.
31. Truswell, A.S., Practical and realistic approaches to healthier diet modifications, *Am. J. Clin. Nutr.* 67, 583S-90S, 1998.

Section III

Cancer

7

Soy–Food and Soy–Drug Interactions in Prevention and Treatment of Cancer

Jin-Rong Zhou

CONTENTS

7.1 Introduction

Dietary modification has long been considered to be an effective regimen for cancer prevention. Epidemiological investigations have suggested that increased consumption of soy products is in part associated with reduced risks of certain types of cancer in Asian populations. Experimental studies have also shown that soybean contains bioactive components that may exert their anticancer activities in different stages of carcinogenesis processes.[1] Among soy bioactive components, the soy isoflavone genistein has been extensively studied for its anticancer activities.[1] Several mechanisms have been proposed for the antitumor activity of genistein, including agonist–antagonist effects on estrogen receptors,[2] stimulation of sex hormone binding globulin synthesis,[2] inhibition of growth factor–associated tyrosine kinase signal transduction,[3] antioxidation,[4] inhibition of DNA topoisomerase,[5,6] antiproliferation,[7] apoptosis induction,[7–9] and antiangiogenisis.[7,9,10] On the other hand, soy contains other bioactive anticancer components such as protease inhibitors, the Bowman-Birk inhibitor, inositol hexaphosphate (phytic acid), lignans, phytosterols, and saponins.[1,11]

It has been realized that cancer incidence and progression may not be reduced to the full extent possible by single agents, and even promising agents usually show significant toxicity at efficacious doses. Therefore the combination of multiple agents based on differences in the mechanisms of cancer inhibition, either by simultaneous or sequential administration, is expected to increase efficacy and/or reduce toxicity.[12] Besides studying the chemopreventive role of soy and its bioactive components, more scientists have focused on studying the role of soy bioactive components in combination with other dietary bioactive components or chemopreventive and chemotherapeutic drugs in cancer prevention and treatment, aiming to discover possible synergistic and/or additive combination regimens.

The objectives of this chapter are to provide an up-to-date review of available evidence on soy–food and soy–drug synergistic combinations, and cancer prevention and treatment, and to identify several critical issues in this research field so that the future research directions can be highlighted.

7.2 Interactive Effects between Soy and Food or Drug

Investigation of the role of soy products in cancer prevention has been one of the priorities in cancer prevention research. Previous research has indicated that soy contains several types of cancer-preventive components. In addition to research on the cancer preventive activities of soy food and individual soy components, some investigators have studied the combination effects of soy bioactive components and other food components as possible synergistic regimens for cancer prevention. Because drugs for cancer prevention and treatment are usually associated with side effects and toxicities at efficacious doses, the possible role of soy bioactive components in interactions with drugs to enhance their efficacy and/or reduce toxicity has been actively studied. In this section, we will provide a concise but critical review of the scientific data published on soy–food or soy–drug interactions and cancer prevention. The studies on soy–food interactions and soy–drug interactions in cancer prevention and treatment are summarized in Tables 7.1 and 7.2, respectively.

7.2.1 Soy and Food Components

7.2.1.1 Soy and Tea

The incidences of certain types of cancer, such as breast and prostate, are significantly higher in the U.S. population than that in the Asian population.[13–16] Epidemiological studies suggest that the differences may be due to environmental factors such as lifestyle and diet, since Asian people who adopt a Western lifestyle show increased cancer incidence.[17–22] Among dietary factors, increased consumption of soy or tea, especially green tea, has been shown to be in part associated with a reduced risk of breast or prostate cancer. Asian people consume soy products and drink tea regularly. It is thus possible that some bioactive components in soy and tea may interact to potentiate their anticancer activities. However, current epidemiological studies have tried to identify the association between individual dietary components and cancer risk, but evidence on soy and tea interactions and the risk of specific cancers is very limited. Similarly, a limited number of experimental studies have investigated the possible role of soy and tea combinations in cancer prevention.

We conducted experimental studies to evaluate the combined effects of soy and tea on the growth and progression of breast cancer and prostate cancer in appropriate *in vivo* model systems.[23,24] A mixture of soy phytochemicals (called soy phytochemical concentrate [SPC], representing the composition commonly consumed by humans), black tea, and green tea, were studied for their combination effects on tumor growth and/or metastasis. In the study of SPC–tea combinations and breast tumor growth,[24] we found that while SPC (0.1%), black tea (1.5% as tea infusion), and green tea (1.5% as tea infusion) alone inhibited the growth of breast tumor by 23% ($p > .05$), 26% ($p > .05$), and 56% ($p < .05$), respectively, the combination of SPC with either black tea or green tea synergistically reduced tumor growth by 54% ($p < .05$) and 72% ($p < .005$), respectively. Further, *in vivo* mechanistic studies indicated that the combined inhibitory effects on tumor angiogenesis and ER-α protein and blood IGF-I levels were in part responsible for the synergistic antitumor growth activities of SPC and tea.[24] In the study of SPC–tea combinations and prostate tumor growth,[23] we applied a clinically relevant

TABLE 7.1

Soy and Food Interactions in Cancer Prevention and Treatment

Study	Ref.	Soy components	Food components	Cancer type	Interactions
In Vitro Studies					
Kumi-Diaka et al.	42	Genistein	β-Lapachone	Prostate cancer cells	Synergistic inhibition of cell growth and proliferation
Nakagawa et al.	43	Genistein	Eicosapentaenoic acid (EPA)	Breast cancer cells (estrogen-dependent and independent)	Synergistic inhibition of cell growth
Rao et al.	32	Genistein	1,25-$(OH)_2D_3$	Prostate epithelial cells and prostate cancer cells	Synergistic inhibition of cell growth
Sakamoto et al.	25	Genistein	Thearubigin	Prostate cancer	Synergistic inhibition of cell growth
Shen et al	40	Genistein	Quercetin	Ovarian cancer cells	Synergistic inhibition of cell growth
Verma et al.	41	Genistein	Curcumin	Breast cancer cells (estrogen-dependent)	Synergistic inhibition of cell growth
Animal Studies					
Cross et al.	29	Soybean meal	Calcium	Mouse colonocytes	Soybean meal inhibited low calcium-induced colon cell proliferation
Zhou et al.	24	Soy phytochemical concentrate (SPC) (0.1%)	Black tea or green tea infusion (1.5%)	Estrogen-dependent MCF-7 breast tumor	Synergistic inhibition of tumor growth
Zhou et al.	23	SPC (0.5%)	Black tea or green tea infusion (1.5%)	Androgen-sensitive LNCaP prostate tumor	Synergistic inhibition of tumorigenicity, final tumor weight, and lymph node metastases (black tea) Synergistic reduction in final tumor weight and lymph node metastases (green tea)

Abbreviations: EPA, eicosapentaenoic acid; SPC, soy phytochemical concentrate.

TABLE 7.2

Soy and Drug Interactions in Cancer Prevention and Treatment

Study	Ref.	Soy components	Drugs	Cancer type	Interactions
In Vitro Studies					
Attalla et al.	91	Genistein	2,6-bis ((3,4-dihydroxyphenyl)-methylene) cyclohexanone (BDHPC)	Estrogen-dependent breast cancer	Synergistic inhibition of cell growth
Jones et al.	86	Genistein	TAM	Estrogen-dependent breast cancer	Genistein negated TAM effect
Ju et al.	85	Genistein	TAM	Estrogen-dependent breast cancer	Genistein negated TAM effect
Khoshyomn et al.	89	Genistein	Cisplatin	Medulloblastoma	Synergy on growth inhibition and cytotoxicity of medulloblastoma cells
Khoshyomn et al.	90	Genistein	1,3-bis (2-chloroethyl)-1-nitrosourea (BCNU)	Glioma	Synergy on growth inhibition and cytotoxicity of medulloblastoma cells
Li et al.	92	Genistein	Tiazofurin	Leukemia	Synergistic inhibition of leukemic cell growth
Li et al.	93	Genistein	Tiazofurin	Ovarian cancer	Synergistic inhibition of ovarian cancer cells growth
Monti et al.	44	Genistein	Adriamycin	Breast cancer	Synergistic inhibition of cancer cell growth
Park et al.	94	Genistein	Dexamethasone	Liver and colon cancers	Synergistic inhibition of hepatic and colon cancer cell growth
Shen et al.	83	Genistein	TAM	Estrogen-independent breast cancer cells	Synergistic cytotoxicity and inhibition of breast cancer cell proliferation
Tanos et al.	82	Genistein	TAM	Dysplastic, and breast cancer cells (estrogen-dependent and independent)	Synergistic inhibition of dysplastic breast cell growth Additive inhibition of breast cancer cell growth

TABLE 7.2 (Continued)

Soy and Drug Interactions in Cancer Prevention and Treatment

Study	Ref.	Soy components	Drugs	Cancer type	Interactions
Animal Studies					
Constantinou et al.	84	Soy protein isolate	TAM	DMBA-induced mammary tumor	Synergistic inhibition of the growth of DMBA-induced mammary tumors
Gotoh et al.	57	Miso	TAM	NMU-induced mammary tumor	Synergistic inhibition of mammary tumorigenesis.
Ju et al.	85	Genistein	TAM	MCF-7 breast tumor	Genistein negated TAM effect.
Wietrzyk et al.	95	Genistein	Cyclophosphamide	Melanoma and Lewis lung carcinoma	Synergistic inhibition of the growth and metastasis of melanoma and Lewis lung carcinoma
Zhou et al.	87	SPC	TAM	MCF-7/TAM-nonresponsive breast tumor	Synergistic inhibition of the growth of TAM-nonresponsive breast tumors
Zhou et al.	88	Genistein	TAM	MCF-7 breast cancer	Synergistic inhibition of the growth of estrogen-dependent breast tumors

Abbreviations: BCNU, 1,3-bis (2-chloroethyl)-1-nitrosourea; BDHPC, 2,6-bis ((3,4-dihydroxyphenyl)-methylene) cyclohexanone; DMBA, 7,12-dimethylbenz (a) anthracene; NMU: *N*-nitroso-*N*-methylurea; SPC, soy phytochemical concentrate.

orthotopic prostate tumor model and studied the combined effects between SPC and tea on tumorigenicity, tumor growth, and metastasis. We found that the combination of SPC and black tea synergistically inhibited prostate tumorigenicity, final tumor weight, and metastases to lymph nodes, and the combination of SPC and green tea synergistically inhibited final tumor weight and metastasis.[23]

Although it is still unknown which combinations of bioactive components in soy and tea are responsible for the synergistic effects, the interactions of soy isoflavones and tea polyphenols may in part be responsible. Indeed, the combination of black tea polyphenol thearubigin and soy isoflavone genistein synergistically inhibited growth of PC-3 human prostate cancer cells and induced PC-3 cell cycle at G2/M phase *in vitro*.[25] Our *in vivo* studies, together with other investigations, suggest that future research should focus on the combinations of soy and tea components as cancer chemopreventive regimens.[23,24]

7.2.1.2 Soy and Vitamin D

The chemopreventive role of vitamin D and analogs, especially 1,25-dihydroxyvitamin D_3 (1,25-$(OH)_2D_3$), in cancer prevention has been well studied.[26–29] Vitamin D acts through binding to the vitamin D receptor (VDR), which is a ligand activated transcriptional factor, and modulates expression of target genes. Both *in vitro* and *in vivo* animal studies have shown that 1,25-$(OH)_2D_3$ and/or its analogs inhibit proliferation, promote differentiation, and induce apoptosis in many cancer cells. Epidemiological investigations have shown that prostate cancer patients have lower blood levels of 1,25-$(OH)_2D_3$[30] and that a polymorphism of VDR is associated with an increased risk for prostate cancer development.[31]

The interactive effect between the soy isoflavone genistein and vitamin D has been studied primarily in *in vitro* systems. A combination of genistein and 1,25-$(OH)_2D_3$ synergistically inhibited the growth of prostate cancer cells *in vitro*.[32] Furthermore, *in vitro* mechanistic studies indicate that genistein may enhance vitamin D activity in cancer cells through multiple mechanisms. The first synergistic mechanism may be related to the role of genistein in increasing intracellular vitamin D levels by increasing vitamin D synthesis and/or reducing vitamin D catabolism. The availability of 1,25-$(OH)_2D_3$ is determined through the activity of the two enzymes, 25-hydroxyvitamin D-24-hydroxylase (CYP24) and 25-hydroxyvitamin D-1α-hydroxylase (CYP27B1), which are responsible for catabolism and synthesis of 1,25-$(OH)_2D_3$, respectively. These enzymes were present not only in kidney, but also in mammary cells, prostate cells, and colonocytes.[29] In human cancer cells, CYP24 expression was enhanced and/or CYP27B1 expression was reduced, resulting in lower intracellular vitamin D_3 levels. Genistein inhibited the expression of CYP24 and/or increased expression of CYP27B1 in prostate cancer cells,[29,33–36] breast cancer cells,[29] and colon cancer cells *in vitro*.[29,37] The effect of genistein on vitamin D metabolizing enzyme activity was also confirmed *in vivo*. Mice supplemented with genistein or soy food had elevated CYP27B1 and decreased CYP24 expression in the colon, and inhibited low-calcium-induced proliferation of colonocytes.[29] It is thus suggested that an observed inverse correlation of soy product consumption with colon tumor incidence may be consequent to enhanced colonic synthesis of vitamin D by soy bioactive components.[38] The second synergistic mechanism may be related to up-regulation of the vitamin D receptor by the soy isoflavone genistein. Genistein up-regulated expression of the vitamin D receptor in prostate cancer cells[29,39] and in colon cancer cells.[37]

This finding of a synergistic anticancer effect between genistein and vitamin D, although preliminary and not confirmed *in vivo*, may have significant impact on vitamin D application to cancer prevention. Though $1{,}25(OH)_2D_3$ has an antimitotic as well as a differentiating action, therapeutic application in tumor patients is still precluded because of their hypercalcemic action at the necessary concentrations. Supplementation of soy bioactive components may improve antitumor activity of vitamin D by enhancing intracellular active vitamin D levels without increasing systematic level of vitamin D. However, this synergistic combination needs to be confirmed in proper animal models before any clinical application can be considered.

7.2.1.3 Soy and Other Food Components

Some studies also investigated the interactive effects between soy and other dietary bioactives on cancer prevention. Genistein was used in most studies as a major bioactive component of soy, and most studies were conducted *in vitro*. It is hypothesized that the combination of different agents that target cancer cells with different mechanisms would be more effective than any single treatment alone. Genistein has been shown to alter cell cycle progression by G2/M arrest and induces apoptosis in most cancer cells *in vitro*. The combination of genistein with quercetin, a dietary flavonoid and an anticancer agent that arrests cells at G1 phase, synergistically inhibited the growth of ovarian carcinoma cells *in vitro*, suggesting that the synergistic action of quercetin and genistein may be of interest in clinical treatment of human ovarian carcinoma.[40] Curcumin is a bioactive component from turmeric and curry and is one of the promising chemopreventive agents. The combination of curcumin and genistein synergistically inhibited the estrogen-induced growth of estrogen-dependent MCF-7 human breast cancer cells *in vitro*, suggesting that the combination of curcumin and genistein in the diet may have the potential to reduce the proliferation of estrogen-positive cells.[41] β-Lapachone (3,4-dihydro-2,2-dimethyl-2H-naphto[1,2-β]pyran-5,6-dione) is a natural phytochemical in the lapacho tree. It is a topoisomerase I inhibitor, and an inductor of apoptosis. β-Lapchone acts at the G1/S phase checkpoint in the cell cycle. The combination of genistein and β-lapachone had a synergistic inhibitory effect on growth and proliferation in both androgen-sensitive and androgen-independent human prostate cancer cells *in vitro*.[42] Genistein and the long chain n-3 fatty acid eicosapentaenoic acid (EPA) synergistically inhibited the growth of both estrogen-dependent MCF-7 and estrogen-independent MDA-MB-231 human breast cancer cells *in vitro*, suggesting that dietary intake of soy product or genistein in combination with EPA may be beneficial for breast cancer control.[43]

Results from these *in vitro* studies suggest that because they target different mechanisms of action the combinations of soy bioactive components such as genistein with other dietary or natural bioactive components may have synergistic effects on cancer inhibition. However, these *in vitro* synergies and the proposed mechanisms of synergistic actions have not been verified in *in vivo* experiments.

7.2.2 Soy and Drugs

Use of chemopreventive and chemotherapeutic drugs is usually associated with limited efficacy and/or unacceptable toxicity. Therefore, the combination of a drug with other agents is considered to be a more effective approach to enhance the efficacy and/or reduce toxicity of drug. The investigation of possible interactions between soy components and chemopreventive and/or therapeutic drugs has become an important research field. In this section, scientific evidence on interactive effects between soy and tamoxifen (TAM), cisplatin or other drugs used for cancer prevention and treatment is reviewed.

7.2.2.1 Soy and TAM Interactions in Breast Cancer Prevention and Treatment

The effect of soy bioactives, especially genistein, on breast cancer has been extensively studied *in vitro* and *in vivo*, and the results are controversial. Most *in vitro*[24,44–54] and animal studies[24,55–66] showed that soy components or genistein had antibreast cancer activities. On the other hand, some studies showed that genistein had biphasic effects on estrogen-dependent breast cancer cells *in vitro*, stimulating breast cancer cell growth at lower concentrations[51–54] and inhibiting breast cancer cell growth at higher concentrations,[51–53] and stimulated the growth of estrogen-dependent breast cancer cells *in vivo*.[67–70]

Explanation of these controversial results is primarily focused on estrogen levels in the system. Clearly estrogen plays a critical role in the growth and development of estrogen-dependent breast cancer. One of the mechanisms by which soy isoflavones and other surrogate estrogen receptor modulators exert their estrogenic–antiestrogenic effect is by competing with endogenous estrogens to bind estrogen receptors.[71] We propose that an animal model or an *in vitro* system with maintained estrogen levels to support growth of MCF-7 cells would have greater clinical relevance than one with depleted estrogen levels for evaluating the effect of genistein on the growth of estrogen-dependent MCF-7 cells. Although estrogen levels in the blood of ovariectomized female mice are comparable to those in postmenopausal women, the growth of MCF-7 estrogen-dependent breast tumors in ovariectomized and even in intact animal models requires estrogen supplements.[72] Conversely, estrogen-dependent breast tumors develop and progress in postmenopausal women, suggesting that estrogen levels in postmenopausal women are sufficient to support growth of estrogen-dependent breast tumors. If this effect indicates that tumor-stimulating estrogen bioactivity in animals might be lower than that in humans, then clinically relevant animal models of estrogen-dependent breast cancer should contain estrogen levels adequate to support tumor growth.

By applying the animal model with maintained estrogens, we[24] and other investigators[73] showed that soy phytochemicals and genistein inhibited the growth of MCF-7 tumors in a dose- and time-dependent manner, whereas in an estrogen-depleted breast tumor model, genistein supplementation stimulated MCF-7 tumor growth.[67–70] Similar to the animal studies, a cell culture system with a maintained estrogen level would be more relevant than one with a depleted estrogen level for evaluating the effects of estrogenic–antiestrogenic compounds on estrogen-dependent breast cancer cells. Indeed, although genistein showed estrogenic activity and stimulated proliferation of MCF-7 cells and enhanced expression of the estrogen-responsive pS2 gene in an estrogen-depleted cell culture system, it inhibited estrogen-induced proliferation of MCF-7 cells[24,45,54] and pS2 expression in an estrogen-maintained system.[45,54]

TAM is an estrogen antagonist that blocks activity of estrogens in most tissues that are sensitive to estrogens. TAM has become the standard treatment for breast cancer at all stages of the disease in both pre- and postmenopausal women.[74] Its potential benefits for prevention has also been investigated, and it has been found that TAM reduced breast cancer risk by 50% among women who had a high risk of breast cancer.[75] While TAM has demonstrated efficacy in the prevention and treatment of estrogen-dependent breast tumors, it has no significant effect on estrogen receptor (ER)–negative breast tumors.[75,76] TAM also possesses partial estrogenic activity in breast cancer tissue,[77] thus limiting its therapeutic potential for the treatment of breast cancer in women. In fact, although 50 to 70% breast tumors are ER positive, about 40% of them do not respond to TAM despite the presence of ER in malignant tissues.[78,79] Moreover, the positive response is usually of short duration,[80] and most tumors eventually develop TAM-resistance in 2 to 5 years.[81] Therefore, more effective regimens are urgently needed to improve the efficacy of TAM on the prevention and treatment of estrogen-dependent breast tumors, to delay the occurrence of TAM-resistant tumors, and to effectively treat TAM-resistant and estrogen-independent breast tumors.

The interaction between soy and TAM has been studied in both *in vitro* and *in vivo* systems. Genistein inhibited the growth of dysplastic, estrogen-dependent, and estrogen-independent human breast cancer cells *in vitro*, and the addition of TAM had a synergistic-additive inhibitory effect.[82] Shen and coworkers found that genistein and TAM had a synergistic inhibitory effect on proliferation and cytotoxicity of estrogen-independent human breast cancer cells *in vitro*.[83] Animal studies showed that miso was synergistic with TAM in inhibiting *N*-nitroso-*N*-methyl-urea (NMU)–induced mammary tumorigenesis in female rats,[57] and soy protein isolate (16% of the diet) and TAM combination resulted in a significantly greater inhibition on dimethylbenz(a)anthracene (DMBA)-induced mammary tumor development in female rats.[84] On the other hand, some *in vitro* and animal studies found that genistein might antagonize the effect of TAM on estrogen-dependent breast cancer cells.[85,86]

We have studied the effects of genistein and TAM combinations on the growth of estrogen-dependent MCF-7 human breast tumors and TAM-nonresponsive (MCF-7/TAM-NR) human breast tumors in clinically relevant animal models. In the study of MCF-7/TAM-NR tumors, we found that soy phytochemical concentrate (SPC), but not TAM, inhibited the growth of MCF-7/TAM-NR tumors, and the combination of TAM and SPC further potentiated the inhibitory effect of SPC.[87] We also evaluated the effect of genistein and TAM combination on the growth of estrogen-dependent MCF-7 tumors *in vivo*, and found that both genistein and TAM inhibited the growth of MCF-7 tumors and the combination of genistein with TAM showed a synergistic effect on inhibiting tumor growth.[88] These results suggest that application of TAM and soy combination for breast cancer prevention deserves further investigation.

7.2.2.2 Genistein and Other Chemotherapeutic Drugs

Another active research area is to investigate the possible effect of soy bioactive components on interacting with chemotherapeutic drugs to enhance the efficacy and/or reduce the side effect of therapeutic drugs. Cisplatin is a commonly used drug for cancer therapy. Genistein at typical dietary plasma levels synergistically enhanced the antiproliferative and cytotoxic action of cisplatin to medulloblastomas cells *in vitro*,[89] and synergistically enhanced the antiproliferative and cytotoxic action of 1,3-bis (2-chloroethyl)-1-nitrosourea (BCNU) to glioma cells *in vitro*.[90] Estrogen exerts its activity via binding with a high-affinity to estrogen receptor as well as with a low affinity to estrogen type II binding site (EBS-II). An analog of an endogenous ligand for EBS-II, 2,6-bis ((3, 4-dihydroxyphenyl)-methylene) cyclohexanone (BDHPC) binds to EBS-II and inhibits growth of breast cancer cells via G1 arrest and apoptosis *in vitro*.[91] Genistein and BDHPC synergistically inhibited growth of estrogen-dependent human breast cancer cells *in vitro*.[91] Tiazofurin (2-R-D-ribofuranosylthiazole-4-carboxamide) is an oncolytic C-nucleoside and is effective in causing complete or partial remissions in patients with chronic granulocytic leukemia in blast crisis. A combination of genistein with tiazofurin synergistically inhibited the growth of human leukemic cells[92] and ovarian cancer cells[93] *in vitro* via synergistic modulations on cell differentiation and cell cycle progression.[92] The combination of genistein with adriamycin, an anthracycline anticancer drug, produced additive to synergistic inhibitory effects on the growth of breast cancer cells, especially hormone-independent and multidrug resistant breast cancer cells *in vitro*.[44] The combination of genistein and dexamethasone, a synthetic glucocorticoid, acted in a synergistic fashion to inhibit the growth of both liver and colon cancer cells *in vitro* in part via synergistic induction of p21 expression.[94] In an animal study, genistein and cyclophosphamide combination synergistically inhibited the growth and metastasis of melanoma and Lewis lung carcinoma.[95]

Results of above discussed *in vitro* studies suggest that lower drug concentrations may be employed in combination with genistein in treatment, thus decreasing potential side effects, because the cytotoxicity of these drugs can be synergistically and/or additively enhanced by genistein. However, despite promising *in vitro* findings, most of these combination effects have not been confirmed in animal studies. Verification of these synergistic and/or additive effects of genistein and drugs *in vivo* should be one of the main focuses of cancer prevention research in the future.

7.3 Critical Issues and Future Directions in Research on Soy–Food or Soy–Drug Interactions

Previous research has indicated that synergistic combinations of soy bioactive components with other dietary bioactives or chemopreventive–therapeutic drugs may play a significant role in cancer prevention and treatment. On the other hand, research in this exciting field is still preliminary. There are large gaps in the data from *in vitro*, animal, and human studies that are barriers to advancing the soy–food or soy–drug synergy and cancer prevention hypothesis. Identification of these critical issues will provide the directions of future research priorities in this field.

7.3.1 Identification of Other Soy Components That May Have Synergistic Effect with Other Foods/Drugs: Effects of Whole Soy Food vs. Supplements

Soybeans, like other foods, contain a diverse array of components. Although some components are "bioactive" and the others are "inactive," it is possible that the presence of these active components may exert an additive or even synergistic action. It is also possible that some "inactive" components are required for the "active" components to be active. Food processing may result in concentration of certain types of bioactive components, but may remove other bioactive and/or cofactors. Although genistein is one of the major bioactives in soy, other soy components may also interact with other food bioactives or drugs. Therefore, effective application of soy–food or soy–drug synergy requires careful evaluation of the combined effects between individual soy components or whole soy food and other food bioactives and/or drugs.

One of the future research priorities should be further identification of other soy components that may have synergistic effects with other food components or drugs. Both *in vitro* and animal models should be applied to this investigation. It should be noted that the *in vitro* system may not be appropriate for evaluating the effects of whole soy food or soy products, so animal models should provide the primary modality for evaluation.

7.3.2 Mechanism Elucidation and Mechanism-Based Design of Synergy Strategies for Cancer Prevention and Treatment

Carcinogenesis involves a cascade of processes including initiation, promotion, progression, and metastasis. DNA damage caused by carcinogen exposure and reactive oxygen substances has been suggested to be one of the early steps in carcinogenesis initiation, whereas deregulated cell proliferation, differentiation and apoptosis, and uncontrolled angiogenesis are major cellular modifiers involved in the promotion, progression, and metastasic stages of carcinogenesis.

Though high doses of single bioactive agents may have potent anticancer effects, the chemopreventive properties of the soy–food or soy–drug combinations result from interactions among several components that potentiate the activities of any single constituent and/or reduce side effects. Successful development of a combined cancer chemopreventive and therapeutic strategy is only possible with continuing research into mechanisms of action and thoughtful application of the mechanisms to new design. Several combination strategies can be applied to achieve possible synergistic effects: (1) combinations of agents that target cell cycles at different critical checkpoints to cause cell death; (2) combinations of agents to enhance induced apoptosis and/or necrosis via different signal pathways; (3) combinations of agents that inhibit angiogenesis via modulation of different angiogenic and antiangiogenic factors; and (4) combinations of agents that target simultaneously proliferation, apoptosis, and/or angiogenesis.

Soybean and other bioactive components in foods possess a variety of biological functions in targeting several stages of carcinogenesis.[1] Chemopreventive or therapeutic drugs also have specific targets in the carcinogenesis processes. Therefore, based on the mechanism-oriented multiple-targeting strategies, the effective combinations can be formulated in a synergistic fashion for cancer prevention and treatment. Therefore another priority of future research will be further elucidation of the mechanisms of action. *In vitro* systems will serve as the first line modality for elucidation of the mechanisms and identification of the mechanism-based biomarkers. Traditional methods of analysis of gene expression patterns have imposed a practical limit on the number of candidate genes. Highly parallel technologies exploiting sample hybridization to oligonucleotide or cDNA arrays permit the expression levels of tens of thousands of genes to be monitored simultaneously and rapidly. The application of this technology and/or other advanced technologies such as proteomics will greatly facilitate identification of biomarkers that can be further validated in animal and clinical studies.

Genomics and proteomics techniques will play a critical role in the mechanism research. Proteomes complement current molecular approaches through the analysis of the gene products responsible for the life processes within the cells and tissue under various physiological conditions, and thus can be applied to compare various protein expression patterns that are responsible for the combined synergy strategy. More complex than genomics, proteomics not only studies the number of proteins, but the many possible interactions those proteins may form. Proteomics is therefore a global analysis of changes in the quantities and posttranslational modifications of all the proteins in cells. A major application of proteomics is the identification, at a protein level, of early changes involved in carcinogenesis and tumorigenesis due to effective intervention.

7.3.3 Systematic Evaluation of Synergistic Combinations and Identification of Biomarkers

The mechanism-based multitargeting strategy will facilitate identification of possible synergistic combinations for cancer chemoprevention and treatment. On the other hand, a large body of data on the chemopreventive and therapeutic potency of an agent and the mechanism of action is derived from *in vitro* studies, and there are substantial differences between *in vitro* and *in vivo* systems; therefore the candidate combinations identified from *in vitro* investigations need to be verified in a series of *in vivo* testing systems. Well-designed *in vivo* efficacy, safety, and mechanism studies are required to identify the effective combinations and verify responsive biomarkers before clinical applications can be considered.

A series of animal models that represent the different stages of carcinogenesis such as initiation, promotion, progression, and metastasis should be used for evaluation. Chemical carcinogen–induced carcinogenesis animal models are commonly used to evaluate the effects of agents on different stages of carcinogenesis. Genetically engineered mouse tumor models have been established for certain types of cancers to evaluate the efficacy of a preventive and treatment regimen in the different stages of carcinogenesis and/or tumorigenesis processes. Xenograft tumor models are the most commonly used model systems for efficacy and safety evaluation, biomarker verification, and elucidation of mechanisms. The tumor microenvironment and tumor–stromal interactions play a critical role in tumorigenesis and may influence the treatment outcomes. Therefore clinically relevant tumor models, such as orthotopic tumor models that mimic the microenvironment of a particular organ should be preferably utilized for evaluation.

Animal studies also provide excellent *in vivo* systems to validate the biomarkers that are responsible for effective treatments. Both conventional molecular biology techniques as well as genomic and/or proteomic approaches should be applied for biomarker validation and for exploration of possible new biomarkers *in vivo*. When biological samples are collected for determination, it is important to evaluate both time- and dose-dependent responses of biomarkers to the treatment because some biomarker changes are responsible for the efficacy of treatment, and others may be secondarily associated with the effective treatment. It is important to appropriately isolate tumor tissues from adjacent normal tissues so that the expression levels of biomarkers in those tissues can be differentiated.

7.3.4 Individual Responses to Chemopreventive and Treatment Combinations

Genetic and environmental factors contribute to a wide inter- and intraindividual variability in bioactive and drug metabolism and thus to different responses to combination regimens. Careful investigation of interactions between genetic background and molecular characteristics of the disease and intervention outcomes should provide critical information on identifying specific subgroups that may be most beneficial to an intervention regimen. Systematic *in vitro* and animal studies should be conducted to evaluate the responses of cell lines and animal models with different genetic backgrounds to specific combination regimens so that a synergistic combination regimen can be identified for individuals with unique genetic and/or molecular background.

With identification of synergistic combinations and biomarker verification in animal studies, intervention studies are an appropriate consideration to assess the clinical effects of these combinations. The golden standard is still the randomized, double-blind, and placebo-controlled intervention trial. Because of high-cost and long-duration of this type of trial, alternative trials with short and intermediate duration using smaller cohorts of a subgroup of cancer patients may provide excellent and cost-effective approaches for efficacy testing.

Prostate cancer is a prime candidate for a strategy aimed at prevention because of its extremely high prevalence rate, rising annual incidence, and long latent interval between the cancer-initiating events and the development of invasive disease.[96] Subjects that are usually at "high risk" of developing cancer are suitable candidates for intervention trials, and biomarkers that would reflect the cancer risk and respond to treatment should be used to evaluate the effectiveness of intervention. Premalignant epithelial changes such as prostate intraepithelial neoplasia (PIN) are highly associated with prostate cancer and share many molecular features of invasive cancer. Subjects with high-grade PIN are a group of candidates for prostate cancer intervention trials. Alternatively, cancer patients that have undergone treatments (chemotherapy, surgery, and/or radiation therapy) are another subgroup for secondary prevention trials to determine the effect of intervention regimen on tumor recurrence and progression, and biomarkers that are related to tumor progression may be used as intermediate endpoints to evaluate the effectiveness of treatment.

Caution is needed in selection of these subjects with different genetic backgrounds for clinical intervention trials. Although they may have similar high risk of developing cancer or have the similar disease stages, the associated risk factors may be different and their responses to the treatment may vary significantly.

7.3.5 Safety Issues Related to Synergistic Combination Strategies

Ideally, synergistic combinations of agents for enhancing the efficacy at lower doses should also result in reduced side effects and toxicity of any treatment alone in which higher doses are required to achieve the similar effects. However, whether a particular combination has less or more side effects than the single treatment alone needs to be carefully determined because of the complexity of the *in vivo* system. It is therefore imperative to evaluate the efficacy and safety of any combinations simultaneously in the related systems, and weigh both efficacy and safety equally as criteria for selection of candidate preventive–therapeutic combinations.

7.4 Conclusions

Data reviewed in this chapter clearly indicate that soybeans contain bioactive anticancer components, and the soy–food and soy–drug combinations provide synergistic regimens for cancer prevention and treatment. Identification of more effective synergistic combinations and verification of their efficacy and safety will be one of the priorities of cancer researchers in the future. The synergistic combination of soy with other Asian foods such as tea may be one of the mechanisms by which the risks of certain types of cancers are significantly lower in the Asian population than in the Western population. On the other hand, not all soy products or supplements are created equal. Different soy components may have different bioactivities, and their combinations with other foods and drugs may result in different activities. Much research is required to determine the interactions of a particular soy product with other foods and drugs so that the efficacy and safety of individual combinations can be clearly elucidated. Caution should be exercised for potential adverse effects of food–drug interactions. For the general public, increased consumption of soy food or whole soy based products is recommended. In addition, people should incorporate other healthy dietary habits and lifestyles, such as increased consumption of fruits, vegetables, and tea, increased exercise; and reduced fat intake. It is believed that supplementation of human diets with certain soy–food or soy–drug combinations, together with a healthy dietary pattern and lifestyle, could markedly reduce the risk and the mortality rate of human cancers.

References

1. Messina, M.J. et al., Soy intake and cancer risk: a review of the in vitro and in vivo data, *Nutr. Cancer,* 21, 113, 1994.
2. Adlercreutz, C.H. et al., Soybean phytoestrogen intake and cancer risk, *J. Nutr.*, 125, 757s, 1995.
3. Akiyama, T. et al., Genistein, a specific inhibitor of tyrosine-specific protein kinases, *J. Biol. Chem.*, 262, 5592, 1987.
4. Naim, M. et al., Antioxidative and antihemolytic activities of soybean isoflavones, *J. Agric. Food Chem.*, 24, 1174, 1976.
5. Okura, A. et al., Effect of genistein on topoisomerase activity and on the growth of [Val 12]Ha-ras-transformed NIH 3T3 cells, *Biochem. Biophys. Res. Comm.*, 157, 183, 1988.
6. Markovits, J. et al., Inhibitory effects of the tyrosine kinase inhibitor genistein on mammalian DNA topoisomerase II, *Cancer Res.*, 49, 5111, 1989.
7. Zhou, J.-R. et al., Soybean phytochemicals inhibit the growth of transplantable human prostate carcinoma and tumor angiogenesis in mice, *J. Nutr.*, 129, 1628, 1999.
8. Kyle, E. et al., Genistein-induced apoptosis of prostate cancer cells is preceded by a specific decrease in focal adhesion kinase activity, *Mol. Pharmacol.*, 51, 193, 1997.
9. Zhou, J.-R. et al., Inhibition of orthotopic growth and metastasis of androgen-sensitive human prostate tumors in mice by bioactive soybean components, *Prostate*, 53, 143, 2002.
10. Fotsis, T. et al., Flavonoids, dietary-derived inhibitors of cell proliferation and in vitro angiogenesis, *Cancer Res.*, 57, 2916, 1997.
11. Kennedy, A.R., The evidence for soybean products as cancer preventive agents, *J. Nutr.*, 125, 733S, 1995.
12. Chemoprevention Working Group, Prevention of cancer in the next millennium: report of the chemoprevention working group to the American Association for Cancer Research, *Cancer Res.*, 59, 4743, 1999.
13. Henderson, B.E. and Bernstein, L., The international variation in breast cancer rates: an epidemiological assessment, *Breast Cancer Res. Treat.*, 18, S11, 1991.
14. Landis, S.H. et al., Cancer statistics, *CA Cancer J. Clin.*, 49, 8, 1999.
15. Muir, C.S., Nectoux, J., and Staszewski, J., The epidemiology of prostate cancer. Geographic distribution and time-trends, *Acta Oncol.*, 30, 133, 1991.
16. Parkin, D.M., Pisani, P., and Ferlay, J., Global cancer statistics, *CA Cancer J. Clin.*, 49, 33, 1999,
17. Ziegler, R.G. et al., Migration patterns and breast cancer risk in Asian-American women, *J. Natl. Cancer Inst.*, 85, 1819, 1993.

18. Boyle, P. et al., Trends in diet-related cancers in Japan: a conundrum? *Lancet*, 342, 752, 1993.
19. Morton, M.S., Griffiths, K., and Blacklock, N., The preventive role of diet in prostatic disease, *Brit. J. Urol.*, 77, 481, 1996.
20. Stellman, S.D. and Wang, Q.S., Cancer mortality in Chinese migrants to New York City. Comparison with Chinese in Tianjin and with United States-born whites, *Cancer (Phila.)*, 73, 1270, 1994.
21. Cook, L.S. et al., Incidence of adenocarcinoma of the prostate in Asian immigrants to the United States and their descendants, *J. Urol.*, 161, 152, 1999.
22. Whittemore, A.S. et al., Prostate cancer in relation to diet, physical activity, and body size in blacks, whites, and Asians in the United States and Canada, *J. Natl. Cancer Inst.*, 87, 652, 1995.
23. Zhou, J.-R. et al., Soy phytochemicals and tea bioactive components synergistically inhibit androgen-sensitive human prostate tumors in mice, *J. Nutr.*, 133, 516, 2003.
24. Zhou, J.-R. et al., Combined inhibition of estrogen-dependent human breast carcinoma by soy and tea bioactive components in mice, *Int. J. Cancer*, 108, 8, 2004.
25. Sakamoto, K., Synergistic effects of thearubigin and genistein on human prostate tumor cell (PC-3) growth via cell cycle arrest, *Cancer Lett.*, 151, 103, 2000.
26. Blutt, S.E. and Weigel, N.L., Vitamin D and prostate cancer, *Proc. Soc. Exp. Biol. Med.*, 221, 89, 1999.
27. Bortman, P. et al., Antiproliferative effects of 1,25-dihydroxyvitamin D3 on breast cells: a mini review, *Braz. J. Med. Biol. Res.*, 35, 1, 2002.
28. Garland, C.F., Garland, F.C., and Gorham, E.D., Calcium and vitamin D. Their potential roles in colon and breast cancer prevention, *Ann. N.Y. Acad. Sci.*, 889, 107, 1999.
29. Cross, H.S. et al., Phytoestrogens and vitamin D metabolism: a new concept for the prevention and therapy of colorectal, prostate, and mammary carcinomas, *J. Nutr.*, 134, 1207S, 2004.
30. Corder, E. et al., Vitamin D and prostate cancer: a prediagnostic study with stored sera, *Cancer Epidemiol. Biomarkers Prevention*, 2, 467, 1993.
31. Ingles, S. et al., Association of prostate cancer risk with genetic polymorphisms in vitamin D receptor and androgen receptor, *J. Natl. Cancer Inst.*, 89, 166, 1997.
32. Rao, A. et al., Genistein and vitamin D synergistically inhibit human prostatic epithelial cell growth, *J. Nutr.*, 132, 3191, 2002.
33. Farhan, H. and Cross, H.S., Transcriptional inhibition of CYP24 by genistein, *Ann. N.Y. Acad. Sci.*, 973, 459, 2002.
34. Farhan, H. et al., Isoflavonoids inhibit catabolism of vitamin D in prostate cancer cells, *J. Chromatogr. B Analyt. Technol. Biomed. Life Sci.*, 777, 261, 2002.
35. Farhan, H., Wahala, K., and Cross, H.S., Genistein inhibits vitamin D hydroxylases CYP24 and CYP27B1 expression in prostate cells, *J. Steroid Biochem. Mol. Biol.*, 84, 423, 2003.
36. Cross, H.S. et al., Regulation of extrarenal vitamin D metabolism as a tool for colon and prostate cancer prevention, *Recent Results Cancer Res.*, 164, 413, 2003.
37. Lechner, D. and Cross, H.S., Phytoestrogens and 17beta-estradiol influence vitamin D metabolism and receptor expression-relevance for colon cancer prevention, *Recent Results Cancer Res.*, 164, 379, 2003.
38. Kallay, E. et al., Phytoestrogens regulate vitamin D metabolism in the mouse colon: relevance for colon tumor prevention and therapy, *J. Nutr.*, 132, 3490S, 2002.

39. Rao, A. et al., Vitamin D receptor and p21/WAF1 are targets of genistein and 1,25-dihydroxyvitamin D3 in human prostate cancer cells, *Cancer Res.*, 64, 2143, 2004.
40. Shen, F. and Weber, G., Synergistic action of quercetin and genistein in human ovarian carcinoma cells, *Oncol. Res.*, 9, 597, 1997.
41. Verma, S.P., Salamone, E., and Goldin, B., Curcumin and genistein, plant natural products, show synergistic inhibitory effects on the growth of human breast cancer MCF-7 cells induced by estrogenic pesticides, *Biochem. Biophy. Res. Commun.*, 233, 692, 1997.
42. Kumi-Diaka, J., Chemosensitivity of human prostate cancer cells PC3 and LNCaP to genistein isoflavone and beta-lapachone, *Biol. Cell.*, 94, 37, 2002.
43. Nakagawa, H. et al., Effects of genistein and synergistic action in combination with eicosapentaenoic acid on the growth of breast cancer cell lines, *J. Cancer Res. Clin. Oncol.*, 126, 448, 2000.
44. Monti, E. and Sinha, B.K., Antiproliferative effect of genistein and adriamycin against estrogen-dependent and -independent human breast carcinoma cell lines, *AntiCancer Res.*, 14, 1221, 1994.
45. So, F.V. et al., Inhibition of proliferation of estrogen receptor-positive MCF-7 human breast cancer cells by flavonoids in the presence and absence of excess estrogen, *Cancer Lett.*, 112, 127, 1997.
46. Hoffman, R., Potent inhibition of breast cancer cell lines by the isoflavonoid kievitone: comparison with genistein, *Biochem. Biophys. Res. Commun.*, 211, 600, 1995.
47. Peterson, G. and Barnes, S., Genistein inhibits both estrogen and growth factor-stimulated proliferation of human breast cancer cells, *Cell Growth Differentiation*, 7, 1345, 1996.
48. Shao, Z.M. et al., Genistein inhibits proliferation similarly in estrogen receptor-positive and negative human breast carcinoma cell lines characterized by P21WAF1/CIP1 induction, G2/M arrest, and apoptosis, *J. Cell. Biochem.*, 69, 44, 1998.
49. Pagliacci, M.C. et al., Growth-inhibitory effects of the natural phyto-oestrogen genistein in MCF-7 human breast cancer cells, *Eur. J. Cancer*, 30A, 1675, 1994.
50. Clark, J.W. et al., Effects of tyrosine kinase inhibitors on the proliferation of human breast cancer cell lines and proteins important in the ras signaling pathway, *Int. J. Cancer*, 65, 186, 1996.
51. Zava, D.T. and Duwe, G., Estrogenic and antiproliferative properties of genistein and other flavonoids in human breast cancer cells in vitro, *Nutr. Cancer*, 27, 31, 1997.
52. Dees, C. et al., Dietary estrogens stimulate human breast cells to enter the cell cycle, *Environ. Health Persp.*, 3, 633, 1997.
53. Wang, C. and Kurzer, M.S., Phytoestrogen concentration determines effects on DNA synthesis in human breast cancer cells, *Nutr. Cancer*, 28, 236, 1997.
54. Wang, T., Sathyamoorthy, N., and Phang, J.M., Molecular effects of genistein on estrogen receptor mediated pathways, *Carcinogenesis*, 17, 271, 1997.
55. Badger, T.M., Ronis, M.J., and Hakkak, R., Developmental effects and health aspects of soy protein isolate, casein, and whey in male and female rats, *Int. J. Toxicol.*, 20, 165, 2001.
56. Fritz, W.A. et al., Dietary genistein: perinatal mammary cancer prevention, bioavailability and toxicity testing in the rat, *Carcinogenesis*, 19, 2151, 1998.

57. Gotoh, T. et al., Chemoprevention of N-nitroso-N-methylurea-induced rat mammary carcinogenesis by soy foods or biochanin A, *Japan. J. Cancer Res.*, 89, 137, 1998.
58. Hakkak, R. et al., Diets containing whey proteins or soy protein isolate protect against 7,12-dimethylbenz(a)anthracene-induced mammary tumors in female rats, *Cancer Epidemiol. Biomarkers Prev.*, 9, 113, 2000.
59. Ohta, T. et al., Inhibitory effects of bifidobacterium-fermented soy milk on 2-amino-1-methyl-6-phenylimidazo[4,5-b]pyridine-induced rat mammary carcinogenesis, with a partial contribution of its component isoflavones, *Carcinogenesis*, 21, 937, 2000.
60. Constantinou, A.I. et al., Chemopreventive effects of soy protein and purified soy isoflavones on DMBA-induced mammary tumors in female Sprague-Dawley rats, *Nutr. Cancer*, 41, 75, 2001.
61. Cohen, L.A. et al., Effect of intact and isoflavone-depleted soy protein on NMU-induced rat mammary tumorigenesis, *Carcinogenesis*, 21, 929, 2000.
62. Gallo, D. et al., Chemoprevention of DMBA-induced mammary cancer in rats by dietary soy, *Breast Cancer Res. Treat.*, 69, 153, 2001.
63. Jin, Z. and MacDonald, R.S., Soy isoflavones increase latency of spontaneous mammary tumors in mice, *J. Nutr.*, 132, 3186, 2002.
64. Yang, X. et al., Hormonal and dietary modulation of mammary carcinogenesis in mouse mammary tumor virus-c-erbB-2 transgenic mice, *Cancer Res.*, 63, 2425, 2003.
65. Yuan, L. et al., Inhibition of human breast cancer growth by GCP (genistein combined polysaccharide) in xenogeneic athymic mice: involvement of genistein biotransformation by beta-glucuronidase from tumor tissues, *Mutat Res*, 523–524, 55, 2003.
66. Yan, L., Li, D., and Yee, J.A., Dietary supplementation with isolated soy protein reduces metastasis of mammary carcinoma cells in mice, *Clin. Exp. Metastasis*, 19, 535, 2002.
67. Hsieh, C.-Y. et al., Estrogenic effects of genistein on the growth of estrogen receptor-positive human breast cancer (MCF-7) cells in vitro and in vivo, *Cancer Res.*, 58, 3833, 1998.
68. Ju, Y.H. et al., Physiological concentrations of dietary genistein dose-dependently stimulate growth of estrogen-dependent human breast cancer (MCF-7) tumors implanted in athymic nude mice, *J. Nutr.*, 131, 2957, 2001.
69. Allred, C.D. et al., Dietary genistin stimulates growth of estrogen-dependent breast cancer tumors similar to that observed with genistein, *Carcinogenesis*, 22, 1667, 2001.
70. Allred, C.D. et al., Soy diets containing varying amounts of genistein stimulate growth of estrogen-dependent (MCF-7) tumors in a dose-dependent manner, *Cancer Res.*, 61, 5045, 2001.
71. Messina, M.J. and Loprinzi, C.L., Soy for breast cancer survivors: a critical review of the literature, *J. Nutr.*, 131, 3095S, 2001.
72. Soule, H.D. and McGrath, C.M., Estrogen responsive proliferation of clonal human breast carcinoma cells in athymic mice, *Cancer Lett.*, 10, 177, 1980.
73. Shao, Z.-M. et al., Genistein exerts mutiple suppressive effects on human breast carcinoma cells, *Cancer Res.*, 58, 4851, 1998.
74. Fisher, B. et al., Five vs more than five years of tamoxifen therapy for breast cancer patients with negative lymph nodes and estrogen receptor-positive tumors, *J. Natl. Cancer Inst.*, 88, 1529, 1996.

75. Fisher, B. et al., Tamoxifen for prevention of breast cancer: report of the National Surgical Adjuvant Breast and Bowel Project P-1 Study, *J. Natl. Cancer Inst.*, 90, 1371, 1998.
76. Early Breast Cancer Trialists' Collaborative Group, Tamoxifen for early breast cancer: an overview of the randomized trials, *Lancet*, 351, 1451, 1998.
77. Gottardis, M.M. et al., Inhibition of tamoxifen-stimulated growth of an MCF-7 tumor variant in athymic mice by novel steroidal antiestrogens, *Cancer Res.*, 49, 4090, 1989.
78. Karamura, I. et al., Antiestrogenic and antitumor effects of droloxifene in experimental breast carcinoma, *Arzneimittelforschung*, 39, 889, 1989.
79. Jaiyesimi, I.A. et al., Use of tamoxifen for breast cancer: twenty-eight years later, *J. Clin. Oncol.*, 13, 513, 1995.
80. Mouridsen, H. et al., Tamoxifen in advanced breast cancer, *Cancer Treat. Rev.*, 5, 131, 1978.
81. Muss, H.B., Endocrine therapy for advanced breast cancer: a review, *Breast Cancer Res. Treat.*, 21, 15, 1992.
82. Tanos, V. et al., Synergistic inhibitory effects of genistein and tamoxifen on human dysplastic and malignant epithelial breast cells in vitro, *Eur. J. Obstet. Gynecol. Reprod. Biol.*, 102, 188, 2002.
83. Shen, F., Xue, X., and Weber, G., Tamoxifen and genistein synergistically down-regulate signal transduction and proliferation in estrogen receptor-negative human breast carcinoma MDA-MB-435 cells, *AntiCancer Res.*, 19, 1657, 1999.
84. Constantinou, A.I. et al., Consumption of soy products may enhance the breast cancer-preventive effects of tamoxifen, *Proc. Am. Assoc. Cancer Res.*, 42, 826 (abst #4440), 2001.
85. Ju, Y.H. et al., Dietary genistein negates the inhibitory effect of tamoxifen on growth of estrogen-dependent human breast cancer (MCF-7) cells implanted in athymic mice, *Cancer Res.*, 62, 2474, 2002.
86. Jones, J.L. et al., Genistein inhibits tamoxifen effects on cell proliferation and cell cycle arrest in T47D breast cancer cells, *Am. Surg.*, 68, 575, 2002.
87. Zhou, J.-R., Mai, Z., and Blackburn, G.L., Soy phytochemicals potentiate the efficacy of tamoxifen treatment to tamoxifen-nonresponsive, ER-positive human breast tumor in a mouse model, *FASEB J.*, 17, Abst. #872.7, 2003.
88. Zhou, J.-R. et al., Soy isoflavone genistein potentiates the efficacy of tamoxifen treatment to estrogen-dependent human breast tumor in a mouse model, *FASEB J.*, 18, A1110 (abst. #728.1), 2004.
89. Khoshyomn, S. et al., Synergistic action of genistein and cisplatin on growth inhibition and cytotoxicity of human medulloblastoma cells, *Pediatr. Neurosurg.*, 33, 123, 2000.
90. Khoshyomn, S. et al., Synergistic effect of genistein and BCNU on growth inhibition and cytotoxicity of glioblastoma cells, *J. Neurooncol.*, 57, 193, 2002.
91. Attalla, H. et al., 2,6-Bis((3,4-dihydroxyphenyl)-methylene)cyclohexanone (BDHPC)-induced apoptosis and p53-independent growth inhibition: synergism with genistein, *Biochem. Biophys. Research Commun.*, 239, 467, 1997.
92. Li, W. and Weber, G., Synergistic action of tiazofurin and genistein on growth inhibition and differentiation of K-562 human leukemic cells, *Life Sci.*, 63, 1975, 1998.
93. Li, W. and Weber, G., Synergistic action of tiazofurin and genistein in human ovarian carcinoma cells, *Oncol. Res.*, 10, 117, 1998.

94. Park, J.H. et al., Synergistic effects of dexamethasone and genistein on the expression of Cdk inhibitor p21WAF1/CIP1 in human hepatocellular and colorectal carcinoma cells, *Int. J. Oncol.*, 18, 997, 2001.
95. Wietrzyk, J. et al., Antitumour and antimetastatic effect of genistein alone or combined with cyclophosphamide in mice transplanted with various tumours depends on the route of tumour transplantation, *In Vivo*, 14, 357, 2000.
96. Kelloff, G. et al., Agents, biomarkers, and cohorts for chemopreventive agent development in prostate cancer, *Urology*, 57, 46, 2001.

8

Flaxseed, Lignans, n-3 Fatty Acids, and Drug Synergy in the Prevention and Treatment of Cancer

Lilian U. Thompson

CONTENTS

8.1 Introduction

Current evidence suggests that increased intake of plant foods may reduce the risk of certain types of cancer; this has been attributed in part to their many phytochemicals.[1,2] To determine their beneficial effects on health, the effects of specific plant foods or food components have been studied in isolation. However, foods are not consumed in isolation but in combination with other foods. An effect of a specific component in a food may not necessarily be equivalent to the effect of the specific food because a component may act either synergistically or antagonistically with other components of the same food. It is therefore important to understand whether food components act in a complementary or adverse manner. Similarly it is of interest to determine whether different foods with the same or complementary mechanisms of action will interact in such a way that the results are more beneficial to health than the intake of the single food alone.

Patients taking drugs to control tumor growth and metastasis often change their diets to assist in their treatment. However, there is little known regarding the interactions of foods with cancer drugs. Combining certain foods or food components with drugs may result in reduced drug dose requirement or toxicity, or there may be an adverse effect.

In this chapter, the synergistic interaction of components within the food, among foods, and between cancer drugs and foods or food components are discussed with specific emphasis on flaxseed (FS), sesame seed, and fish oil and their component lignans (i.e., in FS and sesame seed) and fatty acids, particularly n-3 fatty acids.

8.2 Food Synergy

8.2.1 Flaxseed

FS is an oilseed that contains an exceptionally high concentration of lignans (75 to 800 times higher than other plant foods) and α-linolenic acid (ALA), an n-3 fatty acid (FS contains about 40% oil and 57% is ALA).[3,4] Lignans are dimeric compounds formed by the coupling of two monomeric C_6C_3 moieties derived from the phenylpropanoid pathway. Some plant lignans are metabolized by the bacterial flora in the colon of humans and animals to the mammalian lignans enterolactone (EL) and enterodiol (ED)[5] (Figure 8.1). It is these mammalian lignan metabolites, rather than the plant lignans, that are thought to have the anticancer effect.[4] Their chemical structural similarity to estrogen suggests that they may interfere with the binding of estrogen to the estrogen receptor (ER) and hence protect against hormone-related cancers. The major plant lignan precursors of ED and EL are secoisolariciresinol

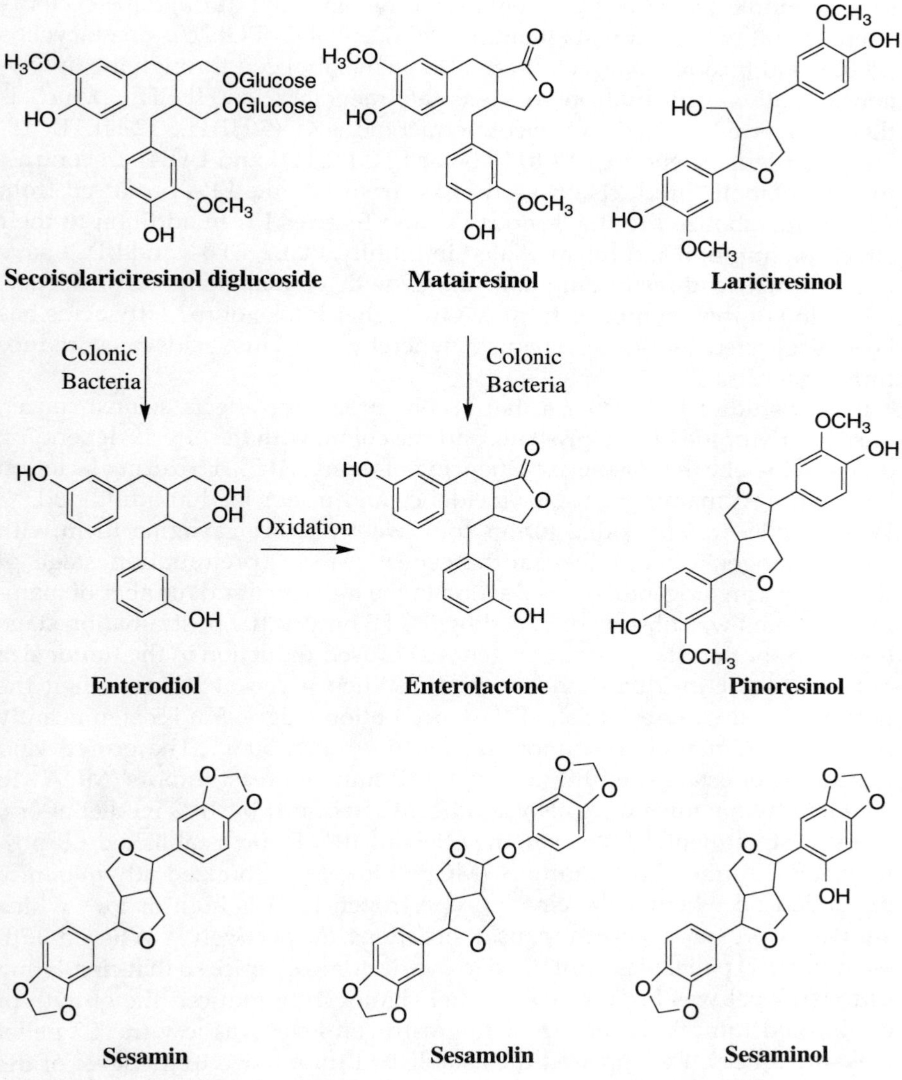

FIGURE 8.1
Plant lignans and their metabolism to mammalian lignans enterolactone and enterodiol.

diglycoside (SDG) and matairesinol[5] (Figure 8.1). Although other precursors of mammalian lignans have recently been identified in rye such as lariciresinol and pinoresinol (Figure 8.1), SDG is known to be the major precursor in FS.[6]

ALA in FS can be metabolized to the longer chain fatty acids eicosapentaenoic acid (EPA;C20:5n3) and docosahexaenoic acid (DHA;C22:6n-3) by the elongation-desaturation pathway; ALA thus competes with linoleic acid (LA; C18:2n-6) for the same enzymes, thus reducing the conversion of LA to arachidonic acid (AA; C20:4n-6).[7] AA is metabolized through the cyclooxygenase pathway to prostaglandins (PGE2, PGD2, PGF2α), prostacyclins (PGI2), and thromboxane A2. It can also be metabolized through the lipoxygenase pathway to hydroperoxy-eicosatetraenoic acid (HPETE), which is then converted to hydroxyl-eicosatetraenoic acid (5-HETE, 12-HETE, 15-HETE) or leukotrienes (LTA4 to LTB4 or LTC4, LTD4 and LTE4). In contrast to the metabolic products of AA derived from LA, the EPA produced from ALA is metabolized to the 3-series PG and 5 series LT. In addition to their effects on humoral and cell mediated immunity, PGE2, LTB4, and LTC4 have been shown to directly stimulate the growth of malignant cells.[7] Hence, inhibition of their synthesis from AA by higher intake of n-3 fatty acids has been suggested as one mechanism whereby n-3 fatty acids may reduce tumorigenesis.[7]

Recent studies have shown that FS has protective effects against cancer, particularly of the breast, prostate, and the colon, with the effects depending on the stage of carcinogenesis.[4] Offspring of dams fed 5% FS during lactation have reduced mammary tumor incidence and tumor load at adulthood.[8–10] When 5% FS was provided to rats for 4 weeks before gavaging them with the carcinogen dimethylbenzanthracene (DMBA) (preinitiation stage of mammary carcinogenesis), a reduction in the incidence and number of mammary tumors was observed.[11] Feeding 5% FS only at the postinitiation stage (early promotion stage of carcinogenesis) caused reduction in the tumor size but not tumor incidence and number.[11] When given at a time when the tumors are already established (late promotion stage), 5% FS significantly regressed the mammary tumor size by more than 50%.[12] The growth and metastasis of established ER negative (ER) human breast tumors (MDA MB 435) in athymic mice were also significantly reduced by 10% FS diet after 6 weeks of treatment.[13] However, the effect of 10% FS on established ER positive (ER+) human breast tumors (MCF-7) in ovariectomized athymic mice depended on whether the circulating estrogen level is high or low, which simulates pre- or postmenopausal situations, respectively.[14] When a 17β-estradiol (E2) pellet was implanted in ovariectomized mice so that circulating estrogen level was high, a 10% FS diet significantly reduced the growth of established tumors. When circulating estrogen level was low (no E2 pellet was implanted), FS regressed the established tumor size to the level of the ovariectomized control mice and did not act like estrogen by promoting tumor growth.[14] Similar results of FS feeding have been reported in postmenopausal breast cancer patients fed muffins containing 25 g FS between the time of diagnosis to time of surgery in a randomized, double-blind placebo-controlled study. Patients fed the FS had lower tumor cell proliferation and c-erbB2 expression, and higher apoptosis than those fed the placebo muffin.[15]

Similarly, prostate cancer patients awaiting prostatectomy who consumed a low fat (20% kcal or less) diet supplemented with 30 g FS for an average of 34 days had significant reductions in total testosterone, free androgen index, and mean tumor cell proliferation but a higher apoptotic index than the historical controls.[16,17] It cannot be conclusively stated that the effect was due to the FS because historical controls were used instead of a low fat diet group or a placebo group. However, using the transgenic adenocarcinoma mouse prostate (TRAMP) model, a 5% FS diet reduced the number of aggressive tumors, prevalence of lung and lymph node metastasis, and prostatic tissue cell proliferation, but increased the cell apoptotic index after 30 weeks of treatment.[18]

While it is evident that FS has cancer protective effects, it is unclear which specific component is responsible for this effect. The effect of FS could be due to its lignans, ALA, or the synergistic or additive interactions between these components.

8.2.2 α–Linolenic Acid Combined with Flaxseed Lignans

Very few studies have been designed to determine which specific component is responsible for the anticancer effects of FS. When SDG, isolated and purified from FS, was fed at a level equivalent to the amount in a 5% FS diet, the incidence and number of tumors in DMBA-treated rats at the early promotion stage was reduced.[19] This suggests that SDG is one component in FS that has an anticancer effect. In a study where 5% FS, or SDG or flaxseed oil (FO) at levels present in the 5% FS diet, were fed to rats with established DMBA-induced mammary tumors, reductions in tumor size were observed in all treatment groups, indicating that both SDG and FO contributed to the tumor regressing effect of FS.[12] The reduction in tumor size tended to be greater in the 5% FS group than either the SDG or FO groups, indicating that the effect of FS may be due to the combined effect of its lignan and the ALA-rich FO. However, a treatment with combined SDG and FO was not included in the experimental design. Therefore, it cannot be conclusively stated that the effect of FS was primarily due to the combined effect of SDG and FO.

To further address the effect of combined SDG and FO, athymic mice were injected with ER-human breast cancer cells (MDA MB 435) and 8 weeks later when the tumors were established (about 100 m^2 size), they were fed the basal diet (BD; control) or BD supplemented with 10% FS, SDG, FO, or combined SDG and FO for 6 weeks.[20] The levels of SDG and FO were equivalent to the amounts in the 10% FS. Compared with the BD group, the tumor growth rate was significantly reduced in the FS, FO, and combined SDG and FO groups, but not in the SDG group. Metastasis incidence in the lungs, distant lymph nodes, and other organs, and total incidence of metastasis were reduced in all four treatment groups, with the reduction being significant in the FS and SDG + FO groups for lung metastasis, and in the FO group for lymph node metastasis. Metastasis incidence in the other organs (liver, bones, kidneys, and abdominal cavity) was significantly reduced by all treatments when compared with the control. Although the total metastasis incidence in the four treatment groups did not differ significantly from each other, it was lowered significantly only in the SDG + FO group when compared with the control.

In another study with similar experimental design as above, except that the established primary tumor was excised before the treatment diets were provided, the incidence of lung metastasis was significantly reduced by 58.3% and 54.5% with FS and SDG + FO, respectively.[20] Feeding SDG or FO alone did not significantly reduce the incidence of lung metastasis. The mean number of lung tumors per mouse was also the lowest in the FS (0.32) and the SDG + FO (0.43) groups compared with that in the FO (0.85) or SDG (0.85) groups. A similar pattern of metastasis incidence was observed in lymph node and other organs. Overall, the above studies indicate that the combination of SDG and FO was more effective in reducing the growth and metastasis of established tumors than the SDG or FO alone, and that the effect of FS can be largely attributed to these components.

8.2.3 Flaxseed Combined with Soy

High intake of phytoestrogens, particularly isoflavones, has been associated with a reduced risk of breast cancer in some but not in all studies (Chapter 7). Most plant foods contain the phytoestrogen lignans; therefore it is likely that isoflavones are consumed not in isolation but rather in combination with lignans. Failure to consider the intake of both lignans and isoflavones in some epidemiological studies may be one reason why no consistent effect of phytoestrogens on cancer has been observed. The synergistic or additive effects of soy and FS, the richest source of lignans, or their purified isoflavones and lignans on breast cancer were therefore studied in our laboratory.[21–23]

Ovariectomized athymic mice were injected with ER+ MCF-7 human breast cancer cells and implanted with an estradiol (E2) pellet to increase circulating estrogen.[22,23] When the tumors were established (about 40 mm^2), the E2 pellet was removed and the mice were randomized such that their tumor size and body weights were similar among groups. They were then fed a control diet or a diet supplemented with isoflavone-rich soy protein isolate (SPI; 20% SPI with about 2 mg isoflavone/g SPI), 10% FS, or combined SPI and 10% FS. After 24 weeks, the tumors in all treatment groups, except the SPI group, regressed in size and were similar in size to the negative control. While the tumors in mice fed the SPI diet initially regressed, they started to grow again after 12 weeks of treatment. The combination of 10% FS with SPI prevented this late stage tumor growth, indicating a synergistic effect.

8.2.4 Lignans Combined with Genistein

In a study with a similar experimental design as above, mice were gavaged daily with either ED, EL, or genistein alone, or in combination, at a level of

10 mg/kg body weight.[21,23] As was observed with the 10% FS and SPI experiment, after 22 weeks' treatment, regression of all established tumors to the level of the negative control was observed. An exception is the genistein-treated group. The tumors in this group decreased in size after 5 weeks of treatment beyond which no further reduction took place. Combining genistein with ED and EL reduced the tumor size to the level of the negative control.

Overall, the above two studies[21–23] indicate that combining soy and FS or their genistein and lignans, respectively, may be more protective against breast cancer, particularly in postmenopausal women with low circulating estrogen levels.

8.2.5 α-Linolenic Acid Combined with γ-Linolenic Acid

Fatty acid synthase (FAS), an enzyme in the *de novo* biosynthesis of fatty acids in mammals, is sensitive to the regulation of lipogenesis in the liver and adipose tissue.[24,25] Interestingly, high activity and overexpression of FAS has been observed in biologically aggressive human breast cancer, indicating that FAS dependent lipogenesis does not respond to nutritional regulation.[24,25] Menendez et al.[24] determined the role of n-3 and n-6 polyunsaturated fatty acids (PUFA) on the enzymatic activity and protein expression of tumor associated FAS in SK-Br3 human breast cancer cells. ALA reduced FAS in a dose dependent manner up to 61%, DHA reduced it by 37%, while EPA was ineffective. γ-Linolenic acid was most effective with a greater than 75% reduction in FAS activity. The n-3 fatty acid–induced reduction in FAS activities and protein expression caused a cytotoxic effect, which is related to peroxidative mechanisms. Hence, ALA and γ-linolenic acid usually lose their FAS inhibitory effect in the presence of antioxidants such as vitamin E. However, ALA and γ-linolenic acid have an additive effect on FAS inhibition, and this was only partially reversed by vitamin E. This indicates that the combination of an ALA-rich oil such as FO and a γ-linolenic acid–rich oil, such as primrose oil, may have a greater anticancer effect through this mechanism than when consumed alone.

8.2.6 α-Linolenic Acid Combined with Phytosterols

Phytosterols, commonly found in plant oils, seeds, cereals, nuts, and legumes, are well known to have a hypocholesterolemic effect (Chapter 2), but studies also suggest that they have anticancer effects. *In vitro* studies have shown that phytosterols can reduce the growth and/or increase apoptosis in human prostate cancer[26,27] and in MDA MB 231 human breast cancer cell lines.[28] β-Sitosterol lowered the incidence of chemically induced colon tumors in rats and the growth of human breast cancer MDA MB 231 cells,[29] estrogen stimulated MCF-7 tumors,[30] and prostate cancer (PC-3) in SCID mice.[26]

The interaction between dietary phytosterols and ALA on tissue levels of phytosterols and cholesterol in rats has been determined.[31] Rats were fed a diet with sunflower oil (70 g/kg diet) or a mixture of sunflower oil (60 g) and 10 g ALA such that the LA/ALA ratio was 117:1 and 3.6:1, respectively. To both diets was then added 2000 mg phytosterols/kg diet. After 29 days of diet treatment, the ALA-rich diet increased the incorporation of phytosterols into tissues (liver, heart, lung). Because phytosterols have potential anticancer effects, the increased tissue uptake of phytosterols induced by ALA may increase the effectiveness of phytosterols as anticancer agents. However, this has yet to be demonstrated in scientific experiments.

8.2.7 Sesame Seed Lignans, n-3 Fatty Acids, and Tocopherols

Sesame seed (SS) is an oilseed with some similarities with FS. Both contain more than 40% oil, 20% protein, vitamin E primarily as γ-tocopherol, and extremely high amounts of lignans.[32] However, the main lignan in FS is SDG, which is water soluble and found in the nonfat portion of the seed, while the major lignans in sesame seed are sesamin, sesamolin, and sesaminol (Figure 8.1), with the first two primarily fat soluble and found largely in the oil fraction. Sesame seed and its oil have health benefits including antioxidant,[33,34] blood pressure lowering,[35,36] serum lipid lowering,[37–40] and anticarcinogen[41] activities; these benefits have been attributed in part to its plant lignans. In particular, sesamin has been shown to reduce the number of DMBA-induced tumors in rats, which has been ascribed to inhibition of PGE2 synthesis, immunopotentiation, and enhanced antioxidant activity.[41]

The tocopherols have high antioxidant activities, but α-tocopherol has gained more attention than γ-tocopherol because of its higher vitamin E activity. However, γ-tocopherol has properties that make it distinct from α-tocopherol. It can be metabolized to 5-NO_2-γ-tocopherol by the scavenging NO radical, its γ-carboxyethylhydroxychroman (α-CEHC) metabolite has natriuretic activity, and γ-tocopherol but not α-tocopherol has anti-inflammatory properties.[32,42–44]

Previous studies have shown that sesame seed and its lignans can increase the α- and γ-tocopherols in the plasma and tissues of rats.[45,46] The increase in γ-tocopherol was due to the ability of sesame lignans to inhibit the oxidation of the phytyl side chain in the metabolism of γ-tocopherol to γ-CEHC.[47–49] γ-Tocopherol has been shown to act synergistically with lignans (sesamin) in sesame seed to produce vitamin E activity equivalent to that of α-tocopherol.[45] In contrast, FS lignans did not prevent the metabolism of γ-tocopherol to γ-CEHC, and therefore did not cause an increase in γ-tocopherol in the plasma and tissues of rats fed either FS, defatted FS, or FO.[32] When FO was combined with sesamin, the γ-tocopherol concentration was significantly increased by about ninefold. The concentration of thiobarbituric acid reducing substances (TBARS), as an indicator of lipid peroxidation in the plasma and liver of rats, was increased by FS and FO because of their high concentration of the highly oxidizable ALA. However, it was almost completely suppressed by the combination of FO with sesamin. All these indicate that sesame lignans are acting synergistically with the ALA-rich oil in FS in increasing γ-tocopherol concentration and hence antioxidant properties.

Because DHA is another n-3 fatty acid that is susceptible to oxidation, its effect (at 0.5% level) in combination with sesamin or sesaminol (at 0.2% level) on lipid peroxidation in rats fed a low α-tocopherol (10 mg/kg) diet was determined.[50,51] The plasma and liver TBARS concentrations was increased and the α-tocopherol was decreased by DHA alone, but these were suppressed when sesamin or sesaminol were added to the diet. Together, they also caused a significant increase of DHA in the triacylglycerol of plasma. This indicates that sesamin and α-tocopherol can synergistically suppress the lipid peroxidation in rats fed DHA by elevating α-tocopherol.

Sesame lignans (sesamin, sesaminol, sesamolin, and sesamol) have also been shown to inhibit the delta-5 desaturation of n-6 fatty acids in the liver. This caused the accumulation of dihomo-γ-linolenic acid and, consequently, reduction in the formation of AA and inflammatory PGE2.[52–54] On the other hand, the delta saturation index of n-3 fatty acids, i.e., the ratio of EPA to ALA, was increased,[55] indicating that in rat livers sesame lignans can promote the inhibition of delta-5 desaturation of n-6 fatty acids but not that of n-3 fatty acids. This implies that inflammation may be reduced if ALA-rich oil is consumed with sesame lignans. Similar results were observed when sesamin was combined with EPA.[56]

Sesamin and α-tocopherol in combination (both at 0.5% level) decreased the production of AA, C22:5n6, and eicosanoids in various tissues, increased the production of IgA, IgG, and IgM by mesenteric lymph node lymphocytes, and reduced IgE. These changes were not apparent when sesamin and α-tocopherol were fed separately.[57] These results indicate that the combination of sesamin and α-tocopherol acted synergistically in regulating the production of eicosanoids and modifying immune function.

8.3 Food–Drug Synergy

Cancer patients often change their diets to complement their drug treatments. Although much has been written about food–drug interactions and their adverse effects,[58,59] increasing evidence suggests that there are potential health benefits as well. Some of these are summarized in Table 8.1, Table 8.2, and Table 8.3.

8.3.1 Flaxseed and Its Lignans Combined with Tamoxifen

Many breast cancer patients take drugs to prevent the growth or recurrence of tumors. One of the drugs commonly prescribed to breast cancer patients

TABLE 8.1

Interactive Effect of 10% Flaxseed (FS) and Tamoxifen (TAM) in Ovariectomized Athymic Mice in the Presence of High or Low Levels of Estradiol (E2)

	Tumor Volume (mm^3)	Ki-67 Labeling Index (%)	Apoptotic Index (cell number/mm^2)
With E2			
Control	352.37 ± 50.54[a]	49.08 ± 2.17[a]	1.78 ± 0.11[a]
FS	268.54 ± 18.84[b]	34.25 ± 2.08[b]	3.45 ± 0.27[b]
TAM	186.93 ± 19.23[c]	34.55 ± 2.01[b]	3.72 ± 0.30[b]
FS + TAM	170.22 ± 21.99[c]	28.54 ± 1.56[c]	4.02 ± 0.33[b]
Without E2			
Control	5.95 ± 1.53[a]	20.43 ± 1.12[a]	6.27 ± 0.44[a]
FS	8.17 ± 1.35[a]	21.52 ± 2.53[a]	5.28 ± 0.52[a]
TAM	56.94 ± 5.63[b]	33.21 ± 2.05[b]	3.45 ± 0.33[b]
FS + TAM	21.49 ± 3.35[c]	26.22 ± 1.29[a]	5.59 ± 0.30[a]

Note: Data are means ± SEM. Means within a column with different superscripts are significantly different; $p < .05$.

Source: Modified from Chen, J. et al., *Clin. Cancer Res.*, 10, 7703, 2004.

TABLE 8.2

Synergistic Interactions of Food or Food Components with Cancer Drugs or Treatment: *In Vitro* Studies

Food	Drugs	Cancer Cell Model System	Ref.
n-3 PUFA	Doxorubicin	L1210 murine leukemia	83, 84
		Glioblastoma	85
		Small cell lung carcinoma	86
		MDA MB 231 breast	75, 77
		ZR-75-1 breast	87, 88
		Transformed rat fibroblasts	89
		PC-3 prostate	87
		A549 lung	87
		THKE tumorigenic human kidney epithelial	90
EPA	TNP-470	MDA MB 231, T-47D, MCF-7, KPL-1, MKL-F breast	91
EPA, GLA	Doxorubicin	Cisplatin resistant human ovarian	82
n-3 PUFA	5-Fluorouracil	Caco-2 colon	92
GLA, EPA, DHA, ALA	Vincristine	KB-3-1 (vincristine-sensitive)	93
		KB-Ch-8-5 (vincristine resistant)	94
		Human cervical carcinoma (HeLa-variant)	
DHA	Methotrexate (MTX) complex with DHA	T27A murine non-T non-B leukemia	95

PUFA — polyunsaturated fatty acids; EPA — ecosapentaenoic acid; GLA — γ-linolenic acid; ALA — α-linolenic acid; DHA — docosahexaenoic acid

TABLE 8.3
Synergistic Interactions of Food or Food Components with Cancer Drugs or Treatment: Animal Studies

Food	Drugs	Cancer Model System	Ref.
Fish oil	Mitomycin C	Human mammary tumor	80, 96
	Edelfosine	MDA MB 231 human breast tumor	75
	Irinotecan(CPT-11)	MCF-7 human breast tumor	76
	Doxorubicin	A549 human lung tumor	97
	Epirubicin(anthracycline)	Rat mammary tumor	98
	Cyclophosphamide	MX-1 human mammary tumor	81
	Mitomycin	MX-1 human mammary tumors	80
	Cisplatin	Lewis lung carcinoma 2LL	78
	Naproxen	Walker 256 tumor	79
	Clenbuterol		
	Naproxen + clenbuterol		
	Naproxen + clenbuterol + insulin		
Fish oil concentrate	Doxorubicin	MDA MB 231 human breast tumor	99
DHA	*cis*-Diamine dichloro-platinum(II) (CDDP)	Human embryonal carcinoma	100
	Cisplatin		
DHA	Irradiation	MNU induced rat mammary tumors	101
	Paclitaxel (complexed with DHA)el	M109 mouse lung carcinoma	102

DHA-docosahexaenoic acid; MNU-methylnitrosourea

is tamoxifen (TAM), a triphenylethylene derivative with 4 OH-TAM as a main metabolite, with both weak estrogenic and antiestrogenic properties.[60] Its use was originally restricted to women with ER+ breast tumors based on the findings that TAM competes with estrogen for its binding with the ER and therefore inhibits estrogen-mediated events that lead to tumor growth.[60] However, alternate ER-independent mechanisms of action of TAM have also been suggested[61] because of observations that 30% of women bearing ER tumors respond to TAM treatment and 30% of patients with ER+ tumors do not respond to this antiestrogen. Also, TAM has been shown to inhibit the growth of ER breast cancer cell lines such as MDA MB 231 and MDA MB 435.[62] As previously summarized,[60,62,63] ER independent mechanisms for TAM include: (a) inhibition of protein kinase C; (b) up-regulation of c-myc expression; (c) modulation of growth factor (e.g., IGF-1) expression; (d) inhibition of enzymes involved in estrogen synthesis and signal transduction; (e) inhibition of lipid peroxidation; (f) reduction in calcium influx by affecting membrane channels; (g) inhibition of angiogenesis; and (h) increasing apoptosis. Because lignans, like TAM, may protect against breast cancer not only by a nonhormonal mechanism but also by interfering with the binding of estrogen to ER, it was thought that the intake of lignan-rich foods such as FS might interfere with the therapeutic effect of TAM and that this effect is dependent on the circulating estrogen level and whether the breast tumor is ER or ER+. However, recent experiments conducted in our laboratory[14,64] and described in the following paragraphs suggest that the combination of TAM and FS or its lignans do not act antagonistically but rather beneficially in reducing human tumor development (Table 8.1).

8.3.1.1 Athymic Mice Study with ER+ MCF-7 Breast Tumors

One study determined the effect of 10% FS, TAM, and their combination in ovariectomized athymic mice to simulate the low circulating estrogen level in postmenopausal women (Table 8.1).[14] Ovariectomized mice were injected with ER+ MCF-7 cancer cells and implanted with estradiol (E2) pellets to allow tumor growth. When the mean palpable tumor size was about 40 mm^2, the E2 pellet was removed and mice were then randomized to either 10% FS, TAM, or combined 10% FS and TAM treatment groups. The palpable tumor area regressed significantly in all treatment groups except in the TAM group. The tumor area in the 10% FS group did not differ significantly from the negative control group. Palpable tumor areas of mice with TAM treatment alone initially regressed but then started to increase after 4 to 5 weeks of treatment. The increase was reduced when TAM was combined with a 10% FS diet. These results indicate that 10% FS does not exert an estrogenic effect in the presence of low levels of circulating estrogen and that TAM exerts a late stage weak estrogenic effect, which can be counteracted by antiestrogenic components of FS such as the lignans.

In another study with a similar experimental design as the preceding one, the treatments were provided after the old E2 pellet was replaced with a new one.[14] Thus, the circulating estrogen level was high, simulating the high levels of circulating estrogen in premenopausal women. FS and TAM treatments alone significantly retarded the tumor growth to a similar extent. When combined, FS and TAM caused an even greater reduction (47%) in tumor growth compared with the control, and resulted in a 36 and 16% reduction in tumor size than FS or TAM treatment alone, respectively.

In both of the above experiments, the reduction in tumor growth by the treatments was accompanied by decreased tumor cell proliferation and increased apoptosis (Table 8.1), further supporting the effectiveness of the combination of TAM and FS.

8.3.1.2 In Vitro *Study with ER-MDA MB 435 Breast Cancer Cells*

As earlier mentioned, we have shown that 10% FS can significantly reduce the growth and metastasis of the ER-MDA MB 435 breast cancer and this was in part due to the SDG from FS.[13] The metastasis process is a complex one, involving cell adhesion, invasion, and migration steps. *In vitro* studies using these ER human breast cancer cells showed that ED and EL derived from SDG can dose dependently reduce all the steps of metastasis. Moreover, the effects of ED and EL are similar to TAM; however their effects were greater when used in combination than when used singly.[64] For example, ED, EL, and TAM at 1 μM reduced the tumor cell adhesion to a maximum of 20% when used singly. In combination, the reduction increased to 36%. Similarly, when used singly at 1 μM concentration, reduction in tumor cell invasion was a maximum of 23%, but in combination the reduction was 40%. The results observed with another ER human breast cancer cell line, MDA MB 231, followed the same pattern.[64] These findings further indicate that the lignans do not interfere with but rather improve the anticancer action of TAM even in ER-human breast cancer cells.

8.3.2 n-3 Fatty Acids Combined with Cancer Drugs

The ALA from FS can be metabolized to the long chain n-3 fatty acids, EPA, and DHA. Although the conversion is limited and may depend on the intakes of total fat, ALA, EPA, DHA, and LA,[65–68] the interaction of EPA and DHA with drugs is relevant to the understanding of the potential effect of ALA and ALA-rich foods such as FS.

Epidemiologic data on the association between the intake of fish or fish oil, the richest source of EPA and DHA, and the risk of breast, prostate, endometrial, or ovary cancer is inconsistent, with about one-third to one-half of the studies showing significant reductions while the others showed nonsignificant inverse association or no association.[69] Several reasons for this discrepancy have been provided including (a) low intake of n-3 fatty acids in some of the populations; (b) low within-population variability in fish or n-3 fatty acid intake; and (c) the critical period for n-3 fatty acid exposure may be during childhood or early adulthood and yet many of the studies may have provided exposure only during middle or old age.[7] However, there is considerable evidence from experimental studies[70–74] that fish oil, DHA, and/or EPA can inhibit carcinogenesis. Mechanisms for the effect of n-3 fatty acids include (a) suppression of AA-derived eicosanoid biosynthesis, which results in altered immune response to cancer cells and modulation of inflammation, cell proliferation, apoptosis, metastasis, and angiogenesis; (b) effect on transcription activity, gene expression, and signal transduction factor activity, which leads to changes in cell metabolism, cell growth, and differentiation; (c) alteration of estrogen metabolism, which leads to reduced estrogen-stimulated cell growth; (d) increased production of free radicals and reactive oxygen species; and (e) mechanism involving insulin sensitivity and membrane fluidity.[7,72]

Because many of the mechanisms whereby DHA and EPA exert their effects are similar to those of many chemotherapeutic drugs, it was thought that combining cancer drugs with fish oil or the n-3 fatty acids DHA or EPA would increase the efficacy of the drugs. For example, both the n-3 fatty acids and drugs such as edelfosine, CPT-11 (irinotecan), doxorubicin, and epirubicin, and radiation increase lipid peroxidation and hence free radicals in the tumor to cytotoxic levels.[75,76] The mechanism involved lipid peroxidation because the effectiveness of these compounds was reduced when antioxidants such as vitamin E or vitamin C were added to the *in vitro* or *in vivo* system while it was increased when a prooxidant such as iron was added.[77,78] Drugs such as naproxen and clenbuterol can act as inhibitors of inflammatory prostaglandin synthesis, similar to n-3 fatty acids.[79] Also, the n-3 fatty acids can enhance the membrane permeability and thus increase the uptake of drugs such as doxorubicin, mitomycin, and cyclophosphamide.[80–82]

Many *in vitro* studies, summarized in Table 8.2, showed that the n-3 fatty acids act synergistically with chemotherapeutic drugs such as doxorubicin, TNP-470, 5-fluorouracil, vincristine, and methotrexate in reducing the growth of several cancer cell lines, including L1210 murine leukemia cells, small lung carcinoma, MDA MB 231, ZR-75-1 breast cancer, transformed fibroblast, PC-3 prostate, A549 lung, THKE tumorigenic human kidney epithelial, T-47D, MCF-7, KPL-1, MKL-F breast cancer cell, Caco-2 colon cancer, vincristine-sensitive KB-3-1, vincristine-resistant KB-Ch-8-5 human cervical carcinoma (HeLa variant), and T27A murine non-T non-B leukemia cell line.[75,77,82–95]

Likewise, as summarized in Table 8.3, a synergistic effect in reducing tumor growth or regressing tumor size was observed upon feeding fish oil, DHA, or fish oil concentrate (with 34 % EPA, 24% DHA, 10% other n-3 fatty acids primarily ALA) with a variety of chemotherapeutic drugs (mitomycin, cyclophosphamide, edelfosine, irinotecan, doxorubicin, epirubicin, mitomycin, *cis*-platin, *cis*-diamine-dichloro-platinum(II) cisplatin, naproxen, clenbuterol, paclitaxel, irradiation) to athymic mice with human breast, lung, or embryonal carcinoma or rats with carcinogen induced tumors.[75–81,96–102] DHA also sensitized MNU-induced mammary tumors to radiation therapy. This effect was likely mediated by increased oxidative stress.[101]

In addition to increasing the efficacy of cancer drugs, n-3 fatty acids have also been shown to reduce their gastrointestinal, hematological, and cardiac side effects.[76,81,98,103] For example, CPT-11, a water soluble derivative of camptothecin, and a topoisomerase I inhibitor drug, has been used to treat many cancer types, including breast, colorectal, ovarian, lymphoma, gliomas, and small cell and non–small cell lung.[104–106] It was found to be the most effective chemotherapeutic agent when compared with cisplatin, doxorubicin, and topotecan against xenografts of lung (H460, A549, H226), breast (MCF-7, T47-D, MDA MB 231), and colon (SW 620, COLO 205 and HT-29) cancer cell lines in nude mice. Its major side effects include debilitating and delayed diarrhea, which accompanies degeneration and necrosis of intestinal villi and crypt cells, as well as anemia, leukopenia, asthenia, weight loss, and liver enlargement.[103] However, the intestinal mucosal architecture was largely unchanged when the fish oil diet was fed to athymic mice with established MCF-7 human breast carcinoma.[76] An n-3 fatty acid product (INCELL AAFA) containing a total of 55% EPA + DHA also reduced intestinal damage and liver inflammation caused by CPT-11 in mice. It also improved white and red cell blood counts, and maintained normal grooming behavior.[103]

Drug resistance is a major problem that leads to cancer therapy failure.[93] This resistance has been attributed in part to reduction in intracellular accumulation of the drug due to reduced uptake and/or increased efflux. However, n-3 fatty acids reversed drug resistance in tumor cells. *In vitro* experiments where GLA, ALA, EPA, or DHA were added to vincristine showed higher intracellular concentrations of vincristine in HeLA cells, vincristine-sensitive (KB-30-1) and -resistant (KB-Ch-8-5) human cervical cells, and hence, increased cytoxicity, than when vincristine was given alone.[93,94] The incorporation of the n-3 fatty acids to membrane lipids increased the membrane fluidity and enhanced the uptake and reduced the efflux of the drug.

When given either before or after chemotherapy, n-3 fatty acids have also been shown to decrease cancer-related cachexia[79,107–111] and to protect from alopecia.[112] The effect of fish oil in reducing both tumor growth and cachexia in Walker 256 tumor bearing rats was potentiated by cotreatment with naproxen, insulin, and clenbuterol, aβ_2 adrenergic agonist.[79]

Because of the strong interaction between n-3 fatty acids such as DHA and drugs, novel DHA containing anticancer agents have been developed. One is DHA conjugated through an ester bond to the paclitaxel 2 oxygen.[102] Paclitaxel, a complex taxane diterpene, is the active component of Taxol, one of the most effective cancer drugs, and is approved for use in the United States against ovarian, breast, and lung cancers and Kaposi's sarcoma.[102] Conjugation of paclitaxel with DHA has been shown to improve the tumor targeting of the drug, i.e., increased the area under the drug concentration-time curve (AUC) in tumors while decreasing the AUC in normal cells, which then increased the therapeutic index (tumor drug exposure time and cure rate) of the drug in the M109 mouse tumor model.[102] At equitoxic doses, the AUC for DHA–paclitaxel conjugate was 61-fold higher than for paclitaxel alone and at equimolar doses, was 8-fold higher. Studies in patients showed that the conjugate was well-tolerated and about 50% of the 22 patients transitioned from progressive to stable disease.[102]

The second conjugate is a novel phophatidylcholine containing DHA in the sn-1 acyl-chain and methotrexate (MTX) in the sn-2 chain.[95] MTX is a major antimetabolite used for chemotherapy of many different types of cancer. It is an antifolate, which interferes with the ability of the cells to synthesize purines and thymidylic acid needed for DNA synthesis and cell division. Although DHA and MTX alone inhibited the cell proliferation of T27A cells *in vitro*, the conjugate caused an inhibition that was greater than the sum of the inhibition caused by DHA and MTX, indicating a synergistic effect. Covalently linking these two agents ensured concurrent delivery and better targeting of specific cancer cells.

8.4 Safety Aspects

There are concerns regarding the potential adverse effects of FS. ALA in FS is very susceptible to oxidation and may consequently increase oxidative stress, decrease the antioxidant capacity in tissues, and increase the requirement for antioxidants such as vitamin E. Rats fed FO have increased tissue TBARS, an index of lipid peroxidation,[113] and those fed 40% FS for 90 days had lower tissue vitamin E levels than the control.[114] Similarly, reductions in liver and heart vitamin E were observed in rats fed 40% FS or 26% partially defatted FS.[115] Hyperlipidemic subjects fed 50 g partially defatted FS for 3 weeks had reduced serum thiol levels, indicating increased oxidative stress, compared with control.[116] On the contrary, the intakes of FS or FO did not affect the vitamin E or TBARS in the plasma or urine of healthy adults,[117] monkeys, [118] or rats,[119] and an increase in liver vitamin E was observed in rats fed 10% FS. Furthermore, FO and FS did not significantly influence vitamin A status.[115,120,121] Taken in moderation, the natural antioxidants in FS, including the lignans, may counteract the oxidative stress induced by ALA. However, SDG and its oligomers (SDG residues interlinked by 3-hydroxy-3-methyl glutaric acid) at 0.1% in the diet of rats for 27 days caused a twofold reduction in the α- and γ-tocopherol in rat plasma and liver.[122] This was unexpected because phenolic compounds very often act as antioxidants and purified SDG, ED, EL, and secoisolariciresinol have previously been shown *in vitro*[123,124] and in rats[125] to have antioxidant effects. The combination of FO with sesame lignan has also been shown to improve the antioxidant status in rats.[32] Because the data are conflicting, there is a need to further study the relationship between antioxidant status and the intake of FS and its component lignans and FO, alone and in combination.

Several epidemiological studies suggest a positive relationship between ALA intake and the risk of advanced prostate cancer but not of total prostate cancer.[126,127] In contrast, the daily intake of 30 g FS in a low fat diet regimen appears to improve the prognosis of prostate cancer patients when compared with historical controls.[16,17] If the latter was due to other components of FS, such as the lignans, counteracting any tumor promoting effect of the ALA, then it is probably safer to consume FS, which combines both components, rather than ALA-rich FO alone, for reducing prostate cancer risk. In light of the known protective effect of ALA on coronary heart disease[126] and its potential adverse effect on prostate cancer, FO should probably be consumed by prostate cancer patients with caution until such time as the role of ALA on prostate cancer is clarified.

In contrast to ALA, the other n-3 fatty acids, EPA and DHA, particularly rich in fish, were found to be protective not only against cardiovascular disease (Chapter 2) but also against prostate cancer.[127] The intake of fish oil supplements appears to have no adverse effect except for some gastrointestinal effects when taken in large concentration (see Chapter 2). However, there are concerns that the intake of farmed fish such as salmon may increase the risk for cancer because of contaminants such as polychlorinated biphenyls, toxaphene, and dieldrin.[128,129] Hites[129] suggested that on the basis of the U.S. Environmental Protection Agency estimates of 55 g monthly consumption of the most contaminated salmon, cancer risk would increase theoretically by 1 in 100,000 and if cancer risk is linear, the cancer risk will increase at 22 cases per 100,000 with a monthly intake of 1190 g (21 g n-3 fatty acids) salmon. It was also suggested that because of the contaminants, salmon should not be eaten more often than 0.25 to 1 time per month. However, these have been disputed by others,[130,131] who indicated that the risk may be an overestimation, and, considering risk benefit analysis, restrictions should not be recommended.

While n-3 fatty acids have been shown to be protective against many primary cancers, others noted ambiguity over their safety with respect to secondary tumor formation.[132] Rats with experimentally induced colon cancer and fed 20% fish oil diet had 1000-fold more metastases and higher secondary tumor formation than the control group fed a low fat diet or a diet enriched with safflower oil.[133] Also, colon cancer cells treated with DHA had decreased adherence to extracellular matrix proteins, suggesting potential for increased tumor cell motility, survival, and hence metastasis.[134] These effects require further clarification in clinical trials but may need to be taken into consideration when fish oil is consumed with or without cancer drugs.

TAM increased the uterine weight of ovariectomized athymic mice relative to control, but it was prevented when TAM was combined with the feeding of 10% FS.[14] The effect of combined TAM and FS treatment on bone, which is sensitive to hormonal changes, has yet to be determined. The mechanism by which the combination of soy and FS affects the uterus and bone also still needs to be established. If the cancer protective effects of these combinations are achieved without adverse effects on other hormone related organs, then the use of these combinations can be further justified.

Exposure to lignans during gestation or suckling stage has been shown to reduce the risk of breast cancer during adulthood.[8–10] Because the lignans have potential antiestrogenic and estrogenic effects, there are concerns regarding the effect of FS and specifically the lignans on the male and female reproductive function and fetal development. Studies have shown that the lignans can be transferred to the suckling offspring via mother's milk.[135] There was no effect on reproductive indices of the offspring when FS was given to the dams during the lactation stage only.[9,136] Feeding 5 or 10% FS during pregnancy had no adverse effects on the rat dams and offspring except for the lower birth weight in the male offspring of dams fed the 10% FS.[135,137,138] However, there was lengthening of estrous cycles in the female offspring. In a later study, 20 and 40% FS or 13 and 26% partially defatted FS (with lower fat but the same amount of lignans as the 20 or 40% FS) were shown to result in normal pregnancy (fertility, litter size, live birth index, and offspring survival) and birth weight of offspring but affected developmental parameters (gestation length, anogenital distance, puberty onset, estrous cycles) in the offspring.[139,140] Feeding FS lengthened the estrous cycle as well, but the greatest frequency of lengthened cycles were observed in the 26% partially defatted FS. The 40% FS had no effect on gestation length, while the 26% partially defatted FS significantly shortened gestation length. These suggest that at high levels of FS intake, the regulation of the estrous cycle and gestation length depends not only on the hormonal effect of the lignans but also on ALA. The ALA-rich oil appears to provide protection against any estrogenic effect of the lignans in FS. The effect of FS appears to be dependent on the dose, timing, and duration of exposure.[135,137–140]

FS contains the cyanogenic glycosides linustatin, neolinustatin, and methyl ethyl ketone cyanohydrin, which release cyanides upon hydrolysis and may cause a toxic response in certain individuals when consumed raw in very large concentrations (e.g. greater than 50 g).[141] However, when FS is processed or incorporated into baked products, the cyanogens are destroyed and undetectable,[142] and so may not pose a problem. Sesame seed is now widely used not only in Asia but also in North America and Europe. It was noted that the increased consumption of foods containing sesame seed and oil appears to parallel an increase in sesame seed–induced allergic reactions.[143] Individuals with allergies should therefore test their reactions to sesame seed before consuming them in large amounts.

8.5 Conclusions

FS has cancer protective effects that can be attributed to the combined effects of its lignans and ALA-rich oil. γ-Linolenic acid and phytosterols can potentially increase synergistically the anticancer potential of ALA. Sesame lignans act synergistically with the ALA-rich oil to increase γ-tocopherol concentration and hence antioxidant properties. Sesame lignans combined with γ-tocopherol act synergistically to produce vitamin E activity equivalent to that of α-tocopherol. The combination of soy and FS or their isoflavones and lignans is more beneficial than the soy or isoflavone alone in controlling human breast cancer growth under low estrogen levels simulating postmenopausal situations. FS does not interfere but rather enhances the tumor growth inhibitory effect of TAM in the presence of high or low levels of estrogen simulating pre- and postmenopausal situations, respectively. The n-3 fatty acids, particularly EPA and DHA from fish oil, can react synergistically with many drugs in reducing tumor growth and metastasis while reducing undesirable side effects. They can also be conjugated to facilitate the targeting of tumors and further increase their effectiveness.

It is evident from the previous paragraph that (1) foods such as FS, soy, sesame seed, and fish oil, (2) their components such as lignans, isoflavones, and n-3 fatty acids, and (3) drugs can synergistically interact to increase their effectiveness against cancer. These interactions enhance the anticancer effects with no or reduced toxicity in many cases. However, there are certain safety issues that need to be taken into consideration in some cases. Many of the studies have been done primarily using *in vitro* or animal models and more clinical studies are still needed to confirm the effectiveness of the interactions in humans. However, the results so far are promising and further emphasize that foods, food components, and drugs should be studied more in combination than in isolation for their potential effect in the prevention and treatment of cancer.

Acknowledgments

The cited work of the author was funded by the Natural Sciences and Engineering Research Council of Canada, the American Institute for Cancer Research, the Flax Council of Canada, the Saskatchewan Flax Development Commission, U.S. National Institutes of Health, the Program in Food Safety (University of Toronto), and the Canadian Breast Cancer Foundation.

References

1. Slattery, M.L. et al., Plant foods, fiber, and rectal cancer, *Am. J. Clin. Nutr.*, 79, 274, 2004.
2. Swanson, C.A., Vegetables, fruits, and cancer risk: The role of phytochemicals, in *Phytochemicals, a new paradigm*, Bidlack, W.R. et al., Eds., Technomic Publications, Lancaster, 1998, p. 1.
3. Thompson, L.U. et al., Mammalian lignan production from various foods, *Nutr. Cancer*, 16, 43, 1991.
4. Thompson, L.U., Flaxseed, lignans and cancer, in *Flaxseed in human nutrition*, 2nd ed., Thompson, L.U. and Cunnane, S.C., Eds. AOCS Press, Champaign, IL, 2003, p. 194.
5. Setchell, K.D.R., Discovery and potential clinical importance of mammalian lignans, in *Flaxseed in human nutrition*, 1st ed., Cunnane, S.C. and Thompson, L.U., Eds., AOCS Press, Champaign, IL, 1995, p. 82.
6. Heinonen, S. et al., *In vitro* metabolism of plant lignans: new precursor of mammalian lignan enterolactone and enterodiol, *J. Agric. Food Chem.*, 49, 3178, 2001.
7. Larson, S.C. et al., Dietary long-chain n-3 fatty acids for the prevention of cancer: a review of potential mechanism, *Am. J. Clin. Nutr.*, 79, 935, 2004.
8. Ward, W., Jiang, F., and Thompson, L.U., Exposure to flaxseed or purified lignan during lactation influences rat mammary gland structures, *Nutr. Cancer*, 37, 187, 2000.
9. Tan, K. et al., Mammary gland morphogenesis is enhanced by exposure to flaxseed or its major lignan during suckling in rats, *Exp. Biol. Med.*, 229, 147, 2004.
10. Chen, J. et al., Exposure to flaxseed or its purified lignan during suckling inhibits chemically induced rat mammary tumorigenesis, *Exp. Biol. Med. (Maywood)*, 228, 951, 2003.
11. Serraino, M. and Thompson, L.U., The effect of flaxseed supplementation on the initiation and promotional stages of mammary tumorigenesis, *Nutr. Cancer*, 17, 153, 1992.

12. Thompson, L.U. et al., Flaxseed and its lignan and oil components reduce mammary tumor growth at a late stage of carcinogenesis, *Carcinogenesis*, 17, 1373, 1996.
13. Chen, J., Stavro, P., and Thompson, L.U., Dietary flaxseed inhibits human breast cancer growth and metastasis and downregulates expression of insulin-like growth factor and epidermal growth factor receptor, *Nutr. Cancer*, 43, 187, 2002.
14. Chen, J. et al., Dietary flaxseed enhances the inhibitory effect of tamoxifen on the growth of estrogen-dependent human breast cancer (MCF-7) in nude mice, *Clin. Cancer Res.*, 10, 7703, 2004.
15. Thompson, L.U. et al., Dietary flaxseed alters tumor biological markers in postmenopausal breast cancer, *Clin. Cancer Res.*, 2005, in press.
16. Demark-Wahnefried, W. et al., Pilot study of dietary fat restriction and flaxseed supplementation in men with prostate cancer before surgery: Exploring the effects on hormonal levels, prostate-specific antigen, and histopathologic features, *Urology*, 58, 47, 2001.
17. Demark-Wahnefried, W. et al., Pilot study to explore effects of low-fat, flaxseed-supplemented diet on proliferation of benign prostatic epithelium and prostate-specific antigen, *Urology*, 63, 900, 2004.
18. Lin, X. et al., Effect of flaxseed supplementation on prostatic carcinoma in transgenic mice, *Urology*, 60, 919, 2002.
19. Thompson, L.U. et al., Antitumorigenic effect of a mammalian lignan precursor from flaxseed, *Nutr. Cancer*, 26, 159, 1996.
20. Wang, L., Chen, J., and Thompson, L.U., The inhibitory effect of flaxseed on the growth and metastastis of human breast cancer is attributed to its lignan and oil components, *Int. J. Cancer*, 2005, in press.
21. Power, K. et al., Lignans (enterolactone and enterodiol) negate the proliferative effect of isoflavone (genistein) on MCF-7 breast cancer cells in vitro and in vivo, *Proc. Am. Assoc. Cancer Res.*, 45, 878, 2004.
22. Saarinen, N. et al., Flaxseed attenuates the tumor promoting effect of soy in ovariectomized athymic mice with breast cancer xenografts, *Proc.Am. Assoc. Cancer Res.*, 45, 878, 2004.
23. Power, K. et al., Interactive effects of flaxseed and soy on human breast cancer, *Proc. U.S. Flax Inst.*, 60, 80, 2004.
24. Menendez, J.A. et al., Overexpression and hyperactivity of breast cancer-associated fatty acid synthase (oncogenic antigen 519) is insensitive to normal arachidonic acid fatty acid-induced suppression in lipogenic tissue but it is selectively inhibited by tumoricidal alpha linolenic and gamma linolenic fatty acids: a novel mechanism by which dietary fat can alter mammary tumorigenisis, *Int. J. Oncol.*, 24, 1369, 2004.
25. Menendez, J.A. et al., Novel signaling molecules implicated in tumor-associated fatty acid synthase-dependent breast cancer cell proliferation and survival: Role of exogenous dietary fatty acids, p53-p21WAF1/C1P1, ERK1/2MAPK, p27KIP1, BRCA1, and NF-kappaB, *Int. J. Oncol.*, 24, 591, 2004.
26. Awad, A.B. et al., *In vitro* and *in vivo* (SCID mice) effects of phytosterols on the growth and dissemination of human prostate cancer PC-3 cells, *Eur. J. Cancer Prev.*, 10, 507, 2001.
27. von Holtz, R.L., Fink, C.S., and Awad, A.B., Beta sitosterol activates the sphingomyelin cycle and induces apoptosis in LNCaP human prostate cancer cells, *Nutr. Cancer*, 32, 8, 1998.

28. Awad, A.B., Roy, R., and Fink, C.S., Beta sitosterol, a plant sterol induces apoptosis and activates key caspases in MDA MB 231 human breast cancer cells, *Oncol. Rep.*, 10, 497, 2003.
29. Awad, A.B. et al., Dietary phytosterols inhibit the growth and metastasis of MDA MB 231 human breast cancer cells grown in SCID mice, *Anticancer Res.*, 20, 821, 2000.
30. Ju, Y.H. et al., Beta-sitosterol, beta-sitosterol glucoside and a mixture of beta-sitosterol and beta- sitosterol glucoside modulate the growth of estrogen-responsive breast cancer cells *in vitro* and *in vivo* in ovariectomized athymic mice, *J. Nutr.*, 134, 1145, 2004.
31. Oen, J., Li, D., and Sinclair, A.J., Effect of dietary alpha-linolenic acid on incorporation of phytosterols into tissues in rats, *Asia Pac J. Clin. Nutr.*, 12 Suppl, S59, 2003.
32. Yamashita, K., Ikeda, S., and Obayashi, M., Comparative effects of flaxseed and sesame seed on vitamin E and cholesterol levels in rats, *Lipids*, 38,1249, 2003.
33. Ikeda, S., Tohyama, T., and Yamashita, K., Dietary sesame seed and its lignans inhibit 2,7,8-trimethyl-2(2′-carboxylethyl-6 hydroxychroman excretion into urine of rats fed gamma-tocopherol, *J. Nutr.*, 132, 961, 2002.
34. Kang, M.H. et al., Sesamolin inhibits lipid peroxidation in rat liver and kidney, *J. Nutr.*, 128, 1018, 1998.
35. Matsumura, Y. et al., Antihypertensive effect of sesamin. I. Protection against deoxycorticosterone acetate-salt induced hypertension and cardiovascular hypertrophy, *Bio. Pharm. Bull.*, 18, 1016, 1995.
36. Matsumura, Y. et al., Antihypertensive effect of sesamin. II. Protection against development and maintenance of hypertension in stroke prone spontaneously hypertensive rats, *Bio. Pharm. Bull.*, 21, 469, 1998.
37. Hirose, Y. et al., Inhibition of cholesterol absorption and synthesis in rats by sesamin, *J. Lipid Res.*, 32, 629, 1991.
38. Ogawa, H., et al., Sesame lignans modulate cholesterol metabolism in the stroke prone spontaneously hypertensive rat, *Clin. Exp. Pharm. Phys.* 22 (Suppl 1), S310, 1995.
39. Ide, T. et al., Interaction of dietary fat type and sesamin on hepatic fatty acid oxidation in rats, *Biochim. Biophys. Acta*, 1682, 80, 2004.
40. Sirato-Yasumoto S. et al., Effect of sesame seed rich in sesamin and sesamolin on fatty acid oxidation in rat liver, *J. Agric. Food Chem.*, 49, 2647, 2001.
41. Hirose, N. et al., Suppressive effect of sesamin against 7,12 dimethylbenzanthracene induced rat mammary carcinogenesis, *Anticancer Res.*, 12, 1259, 1992.
42. Jiang, Q, et al., Gamma tocopherol and its major metabolite in contrast to alpha tocopherol, inhibit cyclooxygenase activity in macrophages and epithelial cells, *Proc. Natl. Acad. Sci. U.S.A.*, 97, 11494, 2000.
43. Cooney, R.V. et al., Gamma tocopherol detoxification of nitrogen dioxide: Superiority to alpha tocopherol, *Proc. Natl. Acad. Sci. U.S.A.*, 90, 1771, 1993.
44. Christen, S. et al., Gamma tocopherol traps mutagenic electrophiles such as NOx and complements alpha tocopherol: Physiological implications, *Proc. Natl. Acad. Sci. U.S.A.*, 94, 3217, 1997.
45. Yamashita, K. et al., Sesame seed lignans and gamma tocopherol act synergistically to produce vitamin E activity in rats, *J. Nutr.*, 122, 2440, 1992.
46. Yamashita, K. et al., Sesame seed and its lignans produce marked enhancement of vitamin E activity in rats fed a low alpha tocopherol diet, *Lipids* 30, 1019, 1995.

47. Parker, R.S., Sontag, R.S., and Swanson, J.E., Cytochrome P4503A-dependent metabolism of tocopherols and inhibition by sesamin, *Biochem. Biophys. Res. Commun.*, 277, 531, 2000.
48. Sontag, T.J. and Parker, R.S., Cytochrome P450 omega-hydroxylase pathway of tocopherol catabolism. Novel mechanism of regulation of vitamin E status, *J. Biol. Chem.*, 277, 2590, 2002.
49. Ikeda, S., Tohyama, T., and Yamashita, K., Dietary sesame seed and its lignan inhibit 2,7,8-trimethyl-2(2 carboxyethyl) 6-hydroxychroman excretion into urine of rats fed gamma tocopherol, *J. Nutr.*, 132, 961, 2002.
50. Yamashita, K. et al., Sesamin and alpha-tocopherol synergistically suppress lipid peroxide in rats fed a high docosahexaenoic acid diet, *Biofactors.*, 11, 11, 2000.
51. Ikeda, S. et al., Dietary sesame lignans decrease lipid peroxidation in rats fed docosahexaenoic acid, *J. Nutr. Sci. Vitaminol (Tokyo)*, 49, 270, 2003.
52. Chavali, S.R. and Forse, R.A., Decreased production of interleukin-6 and prostaglandin E2 associated with inhibition of delta-5 desaturation of omega 6 fatty acids in mice fed safflower oil diets supplemented with sesamol, *Prost. Leuk. Essent. Fatty Acids*, 61, 347, 1999.
53. Shimizu, S. et al., Sesamin is potent and specific inhibitor of delta 5 desaturase in polyunsaturated fatty acid biosynthesis, *Lipids*, 26, 512, 1991.
54. Chavali, S.R., Zhong, W.W., and Forse, R.A., Dietary alpha linolenic acid increases TNF-alpha, and decreases IL-6 and IL-10 in response to LPS: Effects of sesamin on the delta-5 desaturation of omega 6 and omega 3 fatty acids in mice, *Prost. Leukot. Essent. Fatty Acid*, 58, 185, 1998.
55. Fujiyama-Fujiwara, Y. et al., Effects of sesamin on the fatty acid composition of the liver of rats fed n-6 and n-3 fatty acid-rich diet, *J. Nutr. Sci. Vitaminol. (Tokyo)*, 41, 217, 1995.
56. Umeda-Sawada, R., Takahasi, N., and Igarashi, O., Interaction of sesamin and eisosapentaenoic acid against delta 5 desaturation and n-6/n-3 ratio of essential fatty acids in rat, *Biosci. Biotechnol. Biochem.*, 59, 2268, 1995.
57. Gu, J.Y. et al., Effects of sesamin and alpha tocopherol, individually or in combination, on the polyunsaturated fatty acid metabolism, chemical mediator production, and immunoglobulin levels in Sprague Dawley rats, *Biosci. Biotechnol. Biochem.*, 59, 2198, 1995.
58. Valli, G. and Giardina, E.G., Benefits, adverse effects and drug interactions of herbal therapies with cardiovascular effects, *J. Am. Coll. Cardiol.*, 39, 1083, 2002.
59. Izzo, A.A. and Ernst, E., Interactions between herbal medicines and prescribed drugs: a systematic review, *Drugs*, 61, 2163, 2001.
60. MacGregor, J. and Craig Jordan, V., Basic guide to the mechanisms of antiestrogen action, *Pharmacol. Rev.*, 50,152, 1998.
61. Tormey, D.C. et al., Evaluation of tamoxifen dose in advanced breast cancer: a progress report, *Cancer Treat. Rep.*, 60, 1451, 1976.
62. Charlier, C. et al., Tamoxifen and its active metabolite inhibit growth of estrogen receptor negative MDA-MB435 cells, *Biochem. Pharmacol.*, 49, 351, 1995.
63. Palmieri, C. et al., Estrogen receptor beta in breast cancer, *Endocrine-Related Cancer*, 9, 1, 2002.
64. Chen, J. and Thompson, L.U., Lignans and tamoxifen, alone or in combination, reduce human breast cancer cell adhesion, invasion, and migration *in vitro*, *Breast Cancer Res. Treat.* 80, 163, 2003.

65. Burdge, G., Alpha-linolenic acid metabolism in men and women: nutritional and biological implications, *Curr. Opin. Clin. Nutr. Metab. Care,* 7, 137, 2004.
66. Burdge, G.C. et al., Effect of altered dietary n-3 fatty acid intake upon plasma lipid fatty acid composition, conversion of 13C alpha linolenic acid to longer chain fatty acids and partitioning towards beta-oxidation in older men, *Br. J. Nutr.,* 90, 311, 2003.
67. Emken, E.A., Adlof, R.O., and Gulley, R.M., Dietary linoleic acid influences desaturation and acylation of deuterium-labeled linoleic and linolenic acid in young adult males, *Biochim. Biophys. Acta,* 1213, 277, 1994.
68. Pawlosky, R.J. et al., Physiological compartmental analysis of alpha linolenic acid metabolism in adult humans, *J. Lipid Res.*, 42, 1257, 2001.
69. Terry, P.D., Rohan, T.E., and Wolk, A., Intake of fish and marine fatty acids and the risks of cancers of the breast and prostate and of other hormone-related cancers: a review of the epidemiologic evidence, *Am. J. Clin. Nutr.*, 77, 532, 2003.
70. Roynette, C.E. et al., n-3 polyunsaturated fatty acids and colon cancer prevention, *Clin. Nutr.*, 23,139, 2004.
71. Leitzmann, M.F. et al., Dietary intake of n-3 and n-6 fatty acids and the risk of prostate cancer, *Am. J. Clin. Nutr.*, 80, 204, 2004.
72. Hardman, W.E., Omega-3 fatty acids to augment cancer therapy, *J. Nutr.*, 132, 3508S, 2002.
73. Rose, D.P., and Connely, J.M., Omega-3 fatty acid as cancer chemopreventive agents, *Pharmacol. Ther.*, 83, 217, 1999.
74. Chajes, V. and Bougnoux, P., Omega-6/omega-3 polyunsaturated fatty acid ratio and cancer, *World Rev. Nutr. Diet.*, 92, 133, 2003.
75. Hardman, W.E. et al., Effects of iron supplementation and ET-18-OCH3 on MDA-MB 231 breast carcinomas in nude mice consuming a fish oil diet, *Br. J. Cancer,* 76, 347, 1997.
76. Hardman, W.E., Moyer, M.P., and Cameron, I.L., Fish oil supplementation enhanced CPT-11 (Irinotecan) efficacy against MCF-7 breast carcinoma xenografts and ameliorated intestinal side effects, *Br. J. Cancer,* 81, 440, 1999.
77. Germain, E. et al., Enhancement of doxorubicin cytoxicity by polyunsturaed fatty acids in the human breast tumor cell line MDA-MB-231: relationship to lipid peroxidation, *Int. J. Cancer,* 75, 578, 1998.
78. Yam, D., Peled, A., and Shinitzky, M., Suppression of tumor growth and metastasis by dietary fish oil combined with vitamins E and C and cisplatin, *Cancer Chemother. Pharmacol.*, 47, 34, 2001.
79. Pinto, J.A. et al., Fish oil supplementation in F1 generation associated with naproxen, clenbuterol, and insulin administration reduce tumor growth and cachexia in Walker 256 tumor-bearing rats, *J. Nutr. Biochem.*, 15, 358, 2004.
80. Shao, Y., Pardini, L., and Pardini, R.S., Dietary menhaden oil enhances mitomycin C antitumor activity toward human mammary carcinoma MX-1, *Lipids,* 30, 1035, 1995.
81. Shao, Y., Pardini, L., and Pardini, R.S., Intervention of transplatable human mammary carcinoma MX-1 chemotherapy with dietary menhaden oil in athymic mice; increased therapeutic effects and decreased toxicity of cyclophosphamide, *Nutr. Cancer,* 28, 63, 1997.
82. Plumb, J.A., Luo, W., and Kerr, D.J., Effect of polyunsaturated fatty acids on the drug sensitivity of human tumor cell lines resistant to either cisplatin or doxorubicin, *Br. J. Cancer,* 67, 728, 1993.

83. Guffy, M.M., North, J.A., and Burns, C.P., Effect of cellular fatty acid alteration on adriamycin sensitivity in cultured L1210 murine leukemia cells, *Cancer Res*, 44, 1863, 1984.
84. De Salis, H.M. and Meckling-Gill, K.A., EPA and DHA alter nucleoside drug and doxorubicin toxicity in L1210 cells but not in normal murine S1 macrophages, *Cell Pharmacol.*, 2, 69, 1995.
85. Rudra, P.K. and Krokanm, H.E., Cell-specific enhancement of doxorubicin toxicity in human tumour cells by docohexaenoic acid, *Anticancer Res.*, 21, 29, 2001.
86. Ziljlstra, J.G., Influence of docosahexaenoic acid *in vitro* on intracellular adriamycin concentration in lymphocytes and human adriamycin-sensitive and-resistant small cell lung cancer cell lines, and on cytotoxicty in the tumor cell lines, *Int. J. Cancer*, 90, 850, 1987.
87. Begin, M.E. et al., Differential killing of human carcinoma cells supplemented with n-3 and n-6 polyunsaturated fatty acids, *J. Natl. Cancer Inst.*, 77, 1053, 1986.
88. Begin, M.E., Ellis, G., and Horrobin D.F., Polyunsaturated fatty acid-induced cytoxicity against tumors cells and its relationship to lipid peroxidation, *J. Natl. Cancer Inst.*, 80, 188, 1988.
89. Atkinson, T.G. and Meckling-Gill, K.A., Regulation of nucleoside drug toxicity by transport inhibitors and omega-3 polyunsaturated fatty acids in normal and transformed rat-2 fibroblasts, *Cell. Pharmacol.*, 2, 259, 1995.
90. Maehle, L. et al., Effects of n-3 fatty acids during neoplastic progression and comparison of *in vitro* and *in vivo* sensitivity of two human tumor cell lines, *Br. J. Cancer*, 71, 691, 1995.
91. Yamamoto, D. et al., Synergistic action of apoptosis induced by eicosapentaenoic acid and TNP-470 on human breast cancer cells, *Breast Cancer Res. Treat.*, 55, 149, 1999.
92. Jordan, A. and Stein, J., Effect of an omega-3 fatty acid containing lipid emulsion alone and in combination with 5-fluorouracil (5-FU) on growth of the colon cancer cell line Caco-2, *Eur. J. Nutr.*, 42, 324, 2003.
93. Madhavi, N. and Das, U.N., Effect of n-6 and n-3 fatty acids on the survival of vincristine sensitive and resistant human cervical carcinoma cells *in vitro*, *Cancer Lett.*, 84, 31, 1994.
94. Das, U.N. et al., Can tumour cell drug resistance be reversed by essential fatty acids and their metabolites? *Prostaglandins Leukot. Essent. Fatty Acids*, 58, 39, 1998.
95. Zerouga, M., Stillwell, W., and Jenski, L.J., Synthesis of a novel phosphatidylcholine conjugated to docosahexanoic acid and methotrexate that inhibits cell proliferation, *Anti-Cancer Drugs*, 13, 301, 2002.
96. Borgeson, C.E. et al., Effects of dietary fish oil on human mammary carcinoma and on lipid-metabolizing enzymes, *Lipids*, 24, 290, 1989.
97. Hardman, W.E., Moyer, M.P., and Cameron, I.L., Dietary fish oil sensitizes A549 lung xenografts to doxorubicin chemotherapy, *Cancer Lett.*, 151, 145, 2000.
98. Germain., E. et al., Dietary n-3 polyunsaturated fatty acids and oxidant increase rat mammary tumor sensitivity to epirubicin without change in cardiac toxicity, *Lipids*, 34, S203, 1999.
99. Hardman, W.E. et al., Three percent dietary fish oil concentrate increase efficacy of doxorubicin against MDA-MB 231 breast cancer xenografts, *Clin. Cancer Res.*, 7, 2041, 2001.

100. Timmer- Bosscha et al., Differential effects of all trans–retinoic acid, docosahexaenoic acid, and hexadecylphosphocholine on cisplantin-induced toxicity and apoptosis in a cisplantin-sensitive and resistant human embryonal carcinoma cell line, *Cancer Chemother. Pharmacol.*, 41,469, 1998.
101. Colas, S. et al., Enhanced radiosensitivity of rat autochthonous mammary tumors by dietary docosahexanoic acid, *Int. J. Cancer*, 109, 449, 2004.
102. Bradley M.O. et al., Tumor targeting by conjugation of DHA to paclitaxel, *J. Controlled Release*, 74, 233, 2001.
103. Hardman, W.E., Moyer, M.P., and Cameron, I.L., Consumption of an omega-3 fatty acids product, INCELL AAFA, reduced side effects of CPT-11 (innotecan) in mice, *Br. J. Cancer*, 86, 983, 2002.
104. Rothenberg, M.L., Irinothecan (CPT-11): recent developments and future directions-colorectal cancer and beyond, *Oncologist*, 6, 66, 2001.
105. Gerrits, C.J. et al., Topoisomerase I inhibitors: The relevance of prolonged exposure for present clinical development, *Br. J. Cancer* 76, 952, 1997.
106. Adams, D.J. et al., Campthothecin analogues with enhanced antitumor activity at acidic pH, *Cancer Chemother. Pharmacol.*, 46, 263, 2000.
107. Karmali, R.A., Historical perspective and potential use of n-3 fatty acids in therapy of cancer cachexia, *Nutrition*, 12, S2, 1996.
108. Tisdale, M.J., Mechanism of lipid mobilization associated with cancer cachexia: Interaction between polyunsaturated fatty acid, eicosapentaenoic acid and inhibitory guanine nucleotide-regulatory protein, *Prostaglandins Leukot. Essent. Fatty Acids*, 48, 105, 1993.
109. Barber, M.D. et al., The effect of an oral nutritional supplement enriched with fish oil on weight loss in patients with pancreatic cancer, *Br. J. Cancer*, 81, 80, 1999.
110. Burns, C.P. et al., Phase II Study of high dose fish oil capsules for patients with cancer-related cachexia, *Cancer*, 101, 370, 2004.
111. Jatoi, A. et al., An eicosapentanoic acid supplement versus megestrol acetate versus both for patients with cancer-associated wasting: a North Central Cancer treatment group and National Cancer Institute of Canada Collaborative Effort, *J. Clin. Oncol.*, 22, 2469, 2004.
112. Takahata, K. et al., Protection from chemotherapy-induced alopecia by docosahexaenoic acid, *Lipids*, 34, S105, 1999.
113. L'Abbe, M.R., Trick, K.D., and Beare-Rogers, J.L., Dietary (n-3) fatty acids affect rat heart, liver and aorta protective enzyme activities and lipid peroxidation, *J. Nutr.*, 121, 1331, 1991.
114. Ratnayake, W.M.N. et al., Chemical and nutritional studies of flaxseed (variety Linott) in rats, *J. Nutr. Biochem.*, 3, 232, 1992.
115. Wiesenfeld, P.W. et al., Flaxseed increased alpha linolenic acid and eicosapentanoic acid and decreased arachidonic acid in serum and tissues of rat dams and offspring, *Food Chem. Tox.*, 41, 841, 2003.
116. Jenkins, D.J. et al., Health aspects of partially defatted flaxseed, including effects on serum lipids, oxidative measures, and ex vivo androgen and progestin activity: a controlled crossover trial, *Am. J. Clin. Nutr.*, 69, 395, 1999.
117. Cunnane, S.C. et al., Nutritional attributes of traditional flaxseed in healthy adults, *Am. J. Clin. Nutr.*, 61, 62, 1994.
118. Kaasgard, S.G. et al., Effects of dietary linseed oil and marine oil on lipid peroxidation in monkey liver *in vivo* and *in vitro*, *Lipids*, 27, 740, 1992.

119. Babu, U.S. et al., Nutritional and hematological impact of dietary and defatted flaxseed meal in rats, *Int. J. Food Sci. Nutr.*, 51, 109, 2000.
120. Schweigert, F.J. et al., Plasma and tissue concentrations of beta carotene and vitamin A in rats fed beta carotene in various fats of plant and animal origin, *J. Environ. Pathol. Toxicol. Oncol.*, 19, 87, 2000.
121. Tomassi, G. and Olson, J.A., Effect of dietary essential fatty acids on vitamin A utilization in the rat, *J. Nutr.*, 113, 697, 1983.
122. Frank, J. et al., Dietary secoisolariciresinol diglucoside and its oligomers with 3-hydroxy-3-methhyl glutaric acid decrease vitamin E levels in rats, *Br. J. Nutr.*, 92, 169, 2004.
123. Prasad, K., Hydroxyradical scavenging property of secoisolariciresinol diglucoside (SDG) isolated from flaxseed, *Mol. Cell. Biochem.*, 168, 117, 1997.
124. Kitts, D.D., Antioxidant activity of the flaxseed lignan secoisolariciresinol diglycoside and its mammalian lignan metabolites enterodiol and enterolactone, *Mol. Cell. Biochem.*, 202, 91, 1999.
125. Yuan, Y.V., Rickard, S.R., and Thompson, L.U., Short term feeding of flaxseed or its lignans has minor influence on *in vivo* hepatic antioxidant status in young rats, *Nutr. Res.*, 19, 1233, 1999.
126. Brouwer, I.A., Katan, M.B., and Zock, P.L., Dietary alpha linolenic acid is associated with reduced risk of fatal coronary heart disease, but increased prostate cancer risk: a meta analysis, *J. Nutr.*, 134, 919, 2004.
127. Leitzmann, M.F. et al., Dietary intake of n-3 and n-6 fatty acids and the risk of prostate cancer, *Am. J. Clin. Nutr.*, 80, 204, 2004.
128. Sidhu, K.S., Health benefits and potential risks related to consumption of fish or fish oil, *Reg. Tox. Pharm.*, 38, 336, 2003.
129. Hites, R.A. et al., Global assessment of organic contaminants in farmed salmon, *Science*, 303, 226, 2004.
130. Tuomisto J.T. et al., Risk benefit analysis of eating farmed salmon, *Science*, 305(23 July), 476, 2004.
131. Lund, E. et al., Cancer risk and salmon intake, *Science*, 305 (23 July), 477, 2004.
132. Roynette, C.E. et al., n-3 polyunsaturated fatty acids and colon cancer prevention, *Clin. Nutr.*, 23, 139, 2004.
133. Griffini, P. et al., Dietary omega-3 polyunsaturated fatty acid promote colon carcinoma metastasis in rat liver, *Cancer Res.*, 58, 3312, 1998.
134. Meterissian, S.H. et al., Effect of membrane free fatty acid alterations on the adhesion of human colorectal carcinoma cells to liver macrophages and extracellular matrix proteins, *Cancer Lett.*, 89, 145, 1995.
135. Tou, J., Chen, J., and Thompson, L.U., Flaxseed and its lignan precursor, secoisolariciresinol diglycoside, affect pregnancy outcome and reproductive development in rats, *J. Nutr.*, 128, 1861, 1998.
136. Ward, W., Chen, J., and Thompson, L.U., Exposure to flaxseed or its purified lignan during suckling only or continuously does not alter reproductive indices in male and female offspring, *J. Toxicol. Environ. Health A*, 64, 567, 2001.
137. Tou, J., Chen, J. and Thompson L.U., Dose, timing, and duration of flaxseed exposure affect reproductive indices and sex hormone levels in rats, *J. Toxicol. Environ. Health. A*, 56, 555, 1999.
138. Tou, J. and Thompson, L.U., Exposure to flaxseed or its lignan component during different developmental stages influences rat mammary gland structures, *Carcinogenesis*, 20, 1831, 1999.

139. Sprando, R.L., Collins, T., and Wiesenfeld, P.W., Effect of flaxseed consumption on male and female reproductive function and fetal development, in *Flaxseed in human nutrition,* 2nd ed., Thompson, L.U. and Cunnane, S.C., Eds., AOCS Press, Champaign, IL, 2003, p. 341.
140. Collins, T.F. et al., Effect of flaxseed and defatted flaxseed meal on reproduction and development in rats, *Food Chem. Toxicol.*, 41, 819, 2003.
141. Oomah, B.D., Mazza, G., and Kenaschuk, E.O., Cyanogenic compounds in flaxseed, *J. Agric. Food Chem.* 40, 1346, 1992.
142. Cunnane, S.C. et al., High alpha linolenic acid flaxseed (Linum usitissimum): some nutritional properties in humans, *Br. J. Nutr.*, 69, 443, 1993.
143. Pajno, G.B. et al., Anaphylaxis to sesame, *Allergy,* 55,199, 2000.

9

Whole-Grain Component Synergy and Cancer

Joanne Slavin

CONTENTS

9.1 Introduction

Whole-grain intake is protective against a wide range of cancers. This protection is greater than that seen with any component in whole grains alone, such as dietary fiber, minerals, vitamins, antioxidants, or phytochemicals. We attribute this protectiveness of whole grains to the synergy or additive effect of its components.

9.2 Diet and Cancer

It is estimated that 35% of all cancers are attributable to diet and that up to 90% of colorectal cancer in the United States could be avoidable with alterations in diet.[1] Dietary treatments have been tested as chemopreventive measures in the process of cancer. Establishing a cause-and-effect relationship between diet and cancer is a difficult task. Studies in diet and cancer include ecologic studies where dietary variables are compared across populations. Case-control studies can examine differences in diet between people who have cancer compared to those who do not.

A serious limitation of retrospective studies is the accuracy with which intakes of dietary factors can be established. It is difficult to recall dietary intakes in former years and disease tends to alter diet. A stronger epidemiologic design is the cohort study in which subjects exposed to a particular agent are followed over time and their cancer incidence is compared with those who have not been exposed. These studies are costly and require large numbers of subjects. Intervention studies allow investigators to make a dietary change and then follow the course of disease. Intervention studies are limited by the slow progressive nature of the cancer process and the large number of subjects needed for statistical power.

Strategies to avoid these problems include studying individuals who are at high risk for developing cancer to determine whether a chemopreventive agent can prevent the development of cancer. Secondly, studies use intermediate biomarkers of the cancer process as the end point rather than waiting for the cancer to occur. Chemoprevention trials in high risk individuals with measurement of intermediate biomarkers are commonly used to determine the role of dietary ingredients on cancer causation.

Many studies use animal models to study the relationship between diet and cancer. Animal studies offer greater control of variables, allow for a broader range of interventions, and are generally less expensive than human studies. They suffer from species differences, which for whole grains and dietary fiber is particularly problematic since the gastrointestinal tract of the rat varies significantly from the human.

9.3 Whole Grains

Health aspects of whole grains have long been known. In the 4th century BC, Hippocrates, the father of medicine, recognized the health benefits of whole-grain bread. More recently, physicians and scientists in the early 1800s to mid 1900s recommended whole grains to prevent constipation. The "fiber hypothesis," published in the early 1970s, suggested that whole foods, such as whole grains, fruits, and vegetables, provide fiber along with other constituents that have health benefits.[2]

The major cereal grains include wheat, rice, and corn, with oats, rye, barley, triticale, sorghum, and millet as minor grains. In the United States, the most commonly consumed grains are wheat, oats, rice, corn, and rye, with wheat constituting 66 to 75% of the total. Buckwheat, wild rice, and amaranth are not botanically true grains but are typically associated with the grain family because of their similar composition. All grains have a barklike, protective hull, beneath which are the endosperm, bran, and germ. The germ contains the plant embryo. The endosperm supplies food for the growing seedling. Surrounding the germ and the endosperm is the outer covering or bran which protects the grain from its environment, including weather, insects, molds, and bacteria.

About 50 to 75% of the endosperm is starch, and it is the major energy supply for the embryo during germination of the kernel. The endosperm also contains storage proteins, typically 8 to 18%, along with cell wall polymers. Relatively few vitamins, minerals, fiber, or phytochemicals are located in the endosperm fraction. The germ is a relatively minor contributor to the dry weight of most grains (typically 4 to 5% in wheat and barley). The germ of corn contributes a much higher proportion to the total grain structure than that of wheat, barley, or oats. A whole grain health claim has been approved in the United States. For a whole-grain food to meet the whole grain health claim standards, the food must include 51% whole-grain flour by weight of final product and must contain 1.7 g of dietary fiber.

9.4 Whole-Grain Recommendations

Over the past 20 years, more than a dozen governmental, nonprofit health, and industrial/trade groups have encouraged increased whole-grain consumption. Grain products comprise the base of the U.S. Department of Agriculture (USDA) Food Guide Pyramid, which suggests that several of the recommended 6 to 11 servings of grain products per day should be from whole grains. The 2000 Dietary Guidelines for Americans established a separate guideline for grains with a particular emphasis on eating more whole-grain foods. It is recommended that at least 3 servings, or one-half of grain foods consumed daily, be whole grain.

Americans consume far less than the recommended three servings of whole grains on a daily basis. According to a survey of Americans 20 years and older,[3] total grain intake was 6.7 servings per day with only 1 of these servings being whole grain. Only 8% of the study participants consumed the recommended three servings of whole grains on a daily basis. Another investigation[4] reported that less than 2% of the study population consumed two or more whole-grain servings per day, and 23% consumed no whole grains over the 2-week reporting period. Average whole-grain consumption for this study was 0.5 serving per day. A study of U.S. children and teens reported consumption of whole grains was less than one serving per day.[5] Whole-grain intake studies in other countries find similar results. Except for parts of Scandinavia where whole-grain breads are the norm, whole-grain consumption is low.[6] In the United Kingdom, median consumption of whole grains was less than one serving per day.[6]

9.5 Whole-Grain Components

The bran and germ fractions derived from conventional milling provide most of the biologically active compounds found in a grain. Specific nutrients include high concentrations of B vitamins (thiamin, niacin, riboflavin, and pantothenic acid) and minerals (calcium, magnesium, potassium, phosphorus, sodium, and iron), elevated levels of basic amino acids (e.g., arginine and lysine), and elevated tocol levels in the lipids. Numerous phytochemicals, some common in many plant foods (phytates and phenolic compounds) and some unique to grain products (avenanthramides, avenalumic acid), are responsible for the high antioxidant activity of whole-grain foods.[7]

In developed countries, such as the United States and Europe, grains are generally subjected to some type of processing, milling, heat extraction, cooking, parboiling, or other technique prior to consumption. Commercial cereals are usually extruded, puffed, flaked, or otherwise altered to make a desirable product. Processing of whole grains does not remove biologically important compounds.[8] Analysis of processed breads and cereals indicate that they are a rich source of antioxidants.[7] Processing may open up the food matrix, thereby allowing the release of tightly bound phytochemicals from the grain structure.[9] Studies with rye find that many of the bioactive compounds are stable during food processing, and their levels may even be increased with suitable processing.[10]

9.6 Epidemiological Studies of Whole Grains and Cancer

There is substantial scientific evidence that whole grains as commonly consumed reduce the risk of cancer. In a meta-analysis of whole-grain intake and cancer, whole grains were found to be protective in 46 of 51 mentions of whole-grain intake, and in 43 of 45 mentions after exclusion of 6 mentions with design or reporting flaws or low intake.[11] Odds ratios were less than 1 in 9 of 10 mentions of studies of colorectal cancers and polyps, 7 of 7 mentions of gastric, and 6 of 6 mentions of other digestive tract cancers, 7 of 7 mentions of hormone-related cancers, 4 of 4 mentions of pancreatic cancer, and 10 of 11 mentions of 8 other cancers. The pooled odds ratio was similar in studies that adjusted for few or many covariates. A systemic review of case control studies conducted using a common protocol in northern Italy between 1983 and 1996 indicates that a higher frequency of whole-grain consumption is associated with reduced risk for cancer.[12] Whole grains were consumed primarily as whole-grain bread and some whole-grain pasta in the Italian studies.

Other studies have demonstrated a lower risk for specific cancers, such as stomach,[13] mouth, throat and upper digestive tract,[14] endometrial,[15] and rectal.[16] Epidemiological studies have reported that higher serum insulin levels are associated with increased risk of colon, breast, and possibly other cancers.[17] Reduction of these insulin levels by whole grains may be an indirect way in which the reduction in cancer risk occurs.

Studies on the relationship between dietary fiber and cancer are also relevant to the question of whole grains and cancer. Trock et al.[18] analyzed 37 epidemiologic studies that examined the relationship between colorectal cancer and fiber, vegetables, grains, and fruits, either alone or in combination. Overall, 80% of the studies reported up to that time supported the protective role of dietary fiber in colorectal cancer. Howe et al.[19] conducted a combined analysis of data from 13 case control studies in populations with different colorectal cancer rates and dietary practices. The risk of colorectal cancer decreased incrementally as dietary fiber intake increased. Consumption of more than 31 g of fiber/d was associated with a 50% reduction in risk of colorectal cancer compared to diet incorporating less than 11 g/d. The authors estimate that the risk of colorectal cancer in the U.S. population could be reduced by about 31% from an average increase in fiber intake from food sources of about 13 g/d. In contrast, Giovannucci[20] concluded that more recent epidemiologic studies have not supported a strong influence of dietary fiber or fruits and vegetables on colorectal cancer. Many of the participants in prospective studies have low intakes of dietary fiber, often with even the upper quartiles of intake being below recommended fiber intake levels. Thus, the lack of consistency for the protectiveness of dietary fiber may relate to the usual low intakes.

Peters et al.[21] assessed the relation of fiber intake and frequency of colorectal adenoma within the Prostate, Lung, Colorectal and Ovarian (PLCO) Cancer Screening Trial. High intakes of dietary fiber were associated with lower risk of colorectal adenoma. In this case control study of over 38,000 subjects, subjects with the highest amounts of fiber in their diets (36 g/d) had the lowest incidence of colon adenomas. Their risk of having an adenoma detected by sigmoidoscopy was 27% less than that of the people who ate the least amount of fiber (12 g/d). Fiber from fruits and from grain and/or cereals was significantly associated with lower adenoma risk, while fiber from vegetables and legumes was not.

The data from large cohort studies are not consistent. In the Health Professional Follow-up Study,[22] dietary fiber was inversely associated with risk of colorectal adenoma in men. All sources of fiber (vegetables, fruits, and grain) were associated with decreased risk of adenoma. The Nurses' Health Study found no protective effect of dietary fiber on the development of colorectal cancer in women.[23] In the Iowa Women's Health Study, a weak and statistically nonsignificant inverse association was found between dietary fiber intake and risk of colon cancer.[24]

The European Prospective Investigation into Cancer and Nutrition (EPIC) is a prospective cohort study comparing the dietary habits of more than a half-million people in 10 countries with colorectal cancer incidence.[25] They found that people who ate the most fiber (those with total fiber from food sources averaging 33 g/d) had a 25% lower incidence of colorectal cancer than those who ate the least fiber (12 g/d). The investigators estimated that populations with low average fiber consumption could reduce colorectal cancer incidence by 40% by doubling their fiber intake.

Few epidemiologic studies have collected biomarkers of dietary fiber intake. Cummings et al.[26] collected data from 20 populations in 12 countries and found that average stool weight varied from 72 to 470 g/d and was inversely related to colon cancer risk. Dukas et al.[27] reported that in the Nurses' Health Study, women in the highest quintile of dietary fiber intake (median intake 20 g/d) were less likely to experience constipation than women in the lowest quintile (median intake 7 g/d).

Dietary factors, such as fiber, vitamin B_6, and phytoestrogen intake and lifestyle factors such as exercise, smoking, and alcohol use, which are controlled for in most epidemiologic studies, do not explain the apparent protective effect of whole grains against cancer, again suggesting it's the whole-grain "package" that is effective. Several theories have been offered to explain the protective effects of whole grains. Because of the complex nature of whole grains, there are many potential mechanisms that could be responsible for their protective properties.

9.7 Mechanistic Studies of Whole Grains

Potential mechanisms for the protective nature of whole grains against cancer are listed in Table 9.1. Fermentation of carbohydrate in the colon produces short chain fatty acids that help maintain the integrity of the gut.[28] Butyrate may regulate colonic cell proliferation and serve as an energy source for colonic cells. Besides dietary fiber, whole grains contain a variety of anticarcinogenic compounds.

The wide range of protective components in whole grains and potential mechanisms for protection has been described.[2] To conduct feeding studies in human subjects, whole grains must be fed in a form acceptable to participants. Often feeding studies use processed whole grains for the dietary intervention. Additionally, epidemiologic studies that find protection with

TABLE 9.1

Mechanisms by which Whole Grains Can Protect against the Development of Cancer

Increased stool bulk
Decreased transit time
Dilution of carcinogens
Binds with bile acids or other potential carcinogens
Lower fecal pH
Inhibit bacterial degradation of normal food constituents to potential carcinogens
Changes in microflora
Fermentation by fecal flora to short chain fatty acids
Decrease in colonic pH
Inhibition of carcinogens
Increase in lumenal antioxidants
Peptide growth factors
Alteration of sex hormone status
Change in satiety resulting in lowered body weight
Alterations in insulin sensitivity and/or glucose metabolism

consumption of processed whole-grain products, such as breads, cereals, and brown rice.

9.7.1 Large Bowel Effects of Whole Grains

Whole grains are rich sources of fermentable carbohydrates including dietary fiber, resistant starch, and oligosaccharides. Undigested carbohydrate that reaches the colon is fermented by intestinal microflora to short chain fatty acids and gases. Short chain fatty acids include acetate, butyrate, and propionate, with butyrate being a preferred fuel for the colonic mucosa cells. Short chain fatty acid production has been related to lowered serum cholesterol and decreased risk of cancer. Undigested carbohydrates increase fecal wet and dry weight and speed of intestinal transit.

Comparing dietary fiber content of various whole grains, oats, rye, and barley contain about one-third soluble fiber and the rest insoluble fiber. Soluble fiber is associated with cholesterol-lowering and improved glucose response, while insoluble fiber is associated with improved laxation. Wheat is lower in soluble fiber than most grains while rice contains virtually no soluble fiber. Refining of grains removes proportionally more of the insoluble fiber than soluble fiber, although refined grains are low in total dietary fiber.

Disruption of cell walls can increase fermentability of dietary fiber. Coarse wheat bran has a greater fecal bulking effect than finely ground wheat bran when fed at the same dosage,[29] suggesting that the particle size of the whole grain is an important factor in determining physiological effect. Coarse bran delayed gastric emptying and accelerated small bowel transit. The effect seen with coarse bran was similar to the effect of inert plastic particles, suggesting that the coarse nature of whole grains as compared with refined grains has a unique physiological effect beyond composition differences between whole and refined grains.[30]

Not all starch is digested and absorbed during gut transit. Factors that determine whether starch is resistant to digestion include the physical form of grains or seeds in which starch is located, particularly if these are whole or partially disrupted, size and type of starch granules, associations between starch and other dietary components, and cooking and food processing, especially cooking and cooling.

Juntunen et al.[31] evaluated what factors in grain products affected human glucose and insulin responses. They fed the following grain products: whole-kernel rye bread, whole-meal rye bread containing oat β-glucan concentrate, dark durum wheat pasta, and wheat bread made from white wheat flour. Glucose responses and the rate of gastric emptying after consumption of the two rye breads and pasta did not differ from those after consumption of white wheat bread. Insulin, glucose-dependent insulinotropic polypeptide, and glucagonlike peptide 1, were lower after consumption of rye breads and pasta than after consumption of white wheat bread. These results support that postprandial insulin responses to grain products are determined by the form of food and botanical structure rather than by the amount of fiber or the type of cereal in the food.

9.7.2 Antioxidants in Whole Grains

The primary protective function of antioxidants in the body is their reaction with free radicals. Free radical attack on DNA, lipids, and protein is thought to be an initiating factor for several chronic diseases.[7] Cellular membrane damage from free radical attack and peroxidation is thought to be a primary causative factor. Cellular damage causes a shift in net charge of the cell, changing osmotic pressure, leading to swelling and eventual cell death. Free radicals also contribute to general inflammatory response and tissue damage. Antioxidants also protect DNA from oxidative damage and mutation, which lead to cancer. Free radical compounds result from normal metabolic activity as well as from the diet and environment. The body has defense mechanisms to prevent free radical damage and to repair damage, but when the defense is not sufficient, disease may develop. It follows that if dietary antioxidants reduce free radical activity in the body, then disease potential is reduced.

Whole-grain products are relatively high in antioxidant activity. Antioxidants found in whole-grain foods are water-soluble, fat-soluble, and insoluble (approximately half). Soluble antioxidants include phenolic acids, flavonoids, tocopherols, and avenanthramides in oats. A large part of insoluble antioxidants are bound as cinnamic acid esters to arabinoxylan side chains of hemicellulose. Wheat bran insoluble fiber contains approximately 0.5 to 1.0% phenolic groups. Covalently bound phenolic acids are good free radical scavengers. About two-thirds of whole-grain antioxidant activity is not soluble in water, aqueous methanol, or hexane. Antioxidant activity is an inherent property of insoluble grain fiber. In the colon, hydrolysis by microbial enzymes frees bound phenolic acids.[32] Colon endothelial cells may absorb the released phenolic acids and gain antioxidant protection, and these phenolic acids may enter the portal circulation. In this manner, whole-grain foods provide antioxidant protection over a long period through the entire digestive tract.

In addition to natural antioxidants, antioxidant activity is created in grain-based foods by browning reactions during baking and toasting processes that increases total activity in the final product as compared with the raw ingredients. For example, the crust of white bread has double the antioxidant activity of the starting flour or of the crust free bread. Reductone intermediates from Maillard reactions may explain the increase in antioxidant activity. The total antioxidant activity of whole-grain products is similar to that of fruits or vegetables on a per serving basis.[7]

Adom and Liu[33] suggest that the antioxidant activity of grains reported in the literature has been underestimated since only unbound antioxidants are usually studied. They report that in wheat 90% of the antioxidants are bound. Bound phytochemicals could survive stomach and intestinal digestion, but would then be released in the large intestine and potentially play a protective role. When they compared antioxidant activity of various grains, corn had the highest total antioxidant activity, followed by wheat, oats, and then rice.

Phytic acid, concentrated in grains, is a known antioxidant. Phytic acid forms chelates with various metals, which suppresses damaging iron-catalyzed redox reactions. Colonic bacteria produce oxygen radicals in appreciable amounts and dietary phytic acid may suppress oxidant damage to intestinal epithelium and neighboring cells.

Vitamin E is another antioxidant present in whole grains that is removed in the refining process. Vitamin E is an intracellular antioxidant that protects polyunsaturated fatty acids in cell membranes from oxidative damage. Another possible mechanism for vitamin E relates to its capacity to keep selenium in the reduced state. Vitamin E inhibits the formation of nitrosamines, especially at low pH.

9.7.3 Lignans

Hormonally active compounds in grains called lignans may protect against hormonally mediated diseases.[34] Lignans are compounds possessing a 2,3-dibenzylbutane structure and exist as minor constituents of many plants where they form the building blocks for the formation of lignin in the plant cell wall. The plant lignans secoisolariciresinol and matairesinol are converted by human gut bacteria to the mammalian lignans, enterolactone and enterodiol. Limited information exists on the concentration of lignans and their precursors in food. Because of the association of lignan excretion with fiber intake, it is assumed that plant lignans are contained in the outer layers of the grain. Concentrated sources of lignans include whole-grain wheat, whole-grain oats, and rye meal. Seeds are also concentrated sources of lignans including flaxseed seeds (the most concentrated source), pumpkin seeds, caraway seeds, and sunflower seeds. This compositional data suggests that whole-grain breads and cereals are the best ways to deliver lignans in the diet.

Grains and other high fiber foods increase urinary lignan excretion, an indirect measure of lignan content in foods.[35] Mammalian lignan production of plant foods was studied by Thompson et al.[36] using an *in vitro* fermentation method with human fecal microbiota. Oilseeds, particularly flaxseed flour and meal, produced the highest concentration of lignans, followed by dried seaweeds, whole legumes, cereal brans, whole-grain cereals, vegetables, and fruits. Lignan concentration produced from flaxseed was approximately 100 times greater than that produced from most other foods.

Differences in metabolism of phytoestrogens among individuals have been noted. Adlercreutz et al.[37] found total urinary lignan excretion in Finnish women to be positively correlated with total fiber intake, total fiber intake per kilogram of body weight and grain fiber intake per kilogram body weight. Similarly, the geometric mean excretion of enterolactone was positively correlated with the geometric mean intake of dietary grain products (kilocalories per day) of five groups of women ($r=0.996$).

Due to the association of lignan excretion with fiber intake, plant lignans are probably concentrated in the outer layers of the grain. Because current processing techniques eliminate this fraction of the grain, lignans may not be found in processed grain products on the market and would only be found in whole-grain foods.

Serum enterolactone was measured in a cross-sectional study in Finnish adults.[38] In men, serum enterolactone concentrations were positively associated with consumption of whole-grain products. Variability in serum enterolactone concentration was great, suggesting the role of gut microflora in the metabolism of lignans may be important. Kilkkinen et al.[39] also report that intake of lignans is associated with serum enterolactone concentration in Finnish men and women. They suggest that serum enterolactone is a feasible biomarker of lignan intake. Jacobs et al.[40] found similar results in a U.S. study. Subjects were fed either whole-grain or refined-grain foods for 6 weeks. Most of the increase in serum enterolactone when eating the whole-grain diet occurred within 2 weeks, though the serum enterolactone difference between whole-grain and refined-grain diets continued to increase throughout the 6-week study.

9.7.4 Antinutrients

Antinutrients found in grains include digestive enzyme (protease and amylase) inhibitors, phytic acid, hemagglutinins and phenolics and/or tannins. Protease inhibitors, phytic acid, phenolics and saponins have been shown to reduce the risk of cancer of the colon and breast in animals. Phytic acid, lectins, phenolics, amylase inhibitors, and saponins have also been shown to lower the plasma glucose, insulin and/or plasma cholesterol and triglycerides.[41] In grains protease inhibitors make up 5 to 10% of the water soluble protein and are concentrated in the endosperm and embryo.

9.8 Feeding Studies with Whole Grains with Cancer Biomarkers

9.8.1 Dietary Fiber Interventions

Several randomized intervention studies with high fiber diets as a component of chemoprevention have been published. Alberts et al.[42] studied the effects of wheat bran fiber (an additional 13.5 g/d as wheat bran cereal) on rectal epithelial cell proliferation in patients with resection for colorectal cancers. They found that the wheat bran fiber cereal inhibited DNA synthesis and rectal mucosal cell proliferation in this high-risk group, which they argued should be associated with reduced cancer risk. They suggested that such a fiber regimen might be used as chemopreventive agent for colorectal cancers. The study is weakened by poor compliance to the intervention over the 4 years of the study.

In a randomized trial of intake of fat, fiber, and β-carotene to prevent colorectal adenomas, patients on the combined intervention of low fat and added wheat bran had no large adenomas at both 24 and 48 months, a statistically significant finding.[43]

Two intervention studies do not support the protective properties of dietary fiber against colon cancer.[44,45] The studies found no significant effect of high fiber intakes on the recurrence of colorectal adenomas. Both papers described well-planned dietary interventions to determine whether high-fiber food consumption could lower colorectal cancer risk, as measured by a change in colorectal adenomas, a precursor of most large-bowel cancers. Perhaps the fiber interventions were not long enough, the fiber dose was not high enough, and recurrence of adenoma is not an appropriate measure of fiber's effectiveness in preventing colon cancer. Yet the results from the studies are clear. Increasing dietary fiber consumption over 3 years did not alter recurrence of adenomas.

Limited epidemiologic evidence has been published on fiber intake and human breast cancer risk. Since the fat and fiber content of the diet are generally inversely related, it is difficult to separate the independent effects of these nutrients, and most research has focused on the fat and breast cancer hypothesis. International comparisons show an inverse correlation between breast cancer death rates and consumption of fiber-rich foods. An interesting exception to the high-fat diet hypothesis in breast cancer was observed in Finland, where intake of both fat and fiber is high and the breast cancer mortality rate is considerably lower than in the United States and other Western countries where the typical diet is high in fat. The large amount of fiber in the rural Finnish diet may modify the breast cancer risk associated with a high-fat diet.

A meta-analysis of 12 case control studies of dietary factors and risk of breast cancer found that high dietary fiber intake was associated with reduced risk of breast cancer.[46] Dietary fiber intake has also been linked to lower risk of benign proliferative epithelial disorders of the breast.[47] Not all studies find a relationship between dietary fiber intake and breast cancer incidence, including a prospective cohort study reported by Willett and colleagues.[48] Jain et al.[49] also found no association among total dietary fiber, fiber fractions, and risk of breast cancer. Still, nutrition differences, including dietary fiber intake, appear to be important variables that contribute to the higher rate of breast cancer experienced by younger African-American women.[50]

Few studies have examined the effects of dietary fiber on hormone metabolism while fat content of the diet was held constant. Rose and colleagues[51] reported that when wheat bran was added to the usual diet of premenopausal women, it significantly reduced serum estrogen concentrations, whereas neither corn bran nor oat bran had an effect. Goldin and associates[52] reported that a high-fiber, low-fat diet significantly decreased serum concentrations of estrone, estrone sulfate, testosterone, and sex hormone binding globulin in premenopausal women. Dietary fiber also caused prolongation of the menstrual cycle by 0.72 d and of the follicular phase by 0.85 d, changes thought to reduce overall risk of developing breast cancer. Rock et al.[53] found that a high-fiber, low-fat diet intervention in women with a history of breast cancer reduced serum estrodiol concentrations.

Few studies have been reported on dietary fiber intake and other cancer sites. Studies of dietary fiber and endometrial cancer have reported both increases and decreases in risk.[54–56] Ovarian cancer risk is decreased with higher intakes of dietary fiber.[57] No significant relationships have been reported between dietary fiber intake risk of prostate cancer.

9.8.2 Whole-Grains Interventions

Few feeding studies in human subjects have been completed for whole grains and cancer biomarkers. McIntosh et al.[58] fed rye and wheat foods to overweight middle-aged men and measured markers of bowel health. The men were fed low-fiber cereal grains foods providing 5 g of dietary fiber for the refined-grain diet and 18 g of dietary fiber for the whole-grain diet, either high in rye or wheat. This was in addition to a baseline diet that contained 14 g of dietary fiber. Both the high-fiber rye and wheat foods increased fecal output by 33 to 36% and reduced fecal β-glucuronidase activity by 29%. Postprandial plasma insulin was decreased by 46 to 49% and postprandial plasma glucose by 16 to 19%. Rye foods were associated with significantly increased plasma enterolactone and fecal butyrate, relative to wheat and low-fiber diets. The authors conclude that rye appears more effective than wheat in overall improvement of biomarkers of bowel health.

Dietary fiber sources such as wheat bran are complex matrices, and attempts have been made to isolate the effects of chemical components of wheat bran. In an animal study, rats were fed wheat bran, dephytinized wheat bran, and phytic acid alone and aberrant crypt foci were measured after treatment with azoxymethane.[59] Wheat bran without phytic acid was less protective than intact wheat bran suggesting that the protective effects of wheat bran include fiber and phytic acid.

9.9 Conclusions

Epidemiologic studies find that whole-grain intake protects against cancer. Whole grains are rich in nutrients and phytochemicals with known health benefits. Whole grains are concentrated in dietary fiber, resistant starch, and oligosaccharides. Whole grains are rich in antioxidants, including trace minerals and phenolic compounds, and these compounds have been linked to cancer prevention. Other protective compounds in whole grains include phytate, phytoestrogens such as lignan, plant stanols and sterols, and vitamins and minerals. Whole-grain feeding studies report improvements in biomarkers with whole-grain consumption, such as weight loss, increased stool weight, antioxidant protection, and changes in fecal enzymes and serum enterolactone. Although it is difficult to separate the protective properties of whole grains from dietary fiber and other components, the disease protection seen from whole grains in prospective epidemiologic studies far exceeds the protection from isolated nutrients and phytochemicals in whole grains.

The interactions of whole grains with other foods or cancer related drugs have not been reported in the literature. Since whole grains include many nutrients, such as dietary fiber, minerals, vitamins, and phytochemicals, studies that examine the interaction of these nutrients on cancer related drugs would be relevant in evaluating the potential interaction of these components.

References

1. Doll, R. and Peto, R., The causes of cancer: quantitative estimates of avoidable risks of cancer in the United States today, *J. Natl. Cancer Inst.*, 66, 1191, 1981.
2. Slavin, J.L., Whole grains and human health, *Nutr. Res. Rev.*, 77, 99, 2004.
3. Cleveland, L.E., Moshfegh, A., Albertson, A., and Goldman, J., Dietary intake of whole grains, *J. Am. Coll. Nutr.*, 19, 331S, 2000.

4. Albertson, A.M. and Tobelmann, R.C., Consumption of grain and whole-grain foods by an American population during the years 1990 to 1998, in *Whole grain foods in health and disease,* Marquart, L., Slavin, J.L., and Fulcher, R.G., Eds., Eagan Press, St. Paul, MN, 2002.
5. Harnack, L., Walters, S., and Jacobs, D.R., Dietary intake and food sources of whole grains among US children and adolescents: Data from the 1994–1996 continuing survey of food intakes by individuals, *J. Am. Diet. Assoc.,* 103, 1015, 2003.
6. Lang, R. and Jebb, S.A., Who consumes whole grains, and how much? *Proc. Nutr. Soc.,* 62, 123, 2003.
7. Miller, G., Prakash, A., and Decker, E., Whole-grain micronutients, in *Whole grain foods in health and disease,* Marquart, L., Slavin, J.L., and Fulcher, R.G., Eds., Eagan Press, St. Paul, MN, 2002.
8. Slavin, J.L., Jacobs, D., and Marquart, L., Grain processing and nutrition, *Crit. Rev.Biotech.,* 21, 49, 2001.
9. Fulcher, R.G. and Rooney-Duke, T.K., Whole-grain structure and organization: implications for nutritionists and processors, in *Whole grain foods in health and disease,* Marquart, L., Slavin, J.L., and Fulcher, R.G., Eds., Eagan Press, St. Paul, MN, 2002.
10. Liukkonen, K., Katina, K., Wilhelmsson, A., Myllkmaki, O., Lampi, M., Kariluoto, S., Piirronen, V., Heinopen, S., Nurmi, T., Adlercreutz, H., Peltoketo, A., Pihlava, J., Hietaniemi, V., and Poutanen, K., Process-induced changes on bioactive compounds in whole grain rye, *Proc. Nutr. Soc.,* 62, 117, 2003.
11. Jacobs, D.R., Marquart, L., Slavin, J.L., and Kushi, L.H., Whole-grain intake and cancer: An expanded review and meta-analysis, *Nutr. Cancer,* 30, 85, 1998.
12. Chatenoud, L., Tavani, A., La Vecchia, C., Jacobs, D.R., Negri, E., Levi, F., and Franceschi, S., Whole-grain food intake and cancer risk, *Int. J. Cancer,* 77, 24, 1998.
13. Terry, P., Lagergren, J., Ye, W., Wolk, A., and Nyren, O., Inverse association between intake of cereal fiber and risk of gastric cardia cancer, *Gastroenterology,* 120, 387, 2001.
14. Kasum, C.M., Jacobs, D.R., Nicodemus, K., and Folsom, A.R., Dietary risk factors for upper aerodigestive tract cancers, *Int. J. Cancer,* 99, 267, 2002.
15. Kasum, C.M., Nicodemus, K., Harnack, L.J., Jacobs, D.R., and Folsom, A.R., Whole grain intake and incident endometrial cancer: The Iowa Women's Health Study, *Nutr. Cancer,* 39, 180, 2001.
16. Slattery, M.L., Curtin, K.P., Edwards, S.L., and Schaffer, D.M., Plant foods, fiber, and rectal cancer, *Am. J. Clin. Nutr.,* 79, 274, 2004.
17. Giovannucci, E., Insulin and colon cancer, *Cancer Causes Control,* 6, 164, 1995.
18. Trock, B., Lanza, E., and Greenwald, P., Dietary fiber, vegetables, and colon cancer: critical review and meta-analyses of the epidemiologic evidence, *J. Natl. Cancer Inst.,* 82, 650, 1990.
19. Howe, G.R., Benito, E., Castelleto, R., Cornee, J., Esteve, J., Gallagher, R.P., Iscovich, J.M., Deng-ao, J., Kaaka, R., Kune, G.A., Kune, S., L'Abbe, K.A., Lee, H.P., Lee, M., Miller, A.B., Peters, R.K., Potter, J.D., Bivoli, E., Slattery, M.L., Trichopoulos, D., Tuyns, A., Tzonou, A., Whittemore, A.S., Wu-Williams, A.H., and Shu, Z., Dietary intake of fiber and decreased risk of cancers of the colon and rectum: Evidence from the combined analysis of 13 case-control studies, *J. Natl. Cancer Inst.,* 84, 887, 1992.

20. Giovannucci, E., Diet, body weight, and colorectal cancer: a summary of the epidemiologic evidence, *J. Women's Health,* 12, 173, 2003.
21. Peters, L., Sinha, R., Chatterjee, N., Subar, A.F., Ziegler, R.G., Lukdorff, M., Bressalier, R., Weissfeld, J.L., Flood, A., Schatzkin, R., and Hayes, R.B., Dietary fibre and colorectal adenoma in a colorectal cancer early detection programme, *Lancet,* 361, 1491, 2003.
22. Giovannucci, E., Stampfer, M.J., Colditz, G., Rimm, E.B., and Willett, W.C., Relationship of diet to risk of colorectal cancer in men, *J. Natl. Cancer Inst.*, 84, 91, 1992.
23. Willett, W.C., Stampfer, J.M., Colditz, G.A., Rosner, B.A., and Speizer, F.E., Relation of meat, fat, and fiber intake to the risk of colon cancer in a prospective study among women, *N. Engl. J. Med.*, 323, 1664, 1990
24. Steinmetz, K.A., Kushi, L.H., Bostick, R.M., Folsom, A.R., and Potter, J.D., Vegetables, fruit, and colon cancer in the Iowa Women's Health Study, *Am. J. Epidemiol.*, 139, 1, 1994.
25. Bingham, S.A., Day, N.E., Luben, R., Ferrari, P., Slimani, N., Norat, T., Clavel-Chapelon, F., Kesse, E., Nieters, A., Boeing, H., Tjonneland, A., Overvad, K., Martinez, C., Dorronsoro, M., Gonzalez., C.A., Key, T.J., Trichopoulou, A., Naska, A., Vineis, P., Tumino, R., Krogh, V., Bueno-de-Masquita, H., Peeters, P.H.M., Berglund, G., Hallmans, G., Lund, E., Skele, G., Kaaks, R., and Riboll, E., Dietary fibre in food and protection against colorectal cancer in the European Prospective Investigation into Cancer and Nutrition (EPIC): an observational study, *Lancet,* 361, 1496, 2003.
26. Cummings, J.H., Bingham, S.A., Heaton, K.W., and Eastwood, M.A., Fecal weight, colon cancer risk and dietary intake of nonstarch polysaccharides (dietary fiber), *Gastroenterology* 103, 1783, 1992.
27. Dukas, L., Willett, W.C., and Giovannucci, E.L., Association between physical activity, fiber intake, and other lifestyle variables and constipation in a study of women, *Am. J. Gastroenterol.*, 98, 1790, 2003.
28. Topping, D.L., and Clifton, P.M., Short-chain fatty acids and human colonic function: Roles of resistant starch and nonstarch polysaccharides, *Physiol. Rev.*, 81, 1031, 2001.
29. Wrick, K., Robertson, J.B., and Van Soest, P.J., The influence of dietary fiber source on human intestinal transit and stool output, *J. Nutr.*, 113, 1464, 1983.
30. McIntyre, A., Vincent, R.M., Perkins, A.C., and Spiller, R.C., Effect of bran, ispaghula, and inert plastic particles on gastric emptying and small bowel transit in humans: the role of physical factors, *Gut,* 40, 223, 1997.
31. Juntunen, K.S., Niskanen, L.K., Liukkonen, K.H., Poutanen, K.S., Holst, J.J., and Mykkanen, H.M., Postprandial glucose, insulin, and incretin responses to grain products in healthy subjects, *Am. J. Clin. Nutr.*, 75, 254, 2002.
32. Kroon, P.A., Faulds, C.B., Ryden, P., Robertson, J.A., and Williamson, G., Release of covalently bound ferulic acid from fiber in the human colon, *J. Agri. Food Chem.*, 45, 661, 1997.
33. Adom, K.K. and Liu, R.H., Antioxidant activity of grains, *J. Agri. Food Chem.*,50, 6182, 2002.
34. Adlercreutz, H. and Mazur, W., Phyto-oestrogens and western diseases, *Ann. Med.*, 29, 95, 1997.
35. Borriello, S.P., Setchell, K.D., Axelson, M., and Lawson, A.M., Production and metabolism of lignans by the human faecal flora, *J. Appl. Bacter.*,58, 37, 1985.

36. Thompson, L.U., Seidl, M.M., Rickard, S.E., Orcheson, L.J., and Fong, H.H., Antitumorigenic effect of a mammalian lignan precursor from flaxseed, *Nutr. Cancer,* 26, 159, 1996.
37. Adlercreutz, H., Fotsis, T., Bannwart, C., Hamalainen, E., Bloigu, A., and Ollus, A., Urinary estrogen profile determination in young Finnish vegetarian and omnivorous women, *J. Steroid Biochem.,* 24, 289, 1986.
38. Kilkkinen, A., Stumpf, K., Pietinen, P., Valsta, L.M., Tapanainen, H., and Adlercreutz, H., Determinants of serum enterolactone concentration, *Am. J. Clin. Nutr.,* 73, 1094, 2001.
39. Kilkkinen, A., Valsta, L.M., Virtamo, J., Stumpf, K., Adlercreutz, H., and Pietinen, P., Intake of lignans is associated with serum enterolactone concentration in Finnish men and women, *J. Nutr.,* 133, 1830, 2003.
40. Jacobs, D.R., Pereira, M.A., Stumpf, K., Pins, J.J., and Adlercreutz, H., Whole grain food intake elevates serum enterolactone, *Br. J. Nutr.* 88, 111, 2002.
41. Slavin, J.L., Martini, M.C., Jacobs, D.R., and Marquart, L., Plausible mechanisms for the protectiveness of whole grains, *Am. J. Clin. Nutr.,* 70, 459S, 1999.
42. Alberts, D.S., Einspahr, J., Rees-McGee, S., Ramanujam, P., Buller, M.K., Clark, L., Ritenbaugh, C., Atwood, J., Pethigal, P., Earnest, D., Villar, H., Phelps, J., Lipkin, M., Wargovich, M., and Meyskens, F.L., Effects of dietary wheat bran fiber on rectal epithelial cell proliferation in patients with resection for colorectal cancers, *J. Natl. Cancer Inst.,* 82, 1280, 1990.
43. MacLennan, R., Macrae, F., Bain, C., Battistutta, D., Chapuis, P., Gratten, H., Lambert, J., Newland, R.C., Ngu, M., Russell, A., Ward, M., and Wahlqvist, M.L., Randomized trial of intake of fat, fiber, and beta carotene to prevent colorectal adenomas, *J. Natl. Cancer Inst.,* 87, 1760, 1995.
44. Schatzkin, A., Lanza, E., Corle, D., Lance, P., Iber, F., Cann, B., Shike, M., Weissfeld, J., Burt, R., Cooper, M.R., Kikendall, J.W., Cahill, J., and the Polyp Prevention Trial Study Group, Lack of effect of a low-fat, high-fiber diet on the recurrence of colorectal adenomas, *New Engl. J. Med.,* 342, 1149, 2000.
45. Alberts, D.S., Marinez, M.E., Kor, D.L., Guillen-Rodriguez, Marshall, J.R., Van Leeuwen, J.B., Reid, M.E., Ritenbaugh, C., Vargas, P.A., Bhattacharyya, A.B., Earnest, D.L., Sampliner, R.E., and the Phoenix Colon Cancer Prevention Physicians' Network, Lack of effect of a high-fiber cereal supplement on the recurrence of colorectal adenomas, Phoenix Colon Cancer Prevention Physicians' Network, *New Engl. J. Med.,* 324, 1156, 2000.
46. Howe, G.R., Hirohata, T., Hislop, T.G., Iscovich, J.M., Yuan, J.M., Katsouyanni, K., Lubin, F., Marubini, E., Modan, B., and Rohan, T., Dietary factors and risk of breast cancer: Combined analysis of 12 case-control studies, *J. Natl. Cancer Inst.,* 82, 561, 1990.
47. Baghurst, P.A. and Rohan, T.E., Dietary fiber and risk of benign proliferative epithelial disorders of the breast, *Int. J. Cancer,* 63, 481, 1995.
48. Willett, W.C., Hunter, D.J., Stampfer, M.J., Colditz, G., Manson, J.E., Spiegelman, D., Rosner, B., Hennekens, L.H., and Speizer, F.E., Dietary fat and fiber in relation to risk of breast cancer. An 8-year follow-up, *JAMA,* 268, 2037, 1992.
49. Jain, T.P., Miller, A.B., Howe, G.R., and Rohan, T.E., No association among total dietary fiber, fiber fractions, and risk of breast cancer, *Cancer Epidemiol. Biomarkers Prev.,* 11, 507, 2002.
50. Forshee, R.A., Storey, M.L., and Ritenbaugh, C., Breast cancer risk and lifestyle differences among premenopausal and postmenopausal African-American women and white women, *Cancer* 97(1 Suppl), 280, 2003.

51. Rose, D.P., Goldman, M., Connolly, J.M., and Strong, L.E., High-fiber diet reduces serum estrogen concentrations in premenopausal women, *Am. J. Clin. Nutr.*, 54, 520, 1991.
52. Goldin, B.R., Woods, M.N.L., Spiegelman, D., Longscope, C., Morrill-LaBrode, A., Dwyer, J.T., Gualtier, L.J., Hertzmark, E., and Gorbach, S.L., The effect of dietary fat and fiber on serum estrogen concentrations in premenopausal women under controlled dietary conditions, *Cancer,* 74(3 Suppl.), 1125, 1994.
53. Rock, C.L., Flatt, S.W., Thomson, C.A., Stefanick, M.L., Newman, V.A., Jones, L.A., Natarajan, L., Ritenbaugh, C., Hollenbach, K.A., Pierce, J.P., and Chang, R.J., Effects of a high-fiber, low-fat diet intervention on serum concentrations of reproductive steroid hormones in women with a history of breast cancer, *J. Clin. Oncol.*, 22, 2379, 2004.
54. Barbone, F., Austin, H., and Partridge, E.E., Diet and endometrial cancer: A case-control study, *Am. J. Epidemiol.*, 137, 393, 1993.
55. Goodman, M.T., Wilkens, L.R., Hankin, J.H., Lyu, L-C, Wu, A.H., and Kolonel, L.N., Association of soy and fiber consumption with the risk of endometrial cancer, *Am. J. Epidemiol.*, 146, 294, 1997.
56. McCann, S.E., Freudenheim, J.L., Marshall, J.W., Brasure, J.R., Swanson, M.K., and Graham, S., Diet in the epidemiology of endometrial cancer in western New York (United States), *Cancer Causes Control,* 11, 965, 2000.
57. McCann, S.E., Moysich, K.B., and Mettlin, C., Intakes of selected nutrients and food groups and risk of ovarian cancer, *Nutr. Cancer,* 39, 19, 2001.
58. McIntosh, G.H., Noakes, M., Royle, P.J., and Foster, P.R., Whole-grain rye and wheat foods and markers of bowel health in overweight middle-aged men, *Am.J. Clin. Nutr.*, 77, 967, 2003.
59. Jenab, M. and Thompson, L.U., The influence of phytic acid in wheat bran on early biomarkers of colon carcinogenesis, *Carcinogenesis,* 19, 1087, 1998.

10

Synergy and Safety of Antioxidants with Cancer Drugs

Kedar N. Prasad

CONTENTS

10.1 Introduction

It is estimated that in the United States about 1.37 million new cancers may be diagnosed and about 564,000 persons may die of this disease.[1] The incidence of a second primary malignancy among cancer survivors is about 10 to 12% annually. Cancer patients can be divided into three groups:

1. Those receiving standard or experimental therapy;
2. Those that become unresponsive to these therapies;
3. Those in remission and carrying the risk of a second new cancer and nonneoplastic diseases such as aplastic anemia, retardation of growth in some children, and delayed necrosis in some organs such as brain, liver, bone, and muscle.

Standard cancer therapy, which includes radiation therapy, chemotherapy, and surgery (whenever feasible and needed), has been useful in producing increased cure rates in certain tumors including Hodgkin's disease, childhood leukemia, and teratocarcinoma. In addition, acute damage to normal tissue occurs during radiation therapy and chemotherapy, and in some instances, such damage becomes the limiting factor for the continuation of therapy. The efficacy of standard cancer therapy has reached a plateau for most solid tumors in spite of impressive progress in radiation therapy, such as dosimetry, and more efficient methods of delivery of radiation doses to tumors. In chemotherapy, a similar progress has been made, such as the development of novel drugs with diverse mechanisms of action on cell death and proliferation inhibition.

Patients unresponsive to standard or experimental therapies have little option except for poor quality of life. At present, there is no effective strategy to reduce the risk of a second cancer among survivors or improve the quality of life among unresponsive patients. Therefore, additional approaches should be developed to improve the efficacy of current management of cancer.

This chapter discusses the use of antioxidants by patients and the recommendation of antioxidants by oncologists to the patients. It also discusses the synergy and safety of using antioxidants in combination with cancer drugs, and suggests when and how to use them during and after therapy in order to improve the efficacy of drugs.

10.2 Types of Antioxidants and Their Derivatives, Doses, and Treatment Schedule

Antioxidants can be grouped into two groups: those derived from the diet such as vitamins A, C, and E, carotenoids, and phenolic compounds; and those made endogenously in the body such as S-compounds like glutathione, coenzyme Q10, and antioxidant enzymes. The derivatives of α-tocopherol, α-tocopheryl succinate (α-TS), and retinoids, derivatives of vitamin A, have been used in experimental and clinical cancer studies. One of the well-established mechanisms of action of all antioxidants involves scavenging free radicals; however, this mechanism may be predominant at low doses for both normal and cancer cells. At high doses other mechanisms of action of antioxidants may play a dominant role in causing biological effects, and this mechanism may be critical in inhibiting the proliferation of cancer cells, but not of normal cells *in vitro* and *in vivo*.[2,3]

Certain derivatives of antioxidants such as α-TS and retinoic acid can induce differentiation, proliferation inhibition, and apoptosis in cancer cells without affecting normal cells, depending upon the dose, dose schedule, and treatment period. For this review, low doses are referred to as those that do not affect the proliferation of normal or cancer cells. In humans, antioxidant doses of about Recommended Daily Allowance (RDA) amounts can be defined as low dose. In tissue culture, vitamin C doses of up to 50 μg/mL, vitamin E (α-tocopherol) doses of up to 5 μg/mL, *d*-α-tocopheryl succinate (α-TS) doses of up to 2 μg/mL, retinoid doses of up to 5 μg/mL, and β-carotene of up to 1 μg/mL can be defined as low-dose because they do not affect the growth of cancer or normal cells.[2] High doses are referred to as those that inhibit the proliferation of cancer cells but not of normal cells. Based on human studies, oral supplementation with vitamin C up to 10 g/d, vitamin E (α-T or α-TS) up to 1000 IU/d, vitamin A doses of up to 10,000 IU/d, and natural β-carotene doses of up to 60 mg/d can be defined as high dose.

In tissue culture, vitamin C doses of up to 200 μg/mL, vitamin E doses of up to 20 μg/mL, retinoid doses of up to 20 μg/mL, and carotenoid doses of up to 10 μg/mL can be considered high dose.[2] Toxic doses are referred to as those that can inhibit the proliferation of both normal and cancer cells; therefore, they are not relevant to cancer therapy. Although oral retinoic acid doses of 300,000 IU/d, vitamin E doses of 2000 mg/d, β-carotene doses of 150 mg/d, and vitamin C doses of 20 g or more per day have been used in cancer patients; their toxicities are limited to organs such as liver and skin with retinoids, defect in blood clotting with vitamin E, diarrhea with vitamin C, and bronzing of skin with β-carotene.[2]

A treatment schedule with high dose antioxidants is also very important to producing a differential growth-inhibitory effect on normal and cancer cells. A short exposure time (a few hours) even at a high dose may not cause significant reduction in proliferation of cancer cells. Treatment time of at least 24 h or more is needed to observe a significant reduction in proliferation.[2] Therefore, it is essential that high doses of antioxidants and their derivatives be administered daily for the entire treatment period. Dose schedule is equally important for a maximal effect on growth inhibition. Treatment with high dose antioxidants must start a few days before the start of chemotherapy and continue every day thereafter until 1 month after the completion of therapy

10.3 Use of Antioxidants by Cancer Patients and Oncologist's Recommendation to Cancer Patients

Most oncologists do not recommend antioxidants to their patients during standard cancer therapy. Some may recommend a multiple vitamin preparation containing low doses of antioxidants after completion of therapy.[2] On the other hand, over 60% of cancer patients use antioxidants, and the majority combine them with standard therapy mostly without the knowledge of their oncologists.[4] These practices may be harmful for patients. For example, if patients are taking multiple vitamin preparation that contains low doses of endogenously made antioxidants (glutathione-elevating agents such as α-lipoic acid and *n*-acetylcysteine, and antioxidant enzyme-elevating agents such as selenium, which increases glutathione peroxidase activity) or dietary antioxidants[5–8] at low doses may protect cancer cells against damage produced by therapeutic agents. In addition, low doses of individual dietary antioxidants may stimulate the proliferation of some cancer cells.[2] Neither oncologists nor patients are aware of these potential dangers of taking antioxidants without any scientific rationale. Therefore, a scientifically rational nutritional protocol may be proposed in order to prevent the misuse of antioxidants during and after standard therapy.

10.4 Selective Growth-Inhibitory Effect of Individual Dietary Antioxidant and Their Derivatives on Cancer Cells

Dietary antioxidants and their derivatives such as vitamin A (including retinoids), vitamin C, α-TS, and natural β-carotene at high doses can induce differentiation, proliferation inhibition, and apoptosis, depending upon dose and type of antioxidants, treatment schedule, and type of tumor cells, without producing similar effects on most normal cells *in vitro* and *in vivo*. Some cancer cells belonging to the same cancer phenotype exhibit resistance to these antioxidants. These studies have been referenced in several reviews and articles.[9–18] An example of α-TS–induced differentiation of murine melanoma cells (B16) is shown in Figure 10.1.[9] Most of the murine melanoma cells were terminally differentiated; however, α-TS–resistant cells were also present. In contrast to rodent melanoma cells, human melanoma cells exhibited reduced sensitivity to antioxidants except to vitamin C.

10.5 Mechanisms of Action of High-Dose Individual Dietary Antioxidants and Their Derivatives on Cancer Cells

The mechanisms of action of dietary antioxidants and their derivatives on cancer cells may be different from those on normal cells. Even on cancer cells, they may involve more than one mechanism including differential uptake, imbalance in redox status, changes in gene expression, and cell signaling systems.

10.5.1 Differential Accumulation of Dietary Antioxidants and Their Derivatives?

One of the mechanisms of action of dietary antioxidants and their derivatives may involve a differential accumulation of these agents by normal and cancer

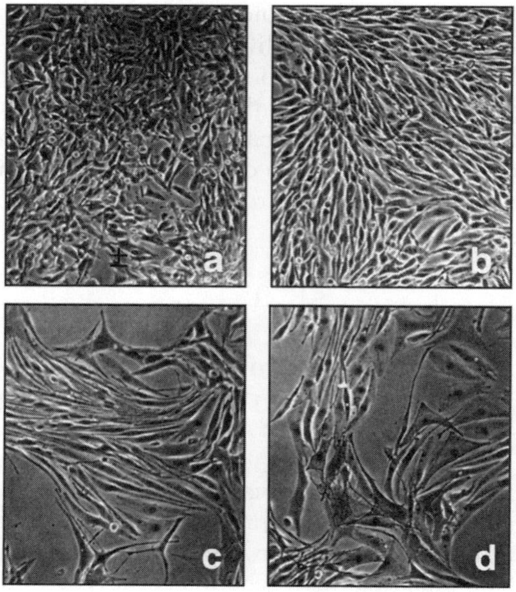

FIGURE 10.1
Vitamin E succinate inhibits growth of B16 murine melanoma cells. Melanoma cells (10^5) were plated in tissue culture dishes (60 mm), and *d*-α-tocopheryl succinate (α-TS) and sodium succinate plus ethanol were added to separate cultures 24 h after plating. Drugs and medium were changed at 2 and 3 d after treatment. Photomicrographs were taken 4 d after treatment. (a) Control cultures showed fibroblastic cells as well as round cells in clumps; (b) cultures treated with ethanol (1%) and sodium succinate (5 to 6 μg/mL) also exhibited fibroblastic morphology with fewer round cells; (c) α-TS-treated cultures 6 μg/mL, and (d) 8 μg/μL showed a dramatic change in morphology. Magnification: ×300. (Prasad, K.N., Kumar, A., Kochupillai, V., and Cole, W.C., *J. Am. Coll. Nutr.*, 18(1), 13–25, 1999.)

cells. For example, tumor cells accumulated more vitamin C than normal tissue following the administration of radioactively labeled vitamin C into animals carrying transplanted tumors.[19] A similar observation was made earlier in patients with leukemia.[2] Thus, increased accumulation of vitamin C by tumor cells following high-dose supplementation may be responsible for its anticancer activity. Our results showed that human cervical cancer cells (HeLa cells) and normal human fibroblasts in culture accumulated similar levels of α-TS within 24 h of treatment,[11] although cancer cells were more sensitive to antioxidants than normal fibroblasts. This suggests that tumor cells acquire increased sensitivity to α-TS during transformation to cancer phenotype.

Basal levels of antioxidants in fresh surgically removed human tumors and their adjacent normal tissues were highly variable[20,21] because of differences in dietary intake, vascularity, and uptake and subsequent intracellular metabolism of antioxidants between normal and cancer cells. Thus, a comparative analysis of the levels of antioxidants in freshly isolated tumor tissues and their adjacent normal tissues may not be suitable to evaluate potential differences between tumor and normal tissues.

10.5.2 Imbalance of Redox Status in Cancer Cells

Some cancer cells, but not normal cells, require increased oxidative stress for proliferation.[22–24] For these cancer cells, a marked reduction or a further enhancement of oxidative stress may lead to proliferation inhibition and/or apoptosis. For example:

Water soluble α-T at high concentrations inhibited the proliferation of cancer cells *in vitro*.[9]

Butylated hydroxyanisole (exhibits antioxidant activity similar to that of vitamin E, but without vitamin E activity) at a concentration of 27.7 μ*M* inhibited proliferation of melanoma cells and NB cells.[9]

Trolox (a water soluble form of vitamin E) at a concentration of 19.9 μ*M* also reduced the growth of both NB cells and melanoma cells in culture[9]; however, at higher concentrations, it can cause apoptosis in human colon cancer cells in culture.[25]

Treatment with a high-dose α-TS reduced the growth of tumors in an animal model.[17,18,25]

Treatment of tumor cells with dietary antioxidants such as vitamin C, β-carotene, and vitamin A also reduced the growth of tumor cells.[2] Thus, antioxidant-induced selective inhibition of growth in cancer cells, but not in normal cells, may in part be explained by imbalances in oxidative stress.

It has been suggested that α-TS–induced inhibition of cell proliferation *in vitro* requires that this molecule remain intact.[26] Because α-TS is not hydrolyzed by cancer cells *in vitro*[11] and because it exhibits strong anticancer activity *in vitro* and *in vivo*,[3,9,10,17,18] the previous suggestion appears to be rational. It has been reported that treatment of cancer cells with α-TS causes mitochondrial damage and increases the levels of free radicals.[27] Thus, α-TS treatment causes proliferation inhibition and/or apoptosis in cancer cells by increasing oxidative stress.

10.5.3 Alteration in Gene Expression, Protein Level, and Protein Translocation in Cancer Cells

When cancer cells are exposed to high dose antioxidants or their derivatives, the genetic responses occur in stages and in a time-dependent manner. An immediate early response (IER) may occur within a few minutes to hours, and changes in gene expression during this period do not require the synthesis of any new proteins because they can utilize already formed proteins, including receptors and transcriptional factors. Once the new IER proteins are translated, they can act as transcriptional regulators triggering new waves of changes in gene expression that may induce proliferation inhibition and/or apoptosis. We have observed that α-TS treatment of neuroblastoma cells at a growth-inhibitory dose alters the expression of several IER genes 30 min after treatment (unpublished observation). It has been proposed that α-TS treatment damages mitochondria, which become the primary source of increased free radicals responsible for apoptosis in cancer cells.[27] We propose that IER genes are the primary targets for the action of α-TS, and that alteration in expression of IER genes may cause damage to mitochondria and may lead to alteration in expression of late genes and their corresponding protein levels associated with proliferation inhibition and/or apoptosis. In addition, the translocation of certain proteins from one cellular compartment to another may occur. Indeed, treatment of cancer cells with high dose retinoic acid, α-TS, or β-carotene markedly alters expression of genes, levels of proteins, and translocation of certain proteins from one cellular compartment to another. These genes and proteins cause differentiation, proliferation inhibition, and apoptosis, depending upon the type and form of antioxidants, treatment schedule, and type of tumor cells. These genetic changes are directly related to proliferation inhibition and apoptosis. These studies have been summarized in recent reviews.[2,3,9,10]

10.6 Effect of Multiple Dietary Antioxidants and Their Derivatives on Cancer Cells

A mixture of dietary antioxidants and their derivatives is more effective in reducing the proliferation of cancer cells than the individual antioxidants or their derivatives. A mixture of retinoic acid, α-TS, vitamin C, and carotenoids produced approximately 50% proliferation inhibition in human melanoma cells in culture at doses that produced no significant effect on proliferation when used individually (Table 10.1).[28] Doubling the dose of vitamin C in the mixture caused a 90 % reduction in proliferation. This synergistic effect of the mixture may occur because each of these antioxidants or their derivatives may a have different mechanism of action in cancer cells.

10.7 Effect of Individual Endogenously Made Antioxidants on Cancer Cells

Endogenously made antioxidants also inhibited the proliferation of cancer cells. For example, over-expression of manganese–superoxide dismutase

TABLE 10.1
Effect of a Mixture of Four Antioxidant Micronutrients on Growth of Human Melanoma Cells in Culture

Treatments	Cell Number (% of Controls)
Vit C (50 μg/mL)	102 ± 5[a]
PC (10 μg/mL)	96 ± 2
α-TS (10 μg/mL)	102 ± 3
RA (7.5 μg/mL)	103 ± 3
Vit C (50 μg/mL) + PC (10 μg/mL) + α-TS (10 μg/mLl) + RA (7.5 μg/mL)	56 ± 3
Vit C (100 μg/mL)	64 ± 3
Vit C (100 μg/mL) + PC (10 μg/mL) + α-TS (10 μg/mL) + RA (7.5 μg/mL)	13 ± 1

PC = Polar carotenoids (PC) originally referred to as β-carotene (Prasad, K.N., Kumar, A., Kochupillai, V., and Cole, W.C., *J. Am. Coll. Nutr.*, 18(1), 13–25, 1999.); Vit C = sodium ascorbate; α-TS = α-tocopheryl succinate; RA = 13-*cis*-retinoic acid

[a] Standard error of the mean

Source: Data were summarized from Prasad, K.N., Hernandez, C., Edwards-Prasad, J., Nelson, J., Borus, T., and Robinson, W.A., *Nutr. Cancer,* 22(3), 233–245, 1994.

(Mn-SOD) reduces the proliferation and suppresses the malignant phenotype of glioma[29] and melanoma cells[30] in culture. Glutathione-elevating agents such as *N*-acetylcysteine (NAC) at high doses inhibit the proliferation of cancer cells *in vitro* and *in vivo*.[31] These data support the idea that cancer cells require increased oxidative stress for proliferation and that inhibition of oxidative stress by endogenous antioxidants may reduce the growth of tumors. However, other mechanisms, such as affecting the expression of genes associated with cell-cycle and apoptosis, may also be involved. The effect of endogenously made antioxidants on proliferation of normal cells has not been investigated.

10.8 Effect of Antioxidant Deficiency on Cancer Cells

Using transgenic mice with brain tumors, investigators reported[32] that a diet deficient in vitamins A and E increased apoptosis by about fivefold and reduced tumor volume by about 50% after 4 months on the diet in comparison to a standard diet or a diet rich in vitamins A and E (twofold more than that in standard diet). No evidence of apoptosis was found in the liver, small intestine, or spleen. The clinical significance of this observation remains uncertain. Deficiency in vitamins A and E may induce irreversible neurological and neuromuscular damage, and other toxicities. Furthermore, such an antioxidant deficient diet before treatment may enhance the effect of x-irradiation or chemotherapeutic agents on both cancer cells and normal cells. These issues should be resolved before considering this approach in the management of human tumors.

10.9 Interaction of Antioxidants and Their Derivatives with Therapeutic Agents

The effects of interaction of antioxidants or their derivatives with cancer drugs depends not only on the type of drugs or type of cancer, but also on the type of antioxidants delivered individually or in combination, dose and dose schedule of antioxidants, and treatment period with antioxidants. Antioxidants may protect both normal cells and cancer cells, may protect only normal cells, or may protect normal cells while enhancing the effect of drugs on cancer cells during therapy, depending upon previously mentioned variables.

10.9.1 Protective Effect of Individual Antioxidants and Their Derivatives on Cancer Cells during Radiation Therapy

Laboratory data show that antioxidants can protect cancer cells when dietary antioxidants are administered at doses low enough that do not affect the proliferation of these cells and only one time shortly before x-irradiation. When administered at a high or low dose only one time shortly before therapeutic agents, endogenously made antioxidants such as glutathione-elevating agents (α-lipoic acid and *N*-acetylcysteine) or antioxidant enzyme-elevating agents such as selenium, a cofactor of glutathione peroxidase, can protect cancer cells. For example, when a single low dose was given shortly before x-irradiation, dietary antioxidants such as vitamin E (α-tocopherol), vitamin C, or *N*-acetylcysteine (NAC), reduced the effectiveness of irradiation in *in vitro* and *in vivo* models.[5–8] The importance of SH-compounds in radiation protection is further demonstrated because mitotic cells, which are most radiosensitive, have the lowest levels of SH-compounds, and S-phase cells, which are the most radioresistant, have the highest level of these compounds.[5] The importance of antioxidant enzyme in radiosensitivity is demonstrated because overexpression of mitochondrial manganese–superoxide dismutase (Mn-SOD-2) enhanced the radioresistance of tumor cells.[33,34] Since one of major mechanisms of cytotoxic effects of x-irradiation is mediated by the generation of excessive amounts of free radicals, oncologists use these data to suggest that antioxidants should not be administered during radiation therapy under any conditions because of the fear that they may protect cancer cells against free radical damage.

10.9.2 Enhancing Effect of Individual Antioxidants and Their Derivatives on Cancer Cells During Chemotherapy: *In Vitro* Studies

Several studies show that individual dietary antioxidants or their derivatives enhance the effect of chemotherapeutic agents on cancer cells while protecting normal cells against some of their toxicities.[9,11,14,27,28] When dietary antioxidants and their derivatives are administered in a single or multiple dose that can inhibit the proliferation of cancer cells, but not of normal cells, several hours to days before therapy and continued every day for the entire treatment period, the viability of cancer cells is markedly reduced in comparison to those treated with antioxidants or therapeutic agents alone.[9,11,28]

The effect of direct interaction between antioxidants and cancer therapeutic agents can initially best be tested on cancer cells in culture. Several studies have revealed that vitamin C, α-TS, α-TA, vitamin A (including retinoids), and polar carotenoids including β-carotene enhance the growth inhibitory effect of most of the chemotherapeutic agents on some cancer cells in culture.[2] Chemotherapeutic agents used in these studies include 5-FU, vincristine, adriamycin, bleomycin, 5-(3,3-dimethyl-1-triazeno)-imidazole-4-carboximide (DTIC), *cis*-platin, tamoxifen, cyclophosphamide, mutamycin, chlorozotocin, and carmustine. The extent of this enhancement depends on the dose and form of antioxidants, treatment schedule, dose and type of chemotherapeutic agent, and type of tumor cell. Some examples of antioxidant-induced enhancement of the effect of chemotherapeutic agents are described below. An aqueous form of vitamin E, α-tocopheryl acetate, enhanced the effect of vincristine on neuroblastoma cells in culture[2] (Figure 10.2). Vitamin C enhanced the effect of 5-fluouracil (5-FU) on neuroblastoma cells in culture[2] (Figure 10.3). Alpha-TS increased the effect of adriamycin on human prostate carcinoma cells in culture.[35] Recently, we have found that α-TS increased the effect of adriamycin on human cervical cancer cells (HeLa) without modifying the effect of adriamycin on normal human fibroblasts in culture (unpublished observation) (Table 10.2). α-TS also enhanced the effect of carmustine on rat glioma cells in culture (unpublished observation).

Mevastatin (a cholesterol-lowering drug), a statin with a closed-ring structure, inhibited the growth of established cancer cells as well as immortalized cells (equivalent to premalignant lesion), whereas statins with an open-ring structure (pravastatin) were ineffective. Retinoic acid, α-TS, or polar carotenoids in combination with mevastatin was more effective in reducing the growth of cancer cells than the individual agents.[36]

10.9.3 Enhancing Effect of Individual Antioxidants and Their Derivatives on Cancer Cells during Chemotherapy: *In Vivo* Studies

A few *in vivo* studies support the concept that antioxidants selectively enhance the effect of chemotherapeutic agents on tumor cells by increasing tumor response. For example, vitamin A (retinyl palmitate) or synthetic β-carotene at doses which were 10-fold higher than the RDA for these nutri-

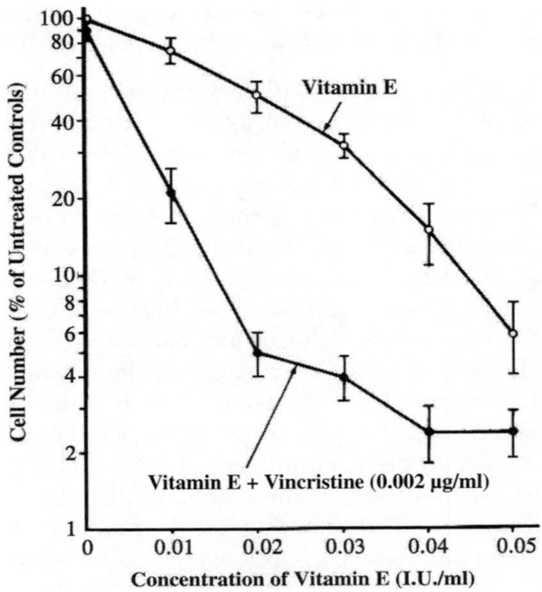

FIGURE 10.2
Combined effects of vitamin E and vincristine. Neuroblastoma cells (NBP2) (50,000 per dish) were plated in tissue culture dishes (60 mm), and vincristine and aqueous preparation of vitamin E (*dl*-α-tocopheryl acetate) were added 24 h later. Drugs and medium were changed 2 d after treatment. The cell number and the number of trypan blue–stained cells were determined 3 d after treatment. The number of stained cells was subtracted from the total number of cells to obtain viable cells per dish. The average of control cultures was considered 100%. Each value represents an average of at least six samples. The bar of each point is standard deviation. The bars not shown in the figure were equal to the sizes of symbol. (Prasad, K.N., Kumar, A., Kochupillai, V., and Cole, W.C., *J. Am. Coll. Nutr.*, 18(1), 13–25, 1999.)

ents, in combination with cyclophosphamide, increased the cure rate from 0 to over 90% in mice with transplanted adenocarcinoma of the breast.[37] A study using a thiol-containing antioxidant, pyrrolidinedithiocarbamate (PDTC), and a water-soluble vitamin E analog (6-hydroxy-2,5,7,8-tetrameythylchroman-2-carboxylic acid; Vitamin E), showed that antioxidant treatment enhanced the antitumor effects of 5-flurouracil (5-FU) in athymic mice with human colorectal cancer.[14] The synthetic retinoid (fenretinide) was effective against a human ovarian carcinoma xenograft and potentiated *cis*-platin activity.[38] A study has reported that NAC at a dose of 1 g/kg of body weight delivered i.p. in combination with doxorubicin reduced tumorigenicity and metastasis following transplantation of B-16 murine melanoma cells in mice.[31] NAC at concentrations greater than 500 mg/person/d increased the urinary excretion of Zn,[39] and thus can induce Zn deficiency. Selenium (sodium selenite) and vitamin E protected against radiation-induced intestinal injury.[40] However, organic selenium at a high dose (0.2 mg/mouse/d or 10 mg/kg body weight/d) enhances the therapeutic efficacy of some chemotherapeutic agents in athymic mice bearing human squamous cell

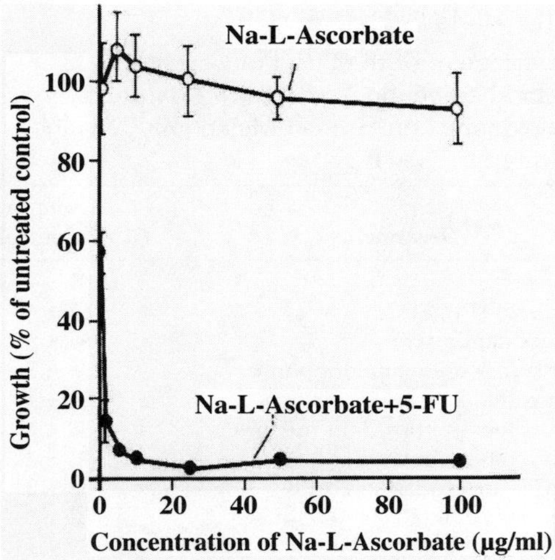

FIGURE 10.3
Effects on growth of P2 mouse neuroblastoma cells by sodium (Na-L) ascorbate with or without 5-FU. Neuroblastoma cells (50,000 per dish) were plated in tissue culture dishes (60 mm), and 5-fluorouracil (5-FU) (0.08 μg/mL) plus sodium ascorbate or sodium ascorbate alone was added 24 h after plating. The drug and medium were changed every day, and the number of cells per dish was determined 3 d after treatment. Each value represents the mean of six to nine samples ± standard deviation (Prasad, K.N., Kumar, A., Kochupillai, V., and Cole, W.C., *J. Am. Coll. Nutr.*, 18(1), 13–25, 1999.)

TABLE 10.2
Modification of Adriamycin Effect on Human Cervical Cancer Cells (HeLa) and Human Normal Skin Fibroblasts in Culture by d-α-Tocopheryl Succinate

Treatment	HeLa Cells	Fibroblasts
Solvent control	99 ± 2.6	104 ± 3.4
Adriamycin (0.1 μg/mL)	57 ± 6.2	77 ± 2.4
Alpha-TS (10 μg/mL)	99 ± 1.6	101 ± 3.7
Adriamycin (0.1 μg/mL) + α-TS (10 μg/mL)	20 ± 7.9	77 ± 1.7
Adriamycin (0.25 μg/mL)	14 ± 2.9	68 ± 1.0
Adriamycin (0.25 μg/mL) + α-TS (10 μg/mL)	5 ± 0.8	62 ± 1.8

Cells (20,000) were plated in 24-well chamber, and adriamycin and α-tocopheryl succinate (α-TS) were added one after another at the same time. Drug, α-TS, and fresh growth medium were changed 2 d after treatment, and the viability of cells was determined by MTT assay. Growth in experimental groups was expressed as percent of the untreated control. Each experiment was repeated at least twice, and each value represents an average of 6 to 9 samples ± SEM (Kumar et al. unpublished observation).

TABLE 10.3

Enhancement of the Effect of Certain Chemotherapeutic Agents by a Mixture of Four Antioxidants[a] on Human Melanoma Cells in Culture

Treatments	Cell Number (% of Controls)
Solvent	101 ± 4
Cisplatin (1 μg/mL)	67 ± 4
Antioxidant mixture	56 ± 3
Cisplatin + antioxidant mixture	38 ± 2
Tamoxifen (2 μg/mL)	81 ± 3
Tamoxifen + antioxidant mixture	30 ± 2
DTIC (100 μg/mL)	71 ± 2
DTIC + antioxidant mixture	38 ± 2
Interferon α2b (10,000 IU/mL)	82 ± 5
Interferon α2b + antioxidant mixture	29 ± 1

Polar carotenoids was originally referred as β-carotene. Vitamin C, 50 μg/mL; polar carotenoids, 10 μg/mL; α-tocopheryl succinate, 10 μg/mL and 13-*cis*-retinoic acid, 7.5 μg/mL were added simultaneously.

[a] Standard error of the mean.

Source: Data were summarized from. Prasad, K.N., Hernandez, C., Edwards-Prasad, J., Nelson, J., Borus, T., and Robinson, W.A., *Nutr. Cancer,* 22(3), 233–245, 1994.

carcinoma of head and neck.[41] This observation could be very exciting if a similar observation is made in human cancer without unacceptable toxicity. It should be pointed out that rodents exhibit a high degree of resistance to most therapeutic agents.

10.9.4 Enhancing Effect of Multiple Antioxidants and Their Derivatives on Cancer Cells during Chemotherapy: *In Vitro* Studies

A mixture of antioxidants containing retinoic acid, vitamin C, α-TS, and polar carotenoids in combination with DTIC, tamoxifen, cisplatin, or interferon-α2b inhibited the proliferation of human melanoma cells in culture more than the growth inhibition produced by the individual agents[28] (Table 10.3). This suggests that multiple antioxidants are also effective in enhancing the effect of certain chemotherapeutic agents on cancer cells. The antioxidant mixture (vitamin C, 100 μg/mL; α-TS, 10 μg/mL; and β-carotene, 10 μg/mL) by itself induced apoptosis in human lung squamous cell carcinoma cells (H520). Paclitaxel treatment 24 h before carboplatin caused 54% apoptosis; however, when cells were treated with a mixture of antioxidants 24 h before chemotherapeutic agents, 89% apoptosis was achieved (Table 10.4).[42]

TABLE 10.4

Flow-Cytometric Analysis of the Effect of Combination of the Agents (Paclitaxel, Carboplatin, and Antioxidant Mixture) on Apoptosis in H520 Cells

Serial No.	Treatment of Cells				Apoptosis (% cells) (Mean ± SE[a]) (Day 5)
	Day 1	Day 2	Day 3	Day 4	
1	Cells plated	—	—	—	20.6 ± 1.2
2	Cells plated	Paclitaxel + carboplatin	—	—	40.3 ± 3.1
3	Cells plated	Paclitaxel	Carboplatin	—	54.3 ± 2.2
4	Cells plated	Vitamins + paclitaxel	Carboplatin	—	70.11 ± 3.7
5	Cells plated	Vitamins	Paclitaxel	Carboplatin	89.15 ± 4.3

Cells were plated on Day 1 and flow-cytometry was performed on Day 5. Control = Serial no. 1. Doses: paclitaxel: 0.05 μmol/mL, carboplatin: 0.5 μg/mL, vitamin C: 100 μg/mL, vitamin E: 10 μg/mL, β-carotene: 10 μg/mL. (Pathak, A.K., Singh, N., Khanna, N., Reddy, V.G., and Prasad, K.N., *J. Am. Cell. Nutr.*, 21(5), 416–421, 2002.)

[a] SE = Standard error. Results are of three separate experiments, each performed in duplicate.

10.10 Protection of Normal Cells against Damage Produced by x-Irradiation and Chemotherapeutic Agents by High-Dose Individual Dietary Antioxidants and Their Derivatives

Treatment with dietary antioxidants reduced the effect of irradiation on normal tissues in patients with small cell lung carcinoma.[43,44] Vitamin E reduces bleomycin-induced lung fibrosis, adriamycin-induced cardiac toxicity, and adriamycin-induced skin necrosis. Vitamin E also reduces doxorubicin-induced toxicity in liver, kidney, and intestinal mucositis. Another study has reported that β-carotene and vitamin A (retinyl palmitate) reduce the adverse effects of cyclophosphamide in mice. Vitamin C has been shown to reduce the adverse effects of some chemotherapeutic agents on normal cells, such as reducing the adverse effects of adriamycin. Vitamin C, α-TS, and 13-*cis*-retinoic acid (RA) reduce bleomycin-induced chromosomal breakage. These studies have been referenced in a recent review.[2] Vitamin E and C supplements reduced the tamoxifen-induced hyperlipidemia in patients with breast cancer.[45]

10.11 Clinical Studies with Multiple Dietary Antioxidants in Combination with Standard Therapy

Eighteen nonrandomized patients with small cell lung cancer received multiple antioxidant treatment with chemotherapy and/or radiation. The median survival time was markedly enhanced, and patients tolerated chemotherapy and irradiation well.[43] Similar observations were made in several private practice settings.[44] A randomized pilot trial (Phase I/II) with high-dose multiple micronutrients including dietary antioxidants and their derivatives (SEVAK, a multiple vitamin preparation, 8 g vitamin C as calcium ascorbate, 800 IU vitamin E as α- TS, and 60 mg natural β-carotene, orally, divided into two doses, half in the morning and half in the evening) in patients with stage 0 to III breast cancer receiving radiation therapy has been completed.[46] There were 25 patients in the radiation arm and 22 patients in the combination arm. A follow-up period of 22 months during which no maintenance supplements were given show that one patient in the radiation arm developed a new cancer in the contralateral breast and another in the same arm developed LCIS (lobular carcinoma *in situ*) in the opposite breast. In the combination arm, no new tumor has developed. A randomized trial with high dose antioxidants (8 g vitamin C as ascorbic acid, 800 IU α-TS, 60 mg β-carotene, 800 μg selenium) in combination with chemotherapeutic agents (cisplatin and paclitaxel) in patients with advanced non–small cell carcinoma of the lung (34 patients in chemotherapy arm and 31 patients in combination arm) reported beneficial effects on tumor response and tolerance to chemotherapeutic agents for a follow-up period of 1 year[47] (Table 10.5). The addition of selenium in this trial may have reduced the efficacy of the protocol. Based on the beneficial effects of multiple antioxidants in combination with standard therapy on two patients with ovarian cancer,[48] Drisko et al. have started a new trial with multiple antioxidants on ovarian cancers. Thus, *in vitro, in vivo* (animal), and human studies suggest that a well-designed trial with multiple antioxidants and their derivatives when

TABLE 10.5

Preliminary Results of a Randomized Clinical Trial Using High Dose Multiple Antioxidants as an Adjunct to Chemotherapy

Treatment and Tumor Response	Chemotherapy Arm (No. of Patients = 29)	Chemo ± Antioxidant Arm (No. of Patients = 28)
Median number of chemotherapy cycles	3	6
Number of patients completing six cycles	11	16
Complete response	0	1
Partial response	9	16
Stable disease	5	4
Progressive disease	15	8
Overall survival at 1 year	7 months	14 months

Daily dose: Ascorbic acid, 6100 mg; *d*-α-tocopherol, 1050 mg; β-carotene, 60 mg; copper sulfate, 6 mg; manganese sulfate, 9 mg; zinc sulfate, 45 mg; and selenium, 900 μg. Antioxidant was started 48 h before chemotherapy and continued 1 month after completion of therapy, and then reduced to half the dose as a maintenance regimen. (Pathak, A.K., Signh, N., Guleria, R., Bal, S., Thulkar, S., Mohanti, B.K., Gupta, S., Khanna, N., Reddy, V.G., Thakur, M.B., Bhamra, D.S., Bhutani, M., Prasad, K.N., and Kochupillai, V., Role of vitamins along with chemotherapy in non small cell lung cancer, in *International Conference on nutrition and cancer,* Montevideo-Uruguay, 2002, p. 28.)

administered before, during, and after standard therapy is urgently needed. Since i.v. vitamin C at very high doses is used by physicians practicing in alternative medicine, the relative value of i.v. vs. oral administration of vitamin C together with other orally administered antioxidants should be evaluated. In addition, how multiple antioxidants and their derivatives at low and high doses affect gene expression in normal and cancer cells should be evaluated because very little is known on this issue.

10.12 Mechanisms of Enhancement of the Effect of Standard Therapeutic Agents on Cancer Cells by High-Dose Dietary Individual Antioxidants and Their Derivatives

The exact reasons for the dietary antioxidant–induced enhancement of damage produced by standard therapeutic agents on cancer cells are unknown. We propose that treatment of tumor cells with high doses of dietary antioxidants before chemotherapy can initiate damage in cancer cells, but not in normal cells. Free radicals generated by chemotherapeutic agents, even if completely quenched by antioxidants, become irrelevant because damaged cancer cells suffer further injuries by mechanisms other than free radicals associated with chemotherapeutic agents.[2] It has been reported that α-TS–induced apoptosis in cancer cells is independent of p53 and p21,[25] whereas 5-FU-induced apoptosis is mediated via p53 and p21.[14] Therefore, the combination of two agents may be more effective than the individual agents. α-TS *in vivo* acts as an antiangiogenesis agent,[18] whereas chemotherapeutic agents do not; therefore, the combination of α-TS with these agents may be more effective than the individual agents. The effect of high dose dietary antioxidants in enhancing the level of damage in cancer cells produced by chemotherapeutic agents may not be due to their antioxidant activity; they may alter expression of genes associated with the cell cycle and apoptosis. These dietary antioxidants and their derivatives do not initiate damage in normal cells before chemotherapy; therefore, when these cells are treated with chemotherapeutic agents, they can be protected by antioxidants through their classical antioxidant activity.

10.13 Enhancement of the Effect of Certain Biological Response Modifiers on Cancer Cells by High-Dose Individual Dietary Antioxidants and Their Derivatives

We have reported that α-TS and polar carotenoids markedly enhanced the levels of cAMP-induced terminal differentiation in neuroblastoma cells and melanoma cells in culture[2] (Figure 10.4). Butyric acid, a four-carbon fatty acid,[49] or its analog, phenylbutyrate,[50,51] exhibit strong anticancer properties on tumor cells in culture. However, clinical studies with these agents produced minimal benefits in cancer patients.[52,53] Therefore, any agent that can enhance the effect of sodium butyrate or phenylbutyrate would enhance the value of these agents in clinical studies. We have reported that α-TS enhanced the growth-inhibitory effect of sodium butyrate on certain tumor cells in culture (Figure 10.5).[54]. Retinoic acid increased the effect of phenylbutyrate on human prostate cancer cell growth and angiogenesis in athymic mice.[55] α-TS[28] and retinoids[56] also enhance the effect of interferon in cell culture and *in vivo*, respectively. In addition, α-TS enhances the antitumor activity of a vaccine (dendritic cells) in an animal tumor model.[57] These data suggest that antioxidants or their derivatives can enhance the growth-inhibitory effect of some biological response modifiers.

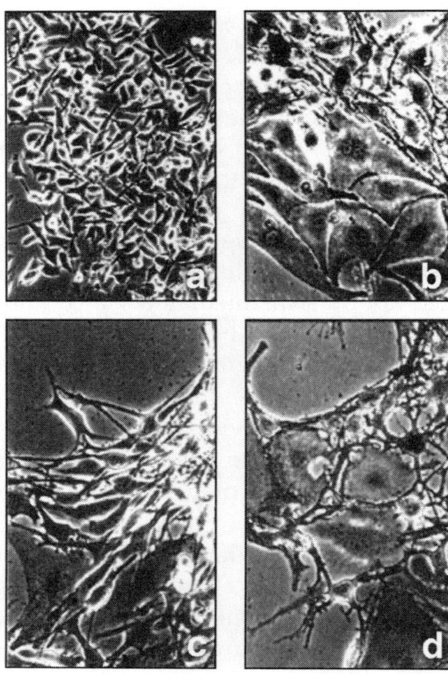

FIGURE 10.4
Combined effect of vitamin E succinate and cAMP elevation on B16 mouse melanoma cells. Photomicrographs of murine melanoma were taken 4 d after treatment. (a) Control cultures contained cells with varied morphology. (b) The melanoma cells treated with vitamin E succinate were elongated, had long cytoplasmic processes, and were arranged alongside each other. (c) Melanoma cells treated with RO20-1724 were large and elongated, had some long processes, and were arranged alongside each other. (d) A combination of RO20-1724 and vitamin E succinate increased the level of morphologic differentiation more than that produced by individual agents. ×450. (Prasad, K.N., Kumar, A., Kochupillai, V., and Cole, W.C., *J. Am. Coll. Nutr.*, 18(1), 13–25, 1999.)

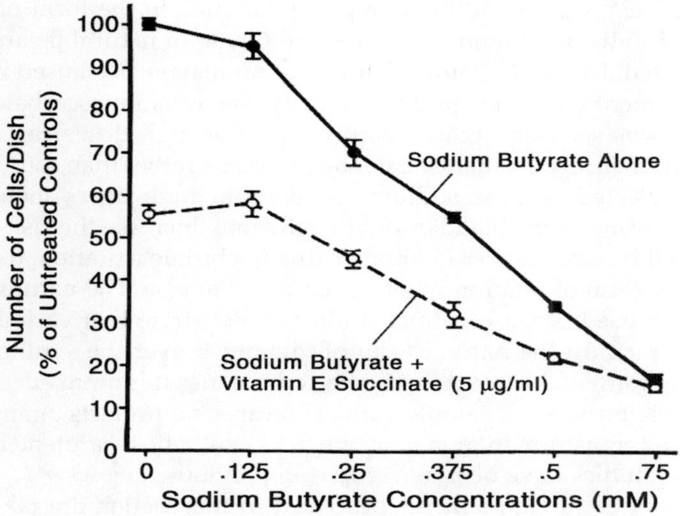

FIGURE 10.5
Effect of *d*-α-tocopheryl succinate (vitamin E succinate) in combination with sodium butyrate on the growth of neuroblastoma cells in culture. Cells (50,000 cells/60 mm dish) were plated in tissue culture dishes, and vitamin E succinate and sodium butyrate were added one after another 24 h later. Fresh growth medium and agents were changed at 2 days after treatment, and growth was determined at 3 days after treatment. Each value represents an average of six samples. The bar at each point is SEM. (Rama, B.N. and Prasad, K.N., Modification of the hyperthermic response on neuroblastoma cells by cAMP and sodium butyrate, *Cancer,* 58(7), 1448–1452, 1986.)

10.14 Proposed Micronutrient Protocols as an Adjunct to Standard Cancer Therapy

The micronutrient supplement protocols are divided into two categories: active cancer treatment protocol and maintenance protocol.

10.14.1 Active Treatment Protocol

This protocol is in clinical trial[46] and contains SEVAK (Premier Micronutrient Corporation, Nashville, Tennessee), which has multiple micronutrients including vitamin A, C, and E, and natural β-carotene, vitamin D, B vitamins, and appropriate minerals but not iron, copper, and manganese, because these three trace minerals interact with vitamin C to produce free radicals. A preparation of multiple micronutrients such as SEVAK is suggested because some of the micronutrients may be depleted during radiation therapy or chemotherapy as a result of extensive cellular death and loss of appetite. In addition to SEVAK, an additional 8 g of vitamin C in the form of calcium ascorbate, 800 IU of vitamin E as α-TS, and 60 mg of natural β-carotene are recommended. Doses of vitamin C at 10 g or more have been used in human cancer treatment without significant toxicity. The calcium ascorbate form of vitamin C was selected because ascorbic acid at high doses can cause an upset stomach in some patients. Calcium ascorbate rather than sodium ascorbate was selected because sodium ascorbate at high doses increases the molarity of urine in the bladder and thereby may increase the risk of chemical-induced bladder cancer in animals due to chronic irritation. α-TS is the most potent form of vitamin E both *in vitro* and *in vivo*. The natural form of vitamin E is used because animal studies demonstrate that various organs selectively pick up the natural form of vitamin E over the synthetic form. The natural form of β-carotene was selected because it is more effective than the synthetic form. For example, natural β-carotene protects against radiation-induced transformation *in vitro*, whereas synthetic β-carotene is ineffective. These studies have been referenced in previous reviews.[2,9]

All micronutrient supplements described in this section are taken orally and in two divided doses, one-half dose in the morning and one-half dose in the evening. The rationale for taking micronutrients twice a day is that the biological half-life of most micronutrients is about 6 to 12 h. Micronutrient supplements can be started at least 48 h prior to standard therapy and should be continued for 1 month after completion of standard therapy.

10.14.2 Maintenance Protocol

A month after therapy, the maintenance protocol begins. This protocol contains SEVAK and an additional 4 g of vitamin C, 400 IU of α-TS, and 30 mg of natural β-carotene. Such maintenance doses of micronutrients may reduce the risk of recurrence of tumors and the development of a second malignancy among survivors. After 5 years, additional doses of vitamin C, α–TS, and β-carotene can be reduced to half, and at this time, other supplements such as coenzyme Q10, NAC (*N*-acetylcysteine), and α-lipoic acid can be added for optimal health, since glutathione and coenzyme Q10 are considered important in reducing oxidative stress. Modifications in diet (low fat and high fiber) and lifestyle (avoiding tobacco smoking or tobacco products, reducing physical and mental stress, exercising moderately) are very important for improving the efficacy of the proposed micronutrient protocol. The efficacy of this protocol has not been tested. The doses are based on safety and scientific data that show that antioxidants are of protective value.

10.15 Conclusions

The analysis of laboratory data (tissue culture and animal tumor models) and limited human studies suggest that the proposed micronutrient protocols when used adjunctively with radiation therapy and/or chemotherapy may enhance their effectiveness by increasing tumor response and decreasing toxicities. In addition, the risk of recurrence of the tumor and development of a new cancer may be reduced by the proposed strategy.

Appropriate doses, dose schedule, type and form of antioxidants, and treatment schedule are essential for improving the efficacy of standard therapy.

Endogenous antioxidants such as glutathione-elevating agents (α-lipoic acid and *N*-acetylcysteine) at any dose, glutathione peroxidase–elevating agents (selenium) at high dose, or dietary antioxidants at low doses are not recommended during standard therapy.

It would be of great public service and scientific value if randomized placebo-controlled clinical trials with appropriate micronutrients including high dose multiple dietary antioxidants such as proposed here are initiated. The fear of oncologists that even high dose multiple dietary antioxidants and their derivatives at appropriate doses, dose schedule, and treatment period may protect cancer cells against damage produced by standard therapeutic agents is not based on scientific evidence.

Acknowledgment

These studies in part have been supported by the Shafroth Memorial Fund.

References

1. Jemal, A., Clegg, L.X., Ward, E., Ries, L.A., Wu, X., Jamison, P.M., Wingo, P.A., Howe, H.L., Anderson, R.N., and Edwards, B.K., Annual report to the nation on the status of cancer, 1975-2001, with a special feature regarding survival, *Cancer,* 101(1), 3–27, 2004.
2. Prasad, K.N., Kumar, A., Kochupillai, V., and Cole, W.C., High doses of multiple antioxidant vitamins: essential ingredients in improving the efficacy of standard cancer therapy, *J. Am. Coll. Nutr.,* 18(1), 13–25, 1999.
3. Neuzil, J., Weber, T., Gellert, N., and Weber, C., Selective cancer cell killing by alpha-tocopheryl succinate, *Br. J. Cancer,* 84(1), 87–89, 2001.
4. Richardson, M.A., Sanders, T., Palmer, J.L., Greisinger, A., and Singletary, S.E., Complementary/alternative medicine use in a comprehensive cancer center and the implications for oncology, *J. Clin. Oncol.,* 18(13), 2505–2514, 2000.
5. Prasad, K.N., *Handbook of Radiobiology,* 2nd ed. CRC Press, Boca Raton, FL, 1995.
6. Salganik, R.I., The benefits and hazards of antioxidants: controlling apoptosis and other protective mechanisms in cancer patients and the human population, *J. Am. Coll. Nutr.* 20 (5 Suppl), 464S–472S; discussion 473S–475S, 2001.
7. Labriola, D. and Livingston, R., Possible interactions between dietary antioxidants and chemotherapy, *Oncology (Huntingt),* 13(7), 1003–1008; discussion 1008, 1011–1012, 1999.

8. Witenberg, B., Kletter, Y., Kalir, H.H., Raviv, Z., Fenig, E., Nagler, A., Halperin, D., and Fabian, I., Ascorbic acid inhibits apoptosis induced by X irradiation in HL60 myeloid leukemia cells, *Radiat. Res.*, 152(5), 468–478, 1999.
9. Prasad, K.N., Kumar, B., Yan, X.D., Hanson, A.J., and Cole, W.C., alpha-Tocopheryl succinate, the most effective form of vitamin E for adjuvant cancer treatment: a review, *J. Am. Coll. Nutr.*, 22(2), 108–117, 2003.
10. Kline, K., Yu, W., and Sanders, B.G., Vitamin E: mechanisms of action as tumor cell growth inhibitors, *J. Nutr.*, 131(1), 161S–163S, 2001.
11. Jha, M.N., Bedford, J.S., Cole, W.C., Edward-Prasad, J., and Prasad, K.N., Vitamin E (d-alpha-tocopheryl succinate) decreases mitotic accumulation in gamma-irradiated human tumor, but not in normal, cells, *Nutr. Cancer*, 35(2), 189–194, 1999.
12. Garewal, H., Beta-Carotene and antioxidant nutrients in oral cancer prevention, in *Nutrients in cancer prevention and treatment*, Prasad, K.N., Santamaria, L., and Williams, R.M., Eds., Humana Press, Totowa, NJ, 1995, pp. 235–247.
13. Meyskens, F.L., Jr., Role of vitamin A and its derivatives in the treatment of human cancer, in *Nutrients in cancer prevention and treatment*, Prasad, K.N., Santamaria, L., and Williams, R.M., Eds., Humana Press, Totowa, NJ, 1995, pp. 349–362.
14. Chinery, R., Brockman, J.A., Peeler, M.O., Shyr, Y., Beauchamp, R.D., and Coffey, R.J., Antioxidants enhance the cytotoxicity of chemotherapeutic agents in colorectal cancer: a p53-independent induction of p21WAF1/CIP1 via C/EBPbeta, *Nat. Med.*, 3(11), 1233–1241, 1997.
15. Cameron, E., Pauling, L., and Leibovitz, B., Ascorbic acid and cancer: a review, *Cancer Res.*, 39(3), 663–681, 1979.
16. Schwartz, J.L., Molecular and biochemical control of tumor growth following treatment with carotenoids or tocopherols, in *Nutrients in cancer prevention and treatment*, Prasad, K.N., Santamaria, L., and Williams, R.M., Eds., Humana Press, Totowa, NJ, 1995, pp. 287–316.
17. Malafa, M.P. and Neitzel, L.T., Vitamin E succinate promotes breast cancer tumor dormancy, *J. Surg. Res.*, 93(1), 163–170, 2000.
18. Barnett, K.T., Fokum, F.D., and Malafa, M.P., Vitamin E succinate inhibits colon cancer liver metastases, *J. Surg. Res.*, 106(2), 292–298, 2002.
19. Agus, D.B., Vera, J.C., and Golde, D.W., Stromal cell oxidation: a mechanism by which tumors obtain vitamin C, *Cancer Res.*, 59(18), 4555–4558, 1999.
20. Piyathilake, C.J., Bell, W.C., Johanning, G.L., Cornwell, P.E., Heimburger, D.C., and Grizzle, W.E., The accumulation of ascorbic acid by squamous cell carcinomas of the lung and larynx is associated with global methylation of DNA, *Cancer*, 89(1), 171–176, 2000.
21. Liede, K.E., Alfthan, G., Hietanen, J.H., Haukka, J.K., Saxen, L.M., and Heinonen, O.P., Beta-carotene concentration in buccal mucosal cells with and without dysplastic oral leukoplakia after long-term beta-carotene supplementation in male smokers, *Eur. J. Clin, Nutr.*, 52(12), 872–876, 1998.
22. Baker, A.M., Oberley, L.W., and Cohen, M.B., Expression of antioxidant enzymes in human prostatic adenocarcinoma, *Prostate*, 32(4), 229–233, 1997.
23. Oberley, T.D. and Oberley, L.W., Antioxidant enzyme levels in cancer, *Histol. Histopathol.* 12(2), 525–535, 1997.
24. Loo, G., Redox-sensitive mechanisms of phytochemical-mediated inhibition of cancer cell proliferation (review), *J. Nutr. Biochem.*, 14(2), 64–73, 2003.

25. Neuzil, J., Weber, T., Schroder, A., Lu, M., Ostermann, G., Gellert, N., Mayne, G.C., Olejnicka, B., Negre-Salvayre, A., Sticha, M., Coffey, R.J., and Weber, C., Induction of cancer cell apoptosis by alpha-tocopheryl succinate: molecular pathways and structural requirements, *FASEB J.*, 15(2), 403–415, 2001.
26. Fariss, M.W., Fortuna, M.B., Everett, C.K., Smith, J.D., Trent, D.F., and Djuric, Z., The selective antiproliferative effects of alpha-tocopheryl hemisuccinate and cholesteryl hemisuccinate on murine leukemia cells result from the action of the intact compounds, *Cancer Res.*, 54(13), 3346–3351, 1994.
27. Weber, T., Dalen, H., Andera, L., Negre-Salvayre, A., Auge, N., Sticha, M., Lloret, A., Terman, A., Witting, P.K., Higuchi, M., Plasilova, M., Zivny, J., Gellert, N., Weber, C., and Neuzil, J., Mitochondria play a central role in apoptosis induced by alpha-tocopheryl succinate, an agent with antineoplastic activity: comparison with receptor-mediated pro-apoptotic signaling, *Biochemistry*, 42(14), 4277–4291, 2003.
28. Prasad, K.N., Hernandez, C., Edwards-Prasad, J., Nelson, J., Borus, T., and Robinson, W.A., Modification of the effect of tamoxifen, cis-platin, DTIC, and interferon-alpha 2b on human melanoma cells in culture by a mixture of vitamins, *Nutr. Cancer*, 22(3), 233–245, 1994.
29. Zhong, W., Oberley, L.W., Oberley, T.D., and St Clair, D.K., Suppression of the malignant phenotype of human glioma cells by overexpression of manganese superoxide dismutase, *Oncogene*, 14(4), 481–490, 1997.
30. Church, S.L., Grant, J.W., Ridnour, L.A., Oberley, L.W., Swanson, P.E., Meltzer, P.S., and Trent, J.M., Increased manganese superoxide dismutase expression suppresses the malignant phenotype of human melanoma cells, *Proc. Natl. Acad. Sci. U.S.A.*, 90(7), 3113–3117, 1993.
31. De Flora, S., D'Agostini, F., Masiello, L., Giunciuglio, D., and Albini, A., Synergism between N-acetylcysteine and doxorubicin in the prevention of tumorigenicity and metastasis in murine models, *Int. J. Cancer*, 67(6), 842–848, 1996.
32. Salganik, R.I., Albright, C.D., Rodgers, J., Kim, J., Zeisel, S.H., Sivashinskiy, M.S., and Van Dyke, T.A., Dietary antioxidant depletion: enhancement of tumor apoptosis and inhibition of brain tumor growth in transgenic mice, *Carcinogenesis*, 21(5), 909–914, 2000.
33. Hirose, K., Longo, D.L., Oppenheim, J.J., and Matsushima, K., Overexpression of mitochondrial manganese superoxide dismutase promotes the survival of tumor cells exposed to interleukin-1, tumor necrosis factor, selected anticancer drugs, and ionizing radiation, *FASEB J.*, 7(2), 361–368, 1993.
34. Sun, J., Chen, Y., Li, M., and Ge, Z., Role of antioxidant enzymes on ionizing radiation resistance, *Free Radic. Biol. Med.* 24(4), 586–593, 1998.
35. Ripoll, E.A., Rama, B.N., and Webber, M.M., Vitamin E enhances the chemotherapeutic effects of adriamycin on human prostatic carcinoma cells *in vitro*, *J. Urol.*, 136(2), 529–531, 1986.
36. Kumar, B., Andreatta, C., Koustas, W.T., Cole, W.C., Edwards-Prasad, J., and Prasad, K.N., Mevastatin induces degeneration and decreases viability of cAMP-induced differentiated neuroblastoma cells in culture by inhibiting proteasome activity, and mevalonic acid lactone prevents these effects, *J. Neurosci. Res.*, 68(5), 627–635, 2002.
37. Seifter, E., Rettura, A., Padawar, J., and Levenson, S.M., Vitamin A and β-carotene as adjunctive therapy to tumor excision, radiation therapy and chemotherapy, in *Vitamins, nutrition and cancer*, Prasad, K.N., Ed., Karger, Basel, 1984, pp. 1–19.

38. Formelli, F. and Cleris, L., Synthetic retinoid fenretinide is effective against a human ovarian carcinoma xenograft and potentiates cisplatin activity, *Cancer Res.*, 53(22), 5374–5376, 1993.
39. Brumas, V., Hacht, B., Filella, M., and Berthon, G., Can N-acetyl-L-cysteine affect zinc metabolism when used as a paracetamol antidote? *Agents Actions*, 36(3–4), 278–288, 1992.
40. Mutlu-Turkoglu, U., Erbil, Y., Oztezcan, S., Olgac, V., Toker, G., and Uysal, M., The effect of selenium and/or vitamin E treatments on radiation-induced intestinal injury in rats, *Life Sci.*, 66(20), 1905–1913, 2000.
41. Cao, S., Durrani, F.A., and Rustum, Y.M., Selective modulation of the therapeutic efficacy of anticancer drugs by selenium containing compounds against human tumor xenografts, *Clin. Cancer. Res.*, 10(7), 2561–2569, 2004.
42. Pathak, A.K., Singh, N., Khanna, N., Reddy, V.G., Prasad, K.N., and Kochupillai, V., Potentiation of the effect of paclitaxel and carboplatin by antioxidant mixture on human lung cancer h520 cells, *J. Am. Coll. Nutr.*, 21(5), 416–421, 2002.
43. Jaakkola, K., Lahteenmaki, P., Laakso, J., Harju, E., Tykka, H., and Mahlberg, K., Treatment with antioxidant and other nutrients in combination with chemotherapy and irradiation in patients with small-cell lung cancer, *Anticancer Res.*, 12(3), 599–606, 1992.
44. Lamson, D.W. and Brignall, M.S., Antioxidants in cancer therapy; their actions and interactions with oncologic therapies, *Altern. Med. Rev.*, 4(5), 304–329, 1999.
45. Babu, J.R., Sundravel, S., Arumugam, G., Renuka, R., Deepa, N., and Sachdanandam, P., Salubrious effect of vitamin C and vitamin E on tamoxifen-treated women in breast cancer with reference to plasma lipid and lipoprotein levels, *Cancer Lett.*, 151(1), 1–5, 2000.
46. Walker, E.M., Ross, D., Pegg, J., Devine, G., Prasad, K.N., and Kim, J.H., Nutritional and high dose antioxidant interventions during radiation therapy for cancer of the breast, in *International conference on nutrition and cancer*, Montevideo-Uruguay, 2002, p. 27.
47. Pathak, A.K., Signh, N., Guleria, R., Bal, S., Thulkar, S., Mohanti, B.K., Gupta, S., Khanna, N., Reddy, V.G., Thakur, M.B., Bhamra, D.S., Bhutani, M., Prasad, K.N., and Kochupillai, V., Role of vitamins along with chemotherapy in non small cell lung cancer, in *International conference on nutrition and cancer*, Montevideo-Uruguay, 2002, p. 28.
48. Drisko, J.A., Chapman, J., and Hunter, V.J., The use of antioxidants with first-line chemotherapy in two cases of ovarian cancer, *J. Am. Coll. Nutr.*, 22(2), 118–123, 2003.
49. Prasad, K.N. and Sinha, P.K., Effect of sodium butyrate on mammalian cells in culture: a review, *In Vitro*, 12(2), 125–132, 1976.
50. Samid, D., Shack, S., and Sherman, L.T., Phenylacetate: a novel nontoxic inducer of tumor cell differentiation, *Cancer Res.*, 52(7), 1988–1992, 1992.
51. Melchior, S.W., Brown, L.G., Figg, W.D., Quinn, J.E., Santucci, R.A., Brunner, J., Thuroff, J.W., Lange, P.H., and Vessella, R.L., Effects of phenylbutyrate on proliferation and apoptosis in human prostate cancer cells *in vitro* and *in vivo*, *Int. J. Oncol.*, 14(3), 501–508, 1999.
52. Thibault, A., Samid, D., Cooper, M.R., Figg, W.D., Tompkins, A.C., Patronas, N., Headlee, D.J., Kohler, D.R., Venzon, D.J., and Myers, C.E., Phase I study of phenylacetate administered twice daily to patients with cancer, *Cancer*, 75(12), 2932–2938, 1995.

53. Carducci, M.A., Bowling, M.K., Eisenberger, M., Sinibaldi, V., Chen, T., Noe, D., Grochow, L., and Donehower, R., Phenylbutyrate (PB) for refractory solid tumors: Phase I clinical and pharmacologic evaluation of intravenor and oral PB, *Anticancer Res.*, 17, 3927, 1997.
54. Rama, B.N. and Prasad, K.N., Modification of the hyperthermic response on neuroblastoma cells by cAMP and sodium butyrate, *Cancer*, 58(7), 1448–1452, 1986.
55. Pili, R., Kruszewski, M.P., Hager, B.W., Lantz, J., and Carducci, M.A., Combination of phenylbutyrate and 13-cis retinoic acid inhibits prostate tumor growth and angiogenesis, *Cancer Res.*, 61(4), 1477–1485, 2001.
56. Lippman, S.M., Kavanagh, J.J., Paredes-Espinoza, M., Delgadillo-Madrueno, F., Paredes-Casillas, P., Hong, W.K., Holdener, E., and Krakoff, I.H., 13-cis-retinoic acid plus interferon alpha-2a: highly active systemic therapy for squamous cell carcinoma of the cervix, *J. Natl. Cancer. Inst.*, 84(4), 241–245, 1992.
57. Ramanathapuram, L.V., Kobie, J.J., Kreeger, M., Payne, C.M., Bearss, D., Trevor, K., and Akporiaye, E.T., Alpha-tocopheryl succinate sensitizes establish tumors to vaccination with immature dendritic cell, *Proc. Am. Assoc. Cancer Res.*, 44, 413a, 2003.

11

Probiotics: Synergy with Drugs and Carcinogens in Diet

Seppo Salminen, Hani El-Nezami, Eeva Salminen, and Hannu Mykkänen

CONTENTS

11.1 Introduction

Humans are exposed to a number of potentially harmful chemicals, some unintentionally ingested via diet, some intentionally used, such as alcohol and drugs. The diet may contain several natural toxins and carcinogens in addition to toxicants formed or added during agricultural and food processing. A number of pharmaceutical products may also interact with food components. This chapter discusses some of the interactions and synergy of probiotics with antibiotics, alcohol, mycotoxins, and food carcinogens. The basic concept is described in Figure 11.1.

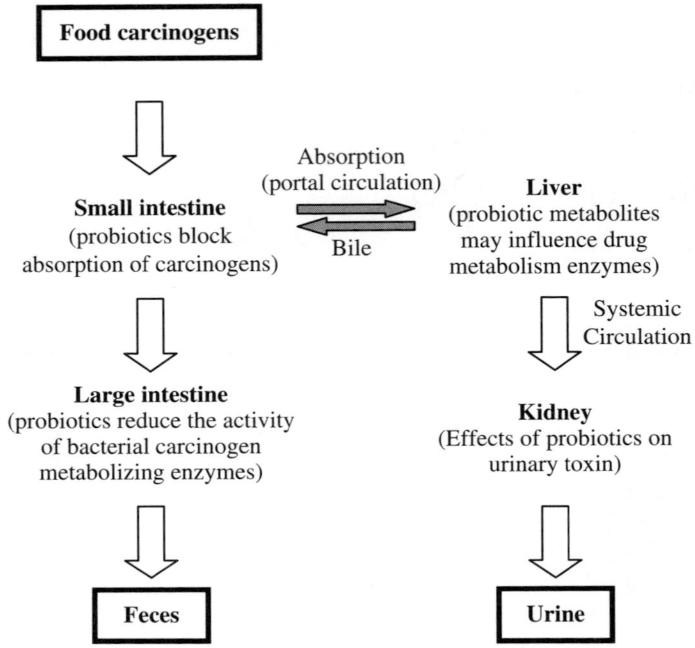

FIGURE 11.1
Potential interactions among food carcinogens, probiotics, and drugs.

11.2 Probiotics and Prebiotics

During recent years a number of research reports have focused on lactic acid bacteria, in particular lactobacilli and bifidobacteria, which are used for the production of yogurt and various fermented milk products.[1] Evidence is accumulating that specific, selected strains of bacteria have scientifically documented health effects in humans.[2–4] These bacteria are called "probiotics," and they are defined as "microorganisms that have a beneficial effect on intestinal function and promote human health." Probiotic bacteria contribute to intestinal mucosal integrity, metabolism, and immune status, both local and systemic. For successful use these bacteria must survive in the environment in which they are intended to act and must reach the small intestine or colon alive. Such bacteria should be safe,[1,4,5] and some may possess health benefits when they are nonviable.[6] Probiotics cannot be assessed as a single group of microbes. Each strain is unique, and the properties of even closely related strains may differ and could be synergistic or, at times, even antagonistic.

The mechanisms of action of probiotics may include intestinal microbiota modification, correction of aberrancies in mucosal or commensal microbiota, impact on immune system through adherence to the intestinal epithelium in the upper gastrointestinal tract, or competition for nutrients and displacement of harmful bacteria in different locations of the gut. Specific probiotics can also interact with drugs and carcinogens in food and water, or in the gastrointestinal tract. Such interactions may include microbiological actions (metabolism or enzymatic conversion of foreign components), physiological binding of foreign components in the gut, or influencing the absorption, enterohepatic circulation, or activation of drugs and carcinogens in the gut (Figure 11.1).

Prebiotics are nonabsorbable carbohydrate components of the diet that are selectively metabolized by beneficial microbes in the gut.[1] They act through promotion of specific microbes (e.g., bifidobacteria) with potential to maintain human health. The prerequisite of this activity is that such microbial strains are already present in the gut. Synbiotics combine the effects of both probiotics and prebiotics.[1] Each probiotic bacterial strain and prebiotic substance has specific effects that have to be evaluated prior to application. Even closely related probiotics and prebiotic components may have completely different microbiota effects, physiological actions, or effects on human health and well-being. Therefore, each probiotic and prebiotic has to be individually studied and the effects characterized.

11.2.1 Role of Intestinal Microbiota in Well-Being

The human intestinal microbiota is important for general health and well-being, and at least some of the over 500 known bacterial species can be divided into health promoting, indifferent (effects potentially not understood), or detrimental.[1] A wide variety of host, diet, and environmental factors, including microbiota composition itself, influence bacterial colonization of the human gastrointestinal tract.[7,8] Intestinal colonization and microbiota succession initiate at birth and continue until the end of life. Thus, there are several stages of microbiota development with potential for different interaction with drugs and carcinogens. Such developments are also potential targets for modifying the microbiota with probiotics and prebiotics.

The infant microbiota is relatively simple but it develops rapidly.[7] The adult intestinal microbiota is a complex community of a great microbial diversity typical to each individual.[7] It can be responsible for a variety of metabolic reactions involving drugs, contaminants, food additives, and dietary carcinogens from both natural and industrial sources. During old age, the microbiota gradually becomes less complex[7] with potential effect on drug and carcinogen metabolism.

The indigenous microbiota of an infant gastrointestinal tract is created through a complicated contact and interaction with the microbiota of the parents and the infant's immediate environment. Nature facilitated initial colonization is enhanced by galacto-oligosaccharides in breast milk and the microbiota of the mother.[9] This process directs the later microbiota succession and health of the infant throughout the life span. Thus, it is important to understand the role of microbiota and probiotic and prebiotic effects during infancy and childhood on metabolism of foreign components during breast-feeding, weaning, and first years of life. This development forms the basis for gut microbiota action in adult years. It has been suggested that organisms such as bifidobacteria, which are regarded as key members of healthy and protective intestinal microbiota, decline in concentration at old age and prior to death[7]; some support for this contention is offered by recent studies using molecular methods for determination of the microbiota composition.[8] However, the intestinal microbiota activity and effects in old age remain largely unknown in terms of their impact on carcinogen and drug metabolism. This is an important area for future studies because the use of different pharmaceutical products generally increases during old age and also several probiotic and prebiotic products have been designed for intestinal microbiota modification during the senior years.

11.2.2 Probiotic Bacteria and Interaction with Antibiotics

The use of oral antibiotics is often associated with mild or even severe side effects including intestinal cramps, vomiting, and diarrhea. Some of these effects are related to antibiotic associated alterations in intestinal microbiota and could be alleviated by dietary manipulation of microbiota using specific probiotics. The success of probiotics in reducing or preventing antibiotic associated diarrhea is strain specific. Clinical intervention studies have been conducted in both healthy volunteers receiving antibiotics and probiotic food products such as yogurt, and populations receiving antibiotics for particular infections randomized to receive either specific probiotics or placebo preparations at the same time.[2]

The incidence of antibiotic associated diarrhea is between 5 and 30%.[10] Several studies have approached the prevention and treatment of antibiotic associated diarrhea through probiotic intake without influencing the efficacy of antibiotics. Siitonen and coworkers[11] assessed the absorption and serum levels of several antibiotics (penicillin, amoxicillin, and erythromycin) in connection with oral intake of *Lactobacillus rhamnosus* strain GG (LGG) (ATCC 53103). No effect on the absorption or serum levels of the antibiotic were observed. However, the gastrointestinal side effects of erythromycin administered to healthy volunteers were significantly reduced, while the reduction in other antibiotic side effects was not observed.[11,12]

A study of 16 healthy volunteers taking erythromycin for 1 week found that coadministration of LGG yogurt reduced the number of days with diarrhea from eight to two, as well as decreasing associated side effects such as abdominal pain from 39 to 23%. Fecal recovery of the administered strain in the feces was seen in 75% of volunteers.[11] Other investigators studied 119 children with a respiratory illness requiring antibiotics and randomized them to receive either LGG or placebo. LGG resulted in a significant decrease in the incidence of diarrhea as compared with placebo (5 vs. 16%). MacFarland and coworkers[13] conducted a double-blind placebo-controlled study of 180 hospitalized patients treated with antibiotics, giving the patients additionally either placebo or *Saccharomyces boulardi*. Over 22% of the placebo treated patients developed diarrhea compared with 9% in the probiotic group. However, a later study concluded that *S. boulardi* was not effective in preventing antibiotic associated diarrhea in an elderly population.[14]

A trial using a combination of *L. acidophilus* and *L. bulgaris* on 79 hospitalized patients treated with ampicillin found that 14% of the placebo group had diarrhea vs. none in the probiotic group.[15] In a double-blind study, 188 children taking a 10-day course of antibiotics were given either LGG or placebo.[16] Administration of LGG decreased the incidence of diarrhea from 26 to 8%, as well as the duration of diarrhea from 5.9 d to 4.7 d. Furthermore the consistency of the stool determined by a visual scoring system was looser in the placebo group. Similar results have been reported in one study in Finland[16] and in another in the United States.[17]

Clostridium difficile diarrhea is associated with microbiota aberrancies and overgrowth by the toxin producing organism in the gut, especially after the use of broad spectrum antibiotics. The target was first described by an early case report of four children with relapsing *C. difficile* that responded to supplement with a probiotic *Lactobacillus* GG.[18] *S. boulardi* has been reported to inhibit the gastroenteritis caused by *C. difficile* toxins A and B, and it has been used in together with standard antimicrobial treatment. The probiotic significantly reduced recurrence in patients with earlier *C. difficile* diarrhea.[19] Several studies have shown that probiotics may prevent side effects during therapy against *Helicobacter pylori*. Other reports indicate that there may even be competitive interaction between some probiotics and *H. pylori*. In a clinical intervention study, these effects were studied with two probiotics.[20] A total of 85 *H. pylori* positive, asymptomatic patients were randomized in four groups to receive probiotic or placebo both during and for 7 days after a 1-week triple therapy scheme (rabeprazole 20 mg bid, clarithromycin 500 mg bid, and tinidazole 500 mg bid). Group I (n = 21) received LGG; group II (n = 22), *S. boulardi*; group III (n = 21), a combination of *Lactobacillus* spp. and bifidobacteria; and group IV (n = 21), placebo. All the probiotics used in this intervention were superior to placebo for side effect prevention.[20] However, the probiotic use was not associated with better compliance with antibiotic therapy.

11.2.3 Probiotics and Alcohol

In the intestinal tract, the bacteriologic pathway for ethanol oxidation leads to high intracolonic levels of the carcinogen acetaldehyde. There is accumulating evidence that the intestinal microbiota can have a major role in the regulation of the intracolonic acetaldehyde concentration, which is toxic and carcinogenic to the liver, thereby influencing the intestinal well-being during high intake of alcohol.[21] Several probiotic lactic acid bacteria and bifidobacteria have been characterized for their intestinal microbiota effects and also their effects on acetaldehyde production.[21] It was proved that several probiotic bacteria decrease high gastrointestinal acetaldehyde levels. LGG has the most significant effect on acetaldehyde levels.[21] It has also been reported that oral antibiotics downregulate the capacity of intestinal microbiota to reduce intestinal acetaldehyde concentration.[22,23] This finding should be further assessed because specific probiotics also normalize the intestinal microbiota during antibiotic treatment and may thus have a beneficial effect during periods of extensive alcohol intake.

It is also noteworthy that LGG has been reported to reduce endotoxemia and alcohol-induced liver injury in the rat model.[23] The interactions of the probiotics with alcohol should be further characterized to clarify their role in correcting intestinal microbiota aberrancies. This may lead to novel possibilities in using probiotics in the management of liver diseases associated with alcohol ingestion.

11.2.4 Probiotics and Carcinogens

Several probiotic bacteria and cultured dairy products made with them have been reported to modify the effects of known chemical mutagens in *in vitro* tests. The antimutagenic effect may not only relate to the probiotic strains alone, but may depend on an interaction between the probotic and milk, or other food components and fermentation products in cultured milks, fermented vegetables, or fermented cereals.[24] The mechanism of the antimutagenicity may partly be related to binding of the mutagens to the cell surface. This has been reported for several mutagens and carcinogens,[25–27] and the binding process and related factors are discussed in detail in the following sections.

The antigenotoxic properties of specific probiotics have been assessed both in the *S. typhimurium* mutagenity assay and in the gastrointestinal tract of laboratory animals. Some tested bacteria and dairy products made with them have shown antimutagenic properties.[28] Hosono and coworkers[29–31] have observed that probiotics and fermented milk products can reduce the mutagenicity of amino acid pyrolysates and *N*-nitroso compounds with reduced fecal mutagen excretion in animal studies. In one report, the viability of the tested probiotic was important to suppress the mutagenicity of nitrosated beef extract.[32] The antigenotoxicity of 10^{10} cells of specific lactic acid bacteria to the mutagens MNNG and DMH was tested in rat colons using the COMET assay; the investigators reported that the tested probiotics prevented DNA damage.[32]

In a Japanese study, the antimutagenic effects of fermented milks on the mutagenicity of 3-amino-1-methyl-5*H*-pyrido[4,3-*b*]indole (Trp P-2), MNNG, B[a]p, AFB2, and AFB1 was investigated by the Ames test.[29] Fermented milks produced by mixed cultures of various kinds of lactic acid bacteria and yeast

(*Lactococcus, Streptococcus, Leuconostoc, Lactobacillus, Bifidobacterium,* and *Saccharomyces*) showed more effective antimutagenic activity over a wider range of mutagens (18 to 75%) than those cultured with a single strain of lactic acid bacteria (0 to 79%). Although the mechanisms were not understood, the antimutagenic activity was proportional to the amount of the fermented milks. Similar findings have been reported in a human intervention study by Lidbeck and coworkers from Sweden.[33]

Oral supplements of *L. acidophilus* in humans have resulted in reduced activities of fecal bacterial enzymes (β-glucuronidase, nitroreductase, azoreductase) involved in procarcinogen activation and reduced the excretion of mutagens in feces and urine.[34]

Moreover, the intestinal bacteria can have an effect on the activity of liver enzymes involved in the biotransformation of xenobiotics. It has been reported that liver enzyme preparations from germ free animals were more effective in activating 2-amino-3,4-dimethyl-3*H*-imidazo[4,5-*f*]quinoline (MeIQ) and Trp-P-2 to bacterial mutagens than enzyme preparation from conventional animals.[35]

Phenol, *p*-cresol, and indican are typical bacterial putrefactive metabolites in the intestine. They are markedly increased in plasma of uremic patients, but oral administration of a mixture of lactic acid bacteria to uremic patients has been reported to be effective in reducing the plasma levels of uremic toxins.[36]

11.3 Probiotics and Carcinogen Binding

There are several studies on the binding of mutagens and carcinogens by lactic acid bacteria. Specifically, effects have been reported on heterocyclic amines and food pyrolysates.[25,27,33] More intensive studies on the binding and mechanisms of binding have been conducted with specific probiotics and mycotoxins.

A number of strains of lactic acid bacteria have been tested for their ability to bind aflatoxin B_1 (AFB_1) *in vitro*. Some strains have proved highly effective, but in a given genus and even within a given species, not all strains were equivalent in terms of toxin binding. The capacity for aflatoxin removal is characteristic of only some species and strains of probiotics, and binding efficacy varies markedly.[27,37–39] The reported studies also indicated that aflatoxins are not removed from solution by bacterial metabolism but rather are bound to the surface of the specific bacteria. Similar results using strains of bifidobacteria were found to bind significant quantities of AFB_1, ranging from 25% to nearly 60% of the added toxin.[40] Several studies have addressed the mechanism by which lactic acid bacteria bind toxins and carcinogens, and point out that strain-specific properties vary and different mechanisms can be identified.[37,41–45]

The above *in vitro* results led to an investigation of the ability of selected strains to bind AFB_1 *in vivo*, and to test whether the strength of binding is sufficient to reduce AFB_1 bioavailability. LGG, *L. rhamnosus* LC705, and *P. freudenreichii* spp *shermanii* JS proved capable of reducing AFB_1 in the luminal content of the 1-week-old chicken.[42] These strains also reduced the uptake of AFB_1 by the intestinal mucosa. The finding was significant in that it indicated a potential reduction in the bioavailability of AFB_1 through a reduction in its absorption via the intestinal mucosa.

A pilot human clinical intervention was carried out in Egypt to investigate the effect of a probiotic mix preparation containing both *L. rhamnosus* LC705 and *P. freudenreichii* spp. *Shermanii* JS on the levels of aflatoxin in human fecal samples.[46] The results suggest that the strains of probiotics used in this trial have the ability to influence the fecal content of AFB_1. Clinical studies are currently underway in China to further assess the possibility of preventing intestinal absorption of ingested aflatoxins by dietary probiotics.

Preliminary studies also suggest that a correlation exists between strong aflatoxin binding and strong adherence to the human intestinal tract; to intestinal epithelial cells; and to mucin secreted by the intestinal mucosa.[38] Bacteria possessing good adherence properties in *in vitro* adhesion models, such as Caco-2 and human intestinal mucus glycoprotein, have been reported to lose this property when aflatoxin is bound.[47] This is important when considering applications in animals and humans because contact with the intestinal mucosa is significantly shortened when either viable or non-viable bacterial cells have bound either aflatoxins or other mycotoxins, facilitating the excretion of the toxins via the feces.

Recent reports have increased the knowledge on bifidobacteria and their ability to bind mycotoxins. This may be an important area of research, especially concerning infants in mycotoxin contaminated areas where even breast milk may contain significant amounts of aflatoxin or other toxins.[48] Because bifidobacteria comprise 60 to 90% of the total healthy infant microbiota, members of this species may offer an important, novel means of decontaminating the diet of breast-fed or formula-fed infants in areas of environmental mycotoxin contamination. Decontamination could take place by the oral treatment of the mother, or by adding inactivated probiotic bacteria to breast milk or treating breast milk with them.

11.4 Probiotics and Cancer

Several studies have investigated the relationship between probiotic administration and cancer.[1,2] The results have not been conclusive, and properly conducted long-term human studies are lacking. However, several potential mechanisms have been identified. These include:

1. Alteration in intestinal microecology (microbiota effects by specific probiotics);
2. Altered intestinal metabolic activity (potential conversion of precarcinogens to carcinogens);
3. Normalized intestinal permeability (decreasing or delaying of carcinogen or toxin absorption);
4. Enhanced intestinal immunity (enhanced immune response);
5. Strengthened intestinal barrier mechanisms (include all previous mechanisms).

Evidence for the antitumor effect of *L. acidophilus* comes from studies conducted by Goldin and Gorbach.[49,50] Oral supplementation of the diet of humans and rats with viable *L. acidophilus* caused a significant decline in the levels of bacterial -glucuronidase, azoreductase, and nitroreductase activities in feces. These enzymes are thought to contribute to the pathogenesis of bowel cancer because of their ability to convert procarcinogens to proximate carcinogens. Fecal levels of carcinogenic amines in rats fed with carcinogen precursors were reduced when diets are supplemented with 10^{10} colony forming units (cfu), indicating viable bacteria of *L acidophilus*.[34] These studies suggest that specific probiotics may have the capacity to suppress the metabolic activity of the colonic microbiota and may reduce the formation of carcinogens in the intestine.

In contrast, Ling and coworkers in studies with human volunteers given *lactobacillus* GG detected no decrease in fecal concentration of nitroreductase, no change in -glucuronidase and azoreductase contents, but an increase in -glucosidase level was reported.[52] Modification of the colonic flora following treatment was observed, however. These results could be explained by differences between the effects of specific probiotic strains used. On the other hand, several reports have observed decreased fecal -glucuronidase, azoreductase, and glycocholic acid hydrolase activity in human volunteers following intake of a yogurt fermented with specific strains of lactic acid bacteria.[12,51]

Goldin and Gorbach[52] performed studies using an animal model of colon cancer induced by the chemical carcinogen, 1,2-dimethylhydrazine (DMH). The carcinogen is activated in the large intestine by the bacterial enzyme -glucuronidase. The authors postulated that enzyme suppression might reduce DMH activation and subsequent tumor formation. Tumor formation was induced with DMH and animals were either given *L. acidophilus* NCFM 10^{10} cfu in powdered form or left untreated. At 20 weeks, 40% of the *L. acidophilus*–treated animals had colonic tumors, compared with 77% of the controls ($p < .02$). After 36 weeks, however, the difference in the incidence of tumors in treatment and control groups was less (73 vs. 83%). Thus, the addition of at least one strain of *Lactobacillus* to the diet can delay tumor formation in rats.

The effect of colonization of *B. breve* YIT 4010 on the induction of colonic aberrant crypt foci (ACF) was examined by ip injection of DMH (20 mg/kg body weight) in F-344 gnotobiotic rats (GB) carrying *E. coli, E. faecium,* four species of *Bacteroides,* and four species of *Clostridium.*[53] The additional colonization of *B. breve* in GB rats resulted in a significant decrease in total number of ACF with four or more crypts per focus and mean number of ACF per focus (crypt multiplicity) compared with *B. breve* free GB rats.

There is no convincing data on effect verified in clinical intervention studies with human subjects. The most interesting documentation is on *L. casei* Shirota. In clinical and multicenter studies carried out in Japan, the prophylactic effects of oral administration of *L. casei* Shirota on the recurrence of superficial bladder cancer have been reported.[54,55] Mechanistic studies on the effects of *L. casei* Shirota report decreased urinary mutagen excretion, probably indicating lesser absorption of the mutagenic compounds from the intestinal tract. Similar results have been reported in an animal study for LGG.[56] Recently, a large Japanese case control study on the habitual intake of lactic acid bacteria and risk reduction of bladder cancer has been conducted in the specific setting of home delivery of the product. This study suggested that the habitual intake of the fermented milk with the strain reduces the risk of bladder cancer in the Japanese population.[57] More studies, also in other countries, are needed to confirm these conclusions. However, the suggested mechanisms deserve closer assessment.

11.5 Probiotics and Toxins

Recent work has focused on the ability of lactic acid bacteria and bifidobacteria to bind heavy metals from the diet. *In vitro* studies show efficacy in such decontamination for specific strains of probiotic bacteria.[44] This new area of potential removal of contaminant from foods and feeds may offer novel means of decontamination when further assessed and characterized. It also emphasizes the potential use of lactic acid bacteria and bifidobacteria in such applications and a need for rapid development of such biotechnology using already accepted food grade microbial ingredients.

11.6 Prebiotics and Other Toxins

Prebiotics have been defined as slowly absorbable or nonabsorbable carbohydrate substrates that enter the colon and are selectively fermented by beneficial intestinal bacteria, such as bifidobacteria, to produce beneficial effects on human health.[1] Prebiotic components are usually plant based carbohydrates such as fructo-oligosaccharides or other complex polysaccharides.[1] Recently, several studies have attempted to assess the effect of prebiotics on intestinal drug and carcinogen metabolism. Because the prebiotics vary, different effects have been reported and even carcinogen activating mechanisms have been identified.[59,60] It is important to recognize that the prebiotic effects are related to microbiota effects. In a recent report, fructo-oligosaccharides were indicated to stimulate unknown intestinal bacteria in an intestinal model system.[61] Because the effects of specific prebiotics on human intestinal microbiota are often not well understood, they need to be further evaluated. Thus, the available evidence may be conflicting, and firm conclusions on the influence of each individual prebiotic on carcinogen and toxin metabolism require further assessment.

A recent assessment of probiotic and carcinogen interactions has been reported in the ILSI Europe working group summary by Rafter and coworkers.[61]

11.7 Conclusions

A large body of evidence indicates that specific probiotics can be used in connection with antibiotics to reduce side effects caused by toxin producing bacteria and their overgrowth during antibiotic treatment. Several specific probiotics also act through modifying the intestinal microbiota in a manner facilitating balanced permeability of the gut epithelium thus preventing the absorption of unwanted components in the diet. There is now also mounting evidence for application of these interactions to food systems with the potential to modify the toxic effects of many contaminants. This area should be the focus for future applications for both food systems and dietary management of disease risk reduction.

References

1. Salminen, S. et al., Functional food science and gastrointestinal physiology and function, *Br. J. Nutr. Suppl.*, 1, 147, 1998.
2. De Roos, N. and Katan, M., Effects of probiotic bacteria on diarrhea, lipid metabolism, and carcinogenesis: a review of papers published between 1988 and 1998, *Am. J. Clin. Nutr.*, 71, 405, 2000.
3. Isolauri, E., Salminen, S., Ouwehand, A., Manipulation of the gut microbiota: probiotics, *Best Practice Res. Clin. Gastroenterol.*, 18, 299, 2004
4. Gueimonde, M., Ouwehand, A., and Salminen, S., Safety of probiotics. *Scand. J. Nutr.*, 26, 16, 2004.
5. Salminen, S. et al., Demonstration of safety of probiotics - a review. *Int. J. Food Microbiol.*, 44, 93, 1998.

6. Ouwehand, A.C. and Salminen, S.J., The health effects of viable and non-viable cultured milks, *Int. Dairy J.*, 8, 749, 1998.
7. Benno, Y. and Mitsuoka, T.M., Development of intestinal microflora in humans and animals, *Bifidobacteria Microflora*, 5, 13, 1986.
8. Hopkins, M.J. and Macfarlane, G.T., Changes in predominant bacterial populations in human faeces with age and with Clostridium difficile infection, *J. Med. Microbiol.*, 51, 448, 2002.
9. Boehm, G. et al., Prebiotics in infant formulas, *J. Clin. Gastroenterol.*, 38, S76, 2004.
10. Salminen, S., Vapaatalo, and H., Gorbach, *S. faecal* colonization with *Lactobacillus* GG during antibiotic treatment, *Proc. Australian Nutr. Soc.*, 14, 132, 1989.
11. Siitonen, S. et al., M Effect of *Lactobacillus* GG yoghurt in prevention of antibiotic associated diarrhea, *Ann. Med.*, 22, 57, 1990.
12. Goldin, B. et al., Survival of *Lactobacillus* species (strain GG) in the human gastrointestinal tract, *Dig. Dis. Sci.*, 37, 121, 1992.
13. McFarland, L.V. et al., Prevention of beta-lactam-associated diarrhea by *Saccharomyces boulardii* compared with placebo, *Am. J. Gastroenterol.*, 90, 439, 1995.
14. Lewis, S.J., Potts, L.F., and Barry, R.E., The lack of therapeutic effect of *Saccharomyces boulardii* in the prevention of antibiotic-related diarrhoea in elderly patients, *J. Infect.*, 36, 171, 1998.
15. Salminen, S., Vapaatalo, H., and Gorbach, S., Faecal colonization with *Lactobacillus* GG during antibiotic treatment, *Proc. Australian. Nutr. Soc.* 14, 132, 1989.
16. Arvola, T. et al., Prophylactic *Lactobacillus* GG reduces antibiotic-associated diarrhea in children with respiratory infections: a randomized study, *Pediatrics*, 104e, 64, 1999.
17. Vanderhoof, J.A. et al., Lactobacillus GG in the prevention of antibiotic-associated diarrhea in children, *J. Pediatr.*, 135, 564, 1999.
18. Gorbach, S.L., Chang, T.W., and Goldin, B., Successful treatment of relapsing Clostridium difficile colitis with Lactobacillus GG, *Lancet*, 26,1519, 1987.
19. Elmer, G.W., Surawicz, C.M., and McFarland, L.V., Biotherapeutic agents. A neglected modality for the treatment and prevention of selected intestinal and vaginal infections, *JAMA*, 275, 870, 1996.
20. Cremonini, F. et al., Effect of different probiotic preparations on anti-helicobacter pylori therapy-related side effects: a parallel group, triple blind, placebo-controlled study, *Am. J. Gastroenterol.*, 97, 2744, 2002.
21. Nosova, T. et al., Acetaldehyde production and metabolism by human indigenous and probiotic *Lactobacillus* and *Bifidobacterium* strains, *Alcohol Alcoholism*, 35,561, 2000.
22. Tillonen, J. et al., Ciprofloxacin decreases the rate of ethanol elimination in humans, *Gut*, 44, 347, 1999.
23. Nanji, A.A., Khettry, U., and Sadrzadeh, S.M., Lactobacillus feeding reduces endotoxemia and severity of experimental alcoholic liver (disease), *Proc. Soc. Exp. Biol. Med.*, 205, 243, 1994.
24. Abdelali, H. et al., Antimutagenicity of components of dairy products, *Mutation Res.*, 331:133, 1995.
25. Orrhage, K. et al., Binding of mutagenic heterocyclic amines by intestinal and lactic acid bacteria, *Mutation Res.*, 311, 239, 1994.
26. Morotomi, M. and Mutai. M., In vitro binding of potent mutagenic pyrolysates by intestinal bacteria, *J. Natl. Cancer Inst.*, 77, 195, 1986.

27. El-Nezami, H., Kankaanpää, P.E., Salminen, S., and Ahokas, J.T., Ability of dairy strains of lactic acidbacteria to bind food carcinogens, *Food Chem. Toxicol.*, 36, 321, 1998.
28. Pool-Zobel, B.L., Bertram, B., Knoll, M., Lambertz, R., Neudecker, C., Schillinger, U., Schmezer, P., and Holzapfel, W.H., Antigenotoxic properties of lactic acid bacteria *in vivo* in the gastrointestinal tract of rats, *Nutr. Cancer,* 20, 271 (1993).
29. Hosono, A., Kashina, T., and Kada, T., Antimutagenic properties of lactic acid-cultured milk on chemical and fecal mutagens, *J. Dairy Sci.*, 69, 2237, 1986.
30. Hosono, A., Wardojo, R., and Otani, H., Inhibitory effects of lactic acid bacteria from fermented milk on the mutagenicities of volatile amines. *Agric. Biol. Chem.*, 54, 1639, 1990.
31. Hosono, A. and Sreekumar, O., Antimutagenic properties of lactic acid bacteria, *Recent Res. Dev. Agric. Biol. Chem.*, 1,173, 1997.
32. Pool-Zobel, B.L. et al., *Lactobacillus* and *Bifidobacterium* mediated antigenotoxicity in the colon of rats, *Nutr. Cancer,* 26, 365, 1996.
33. Lidbeck, A. et al., Effect of *Lactobacillus acidophilus* supplements on mutagen excretion in faeces and urine in humans, *Microb. Ecol. Health Dis.*, 5, 59, 1992.
34. Marteau, P. et al., Effect of chronic ingestion of a fermented dairy product containing *Lactobacillus acidophilus* and *Bifidobacterium bifidum* on metabolic activities of the colonic flora in humans, *Am. J. Clin. Nutr.*, 52, 685, 1990.
35. Bolognani, F., Rumney, C.J., and Rowland, I.R. Influence of carcinogen binding by lactic acid-producing bacteria on tissue distribution and in vivo mutagenicity of dietary carcinogens, *Food Chem. Toxicol.*, 35, 535, 1997.
36. Hida, M. et al., Inhibition of the accumulation of uremic toxins in the blood and their precursors in the feces after oral administration of Lebenin, a lactic acid bacteria preparation, to uremic patients undergoing hemodialysis, *Nephron,* 74, 349, 1996.
37. Kankaanpää, P. et al., Influence of aflatoxin B1 on the adhesion capability of *Lactobacillus rhamnosus* strain GG, *J. Food Prot.*, 63, 412, 2000.
38. Peltonen, K. et al., Binding of aflatoxin B_1 by probiotic bacteria, *J. Sci. Food Agr.*, 80, 1942, 2000.
39. Pieridis, M, et al., Ability of dairy strains of lactic acid bacteria to bind aflatoxin M_1 in a food model, *J. Food Prot.*, 63, 645, 2000.
40. Oatley, J. T. et al., Binding of aflatoxin B_1 to *Bifidobacteria in vitro, J. Food. Prot.*, 63, 1133, 2000.
41. El-Nezami, H.S. et al., Physico-chemical alterations enhance the ability of dairy strains of lactic acid bacteria to remove aflatoxins from contaminated media. *J. Food Prot.* 61, 4661998.
42. El-Nezami, H.S. et al., Removal of common *Fusarium* toxins *in vitro* by strains of *Lactobacillus* and *Propionibacterium, Food Addit. Contam.*, 19, 680, 2002.
43. El-Nezami, H.S. et al., Binding rather than metabolism may explain the interaction of two food grade *Lactobacillus* strains with zearalenone and its derivative zearalenol, *Appl. Environ. Microbiol.*, 68, 3545, 2002.
44. Halttunen, T. et al., Cadmium decontamination by lactic acid bacteria, *Biosci. Microflora*, 22, 93, 2003.
45. El-Nezami, H.S. et al., Ability of *Lactobacillus* and *Propionibacterium* strains to remove aflatoxin B, from the chicken duodenum, *J. Food. Prot.*, 63, 549, 2000.

46. El-Nezami, H.S. et al., The ability of a mixture of Lactobacillus and Propionibacterium examining to influence the faecal recovery of aflatoxins in healthy Egyptian volunteers: A pilot clinical study, *Biosci. Microflora,* 19, 41, 2000.
47. Isolauri, E., Salminen, S., and Ouwehand, A., Manipulation of the gut microbiota: probiotics, *Best Practice Res. Clin. Gastroenterol.*, 18, 299, 2004.
48. El-Nezami, H.S. et al., Aflatoxin M1 in human breast milk samples from Victoria, Australia and Thailandm *Food Chem, Toxicol.*, 33, 173, 1995.
49. Gorbach, S.L., Lactic acid bacteria and human health, *Ann. Med.*, 22, 37, 1990.
50. Goldin, B., The metabolic activity of the intestinal microflora and its role in colon cancer, *Nutr. Today Suppl.*, 31, 24S, 1996.
51. Ling, W.H. et al., Lactobacillus strain GG supplementation decreases colonic hydrolytic and reductive enzyme activities in healthy female adults, *J. Nutr.* 124, 18, 1994.
52. Gorbach, S.L. and Goldin, B.R., The intestinal microflora and the colon cancer connection, *Rev. Infect. Dis.*, 12, S252, 1990.
53. Onoue, M. et al., Specific species of intestinal bacteria influence the induction of aberrant crypt foci by 1,2-dimethylhydrazine in rats, *Cancer Lett.*, 113, 179, 1997.
54. Aso, Y. and Akazan, H. Prophylactic effect of a Lactobacillus casei preparation on the recurrence of superficial bladder cancer. BLP Study Group, *Urol Int.*, 49, 125, 1992.
55. Aso, Y. et al., Preventive effect of a Lactobacillus casei preparation on the recurrence of superficial bladder cancer in a double-blind trial. The BLP Study Group, *Eur. Urol.*, 27, 104, 1995.
56. Lim, B.K. et al., Chemopreventive effect of Lactobacillus rhamnosus on growth of a subcutaneously implanted bladder cancer cell line in the mouse. *Jpn J Cancer Res.*, 93, 36, 2002.
57. Ohashi, Y. et al., Habitual intake of lactic acid bacteria and risk reduction of bladder cancer, *Urol Int.*, 68, 273, 2002.
58. Pajari, A.M. et al., Promotion of intestinal tumor formation by inulin is associated with an accumulation of cytosolic beta-catenin in Min mice, *Int. J. Cancer*, 106, 653, 2003.
59. Mutanen, M., Pajari, A.M., and Oikarinen, S.I. Beef induces and rye bran prevents the formation of intestinal polyps in Apc(Min) mice: relation to beta-catenin and PKC isozymes, *Carcinogenesis*, 21, 1167, 2000.
60. Apajalahti, J. et al., Culture-independent microbial community analysis reveals that inulin in the diet primarily affects previously unknown bacteria in the mouse cecum, *Appl. Environ. Microbiol.*, 68, 4986, 2002.
61. Rafter J. et al., PASSCLAIM — diet-related cancer, *Eu.r J. Nutr.*, 43 (Suppl 2), II47, 2004.

Section IV

Osteoporosis

12

Synergy of Soy, Flaxseed, Calcium, and Hormone Replacement Therapy in Osteoporosis

Wendy E. Ward

CONTENTS

12.1 Introduction

Osteoporosis is a skeletal disorder that is characterized by a low bone mass that ultimately predisposes an individual to an increased risk of fracture. Osteoporosis is a debilitating disease, resulting in significant rates of morbidity and mortality due to fragility fractures. The hip, spine, and forearm are the most prevalent sites of fragility fracture, and the worldwide incidence of hip fracture is steadily increasing.[1] Drug therapies are commonly used to manage osteoporosis with the goal of preventing further bone loss and thereby lowering the risk of fragility fracture. Historically, two of the most common drug therapies are hormone replacement therapy (HRT) or bisphosphonate drugs, and more recently, selective receptor estrogen modulators (SERMs). However, all can be associated with negative side effects.[2–9] To date, findings from the largest study that investigated effects of HRT on multiple health outcomes, the Women's Health Initiative (WHI) Study, demonstrated that while HRT was beneficial at significantly reducing the risk of osteoporotic fracture, the risk of stroke, coronary artery disease, venous thromboembolism, invasive breast cancer, and dementia were significantly increased.[3–5] Consequently, HRT is not as widely accepted or used for prevention or treatment of osteoporosis.[10] Bisphosphonate drugs can also result in complications, namely gastrointestinal disturbances such as ulcers, particularly if there is a preexisting condition or if the strict guidelines for timing of administration are not followed.[6–8] Interest in SERMs for managing osteoporosis is growing with recent reports of effects on maintaining bone mass or reductions in fractures.[11,12] However, some women experience hot flushes with SERMs such as raloxifene, and SERMs can increase the risk of venous thromboembolism.[9]

Interestingly, guidelines set out by various expert panels on prevention and management of osteoporosis advocate that women take supplemental calcium and vitamin D concurrently with drugs aimed at maintaining bone health such as HRT, bisphosphonates, and SERMs.[13,14] The result is that there is great interest in understanding how dietary strategies, or dietary strategies in combination with drugs, may act synergistically to optimize bone health throughout the life cycle. Because there is no ideal drug treatment for maintenance of optimal bone health, particularly during aging, there is considerable interest in whether novel food components with potential estrogenlike activity such as isoflavones in soy and lignans in flaxseed may be potential dietary interventions to slow bone loss and ultimately reduce the risk of fracture.

This chapter discusses the topic of food synergy and food–drug synergy for prevention or management of osteoporosis, focused on the synergy of soy, flaxseed, calcium, and HRT. Due to a paucity of data on this topic, a proportion of this discussion addresses the hypotheses of potential mechanisms by which these combinations of foods interact with each other and with HRT. The data presented in this chapter focuses mainly on postmenopausal women and ovariectomized animal models that are used to understand changes in bone metabolism after estrogen withdrawal.

12.2 Evaluation of Bone Metabolism

Bone is a dynamic tissue, composed predominately of two main components, mineral and matrix proteins, that together contribute to the strength of the skeleton. There are several different ways to assess bone health, and ultimately risk of fragility fracture, in both human and animal feeding studies.

12.2.1 Evaluation of Bone Metabolism in Human Studies

In humans, baseline measures of bone status and responses to dietary or drug treatments can be evaluated by measuring bone mass using dual energy x-ray absorptiometry (DEXA); measuring serum or urinary biochemical markers of bone formation or resorption by radioimmunoassay or enzyme-linked immunoassay; or determining the incidence of a new fragility fracture over a set period. Bone mass measurement involves the determination of the total mineral content of the skeleton, or of a specified skeletal region (termed bone mineral content [BMC]) along with a measurement of the size of the area measured. Bone mineral density (BMD) is an indirect measure of bone mass, derived by expressing BMC as a function of area, thereby accounting for differences in the size of the area measured. Thus, BMD is a measure of the mineral present in a set area. It is possible to measure BMC and/or BMD of the whole skeleton or to perform regional analyses of bone sites at risk of fracture such as the hip, femur neck, and/or spine. The level of exposure to x-rays with a DEXA scan is relatively low, particularly in comparison to exposure from dental x-rays.

Ideally, it would be possible to measure the microarchitecture of the entire skeleton or an individual bone. In other words, to measure how the mineral and matrix proteins interact within a bone, thereby contributing directly to the actual strength of a bone and its ability to withstand a fragility fracture. The term "bone quality" is sometimes used in the literature to describe this.[15–18] It is not yet possible to routinely measure microarchitecture in humans because of technological limitations. Thus, BMD is used as surrogate measure of fracture risk; however this is not without controversy.[19–22] Although not ideal, some long term studies, greater than 2 years in duration, use incidence of new fragility fracture as an indicator of the success of a treatment. Because the bone remodelling cycle takes approximately 6 months for one cycle, only studies that are approximately 2 years or more in duration can adequately evaluate differences in rates of fragility fracture. Thus, studies of short duration may result in transient remodeling that does not necessarily result in a functional benefit such as reduced risk of fragility fracture.[23] Moreover, the sample size required for observing a significant difference in fracture rates among treatment groups is very large.

Biochemical markers of bone turnover can be measured in serum, plasma, or urine depending on which specific marker is being measured.[24–26] In general, bone formation markers are peptides that are released by the osteoblast into the circulation during bone formation, while bone resorption markers are often collagen cross-links that are excreted in the urine as a result of the degradation of bone tissue by osteoclasts during bone resorption. Measurement of biochemical markers can provide useful data regarding changes in the level of bone formation or resorption, particularly in response to treatments. Changes in bone formation and resorption can be observed over relatively short periods, weeks and months, versus greater than 6 months required to observe changes in BMC or BMD. However, to adequately assess long term effects of a treatment, improvements in bone mass should be verified by DEXA.[25,26]

12.2.2 Evaluation of Bone Metabolism in Animal Studies

Using animal models, it is possible to measure the ability of an individual bone to withstand fracture by performing biomechanical testing in which the bone is ultimately fractured. Three commonly performed tests are three point bending of a femur, femur neck fracture, and compression testing of an individual lumbar vertebra.[16,17] The three point bending test is performed at the femur midpoint, a site that contains predominately cortical bone, whereas the femur neck is a more equal mixture of cortical and trabecular bone. The lumbar vertebrae are predominately composed of trabecular rather than cortical bone. Performing tests at multiple sites of the skeleton provides data on how different types of bone, cortical versus trabecular bone, respond to a dietary or drug intervention.

As an overview, biomechanical strength tests are performed using a materials testing system. The bone of interest is placed in (femur neck fracture) or on a customized jig (three point bending at femur midpoint, compression testing of an individual vertebra) and the crosshead travels downward at a constant rate, applying an increasing force to the bone until it is fractured (femur midpoint or neck) or compressed (vertebra).[16,17,27,28] From the load-displacement curve that is generated, several parameters can be interpolated, with peak load, arguably, as the most functionally relevant outcome. Peak load is the maximal force a bone can withstand before fracturing or compressing, and predominately measures the contribution of matrix to bone strength, with a lesser contribution from the mineral content. Comprehensive reviews of biomechanical strength testing and the various outcomes that are obtained are published in the literature.[16–18]

As in human studies, other measurements such as bone mass (BMC, BMD) can be performed by DEXA, albeit very small animals such as mice require measurement on a PIXImus DEXA, designed especially for very small animals and bones. Whole body scans or scans of individual bones can be performed. Moreover, there is a wide variety of species-specific kits that are commercially available for measuring biochemical markers of bone formation or resorption.

12.3 Food Synergy and Osteoporosis

12.3.1 Soy

Epidemiological evidence suggests that diets that are rich in soy protect against bone loss or slow the loss of bone mass that occurs naturally with aging and is expedited after menopause.[29–31] Two main components in soy that may have beneficial effects on bone metabolism include protein and isoflavones (see Chapter 13 for a discussion of protein and bone metabolism). Isoflavones are widely available in the diet, and there is a comprehensive database available on the web (USDA–Iowa State University Database on the Isoflavone Content of Foods).[32] Even though isoflavones are available in the diet, most individuals consume only negligible quantities in their diet, provided they are not following a vegetarian diet or consuming a traditional Asian diet.[33] While soy contains several different isoflavones, genistein and daidzein are predominately believed to mediate biological effects on bone. Some human and animal feeding studies, in postmenopausal women or using ovariectomized animal models, respectively, have demonstrated that isoflavones preserve bone tissue and thereby maintain bone mass after estrogen withdrawal.[27,34–49] While some of these studies fed soy rather than isoflavone extract or purified isoflavones, most studies have shown that only soy with high levels of isoflavones (greater than 50 mg/d) exerts a protective effect on bone tissue, and in studies that measured BMD, it is often the lumbar spine and not other sites that benefit from soy or isoflavones.[41–43,45,49,50]

In contrast, some human and animal feeding trials report weaker or no effects of soy or its isoflavones on bone health.[28,51–59] It is possible that differences in the metabolism of isoflavones among individuals or species may account for some of these discrepant findings. For example, daidzein can be further metabolized by gut microflora to its isoflavone metabolite, equol, a compound that may have greater estrogenic activity.[60] In ovariectomized rats, a direct comparison of feeding equivalent levels of genistein vs. daidzein demonstrated that daidzein had a greater effect on bone tissue.[36] Postmenopausal women who metabolized daidzein to equol experienced preservation of lumbar spine BMD, unlike women who did not produce equol.[49] A study from our laboratory revealed that among four strains of mice, outbred strains such as CD-1 and Swiss Webster mice, produced a significantly greater quantity of equol than inbred strains, C57 and C3H mice.[61] Based on this relatively newer information that the metabolism of daidzein to equol is highly variable within species, more studies investigating effects of soy or isoflavones on bone are including measurements of equol production to verify whether an animal or species produces equol, and if so, the extent of the conversion.

12.3.2 Soy Combined with Calcium

The concept of soy and calcium having a synergistic effect on bone stems from the knowledge that HRT are more effective at improving BMD at multiples sites of the skeleton (forearm, hip, spine) when given in combination with supplemental calcium[62] (discussed further in Section 12.4.1). Mechanisms of the potential synergy between soy isoflavones and high dietary calcium are speculative at present. It is possible that soy isoflavones mediate a hormonal effect on bone, stimulating osteoblastic activity and the production of bone matrix proteins while the supplemental calcium is rapidly used during the mineralization process.[63] Bone, more specifically osteoblasts, have both estrogen receptor-α and estrogen receptor–β receptors, and moreover, isoflavones such as genistein can bind both receptors, acting as weak estrogen agonists at low concentrations.[64–66] At higher concentrations, genistein appears to have effects that are independent of estrogen receptors, possibly with genistein acting through inhibition of tyrosine kinases.[66] Of note is that isoflavones bind estrogen receptor-β with a higher affinity.[65] Using a bone marrow stromal cell culture system, researchers have shown that daidzein stimulates osteogenesis; daidzein stimulated alkaline phosphatase activity, a marker of early osteoblastic differentiation, and led to the formation of nodules, a surrogate measure of bone formation.[63]

Because estrogen (HRT) is known to reduce rates of bone resorption, and thus bone remodeling,[67] it is also possible that isoflavones have a similar effect and that the supplemental calcium in the diet could fill in resorptive pits or remodeling spaces, thereby increasing or preserving BMD. In addition to having an effect on osteoblasts and osteogenesis, when cultured osteoblasts from developing piglets were studied, daidzein appeared to have a role in osteoclastogenesis.[68] Using this cell system, investigators showed that daidzein stimulated production of osteoprotegerin and receptor activator of nuclear factor κβ (RANKL). Osteoprotegrin and RANKL are present on osteoblasts and can both bind to RANKL receptor on the surface of osteoclast precursor cells. If RANKL binds to its receptor, osteoclastogenesis is stimulated, whereas osteoprotegrin acts as decoy, binding the RANKL receptor but not resulting in stimulation of osteoclastogenesis.[67] Ultimately, studies are needed to elucidate the mechanisms by which high calcium may act synergistically with isoflavones.

The benefits of supplemental calcium alone at protecting against bone loss and ultimately fragility fracture in postmenopausal women is well-established in the literature and reported in a recent meta-analysis.[69] Of interest is the finding that calcium supplementation shows greater protection against vertebral fractures, sites rich in trabecular bone that is more metabolically active than cortical bone, compared with fractures at other sites of the skeleton.[69] The Food and Nutrition Board determined the dietary reference intake (DRI) of calcium for women over age 51 to be 1200 mg calcium per day to promote healthy bone.[70] In 2002, Clinical Practice Guidelines for the Diagnosis and Management of Osteoporosis in Canada were published, suggesting a total dietary intake of 1500 mg calcium per day for postmenopausal women.[14] In studies reporting positive effects of soy and isoflavones on preservation of bone mass, the potential synergy of soy and calcium is difficult to tease out because varying levels of dietary calcium were used, and in some studies calcium intakes for some subjects may have been lower than current recommendations.[34,41–43,46,47,71] Thus, it is possible that the effects observed may have been greater if recommended levels of calcium were consumed with soy protein with a high isoflavone content (over 50 mg isoflavones/d). Because of practical considerations and challenges, mainly that calcium supplementation is recommended to all postmenopausal women to help maintain healthy, strong bones, none of these human studies examined the effect of varying the level of dietary calcium.

Using ovariectomized rodents, the synergy of soy isoflavones and high dietary calcium has been studied. In one study, ovariectomized rats were fed a diet rich in isoflavones, in the form of an isoflavone extract containing a mixture of genistein, daidzein, and glycitein, for 8 weeks (Table 12.1).[27] Rats

TABLE 12.1

Effect of an Isoflavone Extract in Combination with High Dietary Calcium on Femur and Lumbar Vertebra (LV1-LV6) Bone Mineral Density (BMD) in Ovariectomized Rats

Dietary Intervention[a]	Femur BMD (mg/cm^2)	LV1-LV6 BMD (mg/cm^2)
Sham — control diet	252 ± 7^a	257 ± 13^a
Ovariectomized — control diet	236 ± 9^b	225 ± 10^c
Ovariectomized — isoflavone diet	229 ± 11^b	218 ± 9^c
Ovariectomized — high calcium diet	229 ± 8^b	224 ± 11^c
Ovariectomized — isoflavone + high calcium diet	249 ± 7^a	239 ± 12^b

Values are expressed as the mean ± SD and values with different superscripts within a column are significantly different ($p < .05$)

[a] Control diet was AIN93G diet with 2 g calcium per kg diet. The other study diets were the control diet with the following modifications: isoflavone diet contained 217 mg genistein, 196 mg daidzein, and 35 mg glycitein per kg diet; high calcium diet contained 25 g calcium per kg diet, and the combination diet contained 217 mg genistein, 196 mg daidzein, 35 mg glycitein, and 25 g calcium per kg diet.

Source: Breitman, P.L. et al., *Bone,* 33, 597, 2003.

fed isoflavones in combination with high calcium had significantly higher BMD at both the femur and the lumbar vertebrae than rats fed high calcium diet alone or isoflavones alone. These findings suggest synergy among isoflavones and supplemental levels of calcium with respect to preservation of bone tissue. Further, these findings suggest that this synergy benefits both cortical and trabecular bone because bone mass of two distinct regions of the skeleton, femur and lumbar vertebrae, were preserved. A companion study in which soy, containing similar levels of isoflavones and calcium as in the aforementioned study, was fed to ovariectomized rats demonstrated similar findings. After 8 weeks of feeding, the combination of soy and high calcium diet resulted in higher lumbar vertebra BMD compared with rats fed high calcium alone or soy alone (Breitman, Fonseca and Ward, unpublished findings). In contrast, soy combined with high calcium did not result in higher femur BMD than either soy or high calcium alone groups. This finding indicates that trabecular bone was more responsive to the combined treatment compared with the femur, which has a higher quantity of cortical bone.

Based on the knowledge that daidzein can be further metabolized to equol, which may have even greater biological effects on bone, a study in ovariectomized mice (C57 strain) was designed.[28] The objective of this study was to determine if purified daidzein in combination with high dietary calcium would have greater protective effects against the loss of BMD and biomechanical bone strength than either treatment alone, and ultimately, if these bone outcomes were preserved to the level of sham mice (Table 12.2). Two different levels of daidzein were studied, 100 mg or 200 mg daidzein per kilogram of diet, both levels attainable by diet alone. As in the two previously discussed studies, the high calcium diet contained 25 g calcium per kilogram of diet. As hypothesized, the combination of the high daidzein and high calcium diet did result in greater preservation of bone mass at the femur and lumbar vertebrae compared with ovariectomized mice fed a control diet. Surprisingly, however, most of this effect was mediated by the high calcium diet. Mice fed a high calcium diet alone or in combination with high or low daidzein had similar femur and lumbar vertebra BMD, and similar peak load of femur midpoint, neck, and LV3 (Table 12.2). Thus, the resistance of a bone to fracture was improved by high dietary calcium in the diet while the daidzein did not confer a measurable benefit.

There are several possible explanations to explain the modest effect of daidzein on bone metabolism, including the level of conversion of daidzein to equol and the dose of daidzein. Significantly higher serum equol indicated that the mice were able to metabolize daidzein to equol, but as discussed previously in Section 12.3.1, a comparative study of four strains of ovariectomized mice indicated that C57 mice produce relatively low levels of equol compared with other strains.[61] The dose of daidzein used may have been too low to observe a biological effect. A study in mice that observed a positive effect of daidzein on bone after ovariectomy used a dose that was several-fold higher, and would be achieved only through supplementation, not the consumption of isoflavone rich foods.[72]

TABLE 12.2

Effect of Daidzein in Combination with High Dietary Calcium on Femurs and Lumbar Vertebrae of Ovariectomized Mice: Bone Mineral Density (BMD) and Peak Load

Dietary Intervention[a]	Femur BMD (mg/cm²)	Femur Midpoint Peak Load (N)	Femur Neck Peak Load (N)	LV1-LV4 BMD (mg/cm²)	LV3 Peak Load (N)
Sham — control diet	64.2 ± 1.3^{a}	21.8 ± 0.8^{a}	17.1 ± 1.3^{ab}	57.5 ± 1.0^{a}	40.1 ± 1.9^{ab}
Ovariectomized — control diet	53.8 ± 0.5^{d}	18.1 ± 0.6^{b}	12.9 ± 0.6^{c}	51.6 ± 1.5^{b}	27.8 ± 1.5^{c}
Ovariectomized — high calcium diet	60.6 ± 0.8^{b}	21.8 ± 0.8^{a}	16.4 ± 0.8^{abc}	59.9 ± 1.8^{a}	48.9 ± 4.8^{a}
Ovariectomized — high daidzein diet	57.2 ± 0.5^{c}	19.8 ± 0.7^{ab}	14.5 ± 0.8^{bc}	51.5 ± 1.3^{b}	29.2 ± 1.3^{bc}
Ovariectomized — high daidzein + high calcium diet	61.5 ± 0.8^{b}	22.1 ± 0.5^{a}	18.5 ± 1.0^{a}	58.8 ± 1.8^{a}	42.2 ± 2.9^{ab}
Ovariectomized — low daidzein	55.8 ± 0.8^{cd}	17.9 ± 0.7^{b}	13.6 ± 1.0^{bc}	52.8 ± 1.0^{b}	31.4 ± 2.7^{bc}
Ovariectomized —low daidzein + high calcium diet	61.0 ± 0.7^{b}	22.3 ± 0.9^{a}	16.5 ± 1.0^{abc}	61.2 ± 1.8^{a}	37.6 ± 3.3^{abc}

Values are expressed as the mean ± SD and values with different superscripts within a column are significantly different ($p<0.05$)

[a] Control diet was AIN93G diet with 2 g calcium per kg diet. The other study diets were control diet with the following modifications: high daidzein diet contained 200 mg daidzein per kg diet; high calcium diet contained 25 g calcium per kg diet; high daidzein + high calcium diet contained 200 mg daidzein and 25 g calcium per kg diet; low daidzein diet contained 100 mg daidzein per kg diet; low daidzein + high calcium diet contained 100 mg daidzein and 25 g calcium per kg diet.

Source: Fonseca, D. and Ward, W.E., *Bone*, 35, 489, 2004.

This study also determined if circulating levels of proinflammatory mediators (interleukin-6 [IL-6], tumor necrosis factor-α [TNF-α], interleukin-1β [IL-1β]) differed among groups because there is discussion in the literature that these mediators are elevated after estrogen withdrawal.[73,74] Only serum IL-1β was elevated among ovariectomized mice fed control diet, suggesting that the daidzein or high calcium in the diet attenuated the rise in IL-1β after ovariectomy.

12.3.3 Flaxseed

Flaxseed is increasingly being incorporated into cereals, breads, and muffins as well as other commonly consumed foods, largely because of the potential health benefits associated with it. Studies that have investigated the effect of flaxseed or its lignan precursor secoisolariciresinol diglucoside on bone metabolism are largely based on the fact that the mammalian lignans, enterodiol and enterolactone, have a similar chemical structure to endogenous estrogen, 17-β-estradiol. Other studies determined if feeding flaxseed could have potential negative effects during critical stages of development because lignans possess antiestrogenic effects in select tissues such as breast (see Chapter 8).

Compared with studies on the effects of soy and isoflavones on bone metabolism, there is a substantially lower number of reports on the effect of flaxseed and/or its lignan component on bone health. Among these studies, two investigated the effects of early exposure to flaxseed or its lignan[75,76] in developing rats while two other studies relate to changes in biochemical markers of bone metabolism in postmenopausal women.[54,77] All of these studies used a level of flaxseed or lignan that is attainable by dietary modification as opposed to consuming supplements. The studies in developing rats demonstrated that although effects of flaxseed or lignan feeding during early stages of life modified some bone strength outcomes, these effects disappeared by adulthood.[75,76] It is hypothesized that the rise in endogenous sex steroid hormones during later life diluted the effects of flaxseed or purified lignan. Both studies in postmenopausal women demonstrated that feeding flaxseed for several months did not alter biochemical markers of bone formation or resorption.[54,77] Overall, these studies suggest that flaxseed does not have either a positive or negative effect when fed during early life or after estrogen withdrawal. A comprehensive review of these flaxseed and lignan feeding studies is available.[78] To date, no studies in humans or animals have combined flaxseed and supplemental levels of calcium.

12.3.4 Soy Combined with Flaxseed

Unpublished findings provide the only insight into the potential synergy of soy and flaxseed (Power and Thompson, unpublished findings). An ovariectomized mouse model (athymic mice) was used to investigate the synergy of soy and flaxseed on carcinogenesis by injecting mice with MCF-7 cells (estrogen receptor positive) and feeding soy, genistein, flaxseed, enterodiol, enterolactone, a combination of soy and flaxseed, or a combination of genistein and the lignans (enterodiol, enterolactone) to elucidate which dietary intervention prevented or slowed the progression of tumors. The levels of soy, genistein, flaxseed, enterodiol, and enterolactone are all attainable by diet alone without taking supplements. Because there is the potential for either soy or flaxseed to have effects, either estrogenic or antiestrogenic, in other tissues, femurs and vertebra were collected, and BMD and biomechanical strength properties determined. Preliminary data indicate that soy or genistein preserved femur BMD whereas combining soy with flaxseed, or genistein with lignans resulted in a lower femur BMD. In addition, positive effects of soy or genistein alone on femur peak load were also attenuated when combined with flaxseed or lignans, respectively. Thus, using this animal model, flaxseed acts contrary to soy or genistein, suggestive of an antiestrogenic effect in bone.

12.3.5 Combination of Soy, Flaxseed, and Calcium

Potential synergy among soy, flaxseed, and high calcium in the diet with respect to bone metabolism is purely speculative. With the potential for flaxseed to attenuate the benefits of soy on BMD in an ovariectomized mouse model, it is likely that minimal synergy would exist in a diet containing soy, flaxseed, and high calcium (Power and Thompson, unpublished findings). In addition, it is interesting that although an antiestrogenic effect was observed in this preliminary study, no negative effect on bone is observed when flaxseed or lignans are fed alone.[54,75–77] There is a definite need for more studies in which multiple components in the diet are studied, not only to evaluate potential synergy, but to also assess potential negative effects of this combination.

12.4 Food–Drug Synergy and Osteoporosis

12.4.1 Calcium and Hormone Replacement Therapy (HRT)

It is well documented that the loss of ovarian estrogen production after menopause leads to the deterioration of bone tissue, and in the most severe cases of bone loss, fragility fractures result.[1,67] Estrogen is believed to inhibit osteoclast formation; therefore this loss of estrogen after menopause leads to elevated rates of bone resorption and turnover. It is not surprising that HRT reduces bone resorption and has a dramatic, positive effect on BMD at multiple skeletal sites (lumbar spine, hip, forearm); however whether HRT ultimately leads to reductions in fragility fractures requires further investigation.[2,11,79]

Clearly, the findings from the Women's Health Initiative (WHI) study raised serious concerns about the safety of long term use of HRT, and in some cases dissuaded clinicians from prescribing HRT and, understandably, deterred women from accepting HRT.[10] However, interest in using lower doses of estrogen, in particular, have led to several investigations that have all shown that substantially lower doses of estrogen can preserve BMD in older women, i.e., over 60 years of age.[80–82] In one study, women over 65 years of age were randomized to placebo or low dose estradiol (0.25 mg estrogen versus 0.625 mg estrogen that is used in many studies, including the WHI study) for 3 years. Subjects who received the low dose estrogen experienced increases in BMD at the femur neck, spine, and hip.[82] Importantly, no adverse effects such as changes in the thickness of the endometrium, breast tenderness, or mammography were observed with low dose estrogen treatment.[82] Studies regarding long-term efficacy, as measured by fracture rates, and safety issues are ongoing. Also, whether low dose estrogen therapy is effective in preventing or managing osteoporosis in younger postmenopausal women without adverse side effects needs to be studied.

Several years before the findings from the WHI study, a review of 31 randomized control trials that reported the effect of HRT, with or without calcium, concluded that HRT results in the biggest improvements in BMD when combined with supplemental calcium.[62] The authors of the study divided the studies into two groups, studies in which calcium supplementation was provided, resulting in a mean calcium intake of 1183 mg that is close to recommended levels of calcium, or studies in which calcium supplementation was not provided, in which mean calcium intakes were 563 mg/d per day, well below recommended intakes. By calculating the percent change in BMD with treatment from baseline, it was determined that the gains in femur neck, lumbar spine, and forearm BMD were higher with the combination of HRT and calcium supplementation. Femur neck BMD increased 0.9 vs. 2.4% per year; lumbar spine BMD increased 1.3 vs. 3.3% per year; and forearm BMD increased 0.4 vs. 2.1% when HRT alone versus HRT in combination with supplemental calcium, respectively were compared. Of note is that many of the studies differed in their characteristics: different bone sites were measured, the duration of the studies varied mostly between 1 and 3 years; different technologies were used to assess BMD and levels of estrogen, and inclusion of progesterone (many of these studies used 0.625 mg conjugated equine estrogen, the same dose and form used in the WHI Study). The fact that an added benefit of calcium could be determined despite the differences in study characteristics, attests to the strength of the synergy between HRT and supplemental calcium.

12.4.2 Soy Combined with HRT

No studies have specifically investigated the potential synergy of soy and HRT. One study that investigated the effect of soy isoflavones on changes in biochemical markers of bone formation, bone specific alkaline phosphatase, and bone resorption, urinary deoxypyridinoline, did include some women who were taking HRT.[41] It was determined that women not receiving HRT benefited the most from the soy intervention. Women receiving soy without concurrent HRT experienced a significant reduction in urinary deoxypryidinoline, suggesting a reduction in bone resorption. No differences in the bone formation marker were observed among women taking or not taking HRT. While it is often speculated that soy isoflavones act like estrogen, and thus would potentially have a similar mechanism of action on bone as HRT, this study suggests that the benefit of HRT to bone cannot be further strengthened with the addition of soy isoflavones. To date, no studies have investigated the potential synergy of flaxseed and HRT.

12.5 Safety Aspects

A common question is what levels of soy (or its isoflavones) or flaxseed (or its lignans) are safe with respect to all aspects of health. Realistically, levels of soy, isoflavones, flaxseed, or lignans that can be achieved by diet alone are thought to be safe. A vegetarian diet or Asian diet could provide a minimum of 50 mg of isoflavones, and in some cases higher levels of isoflavones. Because soy or flaxseed may act as SERMs, thereby acting as an estrogen in some tissues while acting as antiestrogen in others,[83] there should be caution in the consumption of excessive quantities that are achieved only through use of supplements. More research is needed to ultimately determine the level of dietary soy and flaxseed that may pose potential health risks.

Studies using ovariectomized animal models to study the effects of soy or isoflavones on bone metabolism generally include data on uterine weights to monitor for any potential estrogenic, and thus negative, effects on the uterine tissue. To counter the problem of endometrial hyperplasia and thickening in humans, women with an intact uterus are prescribed HRT that contains progesterone in combination with estrogen, whereas women without a uterus are prescribed HRT without progesterone. In the rodent studies that investigated the effect of an isoflavone extract or purified daidzein in combination with high dietary calcium, uterine weight was not negatively affected.[27,28] However, future studies investigating the synergy of soy and low dose HRT will need to diligently include outcome measures of safety, in particular, effects on uterine and breast tissue. Whether soy and HRT act via similar or different mechanisms in some or all tissues needs to be determined to clearly assess safety and identify potential deleterious effects. A study in postmenopausal women suggests that soy does not counter the ability of estrogen to induce changes in the endometrium.[84] Women who received a combination of estrogen and soy for 6 months experienced similar changes in the endometrium as women receiving estrogen alone.[84] The soy intervention, 25 g soy powder per day, provided 120 mg of isoflavones per day, a high level of isoflavones compared with other human feeding studies.

Although this chapter does not specifically discuss effects of progesterone alone on bone metabolism, a recent study reported surprising findings about the combination of progesterone and soymilk on bone metabolism.[49] Postmenopausal women were randomized to placebo, soymilk (providing 76 mg of aglycones/d), progesterone, or soymilk in combination with progesterone for a period of 2 years. Women receiving the combination of soymilk and progesterone experienced a significant loss in BMD at the lumbar spine, whereas progesterone alone or soymilk alone prevented a significant loss in BMD at the lumbar spine.[49] Thus, a food–drug combination that was expected to result in synergy turned out to have a negative effect on bone. This study highlights the importance of investigating food–drug combinations, and although a food or drug may have a positive effect in isolation, the effect of the combination is not necessarily beneficial.

With respect to calcium, upper tolerable limits for women, over 51 years of age, are 2500 mg per day.[70] When designing human feeding studies to investigate synergy with calcium, this level of calcium intake should not be surpassed because of the potential negative effects of high calcium intake (discussed further in Chapter 13).

12.6 Conclusions

Studies on the synergy of soy and its isoflavones, flaxseed and its lignans, supplemental calcium, and HRT are in their infancy. Clearly, long term feeding studies in humans, studies that are a minimum of 2 years in duration, are needed. Additionally, using ovariectomized animal models, investigators can elucidate mechanisms to explain the synergy of soy, flaxseed, calcium, and HRT, particularly low dose estrogen. Based on published studies, it is sensible to recommend that postmenopausal women consume the recommended level of calcium. Further investigation is required to elucidate the dietary levels of soy or isoflavones that will have potential health benefits with respect to lowering risk of fragility fracture. Flaxseed, its lignan precursor (SDG), or the mammalian lignans (enterolactone, enterodiol) appear to have only modest effects on bone. However studies that determine the potential synergy of flaxseed or its lignans with supplemental levels of calcium, and their interaction with soy and its isoflavones are needed. The potential synergy among soy, flaxseed, calcium, and low dose HRT presents an exciting area for future research, based on their potential common and opposing mechanisms of action.

Acknowledgments

The author thanks the Natural Sciences and Engineering Research Council (NSERC) for funding her projects that investigated the synergy of dietary estrogens and calcium on bone mass and biomechanical bone strength in rodents.

References

1. Cummings, S.R. and Melton, L.J., Epidemiology and outcomes of osteoporotic fractures, *Lancet*, 359, 1761, 2002.
2. Nelson, H.D. et al., Postmenopausal hormone replacement therapy: scientific review, *JAMA*, 288, 872, 2002.
3. Writing Group for the Women's Health Initiative Investigators. Risks and benefits of estrogen plus progestin in healthy postmenopausal women: principal results from the Women's Health Initiative randomized controlled trial, *JAMA*, 288, 321, 2002.
4. Shumaker, S.A. et al., Estrogen plus progestin and the incidence of dementia and mild cognitive impairment in postmenopausal women: the Women's Health Initiative Memory Study: a randomized controlled trial, *JAMA*, 289, 2651, 2003.
5. Wassertheil-Smoller, S. et al., Effect of estrogen plus progestin on stroke in postmenopausal women: the Women's Health Initiative: a randomized trial, *JAMA*, 289, 2673, 2003.
6. Thomson, A.B., et al., Role of gastric mucosal and gastric juice cytokine concentrations in development of bisphosphonate damage to gastric mucosa, *Dig. Dis. Sci.* 48, 308, 2003.
7. Graham, D.Y., What the gastroenterologist should know about the gastrointestinal safety profiles of bisphosphonates, *Dig. Dis. Sci.*, 47, 1665, 2002.
8. Donahue, J.G. et al., Gastric and duodenal safety of daily alendronate, *Arch. Intern. Med.*, 62, 936, 2002.
9. Cosman F., Selective estrogen-receptor modulators, *Clin. Geriatr. Med.*, 19, 371, 2003.
10. Ettinger, B. et al., Effect of the Women's Health Initiative on women's decisions to discontinue postmenopausal hormone therapy, *Obstet. Gynecol.*, 102, 1225, 2003.
11. Cranney, A. et al., Meta-analyses of therapies for postmenopausal osteoporosis. IX: Summary of meta-analyses of therapies for postmenopausal osteoporosis, *Endocr. Rev.*, 23, 570, 2002.
12. Stepan, J.J. et al., Mechanisms of action of antiresorptive therapies of postmenopausal osteoporosis, *Endocr. Regul.*, 37, 225, 2003.
13. Osteoporosis prevention, diagnosis, and therapy, *NIH Consensus Statement*, 17, 1, 2000.
14. Brown, J.P. and Josse, R.G., 2002 clinical practice guidelines for the diagnosis and management of osteoporosis in Canada, *Can. Med. Assoc. J.*, 167, S1, 2002.

15. Weinstein, R.S., True strength, *J. Bone Miner. Res.*, 15, 621, 2000.
16. Turner, C.H. and Burr, D.B., Basic biomechanical measurements of bone: a tutorial, *Bone*, 14, 595, 1993.
17. Turner, C.H., Biomechanics of bone: determinants of skeletal fragility and bone quality, *Osteoporos. Int.* 13, 97, 2002.
18. Cullinane, D. and Einhorn, T.A., Biomechanics of bone, in *Principles of Bone Biology*, 2nd ed., Bilezikian, J.P., Raisz, L.G., and Rodan, G.A., Eds., Academic Press, New York, 2002, p. 17.
19. Wilkin, T.J. and Devendra, D., Bone densitometry is not a good predictor of hip fracture, *Br. Med. J.*, 323, 795, 2001.
20. Dequeker, J. and Luyten, F.P., Bone densitometry is not a good predictor of hip fracture, *Br. Med. J.*, 323, 797, 2001.
21. Cummings, S.R. et al., Bone density at various sites for prediction of hip fractures. The Study of Osteoporotic Fractures Research Group, *Lancet*, 341, 72, 1993.
22. Cummings, S.R., Bates, D., and Black, D.M., Clinical use of bone densitometry: scientific review, *JAMA*, 288, 1889, 2002.
23. Heaney, R.P., The bone-remodeling transient: implications for the interpretation of clinical studies of bone mass change, *J. Bone Miner. Res.*, 9, 1515, 1994.
24. Hammett-Stabler, C.A., The use of biochemical markers in osteoporosis, *Clin. Lab. Med.*, 24, 175, 2004.
25. Gundberg, C.M., Biochemical markers of bone formation, *Clin. Lab. Med.*, 20, 489, 2000.
26. Looker, A.C., et al., Clinical use of biochemical markers of bone remodeling: current status and future directions, *Osteoporos. Int.*, 11, 467, 2000.
27. Breitman, P.L. et al., Isoflavones with supplemental calcium provide greater protection against the loss of bone mass and strength after ovariectomy compared to isoflavones alone, *Bone*, 33, 597, 2003.
28. Fonseca, D. and Ward, W.E,. Daidzein together with high calcium preserve bone mass and biomechanical strength at multiple sites in ovariectomized mice, *Bone*, 35, 489, 2004.
29. Ho, S.C. et al., Soy intake and the maintenance of peak bone mass in Hong Kong Chinese women, *J. Bone Miner. Res.*, 16, 1363, 2001.
30. Nagata, C. et al., Soy product intake and serum isoflavonoid and estradiol concentrations in relation to bone mineral density in postmenopausal Japanese women, *Osteoporos. Int.*, 13, 200, 2002.
31. Ho, S.C. et al., Soy protein consumption and bone mass in early postmenopausal Chinese women, *Osteoporos. Int.*, 14, 835, 2003.
32. http://www.nal.usda.gov/fnic/foodcomp/Data/isoflav/isoflav.html
33. Greendale, G.A. et al., Dietary soy isoflavones and bone mineral density: results from the study of women's health across the nation, *Am. J. Epidemiol.*, 155, 746, 2002.
34. Morabito, N. et al., Effects of genistein and hormone-replacement therapy on bone loss in early postmenopausal women: a randomized double-blind placebo-controlled study, *J. Bone Miner. Res.*, 17, 1904, 2002.
35. Picherit, C. et al., Dose-dependent bone-sparing effects of dietary isoflavones in the ovariectomised rat, *Br. J. Nutr.*, 85, 307, 2001.
36. Picherit, C. et al., Daidzein is more efficient than genistein in preventing ovariectomy-induced bone loss in rats, *J. Nutr.*, 130, 1675, 2000.

37. Fanti, P. et al., The phytoestrogen genistein reduces bone loss in short-term ovariectomized rats, *Osteoporos. Int.*, 8, 274, 1998.
38. Arjmandi, B.H. et al., Bone-sparing effect of soy protein in ovarian hormone-deficient rats is related to its isoflavone content, *Am. J. Clin. Nutr.*, 68, 1364S, 1998.
39. Arjmandi, B.H. et al., Role of soy protein with normal or reduced isoflavone content in reversing bone loss induced by ovarian hormone deficiency in rats, *Am. J. Clin. Nutr.*, 68, 1358S, 1998.
40. Arjmandi, B.H. et al., Dietary soybean protein prevents bone loss in an ovariectomized rat model of osteoporosis. *J. Nutr.*, 126, 161, 1996.
41. Arjmandi, B.H. et al., Soy protein has a greater effect on bone in postmenopausal women not on hormone replacement therapy, as evidenced by reducing bone resorption and urinary calcium excretion, *J. Clin. Endocrinol. Metab.*, 88, 1048, 2003.
42. Potter, S.M. et al., Soy protein and isoflavones: their effects on blood lipids and bone density in postmenopausal women, *Am. J. Clin. Nutr.*, 68, 1375S, 1998.
43. Alekel, D.L. et al., Isoflavone-rich soy protein isolate attenuates bone loss in the lumbar spine of perimenopausal women, *Am. J. Clin. Nutr.*, 72, 844, 2000.
44. Blum, S.C. et al., Dietary soy protein maintains some indices of bone mineral density and bone formation in aged ovariectomized rats, *J. Nutr.*, 133, 1244, 2003.
45. Scheiber, M.D. et al., Dietary inclusion of whole soy foods results in significant reductions in clinical risk factors for osteoporosis and cardiovascular disease in normal postmenopausal women, *Menopause*, 8, 384, 2001.
46. Yamori, Y. et al., Soybean isoflavones reduce postmenopausal bone resorption in female Japanese immigrants in Brazil: a ten-week study, *J. Am. Coll. Nutr.*, 21, 560, 2002.
47. Uesugi, T., Fukui, Y., and Yamori, Y., Beneficial effects of soybean isoflavone supplementation on bone metabolism and serum lipids in postmenopausal Japanese women: a four-week study, *J. Am. Coll. Nutr.*, 21, 97, 2002.
48. Uesugi, T. et al., Comparative study on reduction of bone loss and lipid metabolism abnormality in ovariectomized rats by soy isoflavones, daidzin, genistin, and glycitin, *Biol. Pharm. Bull.*, 24, 368, 2001.
49. Lydeking-Olsen, E. et al., Soymilk or progesterone for prevention of bone loss. A 2 year randomized, placebo-controlled trial, *Eur. J. Nutr.*, 43, 246, 2004.
50. Atkinson, C. et al., The effects of phytoestrogen isoflavones on bone density in women: a double-blind, randomized, placebo-controlled trial. *Am. J. Clin. Nutr.*, 79, 326, 2004.
51. Kreijkamp-Kaspers, S. et al., Effect of soy protein containing isoflavones on cognitive function, bone mineral density, and plasma lipids in postmenopausal women: a randomized controlled trial, *JAMA*, 292, 65, 2004.
52. Schult, T.M. et al., Effect of isoflavones on lipids and bone turnover markers in menopausal women, *Maturitas*, 48, 209, 2004.
53. Register, T.C., Jayo, M.J., and Anthony, M.S., Soy phytoestrogens do not prevent bone loss in postmenopausal monkeys, *J. Clin. Endocrinol. Metab.*, 88, 4362, 2003.
54. Brooks, J.D. et al., Supplementation with flaxseed alters estrogen metabolism in postmenopausal women to a greater extent than does supplementation with an equal amount of soy, *Am. J. Clin. Nutr.*; 79, 318, 2004.
55. Wangen, K.E. et al., Effects of soy isoflavones on markers of bone turnover in premenopausal and postmenopausal women, *J. Clin. Endocrinol. Metab.*, 85, 3043, 2000.

56. Dalais, F.S. et al., The effects of soy protein containing isoflavones on lipids and indices of bone resorption in postmenopausal women, *Clin. Endocrinol. (Oxf).*, 58, 704, 2003.
57. Dalais, F.S. et al., Effects of dietary phytoestrogens in postmenopausal women, *Climacteric,* 1, 124, 1998.
58. Cai, D.J. et al., Comparative effects of soy isoflavones, soy protein and 17beta-estradiol on calcium and bone metabolism in adult ovarectomized rats — analysis of calcium balance, bone densitometry and mechanical strength, *J. Bone Min. Res.*, 16, S531, 2001.
59. Wang, C. and Zhang, Y., Effects of protein source and soy isoflavone on bone mineral content and bone density of ovariectomized rats, *FASEB J.*,16, A623, 2002.
60. Setchell, K.D., Brown, N.M., and Lydeking-Olsen, E., The clinical importance of the metabolite equol — a clue to the effectiveness of soy and its isoflavones, *J. Nutr.*, 132, 3577, 2002.
61. Ward, W.E. et al., Serum equol, bone mineral density, and biomechanical bone strength differ among four mouse strains, *J. Nutr. Biochem.*, 2005, in press.
62. Nieves, J.W. et al., Calcium potentiates the effect of estrogen and calcitonin on bone mass: review and analysis, *Am. J. Clin. Nutr.*, 67, 18, 1998.
63. Dang, Z. and Lowik, C.W., The balance between concurrent activation of ERs and PPARs determines daidzein-induced osteogenesis and adipogenesis, *J. Bone Miner. Res.*, 19, 853, 2004.
64. Onoe, Y. et al., Expression of estrogen receptor beta in rat bone, *Endocrinology,* 138, 4509, 1997.
65. Kuiper, G.G. et al., Interaction of estrogenic chemicals and phytoestrogens with estrogen receptor beta, *Endocrinology,* 139, 4252, 1998.
66. Rickard, D.J. et al., Phytoestrogen genistein acts as an estrogen agonist on human osteoblastic cells through estrogen receptors alpha and beta, *J. Cell. Biochem.*, 89, 633, 2003.
67. Pacifici, R. Mechanisms of estrogen action in bone, in *Principles of Bone Biology,* 2nd ed., Bilezikian, J.P., Raisz, L.G., and Rodan, G.A., Eds., Academic Press, New York, 2002, p. 693.
68. De Wilde, A. et al., A low dose of daidzein acts as an ERbeta-selective agonist in trabecular osteoblasts of young female piglets, *J. Cell. Physiol.* 200, 253, 2004.
69. Shea, B. et al., Meta-analyses of therapies for postmenopausal osteoporosis. VII. Meta-analysis of calcium supplementation for the prevention of postmenopausal osteoporosis, *Endocr. Rev.*, 23, 552, 2002.
70. Food and Nutrition Board, *Dietary Reference Intakes for Calcium, Magnesium, Phosphorus, Vitamin D and Fluoride,* Institute of Medicine, National Academy Press, Washington, D.C., 1997.
71. Chen, Y.M. et al., Soy isoflavones have a favorable effect on bone loss in Chinese postmenopausal women with lower bone mass: a double-blind, randomized, controlled trial, *J. Clin. Endocrinol. Metab.*, 88, 4740, 2003.
72. Ohta, A. et al., A combination of dietary fructooligosaccharides and isoflavone conjugates increases femoral bone mineral density and equol production in ovariectomized mice, *J. Nutr.*, 132, 2048, 2002.
73. Romas, E. and Martin, T.J., Cytokines in the pathogenesis of osteoporosis, *Osteoporos. Int.*, 7, S47, 1997.
74. Pfeilschifter, J. et al., Changes in proinflammatory cytokine activity after menopause, *Endocr. Rev.*, 23, 90, 2002.

75. Ward, W.E. et al., Exposure to flaxseed and its purified lignan reduces bone strength in young but not older male rats, *J. Toxicol. Environ. Health*, 63, 53, 2001.
76. Ward, W.E. et al., Exposure to purified lignan from flaxseed (Linum usitatissimum) alters bone development in female rats, *Br. J. Nutr.*, 86, 499, 2001.
77. Lucas, E.A. et al., Flaxseed improves lipid profile without altering biomarkers of bone metabolism in postmenopausal women, *J. Clin. Endocrinol. Metab.*, 87, 1527, 2002.
78. Ward, W.E., Effect of flaxseed on bone metabolism and menopausal symptoms, in *Flaxseed in Human Nutrition*, 2nd ed., Thompson, L.U. and Cunnane, S.C., Eds., American Oil Chemists' Society Press, Champaign, IL, 2003, p. 319.
79. Wells, G. et al., Meta-analyses of therapies for postmenopausal osteoporosis. V. Meta-analysis of the efficacy of hormone replacement therapy in treating and preventing osteoporosis in postmenopausal women, *Endocr. Rev.*, 23, 529, 2002.
80. Heikkinen, J. et al., Long-term continuous combined hormone replacement therapy in the prevention of postmenopausal bone loss: a comparison of high- and low-dose estrogen-progestin regimens, *Osteoporos. Int.*, 11, 929, 2001.
81. Ettinger, B., Unopposed ultra-low-dose estradiol: A new approach to osteoporosis prevention, *J. Fam. Pract.*, 53, S17, 2004.
82. Prestwood, K.M. et al., Ultralow-dose micronized 17beta-estradiol and bone density and bone metabolism in older women: a randomized controlled trial, *JAMA*, 290,1042, 2003.
83. Setchell, K.D., Soy isoflavones — benefits and risks from nature's selective estrogen receptor modulators (SERMs), *J. Am. Coll. Nutr.*, 20, 354S, 2001.
84. Murray, M.J. et al., Soy protein isolate with isoflavones does not prevent estradiol-induced endometrial hyperplasia in postmenopausal women: a pilot trial, *Menopause*, 10, 456, 2003.

13

Synergy of Protein, Fats, and Calcium; Potential Synergies with Drugs for Osteoporosis

Marlena C. Kruger and Raewyn C. Poulsen

CONTENTS

13.1 Introduction

Osteoporosis is defined as a systemic skeletal disease characterized by low bone mass and microarchitectural deterioration of bone tissue with consequent increase in bone fragility and susceptibility to fracture.[1] Osteoporosis has become the focus of much interest, and as a result of extensive research, there is a wealth of information available on bone health. Osteoporotic fractures are a major public health problem. In the United States, 10 million individuals have osteoporosis, while another 18 million more individuals have low bone mass and therefore they are susceptible to the disease.[2] Total expenditure for health care attributable to osteoporotic fractures in 1995 was estimated to be $13.8 billion.[3]

The development of osteoporosis is not associated with specific symptoms, and it is therefore quite difficult to diagnose until a large amount of bone has been lost. Bone mineral density measurements and dual energy x-ray absorptionmetry (DEXA) are the gold standard for diagnosis. The specific risk factors for osteoporosis, as well as its prevention and management, are better understood now as a result of increased interest, new technology for measurement of bone mass such as DEXA, and the availability of biochemical markers to monitor bone formation, turnover, and resorption. Low bone mass is the main factor underlying osteoporotic fracture. Bone mass later in life depends on the peak bone mass (PBM) achieved during growth and the rate of age-related bone loss later in life.[4] Bone is a living dynamic tissue, and bone continually remodels as part of the process of renewal and repair.[5] Two main strategies for the prevention of osteoporosis are (1) the development of maximal bone mass during growth and (2) reduction of bone loss later in life.[6] Any factor, therefore, that will influence the attainment of peak bone mass as well as the rate of bone loss later in life will affect bone density and fracture risk.[7]

Up to 80% of bone strength, bone density, and quality are genetically determined, but many other nutritional and lifestyle factors play a role.

Another very important determining factor for bone health is the person's physiological condition. This includes age, weight, fat, and muscle mass as well as hormonal status (including sex hormone and vitamin D status as well as parathyroid hormone levels).

Nutrition is an important factor in the development and maintenance of bone, and it can be modified and adapted to be bone protective. In general, calcium and phosphorous are considered to be the most important minerals for the maintenance of bone, but there are many other minerals that are also required. These include magnesium, fluoride, zinc, copper, iron, and selenium. Several vitamins are also thought to play an important role; they include vitamins D, A, C, K, and folate. Protein is crucial and is incorporated in the organic matrix of bone for collagen formation. Protein may also regulate the absorption of calcium.[8] Other diet-related factors that may have an effect on bone are total energy consumption and fat, carbohydrate, and fiber intake.[9]

Many nutrients are codependent and also under the influence of genetic and hormonal factors, and in interaction with various lifestyle modifiers.[9] In addition, many bone-active agents interact with nutrients. For the various agents to improve bone mass optimally, adequate nutrition is essential.[10] For example, the skeletal response of postmenopausal women to estrogen is augmented by calcium and vitamin D.[10] Furthermore, bisphosphonates and selective estrogen receptor modulators have all been tested in the presence of adequate calcium and vitamin D. In addition, protein is bone protective in the elderly, and adequate intake is necessary for recovery of fractures.[9] Illich et al.[9] showed some significant associations between various nutrients and bone parameters in a cross-sectional study of 136 healthy Caucasian postmenopausal women. The nutrient intakes were estimated using 3-d dietary records. Some of the nutrients were significantly correlated such as calcium and phosphorous ($r = 0.825$), calcium and magnesium ($r = 0.618$), calcium and vitamin D ($r = 0.621$), and protein and phosphorous ($r = 0.718$). Protein and calcium were also correlated ($r = 0.607$). Further associations were made between bone mineral density and some nutrients. The most significant correlations were found to be with calcium, protein, and energy intake, and these correlations were consistently significant for all measured skeletal sites.[9] In addition; a lower BMD and mineral content were associated with low intakes of calcium and protein. A subgroup analysis by the same authors also showed that higher calcium intake was associated with higher BMD irrespective of energy intake, and a similar relationship existed between protein and calcium and BMD of various skeletal sites. The interaction between calcium and protein is discussed elsewhere in this chapter. This chapter discusses interactions and synergies between protein and calcium, as well as among calcium, protein, and lipids in the following: effects on calcium absorption, calcium retention, and bone mineral density and also possible synergy with specific drugs prescribed for osteoporosis.

13.2 Calcium and Bone Health

Calcium is the most likely to be inadequate in terms of dietary intake.[6] Plasma calcium is tightly regulated by interactions between various hormones. These include parathyroid hormone (PTH), 1,25 dihydroxycholecalciferol (1,25 $(OH)_2D_3$) and calcitonin. These hormones all target the same tissues, namely bone, intestine, and the kidney. These three hormones interact to tightly regulate calcium absorption and excretion and also control entry of calcium into the extracellular space. The plasma concentration of ionized calcium controls the secretion of these hormones. A negative feedback system exists: PTH and 1,25 $(OH)_2D_3$ are secreted when plasma calcium is low and calcitonin is secreted when plasma calcium is high.[6,10,11]

Calcium is required for normal growth and development of the skeleton.[11] The accumulation of calcium by the skeleton changes with aging; it is high during growth until after adolescence (150 mg/d), reaching equilibrium during maturity, and then it is lost from the skeleton from the age of about 50 in men and at menopause in women.[4] Calcium intake can affect and modify both these processes. Positive effects of calcium on bone health in various age groups have been reported. Studies by Johnston et al. in 1992 and Dawson-Hughes in 1996 reported positive effects of calcium on bone health in children.[12,13] A meta-analysis by Welten et al. (1995) reported that there is an association between calcium intake and bone mass in premenopausal women.[14] Calcium is not able to prevent bone loss in postmenopausal women but is able to slow the rate of loss to some extent. Studies have indicated that the effectiveness of calcium is dependent on the subject's habitual calcium intake and also varies by skeletal site and menopausal age.[4]

The first 5 years after menopause is the period when most bone is lost and loss occurs at a rapid pace. Supplementation with calcium in this age group is not effective in slowing bone loss in trabecular regions of the skeleton.[15] Some results, however, indicate that supplemental calcium during menopause may slow cortical bone loss.[15–17] Older women, more than 5 years past menopause, seem to be more responsive to supplemental calcium. Again, baseline or habitual calcium intake is a determining factor of the response to extra calcium.[15] Spinal bone density is not affected by an increased calcium intake in this population of women[18,19]; results of studies show that an effect is only elicited if habitual intake is low (450 to 620 mg/d).[19] In contrast, a study of 3270 institutionalized women in France who were treated with 1200 mg/d of calcium and 800 IU/d of vitamin D for 3 years, indicated a reduction in the risk of hip fracture of 30% compared with that of a placebo group.[20] Habitual intake in more than 50% of the volunteers was less than 500 mg/d for calcium and 200 IU/d of vitamin D.

The need for calcium is determined by the development and maintenance of bone. In the case of calcium, the optimal reserve in the skeleton needs to be maintained and is not a metabolic function. Calcium is also a threshold substance; that means that the ability to store calcium is limited at suboptimal

TABLE 13.1

Recommended Dietary Reference Intakes for Calcium and Vitamin D by Age Group

Age group, year	Adequate intake of calcium, mg/day	Adequate intake of vitamin D, μg/d (IU/day)
9–18	1300	5 (200)
19–30	1000	5 (200)
31–50	1000	5 (200)
51–70	1200	10 (400)
> 70	1200	15 (600)

Source: Information from Food and Nutrition Board, Institute of Medicine, *Dietary Reference Intakes: Calcium, Phosphorous, Magnesium, Vitamin D and Fluoride*, National Academy Press; Washington, DC, 1997, chap. 4

intake but increasing intake above requirement for genetic purposes does not result in more calcium being stored.[21,22] Therefore, increased calcium intake above what is needed to optimize bone mass will not result in more bone. Several genetic and environmental factors influence calcium requirement. These include responsiveness of bone to hormones as well as bone architecture and geometry. Environmental influences such as dietary constituents and mechanical loading on the skeleton have their own effects. Dietary factors such as high protein or sodium effectively increase the daily calcium requirement.[4,21] Other nutrients may, however, lower the daily calcium requirement (Table 13.1) because of positive interactions with either calcium absorption or reduction of calcium excretion. These include dietary lipids, essential fatty acids, and vitamin D.

13.2.1 Dairy Products as a Source of Calcium

Milk and milk products are good sources of the nutrients needed for bone development and maintenance.[23] Milk and dairy products, however, contain sodium and protein, which some have argued negate the benefit of dairy calcium. Studies show that the negative effects of sodium and protein are apparent only at low calcium intakes, and even then the ratio of the calcium in milk to its sodium and protein content is so high that it offsets any calciuric effects. Milk products are rich sources of calcium, phosphorous, magnesium, potassium, zinc, and protein, more so than any other typical food in the diet.[23] Barger-Lux and Heaney analyzed the diets of premenopausal female volunteers and found that women with a low calcium intake also had deficiencies of other key nutrients, and this deficiency could be corrected by one or two servings of dairy product per day.[24]

13.2.2 Calcium Bioavailability: Effects of Other Nutrients

Improving calcium intakes and bioavailability in a population may prove to be challenging. Changing eating habits to encourage increased intake of dairy product may not be feasible. Alternatively, foods eaten by target groups could be fortified with calcium. Because the absorption of calcium is a critical factor in determining the availability of calcium for bone development and maintenance, there is a need to identify food components or food ingredients that may influence calcium absorption in a positive way. Several food constituents have been suggested as enhancers of calcium absorption. Milk constituents such as lactose, lactulose, and caseinphosphopeptides have been suggested. There are only a few studies in humans that suggest that caseinphosphopeptides have an effect on absorption of calcium.[25] Similarly, nondigestible oligosaccharides can improve calcium absorption in adolescents and adults.[26,27] Other factors that may influence calcium absorption are protein intake and dietary lipids. The latter two factors are discussed in the rest of this chapter.

It is clear that calcium is the specific nutrient most important for prevention and treatment of osteoporosis, but large proportions of population groups do not meet recommended dietary calcium intakes. These groups should be encouraged to raise their daily calcium intake. Intake of dairy foods should be encouraged, and for the individuals with habitually low dairy product intake, functional foods with high calcium content should be investigated. These foods should also contain other nutrients, which may enhance intestinal calcium absorption and utilization of calcium by the body.

13.3 Protein and Bone Health

Dietary protein affects bone in a variety of ways. Bone matrix comprises about 30% of bone mass, and dietary protein is necessary for bone matrix synthesis. Protein-rich foods contain nutrients important for bone growth and building, and healing of a bone fracture will improve in an elderly person on a diet supplemented with protein.[28]

The question of whether protein is good or destructive to bone was addressed in a symposium held by the American Society for Bone and Mineral Research in 2002. It was proposed that the negative effect of protein on bone is due to sulfur–amino acid content, which leads to an increased glomerular filtration rate and consequently reduced renal reabsorption of calcium, resulting in hypercalciuria and therefore loss of calcium from bone.[29] This proposed loss of calcium over time is often also quoted as a cause of osteoporosis. Studies testing this hypothesis used purified proteins such as casein rather than common sources of protein such as meat and milk. The difference is that the latter contains phosphorous as well, which may blunt the effect of the protein.[30,31] Another confounding factor in many studies was that the studies were not long enough to allow for adaptation to the experimental diets. In a recent study by Roughead,[29] women were given either a low or a high meat diet with an average intake of 600 mg calcium/d. Results showed that the initial renal acid excretion observed with the high meat diet disappeared over time and was not observed after 8 weeks on the diets. This finding suggests that the body can adapt and buffer renal acid load without losing calcium. At moderate levels of protein intake (between 0.8 to 1 g protein/kg) calcium homeostasis and the skeleton remain normal.[32] It has been difficult to show that high protein diets affect bone density. Protein is consumed over the period of a day, and the human diet contains several other components generating acid or alkali, and the renal and respiratory systems have a substantial buffering capacity.

Recent studies suggest that higher protein intakes may be associated with positive effects on bone. A study by Dawson-Hughes in elderly adults reported that higher protein intakes were associated with favorable changes in total bone mineral density.[33] Pawlak reviewed studies of bone mass in vegetarians and omnivores.[7] Several studies reported on bone mass measurements of vegetarians and omnivores, but very few statistical differences were found. A significant difference was found in fiber intake, with the vegetarians having a higher intake. Fiber seems to limit the availability of estrogen for bioactivity, which could have a negative impact on bone. Another interesting observation was that omnivores seem to lose bone faster after menopause, a possible explanation being a reduced glomerular filtration rate by the kidneys due to aging, and therefore an inability to maintain a constant blood pH. The higher acidity in the blood would need constant buffering, which may require calcium. Notwithstanding these observations, overall the results of several studies show that there is no significant difference in BMD between people consuming vegetarian or meat diets. The specific effects of such diets may be more beneficial and may show differences when investigated in an adolescent population still achieving peak bone mass or in women immediately after menopause when bone turnover is high.[7] The NHANES III study showed that higher protein intake is associated with higher BMD. Munger et al. found that older women consuming the highest amount of protein, particularly animal protein, had the lowest risk of hip fracture.[34] Promislow et al. found that for every 15 g/d increase in animal protein intake, BMD increased by 0.016 g/cm^2 at the hip.[35]

The observed positive effects of protein on bone could be due to various factors; firstly dietary protein supplies the substrates for constant formation and remodeling of the matrix of bone consisting of collagen protein fibers; a second possibility is that protein may increase the circulating levels of insulin-like growth factor (IGF-1), which has an effect on bone growth. Milk supplementation in the elderly leads to increases in circulating IGF-1.[36] IGF-1 affects the osteoblast by stimulating proliferation, differentiation, and phosphate transport of these cells. IGF-1 may also modulate some of the anabolic effects of PTH on bone.[37] A third option is an effect on intestinal calcium absorption. This possibility is discussed under interactions between protein and calcium.

There are inconsistencies in epidemiological data with regards to the role of protein on bone health. The total effect of protein on bone should not be considered without considering the whole diet as well. The diet may contain phosphorus when the protein in the diet is from animal origin, and phosphorus is hypocalciuric. Similarly the potassium content of plant protein foods such as legumes and grains may have the same effect of conserving calcium. The effect of animal or plant protein on bone may not be due to the specific protein content but due to the sum of acid–ash and alkali constituents or potential renal acid load.[29,38]

13.4 Protein and Calcium Interactions

The nutritional interaction between protein and calcium has been well documented, more so than for any two other nutrients. There is some evidence that though high protein intake causes urinary loss of calcium, some coingested nutrients may prevent or compensate for the protein-induced calcium loss.

Several studies during the last 70 years have documented that urinary calcium rises as protein intake increases. An increase of about 50% can be expected if protein intake is doubled without any changes in other nutrient intakes. The long-term consequences of a small change in calcium balance are substantial. A 50-mg increase in urinary calcium loss per day will result in an 18.25 g loss per year or 365 g over 20 years. The female skeleton contains about 750 g calcium at its peak, and the loss would then be up to one-half of the stores.[38]

The harm done by ingestion of a high protein diet depends on the intake of calcium. If protein intake is high, a coinciding high intake of calcium may offset the effect of the high protein in the diet.[39] The 1997 recommended intakes for calcium and protein result in a calcium to protein ratio of 20:1 (mg calcium to g protein).[40] This ratio, however, is not achieved by the average women for whom the ratio may be closer to 9:1 up to 12:1.[28] The observation in the NHANES III study was not that the intake of protein was excessively high, but that the dietary intake of calcium was indeed low. In a paper by Recker et al., both calcium and protein were associated with bone gain in women but combining the two nutrients changed the association with bone gain to highly significant.[41]

Heaney suggested that dietary protein does not affect calcium absorption.[42] In his study he examined a threshold effect for protein. The volunteers were women aged 35 to 45 years, and he studied them over a period of 32 years. The result was 567 studies in 191 women. He divided protein intake into high and low groups, but the relative absorption values of calcium were not significantly different. He concluded that protein causes increased urinary calcium loss, and the resulting calcium balance in the body would depend on the amount of calcium in the diet.

In contrast, Kerstetter et al. suggested that increased protein in the diet may affect calcium absorption.[43] In a study in healthy young women, the effect of a low protein diet (0.7 g/kg body weight) and a high protein diet (2.1 g/kg body weight) on calcium absorption was investigated. The low protein diet resulted in lower urinary excretion of calcium and a rise in parathyroid hormone. The latter could be explained by a decrease in intestinal calcium absorption. Parathyroid hormone (PTH) plays a role in the control of calcium homeostasis and controls blood calcium levels. Any change in blood calcium will affect blood parathyroid hormone levels, followed by effects on intestinal calcium absorption and urinary calcium excretion. PTH affects the activity of renal 1- hydroxylase, the enzyme that converts 25-hydroxycholecalciferol to 1,25-dihydroxycholecalciferol, which in turn affects intestinal calcium absorption.[44] This paper is different because various other calcium balance studies have concluded that dietary protein has no, or a very minimal, effect on intestinal calcium absorption.[30,45,46] In contrast, few studies report an increase in intestinal calcium absorption with increased dietary protein.[44,47] The various studies by Kerstetter et al. conclude that a low protein diet may be associated with reduced bone turnover and intestinal absorption, while a high protein intake may suppress PTH by increasing bone resorption and calcium absorption or both. A daily allowance of 1 g/kg protein does not seem to have any detrimental effect on calcium homeostasis.[32,44,48,49] The critical factor with regards to changes in mineral metabolism with respect to protein intake is whether the diet would have any long-term implications for bone, and this question still needs to be answered.

Review of the literature by Kerstetter et al. indicates that for every 50 g increase in dietary protein there is a 1.6 mmol increase in 24-h urinary calcium excretion.[49,50] When protein intake is doubled, while other nutrients remain constant, urinary calcium loss increases by 50%.[44,50] Increased calcium loss could be due to an increased glomerular filtration rate, but high protein also decreases calcium reabsorption from the distal tubes. High protein in the diet increases the acid load in the body that may induce the above mentioned changes in filtration and reabsorption.[38] Alternatively, the fixed acid load due to sulfur containing amino acids are buffered partly from bone, leading to bone resorption.

Calculation of the calcium intake required to offset urinary losses at various protein intakes indicated that at a mean intake of 76 g/d, an intake of 1200 mg calcium would be needed to offset losses and to adjust for absorption. Data from the National Health and Nutrition Examination Survey (NHANES III) indicate that mean protein intake for women aged 16 to 19 and 20 to 29 in the United States is 67 and 69 g/d. Their calcium intake is between 822 and 778 mg/d, and therefore the general effect on calcium homeostasis should be negligible.[51]

In summary, diets moderate in protein are usually associated with normal calcium metabolism. Sustained hypercalciuria due to an increase in obligatory calcium loss is observed in individuals consuming high animal protein diets — whether this calcium is due to increased intestinal absorption or from bone remains to be proven.[22] Low protein diets lead to a rise in PTH and vitamin D. The long term complications of these observations are unknown and should be further investigated.[49,50]

13.5 Lipids and Bone Health

Dietary lipids influence bone density by altering the efficiency of intestinal calcium absorption as well as by regulating the processes of bone remodeling and mineralization. Several epidemiological studies have demonstrated a relationship between fat intake and bone health. NHANES III was an epidemiological study conducted in the United States involving a large number of men and women of all different ages. Data from 14,850 participants were analyzed to determine the relationship between diet and bone density. Total fat intake was negatively associated with hip bone mineral content and density. The effect was evident in both sexes but was more pronounced in men than in women, and most profound when total saturated fat intake was compared with bone mineral measurements.[52] Other studies have also reported a negative association between fat consumption and bone mineral density in pre- and postmenopausal women as well as an increased risk of fracture with increasing fat consumption in postmenopausal women.[52]

13.6 Lipids and Calcium Interaction

13.6.1 Lipids and Intestinal Structure and Function

Dietary lipids influence nutrient absorption by directly affecting the composition of intestinal cell membranes as well as the excretion of various enterotrophic peptides. Fatty acids originating from dietary lipids are incorporated into the phospholipids, which make up the cell membranes of intestinal cells. Polyunsaturated fatty acids are more readily incorporated into membranes than saturated or monounsaturated fatty acids.[53] Of the polyunsaturated fatty acids, the long chain, highly unsaturated fatty acids known as essential fatty acids or EFAs appear to exert the greatest effect on gut health and nutrient absorption.[60]

Humans lack the ability to synthesize fatty acids with a double bond past the carbon-9 position, therefore these fatty acids must be obtained from the diet and hence are termed "essential." EFAs are classified into one of two families designated as n-3 and n-6 depending on the location of the first unsaturated carbon from the methyl terminus.[54] α-Linolenic acid (ALA) (18:3) is the parent compound for the n-3 series of fatty acids, and linoleic acid (LA) (18:2) is the parent compound for the n-6 series. The most common and widely recognized dietary source of n-3 EFAs is fish oil, although ALA acid is present in the chloroplasts of green leafy vegetables and also in some plant oils such as canola and flaxseed. n-6 EFAs are found in many edible oils, and LA is found in the seed oils of most plants.[55] Evening primrose oil and most of the vegetable oils used to make margarine contain n-6 EFAs. EFAs are precursors for various eicosanoids such as prostaglandins and leukotrienes, which have a regulatory role in the body.

EFA deficiency reduces intestinal mucosal mass.[56] Dietary EFAs appear to have a trophic effect on the intestinal mucosa and may aid in promoting mucosal recovery after surgery or injury.[57] The fluidity of intestinal cell membranes also increases as the level of membrane lipid unsaturation increases.[53] Aside from changing the physical structure of the intestinal mucosa, dietary fat can also influence the release of enterotrophic peptides. Bolus dosing of long chain essential fatty acids has been reported to significantly increase the release of the peptide tyrosine-tyrosine and enteroglucagon.[58]

13.6.2 Lipids and Calcium Absorption

Calcium absorption mainly occurs in the duodenum.[59] Both the amount and the type of fat in the diet have a direct effect on calcium balance in the body. In full term infants, the amount of fat in the diet is positively correlated with calcium absorption. Polyunsaturated fats in particular have been implicated as promoters of calcium absorption as incidence of tetany in formula-fed, full-term infants substantially declined when LA–supplemented formula became available.[60]

There are two methods by which dietary calcium is absorbed in the intestine: transport through intestinal cells (transcellular) and passive diffusion or convection between intestinal cells (paracellular).

13.6.2.1 Transcellular Calcium Transport

There are essentially three steps involved in the uptake of calcium by duodenal cells or enterocytes:

1. Calcium enters the enterocyte via channels in the brush border.
2. Calcium is transported across the cell. This process is facilitated by specific calcium-binding proteins such as calbindin.
3. Calcium is released into the bloodstream from the basolateral membrane. This involves the calcium pump Ca^{2+}-ATPase, a Mg^{2+},Ca^{2+}-dependent ATPase and a Ca^{2+}–Na^{+} exchanger driven by $Na^{+}K^{+}$-ATPase.[61]

Activity of $Na^{+}K^{+}$-ATPase, Ca^{2+}-ATPase, Mg^{2+}-ATPase, and Ca^{2+}-transferase is dependent on the amount and type of fatty acid consumed.[62] Estrogen deficiency, such as occurs at menopause in women, is associated with decreased intestinal calcium absorption. This is illustrated by studies in ovariectomized rats (a well-established model for postmenopausal osteoporosis in women) that revealed decreases in mucosal transference of Ca^{2+} of 11.4 to 14.3% following ovariectomy. High dietary fat intake (30%) in ovariectomized rats has also been shown to reduce membrane-associated enzyme activity with the greatest reduction occurring with a high saturated fat diet (11.02 to 15.94%) compared with a high monounsaturated (9.1 to 14.8%) or polyunsaturated (5.0 to 12.1%) fat diet.[63]

13.6.2.2 Paracellular Calcium Transport

Medium-chain fatty acids such as palmitoylcarnitine, capric, and lauric acids may increase intestinal absorption of various nutrients, including calcium, via the paracellular pathway.[64] C10 and C12 fatty acids alter the permeability of tight junctions (the junctions that exist between cells), significantly enhancing the absorption of nutrients and drugs via the paracellular pathway.[65] Whether increased paracellular transport has a significant physiological effect in terms of overall calcium balance in the body is, however, unknown.

Calcium has a tendency to form insoluble complexes or "soaps" in the intestinal lumen through interaction with the sodium salts of fatty acids. Because calcium must be soluble in order for transport across the intestinal cell membranes to occur, this inhibits calcium absorption. Saturated fats have a greater tendency to form calcium soaps than unsaturated fats.[52]

13.6.3 EFAs, Calcium, and Bone Metabolism

13.6.3.1 EFAs and Calcium Absorption

Dietary intake of n-3 and n-6 EFAs is correlated with increased duodenal ion transport. Several mechanisms have been proposed to explain the effect of EFAs on intestinal calcium transport. One possibility is that enhanced membrane fluidity as a result of increased incorporation of EFAs into phospholipids alters the physical environment of membrane-bound enzymes, thereby enhancing their activity.[60]

Another possibility is that EFAs may mimic, or facilitate, the action of vitamin D in promoting calcium absorption. Ca^{2+}-ATPase is the rate-limiting enzyme in active calcium transport. It is up-regulated by the calcium-binding protein calmodulin. Unsaturated fatty acids bind with Ca^{2+}-ATPase, mimicking the action of calmodulin and stimulating Ca^{2+}-ATPase activity.[66] DHA (but not eicosapentaenoic [EA] or arachidonic acid [AA]) has been reported to increase Ca^{2+}-ATPase activity in the absence of calmodulin.[66] In addition, vitamin D receptor (VDR) availability, which is increased by ovariectomy in female rats, is reduced after EFA supplementation.[62] This is possibly indicative of increased vitamin D binding to the receptor.

EFAs may also influence the activity of the various isoforms of protein kinase C, which is responsible for activation via phosphorylation of various enzymes including Ca^{2+}-ATPase.[66] AA, a member of the n-6 family of EFAs, and the n-3 EFAs EPA and docosahexaenoic acid (DHA), inhibit $Na^{+}K^{+}$-ATPase activity.[66,67]

Conjugated linoleic acid (CLA), a n-6 EFA, has been found to increase paracellular (but not transepithelial or transcellular) calcium absorption *in vitro*.[66]

13.6.3.2 EFAs and Calcium Excretion

Results of human studies on the effects of EFAs and their metabolites on calcium excretion are conflicting. The level of prostaglandin E_2 (PGE_2, derived from the n-6 series of EFAs) was positively correlated with both urine flow and calcium excretion in patients with idiopathic hypercalciuria.[60] In some but not all studies, supplementation with either evening primrose oil (n-6 EFAs), fish oil (n-3 EFAs), or a combination resulted in a reported decrease in urinary calcium excretion.[60] It is possible that γ-linolenic acid (GLA, a n-6 EFA) from evening primrose oil and EPA or DHA (n-3 EFAs) from fish oil increase renal calcium reabsorption[60]; however other factors such as dietary calcium, sodium, or protein intake may mask this effect, particularly in healthy individuals. Inhibition of prostaglandin synthesis, which can occur by supplementation with fish oil, has been shown to decrease urinary calcium excretion in rats.[60] It has also been proposed that EFAs (particularly arachidonic acid) or prostaglandins, may have a role in vitamin D–mediated inhibition of renal calcium reabsorption and as a result lead to increased urinary calcium excretion.[60]

Consumption of long chain polyunsaturated fats, whether from the n-3 or n-6 family of EFAs, appears to be beneficial in enhancing calcium absorption, particularly in those habitually consuming a low calcium diet. Saturated fat consumption reduces intestinal calcium absorption. The effect of dietary lipid consumption on calcium excretion is less clear. In healthy individuals with adequate vitamin D status, EFA consumption may have little effect on calcium excretion. In individuals with pathological conditions such as idiopathic hypercalciuria, n-6 EFAs may increase urinary calcium excretion whereas n-3 EFAs may promote renal calcium reabsorption.

13.6.3.3 EFAs and Bone Density

n-3 EFAs appear to influence bone metabolism, particularly in the estrogen-deficient state. Eskimos in Greenland consume a high n-3 fatty acid diet because of their high consumption of fish. The incidence of atherosclerosis, nephrolithiasis, and osteoporosis is low among Greenland Eskimos compared with other countries.[68]

Serum n-6 fatty acid levels have been reported as higher in individuals with bone loss compared to those without.[69] An imbalance between the ratio of n-6 to n-3 EFAs has been suggested as a cause of bone loss during adulthood.[70] The n-6 to n-3 fatty acid ratio may have a role in regulating the site of calcium deposition within the body.

EFA metabolites have also been implicated as regulators of bone metabolism. Intravenous infusion of the n-6–derived prostaglandin PGE_1 is used as a preoperative treatment for infants with congenital heart disease in order to maintain the ductus in an open state pending corrective surgery. A side effect of treatment is rapid bone growth,[60] implicating prostaglandins, particularly those derived from n-6 EFAs, as regulatory factors in bone metabolism.

Several intervention studies involving feeding different combinations of n-3 and n-6 EFAs have been conducted. The majority of these studies have utilized ovariectomized rats. Positive results in terms of decreased levels of bone resorption markers, increased levels of bone formation markers, and/or increased bone density measured by DEXA have generally been obtained. It appears that both n-3 and n-6 EFAs are required for maximal inhibition of loss of bone density postovariectomy. Synergism may exist between the two EFA families; however the optimal ratio of n-3 to n-6 EFAs or the effects of individual n-3 and n-6 EFAs has yet to be determined.

Only three human studies have been published involving EFA supplementation and the measurement of bone parameters. Fish oil supplementation (4 g/d) or a mixture of fish oil and evening primrose oil for 16 weeks in elderly, osteoporotic women increased levels of serum calcium as well as levels of the bone formation marker osteocalcin. Alkaline phosphatase activity (which is associated with bone turnover) decreased, and the ratio of urinary calcium and creatinine increased, compared with subjects receiving 4 g/d of placebo or evening primrose oil. The greatest increase in bone formation markers was achieved with the evening primrose oil–fish oil mixture.[71]

Supplementation of elderly, osteoporotic and/or osteopenic women who had habitually low dietary calcium intakes with 6 g of high EFA oil in conjunction with 600 mg calcium carbonate/d for 18 months resulted in decreased urinary phosphate excretion and maintenance of lumbar spine bone density compared with increased urinary phosphate excretion and a 3.2% decrease in lumbar spine density in subjects receiving 600 mg calcium carbonate and 6 g of coconut oil per day. Combined EFA and calcium supplementation for a further 18-month period resulted in an increase of 3.1% in lumbar spine bone density.[72] EFAs, therefore, appear to be beneficial in treating senile osteoporosis, which is often caused by low dietary calcium intake, a decreased ability to absorb dietary calcium, and decreased vitamin D status as a result of lifestyle and metabolic factors associated with aging.[60]

One trial involving supplementation of pre- and postmenopausal women (age range 25 to 40 and 50 to 65 years, respectively) with a combination of n-3 and n-6 EFAs and calcium for a period of 12 months showed no additional benefit on bone density of EFA supplementation over calcium supplementation alone.[73] However the supplementation period was shorter and the EFA dosing regime (calcium 1 g, evening primrose oil 4 g, and fish oil 440 mg/d) was lower than that employed in trials reporting a positive effect of EFA supplementation. Women in this study were also considerably younger than those in the previous two reported studies and may have been at different stages of menopause. Bone density losses are greatest in the first 5 years following menopause.[74] It is likely that EFAs lack sufficient potency to overcome the effects of estrogen withdrawal during this period.

Intake of n-6 EFAs increases PGE_2, which in turn stimulates synthesis of proinflammatory cytokines such as interleukin-1 (IL-1), interleukin-6 (IL-6), and tumor necrosis factor-α (TNF-α).[54] Interestingly, estrogen deficiency also results in elevation of the levels of these cytokines, and all three cytokines are known to promote bone resorption.[3] n-3 EFAs down-regulate production of all prostaglandins but particularly those derived from n-6 EFAs such as PGE_2. As a result, n-3 EFAs act as antiinflammatory agents, inhibiting cytokine synthesis.

Bone turnover is essential to maintain the structural integrity of bone. The bone turnover cycle commences with bone resorption and is followed by bone formation. Estrogen deficiency results in increased bone resorption as well as formation, although the increase in rate of formation is less than that of resorption. This leads to reduced bone density and osteoporosis. High consumption of n-6 EFAs is becoming increasingly common as people switch from animal sources of fats and oil, such as butter, to plant sources, such as margarine. Although a reduction in intake of animal fat (and therefore, saturated fat) carries many health benefits, choice of the replacement dietary fat is also important. An imbalance between n-6 and n-3 EFAs in the diet may also have health consequences. Modulating the dietary ratio of n-6 to n-3 EFAs may be a means of at least partially compensating for the effects of the estrogen deficiency resulting from postmenopause. More research in this field is required before recommended dietary intakes for n-3 and n-6 EFAs can be proposed. Evidence to date suggests that during estrogen deficiency, a higher consumption of n-3 EFAs, such as can be achieved by increasing consumption of fatty fish, may be beneficial in reducing bone density losses.

13.7 Lipids and Other Nutrients

A high protein diet may affect EFA metabolism by increasing activity of δ-6-desaturase. Conversely the amino acids phenylalanine and tyrosine inhibit δ-6-desaturase activity.[75] Several other dietary and lifestyle factors modify δ-6-desaturase activity. Zinc, magnesium, and vitamins B_6, B_3, C, and E increase δ-6-desaturase activity. Enzyme activity is decreased by alcohol, trans fatty acids, and coffee consumption as well as by the action of insulin.[76] Coincidentally, smoking, diabetes, and high alcohol and protein consumption are also associated with decreased bone mineral density. High zinc, magnesium, and vitamin C intakes are linked with increased bone mineralization.[76] A direct relationship between bone density and lipid–nutrient–lifestyle interactions has yet to be demonstrated; however, it is possible that such interactions may contribute to overall bone health.

13.8 Synergy between Drug and Nutrient Therapies for Osteoporosis

Nutrition and nutritional therapies may modulate levels of drugs in the blood, may have independent effects on risk factors for many conditions, and will interact with a variety of medical therapies. In addition, for drugs to induce bone gain, nutrition must be adequate to provide the building blocks for normal bone. Most of the therapies for osteoporosis, such as hormone replacement therapy (HRT), bisphosphonates, an antiresorptive agent, and selective estrogen receptor modulators (SERMS) have been tested in trials together with a supply of calcium and vitamin D up to the required level, or the levels suggested by the NIH (see Table 13.1). Also, adequate protein intake has been shown to protect bone mass in the elderly.[28,29,32] Some synergy between protein in the diet and bone maintenance or prevention of bone loss is recognized because protein is essential for building the collagen compartment of bone matrix.[37,39]

Because osteoporosis is a multifactorial disease, no single intervention or drug can be expected to treat the problem. Because the relatively fast bone loss at menopause is due to the loss of estrogen, calcium and other nutrients cannot restore lost bone or the organic matrix of bone, but calcium and other nutrients may play a critical role in combination with pharmacologic treatment options. Estrogen, for example, has a two- to threefold greater protective effect when taken together with calcium.[77] Loss of estrogen, in menopause, increases bone resorption, or bone loss, and when replacement estrogen is supplied together with calcium, the antiresorptive effect of estrogen could prevent or slow bone loss while extra calcium in the diet could be available to maintain bone.[10,20,77]

Several of the drugs used to treat osteoporosis now require the intake of high levels of calcium. In adults, before menopause, maintenance of peak bone mass is probably achieved with calcium intakes of 1000 mg/d.[78] The question of how much of a mineral is needed to support bone active agents to add bone to the skeleton is often raised. If new bone is to be built, intake recommended for maintenance may not be adequate. An absorbed amount of calcium greater than the sum of urinary and skin losses may be required.[79] Although calcium intake should be increased above maintenance, the vitamin D requirement for therapeutic support is not different from that required for maintenance.[79] Heaney and Weaver[79] do raise this issue, but there are not many other publications that do recommend a specific intake of calcium and vitamin D in order to support drug treatments of osteoporosis. It can be, however, assumed that adequate calcium and vitamin D is needed to provide synergy with bone active drugs and protect bone against excessive loss of calcium.

The drugs of interest for osteoporosis are estrogen or HRT, SERMs, the bisphosphonates, calcitonin, intermittent PTH (teriparatide), and fluoride. All of these are classified as antiresorptive agents with the exception of PTH and fluoride. The name "antiresorptive" is misleading because the processes of bone resorption and formation are coupled, and the mentioned drugs would decrease the rates of both processes. Antiresorptive drugs decrease bone resorption within weeks, followed by a decrease in formation within months. This difference is due to the time sequence of the bone remodeling cycle.[20]

Fluoride and intermittent PTH act by increasing bone formation. The new bone is formed in areas that have been resorbed or on surfaces that have not been resorbed at all. Increases in bone density due to these drugs is similar to those measured with antiresorptive agents, but the extra bone is laid down on surfaces that have not been resorbed.[20]

13.8.1 Use of Calcium in Combination with Various Drugs

Increases in calcium intake in postmenopausal women reduce bone loss and fracture risk in this population.[80] Because of the large number of women already being diagnosed with osteoporosis, and the even larger number with low bone density, it is important to consider the role of additional calcium in the use of drugs for the prevention and treatment of osteoporosis. Originally, in 1994, the National Institutes of Health Consensus development Conference on Calcium recommended an intake of 1000 mg/d for postmenopausal women on HRT, and 1500 mg/d for women not receiving treatment. The Institute of Medicine in 1997 then reported that evidence does not support a different recommendation for older women.[40] These recommendations have been reviewed and current recommendations by The National Academies[40] are for at least 1200 mg calcium/d for men and women over 50 years of age. One can assume that these requirements would also be justified for a population with low bone mass, and that this level would be supportive of drugs to maintain bone mass.

Bisphosphonates are stable analogs of pyrophosphate. They are deposited in bone at sites of mineralization and have their effect there by affecting the process of bone resorption. The net effect of the bisphosphonates is on the osteoclasts, resorbing bone. The bisphosphonates cause cell death and a decrease in bone resorption.[20] The absorption of bisphosphonates is prevented by food, orange juice, coffee, calcium products, and other medications; patients are therefore recommended to take the bisphosphonates with water on an empty stomach, and to stay upright and consume nothing else for at least 30 min.

Bisphosphonates and raloxifene are routinely prescribed together with calcium, and all trials testing the two drugs used supplemental calcium, often together with some vitamin D.[20,77,78,80,81] It is difficult, however, to estimate the specific effect of the drug if calcium was not prescribed. These two agents suppress bone remodeling and resorption and some bone gain is usually observed. For an increase in bone mass to occur, calcium needs to be absorbed and retained in the body, thus reducing excretion. This may be accomplished only with adequate intake. Calcium binds with etidronate, one of the older generation bisphosphonates, reducing its bioavailability. Patients are generally instructed to avoid calcium supplements while using etidronate.

Heaney et al. suggested that the bisphosphonates and other antiresorptives reduce the response of bone to PTH.[81] The result of this reduction is an increase in circulating PTH, which reduces urinary excretion of calcium, increasing intestinal calcium absorption via vitamin D, and therefore reserving calcium in the body.[79] Most trials with the antiresorptives have raised calcium intake to between 800 and 1000 mg/d and not always with an accompanying increase in vitamin D intake. It is therefore possible that the use of higher levels of calcium plus substantial increases in vitamin D intake can augment the currently measured effects of the bisphosphonates and raloxifene or HRT. Combination therapy with estrogen and the bisphosphonates, such as etidronate, showed that these taken in combination with calcium resulted in a significantly greater increase in bone mineral density than with each therapy alone.[20] The synergy between the use of calcium together with these drugs for prevention of bone loss has therefore been established.

The development of human PTH (teriparatide) as an anabolic agent increased the requirement for calcium and vitamin D to ensure adequate calcium for building bone mass. Trials on teriparatide have shown increases of 9 to 15% in spine bone mineral density per year.[82,83] Increases in bone density such as these would require sufficient calcium and the current average intake of 600 to 800 mg calcium/d would not be sufficient. The study by Neer et al.[83] used supplemental calcium of 1000 mg/d with the addition of 10 to 30 μg vitamin D. The study by Arnaud et al. used supplemental calcium up to a level of 1500 mg/d and showed bone mass increases up to 30% at the lumbar spine and 12% at the hip.[82] In these studies, there was some concern about the occurrence of hypercalcemia. Up to 11% of women on PTH did show hypercalcemia. Reduction in calcium intake usually reduced the incidence, and if not, further halving of the dose of PTH resulted in normalization of the serum calcium. Out of the 500 plus women randomized to take a placebo or the two doses of PTH, only one woman in the placebo group, one in the lower dose and nine in the higher PTH dose were withdrawn because of persistence of elevated serum calcium.[83] An older study by Slovik et al. indicates that the substantial effect of PTH on bone cannot be produced without providing large quantities of calcium, achieved by giving 1,25 $(OH)_2D_3$ in their trial.[84] Calcium therefore seems to be essential to obtain increases in bone mass with PTH, and the synergy of calcium with PTH cannot be overemphasized. The role of vitamin D in acting synergistically with PTH still needs to be explored; there are no data available.

13.8.2 Protein and Phosphorous Required for Bone Maintenance in Combination with Drugs

The relationship between protein intake and bone mass remains controversial. The previous discussion about the role of protein in the maintenance of bone indicates that increased intake of protein is correlated with increased bone mass.[85] The calciuretic effects of a high protein diet could be offset by an increase in dietary calcium, and at high calcium intakes, the absorption of calcium is down-regulated. The implication is that there is a reserve capacity to increase calcium absorption in response to demands such as a high calcium diet–induced calciuria.[85] In the elderly with hip fractures, a raised intake of protein results in improved recovery from hip fracture, reduced stay in hospital, and a return to independent living.[85]

Bone mineral consists predominantly of calcium phosphate. Adequate intake of phosphorous is essential for building of new bone, and lack of phosphorous can inhibit osteoblast function and increase bone resorption by the osteoclasts.[86] Heaney and Weaver[79] suggested that phosphorous intake may become more of importance with therapies such as teriparatide. Phosphorous is not a major factor in bone maintenance, but some older women may have diets low in phosphorous. If these women receive calcium supplements as well, the calcium would bind the phosphorous in the intestine preventing absorption and therefore result in a deficiency of phosphorous. In this population, the concurrent supplementation of calcium and phosphate is probably needed.[79] Both these nutrients have been shown to act synergistically with bone active drugs in supplying the building blocks needed for maintenance of bone.[85,86]

13.8.3 Lipids and Drugs

13.8.3.1 Essential Fatty Acids and Estrogen

One study has identified a synergistic effect between EFAs and exogenously administered estrogen on preventing increases in bone turnover and decreases in bone calcium content in ovariectomized rats.[87] In this study, EFAs had a positive effect by preserving bone mass more effectively than estrogen alone in the ovariectomized female rat. To date, no studies investigating this effect in humans have been published.

Alternative medicines such as supplements are commonly used to treat the symptoms of menopause. They are naturally occurring phytochemicals that exhibit some estrogenic activity. The most common dietary source is the isoflavones found in soy, although many fruits, vegetables, and whole-grain products also contain phytoestrogens. Phytoestrogens are similar in structure to estrogen and are able to interact with estrogen receptors (ERs) albeit with differing, and lower, affinities than animal estrogens. In addition to interaction with the ER, phytoestrogens such as soy isoflavones are also thought to exert nonestrogenic effects, which are purportedly beneficial not only for bone but also for cardiovascular health and in reducing the risk of cancer. (Soy isoflavones are extensively discussed in Chapter 12.) If EFAs are able to synergistically enhance the effect of animal estrogens on bone, it is likely that synergism also exists between phytoestrogens and EFAs. To date, only one study has been published that has explored this possibility. Results from this study were inconclusive as soy protein together with fish oil fed to ovariectomized mice appeared to have a synergistic effect on the distal femur but not the lumbar spine.[54] This is perhaps a result of the differing bone compositions in these two sites, with the femur having a greater proportion of cortical bone than the lumbar spine.

13.8.3.2 Essential Fatty Acids and Statins

Although statins are generally prescribed to lower blood cholesterol levels, they also promote bone formation even in postmenopausal women.[68] Estrogen, statins, and n-3 EFAs appear to have similar effects in the body. They suppress the production of proinflammatory cytokines, stimulate nitric oxide synthesis, increase bone density, and inhibit tumor cell proliferation.[68] Statins also influence the metabolism of polyunsaturated fatty acids.[68] It has been proposed that statins, estrogen, and EFAs may act synergistically if coadministered to not only improve bone density but also potentially reduce atherosclerotic risk.[68,88] More research in this field is required to determine if synergism does exist.

13.9 Safety Issues around a High Intake of Calcium, Protein, and Lipids

Calcium plays a major role in the metabolism of almost all cells in the body, and it also interacts with various other nutrients. Disturbances of calcium metabolism can give rise to a variety of adverse reactions, and excessive changes in extracellular ionized calcium concentrations can cause damage in the function and structure of many organs.

Data on adverse effects of high calcium intake has been collected mostly around supplements; the areas for concern are kidney stone formation, hypercalcemia, and renal insufficiency, as well as interaction of calcium with other essential minerals. Renal stone formation may occur in about 12% of the U.S. population. A variety of dietary factors seem to play a role in determining the incidence of this disease. One factor is increased calcium intake, but stone formation also seems to be associated with higher intake of oxalate, protein, and vegetable fiber. There is also, however, an association between high sodium intake and stone formation, while other minerals such as phosphorous and magnesium are also implicated. Calcium may therefore only play a contributing role and may not be the determinant. In a recent prospective study in young women (Nurses' Health Study II), the association between dietary factors and risk of incident of symptomatic kidney stones was examined. The conclusion was that a higher intake of dietary calcium decreases the risk of kidney stone formation.[89] Earlier studies have indicated that the lowering of renal stone formation with a high calcium diet may be due to the binding of oxalate in the intestines by calcium, and oxalate is a critical component of kidney stones.[90]

Hypercalcemia and renal insufficiency (milk–alkali Syndrome [MAS]) got its name from a diet regime recommended for treatment of peptic ulcer, where high milk intake was recommended together with absorbable antacid intake. A review of reports on MAS indicated that supplemental intakes of calcium needed to be 15 to 16.5 g/d for 2 d to 30 years, and the syndrome was rarely detected in a healthy population.[40]

Mineral interactions are common, and calcium, for example, interacts with iron, zinc, magnesium, and phosphorous. The interactions are usually on the absorption level, where calcium affects the absorption of other minerals. Although calcium has a strong inhibitory effect on iron absorption, data on iron deficiency due to high intake of calcium is not available. Similar conclusions can be reached with regards to interactions between calcium and zinc, magnesium, and phosphorous because deficiency in any of these minerals in the presence of high calcium intake has not been proven.[91]

The upper limit for calcium intake in adults has been set at 2500 mg/d.[40] The human body has been well designed to adapt to high intakes of calcium, and intoxication is unusual. The hunter–gatherer ancestors are estimated to have had a calcium intake of 2 to 4 g/d, well above what is generally consumed now. The body is therefore programmed for the high intakes that it would have had in primitive conditions. Several mechanisms in the body offset high calcium intakes such as poor absorption, dermal losses, and weak renal conservation.[77] Persons at risk of kidney, liver, or parathyroid disorders should however consult with a physician.

13.9.1 Safety and Recommended Intake of Lipids

Recommendations from the World Health Organisation[92] for dietary fat intake for healthy adults are depicted in Table 13.2. Excessive intake of polyunsaturated fats may lead to increased formation of lipid peroxides and place an unnecessary burden on the body's antioxidant defense systems.[93]

13.9.2 Recommended Intakes of Specific Fatty Acids

Recommendations for n-3 EFA intake have been developed by several different countries, as well as multinational groups such as WHO, in

TABLE 13.2

Recommended Daily Intake for Total Fat, Saturated Fat, and Poly- and Monounsaturated Fats

	Minimum	Maximum
Total fat	15% of energy 20% of energy (women of reproductive age)	30% of energy (sedentary individuals) 35% of energy (active individuals)
Saturated fat		< 10% of energy
Polyunsaturated fat	6% of energy	10% of energy
n-6 EFAs	5% of energy	8% of energy
n-3 EFAs	1% of energy	2% of energy
Monounsaturated fat		By difference, i.e., Total fat – saturated fat – polyunsaturated fat = monounsaturated fat.

response to the decreased level of consumption of these EFAs in the typical Western diet. Typically, 0.3 to 0.5 g/d in total of EPA and DHA and 0.8 to 1.1 g/d of ALA is advised for healthy individuals. The U.S. Food and Nutrition Board, Institute of Medicine, National Academies, and Health Canada have jointly put forward an Acceptable Macronutrient Distribution Range (AMDR) for ALA of 0.6 to 1.2% of energy (1.3 to 2.7 g/d based on a 2000 calorie diet) (Table 13.2). The lower limit of these recommendations is based on intake required to prevent EFA deficiency whereas the upper intake represents the highest intake of ALA by individuals in the United States and Canada.[94] These recommendations therefore simply represent a safe range of intake and may not be optimal for health or disease prevention. In terms of actual food intake, consuming a variety of (preferably oily) fish at least twice a week would ensure the recommended intakes of n-3 EFAs are achieved. This is in keeping with the American Heart Association recommendation for reducing the risk of heart disease in a healthy population.[94]

13.9.3 Safety of n-3 EFAs

The U.S. Food and Drug Administration (FDA) has ruled that intakes of up to 3 g/d of marine n-3 oils are generally recognized as safe. The most commonly reported side effects arising from high intakes of n-3 EFAs are gastrointestinal disturbances and nausea.[94] The likelihood of other potential side effects of n-3 EFA consumption are outlined in Table 13.3.

13.9.4 Ratio of n-6:n-3 EFAs

The ratio of n-6 to n-3 EFAs in the diet of early humans has been estimated as being 1:1. WHO recommend the dietary ratio of LA to ALA should be

TABLE 13.3

Risk for Side Effects from Ingestion of ω-3 Fatty Acids

	Gastrointestinal upset	Clinical bleeding	Worsening glycemia[a]	Rise in LDL-C[b]
Up to 1g/d	Very low	Very low	Very low	Very low
1 to 3 g/d	Moderate	Very low	Low	Moderate
>3g/d	Moderate	Low	Moderate	Likely

[a] Usually only in patients with impaired glucose tolerance and diabetes.
[b] Usually only in patients with hypertriglyceridemia.

Source: Reproduced with permission from AHA Scientific Statement (Kris-Etherton, P.M., Harris, W.S. and Appel, L.J., *Circulation* 106, 2747, 2002).

between 5:1 and 10:1. Whether this ratio represents the optimum ratio for bone and vascular health has yet to be determined.

13.10 Sources of Food to Supply Nutrients Required for Maintenance of Bone Health

Specially modified foods generally termed "functional foods" are being developed, all claiming some health benefit. Functional foods are foods that provide health benefits beyond energy and essential nutrients. A food must provide 20% of the daily recommended intake (DRI) to be an excellent source of a nutrient. Alternatively, a good source of a nutrient would need to contain 10% of the DRI or recommended daily allowance (RDA). Examples of functional foods containing calcium are orange juice or chocolate candy fortified with calcium. The 90th percentile of calcium intake (1080 mg for men and women, aged 50 to 70 years), three calcium fortified products per day would be well below the tolerable limits of 2500 mg/d. Therefore, functional foods should be of significant value in assisting elderly people to obtain the recommended calcium and vitamin D intake.[95]

The use of calcium supplements is sometimes also required, but then one has to bear in mind that the various salts all show a similar efficiency for absorption. Vitamin D usually forms part of a calcium supplement. If not, a single supplement of 10 μg per day should result in the required level of 25(OH) D levels in individuals. The best source of calcium is food, specifically dairy foods. Recent research also shows that the benefit of consuming dairy products for bone health is extended beyond the calcium content. Dairy products contain a cluster of nutrients, such as calcium, vitamin D, protein, phosphorous, magnesium, vitamin A, vitamin B_6, and trace elements such as zinc, that are all important for bone health.[96]

13.11 Conclusions

Maintenance and/or building of bone mass must take place in the presence of adequate nutrients, not only carbohydrate, protein, and fat but also in the presence of adequate calcium and vitamin D, and possibly other essential minerals not covered in this chapter. Several published studies support the position that calcium is an important component of a regimen that includes antiresorptive therapy for the prevention and treatment of osteoporosis. It is also possible that women receiving antiresorptive treatments may benefit from an even higher calcium intake than the average women. The intestinal absorption of calcium will be facilitated in the presence of adequate vitamin D. However, research on fatty acids, discussed in this chapter, also suggests that fatty acids may increase absorption and retention of calcium by the body. It is therefore possible that calcium and lipids will act synergistically with drugs for osteoporosis by increasing available calcium to the body, and therefore supporting bone active agents.

Protein comprises 50% of the extracellular material of bone, and optimal protein nutrition is therefore essential for bone maintenance. Some studies have suggested that protein may affect calcium absorption and retention in the body, but the overall conclusion seems to be that in the presence of adequate protein, no adverse effects on absorption or excretion of calcium are observed. It is important to note that protein is essential for bone maintenance, and adequate protein should act in synergy with bone active drugs to build and maintain bone matrix. Nutrition has a lifelong effect on bone, and for optimal bone health, diet is as important as drugs; diet and drugs represent two legs of a three-legged stool,[77] the third is exercise. For optimal response to drugs used in osteoporosis, the support and synergy provided by adequate protein, calcium, vitamin D, and certain lipids are needed.

References

1. Consensus Development Conference, Diagnosis, prophylaxis and treatment of osteoporosis, *Am. J. Med.*, 95, 646, 1993.
2. National Institutes of Health. Osteoporosis Prevention, Diagnosis, and Therapy. NIH Consensus Development Conference Statement 2000. http://odp.od.nih.gov/consensus/cons/111/111_statement.htm
3. Ray N.F. et al., Medical expenditures for the treatment of osteoporotic fractures in the United States in 1995: report from the National Osteoporosis Foundation, *J. Bone Miner. Res.*, 12, 24, 1997.
4. Cashman, K.D., Calcium intake, calcium bioavailability and bone health, *Br. J. Nutr.*, 87, S169, 2002.
5. Prentice, A., Is nutrition important in osteoporosis? *Proc. Nutr. Soc.*, 56, 357, 1997.
6. Weaver, C., The growing years and prevention of osteoporosis in later life, *Proc. Nutr. Soc.*, 59, 303, 2000.

7. Pawlak, R., A comparison of bone mass measurements of vegetarians and omnivores, *Top Clin. Nutr.*, 18(1), 21, 2003.
8. Kerstetter, J.E., O'Brien, K.O., and Insogna, K.L., Dietary protein affects intestinal calcium absorption, *Am. J. Clin. Nutr.*, 68, 859, 1998.
9. Ilich, J.Z., Brownbill, R.A., and Tamborin, L., Bone and nutrition in elderly women: protein, energy, and calcium as main determinants of bone mineral density, *Eur. J. Clin. Nutr.*, 57, 554, 2003.
10. Heaney, R., Constructive interactions among nutrients and bone active pharmacologic agents with principal emphasis on calcium, phosphorous, vitamin D, and protein, *J. Am. Coll. Nutr.*, 20(5), 403S, 2001.
11. Nordin, B.E., Calcium in health and disease, *Food, Nutr. Agric.*, 20, 13, 1997.
12. Johnston, C.C. et al., Calcium supplementation and increases in bone mineral density on children, *New Engl. J. Med.*, 327, 82, 1992.
13. Dawson-Hughes, B., Calcium insufficiency and fracture risk, *Osteoporosis Int.*, 3, S37, 1996.
14. Welten, D et al., A meta-analysis of the effect of calcium and bone mass in young and middle aged females and males, *J. Nutr.*, 125, 2802, 1995.
15. Dawson-Hughes, B. et al., A controlled trial of the effect of calcium supplementation on bone density in postmenopausal women, *New Engl. J. Med.*, 323, 878, 1990.
16. Polley, K.J. et al., Effect of calcium supplementation on forearm bone mineral content in postmenopausal women: a prospective, sequential controlled trial, *J. Nutr.*, 117, 1929, 1987.
17. Elders, P.J.M. et al., Long-term effect of calcium supplementation on bone loss in perimenopausal women, *J. Bone Min. Res., 9, 938, 1994.*
18. Nelson, M.E. et al., A 1-year walking program and increased dietary calcium in postmenopausal women: effects in bone, *Am. J. Clin. Nutr.*, 53, 1304, 1991.
19. Chevalley, T. et al., Effects of calcium supplements on femoral bone mineral density and vertebral fracture rate in vitamin D replete elderly patients, *Osteoporosis Int.*, 4, 245, 1994.
20. Eastell, R., Drug therapy: treatment of postmenopausal osteoporosis, *New Engl. J. Med.*, 338(1), 736, 1998.
21. Heaney, R.P., Nutrient effects: discrepancy between data from controlled trials and observational studies, *Bone*, 21, 469, 1997.
22. Power, M.L. et al., The role of calcium in health and disease, *Am. J. Obstet. Gynecol.*, 181(6), 1560, 1999.
23. Heaney, R.P., Calcium, Dairy products and osteoporosis, *Am. J. Clin. Nutr.*, 19(2), 83S, 2000.
24. Barger-Lux, M.J. et al., Nutritional correlates of low calcium intake, *Clin. Appl Nutr.*, 2, 39, 1992.
25. Hansen, M. et al., Effect of casein phosphopeptides on zinc and calcium absorption from bread meals, *J. Trace Elements Med. Biol.*, 11, 143, 1997.
26. Coudray, C. et al., Effect of soluble or partly soluble dietary fibre supplementation on absorption and balance of calcium, magnesium, iron and zinc in healthy young men, *Eur. J. Clin. Nutr.*, 51, 375, 1997.
27. Abrams, S.A. and Griffin, I.J., Inulin and oligofructose and calcium absorption: Human data. In *Proceedings of the 3rd Orafti Research Conference: Recent Scientific Research on Inulin and Oligofructose*, Orafti Active Food Ingredients, Leatherhead Publishing: Leatherhead, UK, 2001, pp. 26–27.

28. Heaney, R.P., Excess dietary protein may not adversely affect bone, *J. Nutr.*, 128 (6), 1054, 1998.
29. Roughead, Z.K., Is the interaction between dietary protein and calcium destructive for bone? Summary, *J. Nutr.*, 133, 866S, 2003.
30. Hegsted, M. et al., Dietary calcium and calcium balance in young men as affected by level of protein and phosphorous intake, *J. Nutr.*, 111, 553, 1981.
31. Spencer, H. et al., Effect of phosphorous on the absorption of calcium and on the calcium balance in man, *J. Nutr.*, 108, 447, 1978.
32. Kerstetter, J., O'Brien, K.O., and Insogna, K.L., High protein diets, calcium economy and bone health, *Topics Clin. Nutr.*, 19 (1), 75, 2004.
33. Dawson-Hughes, B. and Harris, S.S., Calcium intake influences the association of protein intake with rates of bone loss in elderly men and women, *Am. J. Clin. Nutr.*, 75, 773, 2002.
34. Munger, R.G., Cerhan, J.R, and Chui, B.C., Prospective study of dietary protein intake and risk of hip fracture in postmenopausal women, *Am. J. Clin. Nutr.*, 69, 147, 1999.
35. Promislow, J.H. et al., Protein consumption and bone mineral density in the elderly: The Rancho Bernardo study. *Am. J. Epidemiol.*, 155, 636, 2002.
36. Heaney, R.P. et al., Dietary changes favorably affect bone remodeling in older adults, *J. Am. Diet. Assoc.*, 99, 1228, 1999.
37. Bonjour, J.P. and Rizzoli, R., Inadequate protein intake and osteoporosis: possible involvement of the IGF system, in *Nutritional Aspects of Osteoporosis*, Burckhardt, P. and Heaney, R.P., Eds., Ares-Serono Symposia Publications, Rome, Italy, 1995.
38. Barzel, U.S. and Massey, L.K., Excess dietary protein can adversely affect bone, *J. Nutr.* 128(6), 1051, 1998.
39. Heaney, R.P., Nutritional factors in osteoporosis, *Ann. Rev. Nutr.*, 13, 287, 1993.
40. Food and Nutrition Board, Institute of Medicine, *Dietary Reference Intakes: Calcium, Phosphorous, Magnesium, Vitamin D and Fluoride*, National Academy Press; Washington, DC, 1997, chap. 4.
41. Recker, R.R. et al., Bone gain in young adult women, *JAMA*, 268, 2403, 1992.
42. Heaney, R.P., Dietary protein and phosphorous do not affect calcium absorption, *Am. J. Clin. Nutr.*, 72, 758, 2000.
43. Kerstetter, J.E., O'Brien, K.O. and Insogna K.L., Dietary protein affects intestinal calcium absorption, *Am. J. Clin. Nutr.*, 68, 859, 1998.
44. Kerstetter, J.E. et al., Increased circulating concentrations of parathyroid hormone in healthy, young women consuming a protein-restricted diet, *Am. J. Clin. Nutr.*, 66, 1188, 1997.
45. Draper, H.H., Piche, L.A., and Gibson, R.S., Effects of a high protein intake from common foods on calcium metabolism in a cohort of postmenopausal women, *Nutr. Res., 11, 273, 1991.*
46. Lutz, J., Calcium balance and acid-base status of women as affected by increased protein intake and by sodium bicarbonate ingestion, *Am. J. Clin. Nutr.*, 39, 281, 1984.
47. Pannemans, D.L.E., Schaafsma, G., and Westertrep K.R., Calcium excretion, apparent calcium absorption and calcium balance in young women and elderly subjects: influence of protein intake, *Br. J. Nutr.*, 77, 721, 1997.
48. Kerstetter, J.E. et al., A threshold for low-protein-induced elevations in parathyroid hormone, *Am. J. Clin. Nutr.*, 72, 168, 2000.

49. Kerstetter, J.E., O'Brien, K.O., and Insogna, K.L., Low protein intake: the impact on calcium and bone homeostasis in humans, *J. Nutr.*, 133, 855S, 2003.
50. Kerstetter, J.E., O'Brien, K.O. and Insogna, K.L., Dietary protein, calcium metabolism and skeletal homeostasis revisited, *Am. J. Clin. Nutr.*, 78 (suppl), 584S, 2003.
51. Teegarden, D. et al., Dietary calcium, protein, and phosphorous are related to bone mineral density and content in young women, *Am. J. Clin. Nutr.*, 68, 749, 1998.
52. Corwin, R.L. Effects of dietary fats on bone health in advanced age, *Prostaglandins, Leukot. Essent. Fatty Acids*, 68, 379, 2003.
53. Nano, J.L et al., Effects of fatty acids on the growth of Caco-2 cells, *Prostaglandins, Leukot. Essent. Fatty Acids* 69, 207, 2003.
54. Fernandes, G., Lawrence, R., and Sun, D., Protective role of n-3 lipids and soy protein in osteoporosis, *Prostaglandins, Leukot. Essent. Fatty Acids*, 68, 361, 2003.
55. Albertazzi, P. and Coupland, K., Polyunsaturated fatty acids. Is there a role in postmenopausal osteoporosis prevention? *Maturitas*, 42, 13, 2002.
56. Maxton, D.G. et al., Effect of dietary fat on the small intestinal mucosa, *Gut* 30, 1252, 1989.
57. Hart, M.H. et al., Essential fatty acid deficiency and postsection mucosal adaptation in the rat, *Gastroenterology*, 94, 682, 1988.
58. Jenkins, A.P. et al. Effects of bolus doses of fat on small intestinal structure and release of gastrin, cholecystokinin, peptide tyrosine-tyrosine, and enteroglucagon, *Gut*, 33, 218, 1992.
59. Rosol, T.J., Mammalian calcium metabolism, in *Calcium Metabolism: Comparative Endocrinology*, Danks, J., Dacke, C., Flik, G., and Gay, C., Eds., BioScientifica Ltd, Bristol, England, 1999, pp. 119–130.
60. Kruger, M.C. and Horrobin, D.F., Calcium metabolism, osteoporosis and essential fatty acids: A review. *Prog. Lipid Res.*, 36, 131, 1997.
61. Haag, M. and Kruger, M.C., Upregulation of duodenal calcium absorption by polyunsaturated fatty acids: events at the basolateral membrane, *Med. Hypotheses*, 56, 637, 2001.
62. Leonard, F., Haag, M., and Kruger, M.C., Modulation of intestinal vitamin D receptor availability and calcium ATPase activity by essential fatty acids, *Prostaglandins Leukot. Essent. Fatty Acids*, 64, 147, 2001.
63. Chanda, S. et al., Effects of a high intake of unsaturated and saturated oils on intestinal transference of calcium and calcium mobilization from bone in an ovariectomised rat model of osteoporosis, *Asia Pac. J. Clin. Nutr.*, 8, 115, 1999.
64. Jewell, C. and Cashman, K.D., The effect of conjugated linoleic acid and medium-chain fatty acids on transepithelial calcium transport in human intestinal-like Caco-2 cells, *Br. J. Nutr.*, 89, 639, 2003.
65. Lindmark, T., Kimura, Y., and Artursson, P., Absorption enhancement through intracellular regulation of tight junction permeability by medium chain fatty acids in Caco-2 cells, *J. Pharmacol. Exp. Ther.*, 284, 362, 1998.
66. Haag, M. et al., Omega-3 fatty acids modulate ATPases involved in duodenal Ca absorption, *Prostaglandins, Leukot. Essent. Fatty Acids*, 68, 423, 2003.
67. Haag, M. et al., Effect of arachidonic acid on duodenal enterocyte ATPases, *Prostaglandins*, 66, 53, 2001.
68. Das, U.N., Estrogen, statins and polyunsaturated fatty acids: Similarities in their actions and benefits — is there a common link? *Nutrition*, 18, 178, 2002.

69. Requirand, P. et al., Serum fatty acid imbalance in bone loss: example with periodontal disease, *Clin. Nutr.*, 19, 271, 2000.
70. Horrobin, D.F. et al., Eicosapentaenoic acid and arachidonic acid: collaboration and not antagonism is the key to biological understanding, *Prostaglandins, Leukot. Essent. Fatty Acids*, 66, 83, 2002.
71. van Papendorp, D.H., Coetzer, H., and Kruger, M.C., Biochemical profile of osteoporotic patients on essential fatty acid supplementation, *Nutr. Res.*, 15, 325, 1995.
72. Kruger, M.C. et al., Calcium, gamma-linolenic acid and eicosapentaenoic acid supplementation in senile osteoporosis, *Aging Clin. Exp. Res.*, 10, 385, 1998.
73. Bassey, E.J. et al., Lack of effect of supplementation with essential fatty acids on bone mineral density in healthy pre- and post-menopausal women: two randomized controlled trials of Efacal® v. calcium alone, *Br. J. Nutr.* 83, 629, 2000.
74. Riggs, B.L., Endocrine causes of age-related bone loss and osteoporosis, in *Endocrine Facets of Ageing*. Novartis Foundation Symposium 242, John Wiley & Sons Ltd., West Sussex, England, 2002.
75. Peluffo, R.O. et al., Effect of different amino acid diets on 5, 6 and 9 desaturases, *Lipids*, 19, 154, 1984.
76. Monograph, Gamma-Linolenic acid, *Alt. Med. Rev.*, 9, 70, 2004.
77. Dowd, R., Role of calcium, vitamin D, and other essential nutrients in the prevention and treatment of osteoporosis, *Nursing Clin. N. Am.*, 36(3), 417, 2001.
78. Atkinson, S. and Ward, W.E., Clinical nutrition: 2. The role of nutrition in the prevention and treatment of adult osteoporosis, *Can. Med. Assoc. J.*, 165(11), 1511, 2001.
79. Heaney, R.P. and Weaver, C.M., Calcium and vitamin D, *Endocrinol. Metab. Clin. N. Am.*, 32, 181, 2003.
80. Dawson-Hughes, B., Osteoporosis treatment and the calcium requirement, *Am. J. Clin. Nutr.*, 67, 5, 1998.
81. Heaney R.P., Yates, A.J., and Santora, A.C., II, Bisphosphonate effects and the bone remodeling transient, *J. Bone. Min. Res.*, 12, 1143, 1997.
82. Arnaud, C.D. et al., Two years of parathyroid hormone 1-34 and estrogen produce dramatic bone density increases in postmenopausal osteoporotic women that dissipate only slightly during a third year of treatment with estrogen alone: results from a placebo-controlled randomized trial [abstract], *Bone*, 28, S77, 2001.
83. Neer, R.M. et al., Effect of parathyroid hormone (1034) on fractures and bone mineral density in postmenopausal women with osteoporosis, *N. Engl. J. Med.*, 344(19), 1434, 2001.
84. Slovik, D.M. et al., Restoration of spinal bone in osteoporotic men by treatment with human parathyroid hormone (1034) and 1,25 dihydroxyvitamin D, *J. Bone Min. Res.*, 1, 377, 1986.
85. Heaney, R.P., Constructive interactions among nutrients and bone-active pharmacologic agents with principal emphasis on calcium, phosphorous, vitamin D and protein, *J. Am. Coll. Nutr.*, 20(5), 403S, 2001.
86. Heaney R.P., Nutrients, interactions and foods. The importance of source, in *Nutritional Aspects of Osteoporosis*, 2nd ed., Burckhardt, P., Dawson-Hughes, B., and Heaney, R.P., Eds: Elsevier, San Diego, CA, 2004, pp. 57.

87. Schlemmer, C.K., et al. Oestrogen and essential fatty acid supplementation corrects bone loss due to ovariectomy in the female Sprague Dawley rat, *Prostaglandins, Leukot. Essent. Fatty Acid,s* 61, 381, 1999.
88. Das, U.N., Essential fatty acids as possible mediators of the actions of statins, *Prostaglandins, Leukot. Essent. Fatty Acids,* 65(1) 37, 2001.
89. Curhan, G.C., et al., Dietary factors and the risk of incident kidney stones in younger women, *Arch. Intern. Med.,* 164(8), 885, 2004.
90. Curhan, G.C. et al., Comparison of dietary calcium with supplemental calcium and other nutrients as factors affecting the risk for kidney stones in women, *Ann. Int. Med.,* 126, 497, 1997.
91. Hallberg, L. et al., Calcium and iron absorption: mechanism of action and nutritional importance, *Eur. J. Clin. Nutr.,* 46, 317, 1992.
92. WHO Technical Report Series No. 916 (TRS 916). Diet, Nutrition and the Prevention of Chronic Diseases, Report of the joint WHO/FAO expert consultation, WHO, Geneva, 2003.
93. Eritsland, J., Safety considerations of polyunsaturated fatty acids, *Am. J. Clin. Nutr.,* 71, 197, 2000.
94. Kris-Etherton, P.M., Harris, W.S., and Appel, L.J., AHA Scientific Statement: Fish consumption, fish oil, omega-3 fatty acids and cardiovascular disease, *Circulation,* 106, 2747, 2002.
95. McCabe, B.J., Food and nutrition update, in *Handbook of Food-Drug Interactions,* McCabe, B.J., Frankel, E.H., and Wolfe, J.J., Eds., CRC Press, Boca Raton, FL, 2003, pp. 53.
96. Hoolihan, L., Beyond calcium, *Nutr. Today,* 39(2), 69, 2004.

Section V

Inflammatory Disease, Hypertension, and Obesity

14

Molecular Targets for Antiinflammation and Dietary Component–Drug Synergy

Akira Murakami and Hajime Ohigashi

CONTENTS

14.1 Introduction

Inflammation is a pathophysiological phenomenon that is involved in numerous diseases. Each human organ has the potential for diseases that possess an inflammatory condition essential to their etiology. A considerable proportion of chronic inflammatory diseases display an overlap with the onset and development of cancer, such as ulcerative colitis and Crohn's disease (colorectal cancer), reflux esophagitis, Barrett's esophagus (esophageal carcinoma), and hepatitis (hepatocellular carcinoma).[1] Further, we know that inflammation plays a pivotal role in insulin resistance, obesity, and diabetes,[2] as well as in brain and myocardial infarctions that originate from vascular atherosclerosis.[3] Thus, regulation of inflammatory conditions with food and drugs that are designed from a mechanistic viewpoint should provide great benefit for health promotion and disease prevention.

An understanding of the cellular and molecular mechanisms involved with the occurrence of inflammation is needed for the development of a synthetic drug through discovery of a food phytochemical with antiinflammatory properties. In this chapter, molecular mechanisms underlying the induction and activation of several proinflammatory enzymes as well as their relevance to inflammatory disease onset are described. Subsequently, the antiinflammatory potentials of some synthetic and dietary components, both alone and in combination, are highlighted.

First, we would like to describe the biochemical aspects of inflammatory cell functions. In the process of nonpathologic inflammation, e.g., wound healing, platelets are known to release several mediators that tightly regulate vascular permeability and recruit fibrinogen, leading to the formation of fibrin clots. These activities also induce and produce chemotactic factors, including platelet-derived growth factor, transforming growth factor-β, and interleukin (IL)-1β, which lead to the activation of stromal cells, which are responsible for the release of a cocktail of proteases, such as the matrix metalloproteinases (MMPs) superfamily that can virtually degrade the extracellular matrix. Concurrently, neutrophils and monocytes are maturated and recruited, then infiltrate the inflamed tissue as part of the innate immune machinery, and are well known as biological sources of reactive oxygen and nitrogen species (RONS), prostaglandins (PGs), inflammatory cytokines, and chemokines, as well as others. As indicated in the following sections, RONS, including free radicals, are chemically unstable molecules that are able to modify, denature, and decompose biological components such as lipid membranes, proteins, and DNA. Further, PGE_2 has been shown to induce angiogenesis and plays some notable roles in the growth of fibroblasts, and endothelial and epithelial cells. On the other hand, cytokines and chemokines are systematically activated and released into neighboring tissues in a coordinated manner, after which they circulate in the bloodstream for further activation of the immune system. All of these biological phenomena progress in a concerted fashion toward reepithelialization and resolution of healing.

In pathogenic conditions, most of those processes are shared, though they are sustained and exaggerated in a dysregulated manner. Further, genetic alterations are frequently associated with cases of chronic and pathogenic inflammation. For example, Kubaszek et al. reported an intriguing finding that they discovered the promoter polymorphism of the tumor necrosis factor (TNF)-α (*G-308A*) gene that confers increased TNF-α production, even

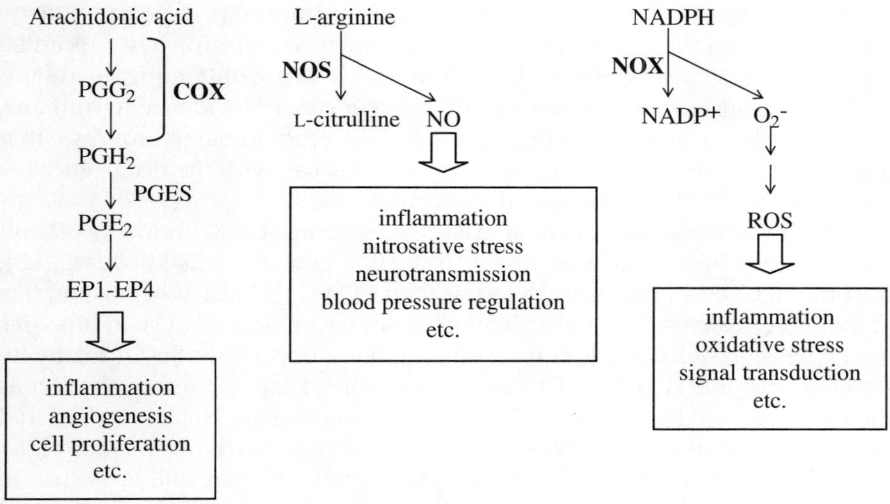

FIGURE 14.1
Enzymatic functions of COX, NOS, and NOX, and their relevance to homeostasis and pathogenesis.

though high concentrations of inflammatory cytokines are risk factors for type-2 diabetes.[4] In addition, Hwang et al. showed evidence indicating that polymorphisms of IL-1β significantly affect its levels in serum.[5] Epigenetic factors are also attributable to the onset of pathologic inflammation. In this context, it is well documented that infection with microorganisms is closely related to inflammation-derived carcinogenesis.[1,6]

14.2 Proinflammatory Enzymes

In order to better understand the rationale for combining synthetic and natural agents, three proinflammatory enzymes important for the progression of inflammation are discussed in this section, as well as their relevance to pathophysiological conditions. See Figure 14.1 for an illustration of the enzymatic functions of the proinflammatory enzymes and their relevance to homeostasis and pathogenesis.

14.2.1 Cyclooxygenase

Cyclooxygenase (PGH_2 synthase = COX) donates two oxygen molecules to arachidonic acid to form PGG_2 by peroxidation, which in turn is reduced to PGH_2. This is the initial step for production of a variety of prostanoids. COX is a well known enzyme and is the molecular target for analgesic and antiinflammatory remedies that have been used for hundreds of years. Nonsteroidal antiinflammatory drugs (NSAIDs), such as aspirin, have received enormous considerable attention for their ability to not only mitigate inflammatory responses, but also potentially prevent cancer incidence in humans, based on the results of several independent epidemiologic surveys that demonstrated a negative association of NSAIDs use with the occurrences of colon,[7] stomach,[8] and esophageal[9] cancers.

The COX enzyme consists of at least two isoforms, COX-1 and COX-2 and the latter has been cloned as a v-*src*-inducible gene.[10] At 22 kilobases (kb), the human *COX-1* gene is much larger than *COX-2* (8.3 kb), whereas the size of the COX proteins are nearly identical at approximately 70 kDa. In humans, the expression of COX-1 is constitutive in many normal tissues at relatively stable levels and is believed to play some housekeeping functions such as the production of PG precursors for thromboxane in platelets,[11] which is vital for the regulation of blood flow. This is a reasonable mechanism since platelets, which have no nuclei, are unable to synthesize inducible enzymes. In the kidney, COX-1 has an essential role of generating vasodilating PGs that maintain renal plasma flow at a normal level and also determine glomerular filtration rate during systemic vasoconstriction conditions. In contrast to COX-1, the COX-2 protein is only slightly expressed in most normal mammalian tissues in response to physical, chemical, and biological stimuli, including UV light exposure, dioxin, and lipopolysaccharide insult. Recently, COX-2 has received the attention of numerous researchers for the relevance of its expression to pathogenesis. In particular, there is ample evidence of the involvement of COX-2 expression in carcinogenesis in many different target organs.

To better understand differences in the characteristics of COX-1 and COX-2, it is important to determine their cellular localization. Morita et al.[12] described COX-1 and COX-2 localization to be in the cytoplasmic and perinuclear compartments, respectively, which generated an attractive hypothesis that PGs derived from these COX proteins confer biochemical signaling via autocrine or paracrine and intracrine loops, respectively. Conversely, PGs have their receptors in both the cellular membrane[13] and the nucleus.[14] In addition, the COX-1– and COX-2–dependent synthesis of PGD_2 utilize arachidonic acid released from secretory and cytoplasmic phospholipase A_2, respectively.[15,16] Further, Takeda et al. proposed that COX-1 expression in intestinal stromal cells secures a basal level of PGE_2 that is able to support polyp growth (less than 1 mm), and that simultaneous induction of both COX-2 and inducible microsomal PGE synthase (mPGES) promotes polyp expansion (greater than 1 mm) by boosting stromal PGE_2 production.[17] Collectively, recent research evidence does not support the notion that COX-1 plays housekeeping functions and is only important for homeostasis, or that inducible COX-2 alone is a remarkable target for antiinflammation and anticarcinogenesis. Rather, the activities of these individual COX isoforms induce different signaling pathways in a concerted fashion, thereby creating various PG profiles that are related to disease onset.

COX-2 mRNA expression is regulated by at least three distinguishable stages in a complex manner. The earliest induction mechanism is related to the finding that COX-2 mRNA contains the AU-rich element (ARE) in its 3-untranslated region (UTR), which has some critical roles in the stability of its mRNA.[18] Several reports of different cell types have shown that activation of p38 mitogen-activated protein kinase (MAPK) led to stabilization of COX-2 mRNA. Next, a substrate for p38 MAPK, i.e., MAPK-activated protein kinase 2 (MAPKAPK-2), phosphorylates certain candidate proteins such as HSP27,[19] heterogeneous nuclear ribonucleoprotein (hnRNP) A0,[20] and Hu antigen R (HuR),[21] which bind to the AREs, thereby contributing to a rapid synthesis of COX-2 protein. In addition, Sully et al. identified several proteins, including AUF-1 [AU-rich element/poly(U)-binding/degradation factor-1], AUF-2, tristetraprolin, HuR, and FBP1 (far-upstream-sequence-element-binding protein 1), that target the conserved region 1 (CR 1) that is located at 3-UTR.[22] However, they concluded that CR-1-mediated COX-2 mRNA decay has no correlation with the binding of those proteins and that another unidentified process may play a critical role in the instability of COX-2 mRNA.

The next stage for COX-2 expression takes place at two different transcriptional levels. In macrophages, lipopolysaccharide (LPS)-triggered induction and activation of signal transduction pathways lead to transcriptional activation of the COX-2 gene. The toll-like receptor (TLR) family, particularly TLR4, is now recognized as the central receptor for LPS.[23] TLR4 has several associated proteins, such as MD2 and Myd88, needed for full activation, after which it stimulates some protein kinases, including phosphatidylinositol 3-kinase (PI3K) and phosphoinositide-dependent kinase (PDK). The phosphorylated protein kinase B (Akt), in turn, activates IkappaB (IκB) kinase (IKK), which is composed of the α, β, and γ subunits, and phosphorylates IκB protein,[24] leading to degradation of this protein. Since IκB is a suppressive protein that binds to the NFκB transcription factor in a normal state, LPS-induced IκB degradation results in the activation of this particular transcription factor for COX-2 mRNA induction. It is essential to understand that NFκB-targeted genes include the IκB gene, and this negative feedback mechanism causes the NFκB-induced COX-2 expression to be intermediate and transient.

For full induction of COX-2, several NFκB-targeted genes play a major role, which is recognized as the third stage. Two of these genes are CCAAT enhancer-binding protein beta (C/EBPβ) and delta (C/EBPδ), which form β/β homodimer and β/δ heterodimer, both of which play crucial roles in late and continuous COX-2 expression, though their suppressive factors have not been identified.[25] In parallel, LPS insult of macrophages also leads to activation of the protein kinase A (PKA) pathway, in which PKA targets cAMP-responsive element-binding protein (CREB), another major transcription factor for the COX-2 gene.[26] It is also interesting to note that COX-2-generated PGE_2 binds to its receptors (EP1–EP4)[13] for the activation of adenylyl cyclase and thereby increases the level of intracellular cAMP. As mentioned above, this leads to the activation of PKA and, thus, CREB transcriptional activity. Collectively, these form a positive feedback loop in PKA-mediated COX-2 expression.

14.2.2 Nitric Oxide Synthase

Nitric oxide synthase (NOS) is an enzyme that catalyzes the conversion of L-arginine into L-citrulline with stoichiometric formation of a gaseous radical, nitric oxide (NO). NOS is classified into subfamilies, according to the location of expression in the body and manner of expression, namely, constitutive or inducible. Constitutive NOS is detected in neuronal tissues (nNOS) and vascular endothelial cells (eNOS), whereas inducible NOS (iNOS) is expressed in many cell types under both normal and pathological conditions, including macrophages, microglial cells, keratinocytes, hepatocytes, astrocytes, and vascular endothelial and epithelial cells. With infectious and proinflammatory stimuli, iNOS protein is highly induced to produce a micromolar range of NO, whereas NO generation from nNOS and eNOS enzymes is constant and within the nanomolar range.

Various NOS forms have essential roles in the maintenance of homeostasis, e.g., regulating blood vessel tone (eNOS), and serving as a neurotransmitter and neuromodulator (nNOS) in nonadrenergic and noncholinergic nerve endings. On the other hand, numerous reports have shown that sustained and/or excess NO generation, most of which is attributable to iNOS expression, is often implicated in pathogenic conditions. In particular, iNOS has drawn considerable attention for its critical functions in inflammation-related disease. For example, exaggerated iNOS expression has been reported in synovial fluid granulocytes from patients with chronic arthritis,[27] primary airway epithelial cells with patients with asthma,[28] and premalignant and malignant colonic epithelial cells,[29] and in tissues associated with inflammatory bowel disease such as ulcerative colitis and Crohn's disease.[30] However, the processes by which NO generation leads to disease onset remain to be fully elucidated. Nonetheless, it is essential to point out that NO is coupled with superoxide anion radical (O_2^-) to form peroxynitrite ($ONOO^-$) in a diffusion-dependent manner that is extremely reactive, as compared with NO or O_2^- alone, because NO has been shown to have the chemical potential to cause DNA damage by nitration, nitrosation, and oxidation.[31]

Many aspects of the signal transduction pathways involved with iNOS induction are overlapped with those for COX-2 induction in macrophages. Lee et al. presented an interesting finding that both NFκB and activator protein (AP)-1 binding sites located on the iNOS promoter are necessary for iNOS induction, whereas the COX-2 gene promoter is composed of NFκB, C/EBP, and CREB binding sites.[32] Activation of the PKA pathway is partly involved in iNOS induction because dibutyryl cyclic adenosine monophosphate, a cell-permeable precursor of cAMP, was found to induce iNOS and

IL-6 expression via the activation of PKA, protein kinase C (PKC), and p38 MAPK,[33] which was later supported by other study results.[34,35] Blanchette et al. reported that Janus kinase 2, MAP kinase kinase (MEK1/2), ERK1/2, and signal transducer and activator of transcription (STAT) 1a, but not NFκB, are key players in the iNOS-induction pathway.[34] Elucidation of the MAPK pathways that contribute to iNOS induction is probably dependent on the stimuli and cell types used. On the other hand, SP600125, a JNK inhibitor, reduced iNOS mRNA half-life from 5 to 2 h,[36] implying that iNOS induction, similar to that of COX-2, is regulated at not only the transcriptional, but also the posttranscriptional level, and that activation of the JNK pathway plays a significant role in destabilization of this mRNA.

14.2.3 NADPH Oxidase

With proinflammatory stimuli, activated leukocytes generate not only NO from iNOS, but also O_2^- from NADPH oxidase (NOX). These processes serve as innate immune systems by exposing the invading microorganisms to the resultant RONS. A representative biological phenomenon regarding RONS generation through NOX is the respiratory burst of neutrophils and macrophages.

NOX comprises a catalytic subunit, gp91phox, and regulatory proteins, including small GTPase RAC1/2, p22phox, p47phox, p40phox, and p67phox.[37] RAC is associated in a constitutive manner with the cellular membrane, as are gp91phox and p22phox, which are collectively termed flavocytochrome b_{558}, whereas others are located in the cytoplasm in a resting state. Among those partner proteins, phosphorylation of p47phox has been recognized as a critical step for the stimuli-induced activation and assembly of this oxidase, and several kinases, including PKC isoforms (βII, δ, ζ), but not α and βI,[38] though another research group has proposed the involvement of PKCα and βII.[39] In addition, the activation of ERK1/2 and p38 MAPK, but not JNK1/2,[40] as well as PI3K/Akt have been shown to be involved in NOX activation.

Recent reports have provided evidence that a homolog of this oxidase, mitogen oxidase (MOX)-1, which is expressed in guinea pig gastric pit cells, also plays central roles in the regulation of spontaneous apoptosis as well as cell proliferation, by generating measurable amounts of reactive oxygen species (ROS).[41] Further, MOX-1 (currently termed NOX-1) has recently been demonstrated to mediate activated and mutated RAS-induced cell proliferation, transformation, and tumorigenesis by producing ROS endogenously.[42] In addition, up-regulation of NOX-1 is associated with the induction of vascular endothelial growth factor (VEGF) and its receptors, thereby directing the cancerous tissue to an angiogenic environment.[43] It is also important to note that ROS derived from angiotensin II-mediated stimulation of NOX-like systems in endothelial cells participate in biological and biochemical events related to cardiovascular diseases.[44]

In some pathological conditions, NOX and related enzymes are overexpressed. For example, a significant up-regulation of gp91 phox in the liver and kidney, but not xanthine oxidase, has been noted in a rat model for chronic renal failure.[45] In addition, experiments with gp91phox-knockout mice have shown that they were less susceptible to renal artery clipping–induced hypertension, which also indicated that the formation of O_2^- by NOX containing endothelial gp91phox accounts for the reduced NO bioavailability, and this may lead to the development of renovascular hypertension and endothelial dysfunction.[46,47] However, it is also important to note that a deficiency in the genes coding the NOX units severely affects the innate immune functions of phagocytes, and thus becomes part of the etiology for chronic granulomatous disease (CGD).[48]

14.3 Antiinflammatory Drugs and Dietary Factors

Inhibition of the catalytic activities of the previously mentioned proinflammatory mediators is anticipated to exert antiinflammatory effects, and a large number of agents have been designed and chemically synthesized for this purpose. On the other hand, certain food components have also shown suppressive and repressive activities toward those enzymes at the transcriptional, posttranscriptional, and posttranslational levels. Next, we focus on some synthetic drugs and food components that target COX-2, iNOS, and NOX. See Figure 14.2 and Figure 14.3 for the structures of synthetic and natural inhibitors, respectively.

14.3.1 Synthetic COX Inhibitors

More than 30 years ago, Vane was the first to demonstrate that the molecular target of aspirinlike drugs is COX.[49] Since then, a great body of evidence for the efficacy of NSAIDs for mitigating inflammatory responses has accumulated, and the results are supported because these drugs are administered widely throughout the world. However, nonspecific COX inhibitors such as aspirin have potential side-effects, including bleeding in the digestive organs because the blockaded activities of COX-1 enzymes, which, as mentioned above, have an important role in the protection of gastrointestinal mucosa. Since the discovery of COX isozymes, strategies for antiinflammatory drug development have been directed toward COX-2–selective inhibition, rather than COX-1 and COX-2 dual inhibition. One representative success in this field is work by Oshima et al., who showed that treatment of *Apc* knockout mice, a model for familial adenomatous polyposis, with a novel COX-2 inhibitor (MF tricyclic) reduced the number of polyps more significantly than sulindac, which inhibits both isozymes.[50] Thereafter, a number of research

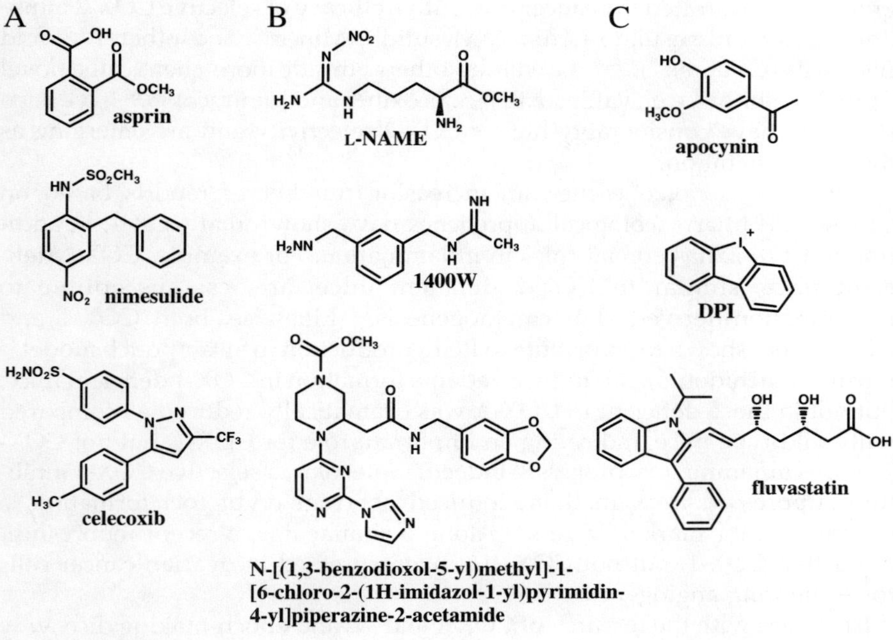

FIGURE 14.2
Structures of inhibitors of **(A)** COX, **(B)** NOS, and **(C)** NOX.

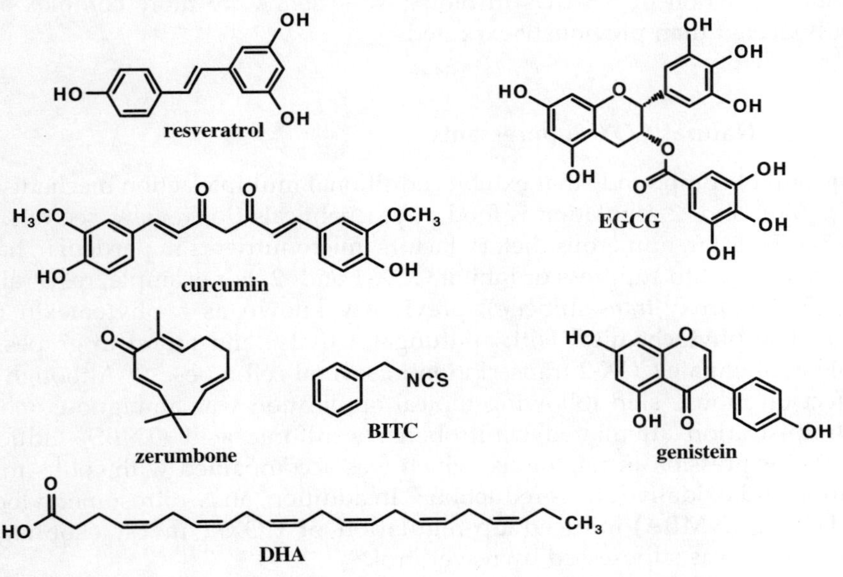

FIGURE 14.3
Structures of natural suppressants of COX, NOS, and NOX.

groups demonstrated the cancer preventive efficacy of selective COX-2 inhibitors such as nimesulide (Aulin™, Mesulid™, Mined™, and others)[51–54] and celecoxib (Celebrex™),[55–59] as well as others. In addition, chemically novel COX-2 inhibitors, e.g., valdecoxib,[60] refecoxib,[61] and lumiracoxib,[62] have been shown to have considerably higher COX-2 selectivity and are emerging as the next generation.

However, as noted earlier, an increasing number of reports based on genetic and pharmacological approaches have shown that COX-1, in addition to COX-2, has crucial roles in inflammation. For example, COX-1 deficient mice, similar to COX-2 deficient mice, are less susceptible to inflammation-derived skin carcinogenesis.[63] Likewise, both COX-1 and COX-2 were shown to contribute to PGE_2 production in an air pouch model.[64] Further, arachidonic acid–induced edema formation in COX-1 deficient mice, but not in those deficient in COX-2, was dramatically reduced as compared with wild-type mice, indicating an important role for COX-1, but not COX-2, in this inflammatory process.[65] Indeed, mofezolac, a selective COX-1 inhibitor, suppressed azoxymethane-induced aberrant crypt foci formation, a putative tumor marker, in rats.[66] Along a similar line, a recent report indicated that COX-1, but not COX-2, is overexpressed in ovarian cancer cells for promoting angiogenesis.[67]

In concert with the research of COX-1 and –2, and epoch-making discovery was that NSAIDs, including celecoxib, exert effects on cell cycle arrest and apoptosis through pathways independent of COX expression status,[68] which are mediated, at least in part, by targeting PDK1 and Akt.[69–71] Thus, the modes of action of NSAIDs in biological systems are more complex and multifaceted than previously expected.

14.3.2 Natural COX Suppressants

A group of compounds that exhibits additional multiple action mechanisms of COX-1 and -2 regulation is food phytochemicals (for review, see refs. 72 to 74). Thus far, numerous dietary factors, micronutrients in particular, have been reported to suppress or inhibit COX-1 and -2. For example, resveratrol (3,4,5-trihydroxy-*trans*-stilbene), previously known as a phytoalexin (an inducible phytochemical with antifungal activity) and found in grapes, is able to attenuate COX-2 transcription in several cell types.[75–77] Although its effect on mouse skin following topical application was ambiguous,[78] oral administration attenuated trinitrobenzenesulfonic acid (TNBS)–induced COX-2 expression in rat colons, which was accompanied with colitis mitigation and oxidative stress reduction.[79] In addition, an *N*-nitrosomethylbenzylamine (NMBA)-induced up-regulation of COX-2 in rat esophagus specimens was suppressed by resveratrol.[80]

Curcumin (diferuloylmethane) is a major yellow pigment in the rhizomes of turmeric (*Curcuma longa* L.) and is a spice used in curry throughout the world. Along with its high potential for cancer prevention,[81] the suppressive efficacy of this compound for COX-2 expression has attracted the attention of a great number of researchers. One of the first research groups to report the marked ability of curcumin to suppress COX-2 expression is Zhang and colleagues, who reported that it decreased chenodeoxycholate– and phorbol ester–mediated induction of COX-2 in several gastrointestinal cell lines.[82] Their findings were later supported by other similar studies using colon cancer cells,[83] leukocytes from healthy volunteers,[84] Kupffer cells,[85] non–small cell lung carcinoma cells,[86] microglial cells,[87] and macrophages.[88] Of note, topical application of curcumin was able to attenuate phorbol ester–induced COX-2 protein expression in mouse skin.[89] In addition, a *Curcuma* extract containing curcumin reduced blood PGE_2 concentration in 15 patients with advanced colorectal cancer, presumably by COX-2 repression.[78] In contrast, curcumin was found to increase COX-2 expression when given without a COX-2-inducer.[88]

Fish oil, which is rich in n-3 fatty acids such as docosahexaenoic acid (DHA), is another reliable and safe food item that is able to regulate COX-2 expression.[90] Plummer et al. demonstrated that feeding rats with high-fat fish oil, but not high-fat corn oil, resulted in a significant decrease in COX-2 expression in both colonic mucosa and tumors.[91] In cellular studies, fish oil and n-3 fatty acids were shown to attenuate COX-2 expression in macrophages[92,93] and smooth muscle cells.[94] On the other hand, a controversial report showed that LPS-induced COX-2 protein levels were increased without a change in COX-2 mRNA levels with n-3 fatty acids pretreatment, suggesting that they may cause a posttranscriptional stabilization of existing COX-2 mRNA.[95] Further, Boudreau et al. reported a surprising finding that a fish oil diet suppressed the growth of colon cancer cells in nude mice through a COX-2-independent pathway,[96] implying that n-3 fatty acids targets other molecules to exhibit anticell proliferating activities.

A green tea polyphenol, (–)-epigallocatechin-3-gallate (EGCG), has emerged as a promising cancer preventive and antiinflammatory agent, based on its antioxidative properties. This polyphenol suppressed 2,2′-azobis (2-amidinopropane) dihydrochloride (AAPH)–induced expression of COX-2 in a human keratinocyte cell line, HaCaT.[97] In addition, Kundu et al. presented interesting data showing that EGCG suppressed phorbol ester–induced COX-2 expression in mouse skin as well as cultured human mammary epithelial cells,[98] while it also attenuated NMBA-induced COX-2 expression and tumor development in rat esophagus tissues.[98] Further, IL-1β–induced COX-2 up-regulation in chondrocytes derived from osteoarthritis cartilage was reduced by EGCG.[99] In contrast, some have found that EGCG increased COX-2 expression via ERK1/2 and tyrosine phosphatase–related pathways in macrophages,[100] and promoted the production of PGE_2 and TNF-α.[101] These contrasting results may be associated with the experimental conditions used, including cell types and the presence or absence of stimuli.

Isothiocyanate-related compounds occur widely in plants in the *Brassica* genus. Sulforaphene, an aliphatic isothiocyanate, was reported to suppress LPS-induced COX-2 expression in macrophages,[102] which appears to be important for a better understanding of the antiinflammatory actions of this compound. We also reported findings in support of those results using benzyl isothiocyanate (BITC), which markedly blocked degradation of IκB and thereby abrogated COX-2 expression.[102] However, it should be kept in mind that a conflicting report showed that oral feeding of 6-phenylhexyl isothiocyanate promoted colon carcinogenesis with increased PGE_2 levels in colonic mucosa, suggesting the enhancement of COX-2 expression by this isothiocyanate.[103,104]

The soybean isoflavonoid genistein is another promising phytochemical for COX-2 suppression, whose ability was highlighted by its characteristic as a tyrosine kinase inhibitor.[105] Thereafter, a number of reports demonstrated COX-2 suppression by genistein in mesangial cells,[106] islet cells,[107] macrophages,[108] pulmonary epithelial,[109] colon cancer,[110] and lung epithelial cells,[110] though its *in vivo* capabilities remain to be demonstrated

Zerumbone, a sesquiterpenoid occurring in the rhizomes of *Zingiber zerumbet* Smith, has been shown to have antiinflammatory[112,113] and anticarcinogenic properties[114–117] in several experimental systems. Further, this compound has demonstrated the ability to attenuate COX-2 expression in macrophages,[109] mouse skin following topical application, and colonic mucosa in rodents, which was accompanied with decreased PGE_2 formation and COX-2 repression with oral feeding.[110]

In contrast to the great number of studies of phytochemicals that suppress or attenuate COX-2 transcription, reports of those that directly inhibit COX enzyme activity are limited. Recently, resveratrol was shown to inhibit COX-1, but not COX-2, catalytic activity via a peroxidase-mediated mechanism, in which it was shown to serve as a substrate for oxidation.[118] Further, EGCG was also reported to inhibit COX-2 activity.[99]

14.3.3 Synthetic NOS Inhibitors

Many iNOS inhibitors are synthetic compounds that are structurally analogous to its substrate, L-arginine, and thus inhibit the functions of nNOS and eNOS. Although some investigators have reported the beneficial effects of nonselective NOS inhibitors,[119,120] an increasing number of articles describe their potential side effects. For instance, rats that received *N*-nitro-L-arginine methyl ester (NAME) showed enhanced mean basal arterial blood pressure levels, decreased heart rate, a greater number of abberrant crypt foxi (ACF), and higher ornithine decarboxylase activity as compared with controls.[121] In addition, it has been well established that blockade of NO generation by nonselective inhibitors often leads to hypertension and reductions in renal function, and intrarenal vascular, tubular, and glomerular.[122]

On the other hand, there is a great body of data showing the additional benefits and lower toxicity of iNOS-selective inhibitors. Chen et al. reported the distinct efficacy of *S,S′*-1,4-phenylene-bis(1,2-ethanediyl)bis-isothiourea (PBIT) for preventing *N*-nitrosomethylbenzylamine (NMBA)-induced tumors in the rat esophagus[123] and Naito et al. demonstrated that a selective iNOS inhibitor, ONO-1714, provided protection from reperfusion-induced intestinal injury by inflammation and oxidative and/or nitrosative stress.[124] Further, GW274150, a novel, potent, and selective inhibitor of iNOS showed antiinflammatory effects in a model of lung injury induced by carrageenan administration[124] and in collagen-induced arthritis.[125] Moreover, a selective iNOS inhibitor, 1400W, but not L-NAME, attenuated *S*-nitroso-acetylpenicillamine (SNAP, an NO donor)–induced proinflammatory cytokine production in colonic mucosa in ulcerative colitis,[126] while 1400W also exhibited 5000- and 200-fold selectivity for eNOS and nNOS, respectively.[127] Those results indicate that selectivity is essential for preventive and therapeutic utility in regards to the homeostatic functions of NO. Recent reports have shown a new class of iNOS inhibitor, whose mechanisms are substantially different from those of substrate analogs.[128] Namely, *N*-[(1,3-benzodioxol-5-yl)methyl]-1-[6-chloro-2-(1*H*-imidazol-1-yl)pyrimidin-4-yl] piperazine-2-acetamide showed a greater than 1000-fold stronger inhibition of iNOS than 1400W, with 1000- and 5-fold greater selectivity as compared with eNOS and nNOS, respectively, and was shown to function by blocking the dimerization of iNOS monomers.[129,130]

14.3.4 Natural NOS Suppressants

Each of the phytochemicals described previously as COX-2 suppressants have been reported to attenuate endotoxin– or phorbol ester–induced iNOS expression in cellular systems and experimental animals. An early work by Tsai et al.[131] showed that resveratrol suppressed LPS-induced iNOS mRNA expression in macrophages, and this was followed by several other investigations,[132] including ours.[94] To the best of our knowledge, the *in vivo* efficacy of resveratrol for iNOS suppression remains to be demonstrated, though it induced the expression of iNOS in mouse hearts when given without stimuli.[133] Chan et al. also reported the *in vivo* efficacy of curcumin, which attenuated LPS-induced iNOS expression in rat livers,[135] while its iNOS-suppressive activity has been shown in mammary glands,[136] macrophages,[137] and melanoma cells.[138] Further, many lines of evidence have established that n-3 fatty acids, including DHA, are a promising group for iNOS suppression, as demonstrated in macrophages[139–141] and colon cancer cells,[142] as well as renal arteries in mice as well. Lin et al. published a pioneering work that showed that certain food phytochemicals have a pronounced ability to suppress iNOS expression, one of which is EGCG.[144] Thereafter, a number of reports supported their findings,[145–147] including *in vivo* and *ex vivo* efficacy results.[148,149] In addition, a recent report noted an intriguing property of EGCG, induction of endothelium-dependent vasodilation, which may be primarily based on rapid activation of eNOS by a phosphatidylinositol 3-kinase–, PKA–, and an Akt–dependent increase in eNOS activity.[150] Organosulfur compounds, including allyl and BITC, were also indicated as a notable group for iNOS suppression in macrophages.[151,152] Further, genistein is believed to exert iNOS suppressive profiles via inhibition of tyrosine kinase,[153] while zerumbone has shown potent suppressive activities toward iNOS expression in macrophages.[101,154]

14.3.5 Synthetic NOX Inhibitors

Recently, sanguinarine, a member of the group of benzo[c]phenanthridine isoquinoline alkaloids, has been suggested to be a direct NOX inhibitor.[154] Diphenylene iodonium chloride (DPI), which targets NADPH but not NADH,[156] is used widely as a potent inhibitor of O_2^- generation.[157,158] Interestingly, fluvastatin, a potent 3-hydroxy-3-methylglutaryl coenzyme A (HMG-CoA) reductase inhibitor, attenuated O_2^- generation from rat peritoneal neutrophils, presumably through inhibition of NOX.[159] In parallel, ML-7, (5-iodonaphthalene-1-sulfonyl)homopiperazine, commonly employed as a myosin light chain kinase (MLCK) inhibitor, showed a similar effect.[160] Additionally, 3-(5′-hydroxymethyl-2′-furyl)-1-benzyl indazole (YC-1), a soluble guanylyl cyclase activator, inhibited formyl-methionyl-leucyl-phenylalanine (fMLP)-induced O_2^- generation in rat neutrophils.[101] Further, Ohashi and colleagues reported that the synthetic protease inhibitor gabexate mesilate prevented O_2^- generation through blockade of the translocation of p47phox, p40phox, and p67phox into the cellular membrane with unknown mechanisms.[162] Thereafter, synthetic peptides, mapped within the near carboxyl-terminal domains of Rac1, were found to be functionally active for suppressing NOX activity in macrophages O_2^-.[163]

14.3.6 Natural NOX Suppressants

Apocynin (4-hydroxy-3-methoxyacetophenone), a natural compound found in the roots of *Picrorhiza kurroa*, prevents NOX assembly via its metabolic activation as a myeloperoxidase-dependent reaction.[164] This phytochemical is currently used as an antioxidative and antiinflammatory agent with pronounced physiological activity.[165] Conversely, it also suppresses O_2^- generation with a concomitant increase in NO bioavailability, thereby improving endothelial functions in human internal mammary arteries and saphenous veins.[46] Another report found that resveratrol decreased NADH/NADPH oxidase activity in rat aortic homogenates,[166] and n-3, but not n-6, polyunsaturated fatty acids were demonstrated to suppress O_2^- generation in neutrophils,[167] whereas DHA hydroperoxide induced radical generation.[168] Further, both n-3 and n-6 fatty acids stimulated the translocation of the proteins PKCα, -βI, -βII, and -ε, and thereby enhanced agonist-induced NOX in macrophages,[169] which was partly supported by the findings of another group,[170] indicating that the effects of n-3 and n-6 polyunsaturated fatty acids toward NOX are dependent on experimental conditions, such as the presence or absence of stimuli and the cell lines used. In contrast to the well known scavenging activity of O_2^- (SOD-like activity),[171] information regarding the effects of EGCG on NOX is limited, though our previous results showed that this catechin may have dual SOD-like and NOX suppressive activities.[154] Miyoshi et al. found that BITC is a potent inhibitor of the activation of NOX in cultured cells and phorbol ester-treated mouse skin,[172] and a number of studies have described the inhibition of NOX activation by genistein through tyrosine kinase inhibition.[172,173] Further, our laboratory has identified food phytochemicals and food items that suppress O_2^- generation via, at least in part, inhibition of NOX activation, some of which also exhibited notable antiinflammatory and antioxidative activities in rodent models.[174–184]

14.4 Combination Effects

While there are a number of reports regarding the antiinflammatory effects of drug–drug, drug–food component, and food component–food component combinations, studies based on the molecular mechanisms of combinations of individual agents are scarce. Following is our classification of published studies on combinatorial antiinflammation into three groups, in which n-3 fatty acids, antioxidants, and antiinflammatory agents are paired. Figure 14.4 provides examples of combinations that inhibit or suppress inflammatory agents.

14.4.1 n-3 Fatty Acids

It is interesting to note that a diet low in arachidonic acid ameliorated clinical signs of inflammation in patients with rheumatoid arthritis and augmented the beneficial effect of fish oil supplementation.[185] Further, those patients improved when given a vegetarian diet or a diet supplemented with fish oil, both of which are rich in n-3 fatty acids. Adam et al. found that 68 patients given an antiinflammatory diet (arachidonic acid intake less than 90 mg/d), but not those given a normal Western diet, demonstrated a remarkable augmentation of the beneficial effects of fish oil supplementation.[186] Tate et al.[187] also documented the rationale for a combination of fish oil (rich in n-3 fatty acids such as EPA) and plant seed oil (rich in γ-linolenic acid [GLA]), and demonstrated that the GLA-enriched diet significantly suppressed the cellular phase of inflammation, though it had little effect on the fluid phase, using a monosodium urate crystals–induced acute inflammation model. In contrast, the EPA-enriched diet suppressed the fluid phase and not the cellular phase of inflammation. Notably, a combined diet of fish oil and plant seed oil reduced both the cellular and fluid phases of inflammation.[187] It is also important to indicate that neutrophils isolated from volunteers fed diets supplemented with γ-linolenic acid and eicosapentaenoic acid synthesized

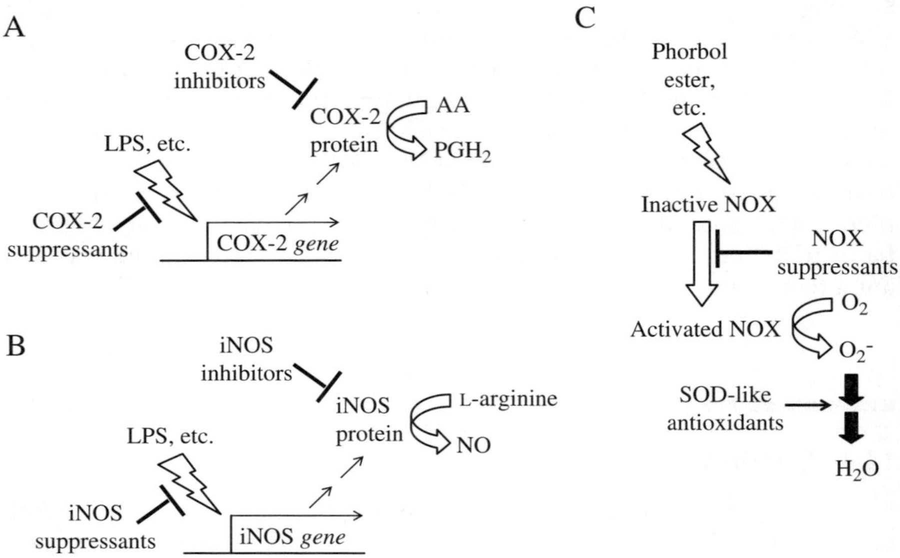

FIGURE 14.4
Examples of the combinations of agents that have shown distinct action mechanisms for the inhibition or suppression of **(A)** COX-2, **(B)** iNOS, and **(C)** NOX.

significantly lower quantities of leukotrienes as compared with neutrophils prior to supplementation, indicating that this combination may be utilized to reduce the synthesis of proinflammatory arachidonate metabolites and, notably, does not induce potentially harmful increases in serum arachidonate levels.[188] In a recent study on the functional interactions between n-3 and n-6 fatty acids, Pischon et al. measured serum sTNF-R1, sTNF-R2, IL-6, and C-reactive protein in 405 healthy men and 454 healthy women, and concluded that n-6 fatty acids do not inhibit the antiinflammatory effects of n-3 fatty acids, while the combination of both types of fatty acids was associated with the lowest levels of inflammation.[189] In addition, it has been proposed that a combination of long-chain polyunsaturated fatty acids and probiotics offers significant protection against atopy[190]; however, supplementation with n-3 fatty acids and α-tocopherol failed to exert antiinflammatory effects in healthy nonsmoking volunteers.[191]

14.4.2 Antioxidants

There are also some examples of antagonistic effects of antioxidant combinations. For example, supplementation with vitamins C and E in a triple antibiotic therapy did not improve the *H. pylori* eradication rate or gastric inflammation, and may even reduce the eradication rate of triple therapy.[192] In contrast, a combined administration of vitamins C and E for 6 months resulted in a successful reduction of the fibrosis scores in patients with nonalcoholic steatohepatitis (NASH).[193] Vitamins A and E, when combined with antibiotics, showed a pronounced reduction in the development of inflammation in an animal model of ascending pyelonephritis,[194] while they were also useful to mitigate survival elongation of the antiinfluenza viral drug, ribavirin, induced in mice, presumably by reducing oxidative damage.[195] Further, supplementation with a natural antioxidants mixture (wheat sprouts 280 mg, aphanizomenon flos-aquae [Klamath Lake algae] 100 mg, *Gingko biloba* at an 8:1 ratio, pycnogenol 10 mg, vitamin E 10 IU, β-carotene 15 mg, green tea 10 mg, and milk thistle 10 mg) for 12 weeks reduced serum concentrations of the endothelium-derived adhesion molecules sICAM-1 and sVCAM-1 in 60 postmenopausal women with high cardiovascular risk profiles.[196] In addition, Hwang et al. identified a synergism of antioxidant activity with alfalfa extract and acerola cherry extract toward LDL oxidation, in which flavonoids in the alfalfa extracts and ascorbic acid in the acerola cherry extract were shown to have an interplay.[197]

Our group is currently investigating strategies that utilize combinations of food chemicals, as well as combinations of food chemicals and drugs, for generating synergistic antioxidative and antiinflammatory effects with low toxicity. As an initial approach, we combined zerumbone (iNOS expression suppressant) and L-NMMA (synthetic NOS inhibitor), and measured nitrite concentrations.[197] When tested at various concentrations (0.2 to 6.3 μ*M* for zerumbone, 3.2 to 200 μ*M* for L-NMMA), the combination effects at relatively higher concentrations were either additive or antagonistic, whereas those at lower ones (less than1.6 μ*M* for zerumbone, less than 25 μ*M* for L-NMMA) generated marked synergistic effects. On the other hand, when combinations of two to four compounds from the group of EGCG, genistein, BITC, and resveratrol were tested, EGCG/genistein, EGCG/BITC, genistein/BITC, and EGCG/BITC/genistein at lower concentrations were shown to be highly synergistic combinations in each setting, though mechanistic insights into the generation of synergy remain to be elucidated. Thus, combinations of agents with different molecular mechanisms might be the key to a synergistic outcome because a combination of the mechanistically identical compounds L-NMMA and L-NIO (another NOS inhibitor) was highly antagonistic at both high and low concentrations.

In phorbol ester–induced O_2^- generation tests using dimethylsulfoxide-differentiated HL-60 cells (a model for neutrophils), we combined SOD, 1-acetoxychavicol acetate (ACA), EGCG, and caffeic acid (CA) to explore the synergistic antioxidation effects. While SOD and ACA[164] have been characterized to selectively scavenge O_2^- and suppress NOX, respectively, both CA and EGCG have dual properties, as the former is rather SOD-like and the latter ACA-like, when determined by measuring SOD-like activity in a xanthine–xanthine oxidase system.[197] We have also observed notable synergistic effects with the combinations of two agents with different properties, e.g., SOD/ACA, SOD/EGCG, and CA/ACA; however, we have not seen these effects in combinations of agents with similar properties such as SOD/CA, EGCG/CA, and EGCG/ACA. Further, synergy was only seen in combinations at lower concentrations,[197] at which each agent alone would exert little antioxidative activity. These data indicate that combinations of NOX suppressants and SOD-like compounds are able to generate a synergistic outcome when combined at relatively lower concentrations.

14.4.3 Antiinflammatory Agents

The combination effects of an aqueous garlic extract with a proton pump inhibitor (omeprazole) on the growth of *Helicobacter pylori*, which plays a significant role in gastritis, were synergistic in 47% of the strains studied.[198] Rovensky et al. demonstrated an intriguing synergism between methotrexate and the probiotic bacteria *Enterococcus faecium* enriched with organic selenium in rats with adjuvant arthritis, in which a combination therapy, in contrast to methotrexate alone, inhibited the reduction of whole body bone mineral density and bone mineral content.[199] Further, the combination of a grape seed proanthocyanidins extract and niacin-bound chromium synergistically reduced atherosclerosis in hamsters fed a hypercholesterolemic diet for 10 weeks.[200] Klivenyi et al. also found that COX-2 inhibitors both alone and in combination with creatine significantly reduced PGE_2 levels in a G93A transgenic mouse model of amyotrophic lateral sclerosis,[201] with similar results obtained in a mouse model of Parkinsons disease.[202]

As noted earlier, the production of both PGE_2 and TNF-α is associated with the inflammatory process, and NSAIDs are effective drugs for mitigation of inflammatory symptoms. Rapid and prolonged PGE_2 production is regulated by COX-2 and NSAIDs, such as aspirin and indomethacin, which are nonselective, while nimesulide is a COX-2 selective inhibitor. Since genistein is capable of suppressing the *de novo* synthesis of COX-2, as described above, we attempted to determine whether COX-2 inhibitors and their suppressants originating from food exhibit synergy.[102] Our results showed that combinations of indomethacin and genistein, and aspirin and genistein generated a synergistic inhibition of PGE_2 production in LPS/IFN-γ–stimulated RAW264.7 macrophages, whereas the combinations nimesulide and genistein, and indomethacin and nimesulide were not successful, suggesting that antiinflammatory effects increase when COX-2 dual inhibitors and their suppressants are paired. As also noted previously, n-3 fatty acids such as DHA are able to attenuate COX-2 expression and celecoxib is a prominent selective COX-2 inhibitor, indicating that they have independent molecular mechanisms. In addition, Swamy et al. reported an important finding that the combined administration of these agents led to a marked synergistic effect on apoptosis and inhibition of cell proliferation.[203]

Surprisingly, EGCG remarkably enhances LPS/IFN-γ–induced COX-2 protein expression, PGE_2 production, and TNF-α release in RAW cells. Therefore, we conducted an investigation of dietary chemicals that can mask these potential proinflammatory effects of EGCG and found that the combinations of EGCG either with genistein, BITC, or resveratrol, all of which were each highly suppressive of those parameters and by individual administration, led to substantial suppression. On the other hand, combinations of genistein and resveratrol, and genistein and BITC were either additive or antagonistic, implying that genistein, BITC, and resveratrol share molecular targets that are distinct from that of EGCG, though the hypothesis remains to be proven.

We also fed zerumbone or nimesulide alone, or both in combination to ICR mice to explore the suppressive effects on dextran sulfate sodium–induced colitis.[113] Of the biochemical and histological parameters relating to inflammation examined, the combination diet showed the highest levels of suppression of IL-1α and IL-1β levels in colonic mucosa, as well as decreased erosion and inflammatory scores, including leukocyte infiltration, along with a marked improvement of tissue regeneration.

14.5 Conclusions

There is an increasing number of publications that have described the amplified efficacy and/or reduced toxicity of combined synthetic and natural agents, though additional results are needed. While combinations of synthetic compounds that selectively act on individual molecular targets appear to be efficient in terms of disease prevention and therapeutic efficacy, those of natural compounds as well as of drugs and natural compounds might be more practical, inexpensive, and acceptable. In general, the action spectrum of dietary components is broad as compared with that of synthetic drugs. Nonetheless, an action mechanism–based combination is a prerequisite for exhibiting a synergistic outcome, which may be partly supported by our data from antioxidative combinations (SOD plus ACA, etc.). Along this line, a recent report of the dramatic synergy between EGCG and vinblastine for inhibiting cell proliferation is quite attractive, because EGCG was shown to inhibit the function of P-glycoprotein, thereby restoring the anticell proliferating activity of vinblastine in a vinblastine-resistant cell line.[204] Those results reinforce the notion that one of the roles of dietary phytochemicals in a combination strategy is drug dose reduction and shortening of the duration of administration.

Acknowledgments

The authors' works cited here were supported by a grant from the Ministry of Agriculture, Forestry, and Fisheries of Japan.

References

1. Coussens, L.M. and Werb, Z, Inflammation and cancer, *Nature*, 420, 860, 2002.
2. Dandona, P., Aljada, A., and Bandyopadhyay, A, Inflammation: the link between insulin resistance, obesity and diabetes, *Trends Immunol.*, 25, 4, 2004.
3. Libby, P. and Ridker, P.M, Inflammation and atherosclerosis: role of C-reactive protein in risk assessment, *Am. J. Med.*, 116, 9S, 2004.
4. Kubaszek, A. et al., Promoter polymorphisms of the TNF-alpha (G-308A) and IL-6 (C-174G) genes predict the conversion from impaired glucose tolerance to type 2 diabetes: the Finnish Diabetes Prevention Study, *Diabetes*, 52, 1872, 2003.
5. Hwang, I.R. et al., Effect of interleukin 1 polymorphisms on gastric mucosal interleukin 1beta production in Helicobacter pylori infection, *Gastroenterology*, 123, 1793, 2002.
6. Peto, J., Cancer epidemiology in the last century and the next decade, *Nature*, 411, 390, 2001.
7. Kune, G.A., Kune, S., and Watson, L.F., Colorectal cancer risk, chronic illnesses, operations, and medications: case control results from the Melbourne Colorectal Cancer Study, *Cancer Res.*, 48, 4399, 1988.
8. Farrow, D.C. et al., Use of aspirin and other nonsteroidal anti-inflammatory drugs and risk of esophageal and gastric cancer, *Cancer Epidemiol. Biomarkers Prev.*, 7, 97, 1998.
9. Thun, M.J. et al., Aspirin use and risk of fatal cancer, *Cancer Res.*, 53, 1322, 1993.
10. Simmons, D.L. et al., Identification of a phorbol ester-repressible v-src-inducible gene, *Proc. Natl. Acad. Sci. U.S.A.*, 86, 1178, 1989.
11. Schafter, A.I., Effects of nonsteroidal antiinflammatory drugs on platelet function and systemic hemostasis, *J. Clin. Pharmacol.*, 35, 209, 1995.
12. Morita, I. Et al., Different intracellular locations for prostaglandin endoperoxide H synthase-1 and –2, *J. Biol. Chem.*, 270, 10902, 1995.
13. Narumiya, S., Prostanoids in immunity: roles revealed by mice deficient in their receptors., *Life Sci.*, 74, 391, 2003.
14. Bocher, V. et al., PPARs: transcription factors controlling lipid and lipoprotein metabolism, *Ann. N.Y. Acad. Sci.*, 967, 7, 2002.
15. Reddy, S.T., and Herschman, H.R., Prostaglandin synthase-1 and prostaglandin synthase-2 are coupled to distinct phospholipases for the generation of prostaglandin D2 in activated mast cells, *J. Biol. Chem.*, 272, 3231, 1997.
16. Pardue, S., Rapoport, S.I., and Bosetti, F., Co-localization of cytosolic phospholipase A2 and cyclooxygenase-2 in Rhesus monkey cerebellum, *Brain Res. Mol. Brain Res.*, 116, 106, 2003.
17. Takeda, H. et al., Cooperation of cyclooxygenase 1 and cyclooxygenase 2 in intestinal polyposis, *Cancer Res.*, 63, 4872, 2003.
18. Xu, K., Robida, A.M., and Murphy, T.J., Immediate-early MEK-1-dependent stabilization of rat smooth muscle cell cyclooxygenase-2 mRNA by Galpha(q)-coupled receptor signaling, *J. Biol. Chem.*, 275, 23012, 2000.
19. Lasa, M. et al., Regulation of cyclooxygenase 2 mRNA stability by the mitogen-activated protein kinase p38 signaling cascade, *Mol. Cell Biol.*, 20, 4265, 2000.
20. Rousseau, S. et al., Inhibition of SAPK2a/p38 prevents hnRNP A0 phosphorylation by MAPKAP-K2 and its interaction with cytokine mRNAs, *EMBO J.*, 21, 6505, 2002.

21. Subbaramaiah, K. et al., Regulation of cyclooxgenase-2 mRNA stability by taxanes: evidence for involvement of p38, MAPKAPK-2, and HuR, *J. Biol. Chem.*, 278, 37637, 2003.
22. Sully, G. et al., Structural and functional dissection of a conserved destabilizing element of cyclo-oxygenase-2 mRNA: evidence against the involvement of AUF-1 [AU-rich element/poly(U)-binding/degradation factor-1], AUF-2, tristetraprolin, HuR (Hu antigen R) or FBP1 (far-upstream-sequence-element-binding protein 1), *Biochem. J.*, 377(Pt 3), 629, 2004.
23. Chow, J.C. et al., Toll-like receptor-4 mediates lipopolysaccharide-induced signal transduction., *J. Biol. Chem.*, 274, 10689, 1999.
24. Karin, M., How NF-kappaB is activated: the role of the IkappaB kinase (IKK) complex, *Oncogene*, 18, 6867, 1999.
25. Caivano, M. and Cohen, P., Role of mitogen-activated protein kinase cascades in mediating lipopolysaccharide-stimulated induction of cyclooxygenase-2 and IL-1 beta in RAW264 macrophages, *J. Immunol.*, 164, 3018, 2000.
26. Caivano, M. et al., The induction of cyclooxygenase-2 mRNA in macrophages is biphasic and requires both CCAAT enhancer-binding protein beta (C/EBP beta) and C/EBP delta transcription factors, *J. Biol. Chem.*, 276, 48693, 2001.
27. Cedergren, J. et al., Inducible nitric oxide synthase is expressed in synovial fluid granulocytes, *Clin. Exp. Immunol.*, 130, 150, 2002.
28. Donnelly, L.E. and Barnes, P.J., Expression and regulation of inducible nitric oxide synthase from human primary airway epithelial cells, *Am. J. Respir. Cell Mol. Biol.*, 26, 144, 2002.
29. Hao, X.P. et al., Inducible nitric oxide synthase (iNOS) is expressed similarly in multiple aberrant crypt foci and colorectal tumors from the same patients, *Cancer Res.*, 61, 419, 2001.
30. Cross, R.K. and Wilson, K.T., Nitric oxide in inflammatory bowel disease, *Inflamm. Bowel Dis.*, 9, 179, 2003.
31. Szabo, C. and Ohshima, H., DNA damage induced by peroxynitrite: subsequent biological effects, *Nitric Oxide*, 1, 373, 1997.
32. Lee, A.K. et al., Inhibition of lipopolysaccharide-inducible nitric oxide synthase, TNF-alpha and COX-2 expression by sauchinone effects on I-kappaBalpha phosphorylation, C/EBP and AP-1 activation, *Br. J. Pharmacol.*, 139, 11, 2003.
33. Chio, C.C. et al., PKA-dependent activation of PKC, p38 MAPK and IKK in macrophage: implication in the induction of inducible nitric oxide synthase and interleukin-6 by dibutyryl cAMP, *Cell Signal.*, 16, 565, 2004.
34. Blanchette, J., Jaramillo, M., and Olivier, M., Signalling events involved in interferon-gamma-inducible macrophage nitric oxide generation, *Immunology*, 108, 513, 2003.
35. Lahti, A. et al., c-Jun NH2-terminal kinase inhibitor anthra(1,9-cd)pyrazol-6(2H)-one reduces inducible nitric-oxide synthase expression by destabilizing mRNA in activated macrophages, *Mol. Pharmacol.*, 64, 308, 2003.
36. Lambeth, J.D., NOX enzymes and the biology of reactive oxygen, *Nat. Rev. Immunol.*, 4, 181, 2004.
37. Sergeant, S. and McPhail, L.C., Opsonized zymosan stimulates the redistribution of protein kinase C isoforms in human neutrophils, *J. Immunol.*, 159, 2877, 1997.
38. Nixon, J.B. and McPhail, L.C., Protein kinase C (PKC) isoforms translocate to Triton-insoluble fractions in stimulated human neutrophils: correlation of conventional PKC with activation of NADPH oxidase, *J. Immunol.*, 163, 4574, 1999.

39. El Benna, J. et al., Activation of p38 in stimulated human neutrophils: phosphorylation of the oxidase component p47phox by p38 and ERK but not by JNK, *Arch. Biochem. Biophys.*, 334, 395, 1996.
40. Chen, Q. et al., Akt phosphorylates p47phox and mediates respiratory burst activity in human neutrophils, *J. Immunol.*, 170, 5302, 2003.
41. Teshima, S. et al., Regulation of growth and apoptosis of cultured guinea pig gastric mucosal cells by mitogenic oxidase 1, *Am. J. Physiol. Gastrointest. Liver. Physiol.*, 279, G1169, 2000.
42. Mitsushita, J., Lambeth, J.D., and Kamata, T., The superoxide-generating oxidase Nox1 is functionally required for Ras oncogene transformation, *Cancer Res.*, 64, 3580, 2004.
43. Arbiser, J.L. et al., Reactive oxygen generated by Nox1 triggers the angiogenic switch, *Proc. Natl. Acad. Sci. U.S.A.*, 99, 715, 2002.
44. Cai, H., Griendling, K.K., and Harrison, D.G., The vascular NAD(P)H oxidases as therapeutic targets in cardiovascular diseases., *Trends Pharmacol. Sci.*, 24, 471, 2003.
45. Vaziri, N.D. et al., Oxidative stress and dysregulation of superoxide dismutase and NADPH oxidase in renal insufficiency, *Kidney Int.*, 63, 179, 2003.
46. Hamilton, C.A. et al., NAD(P)H oxidase inhibition improves endothelial function in rat and human blood vessels, *Hypertension*, 40, 755, 2002.
47. Jung, O. et al., gp91phox-containing NADPH oxidase mediates endothelial dysfunction in renovascular hypertension, *Circulation*, 109, 1795, 2004.
48. Heyworth, P.G., Cross, A.R., and Curnutte, J.T., Chronic granulomatous disease, *Curr. Opin. Immunol.*, 15, 578, 2003.
49. Vane, J.R., Inhibition of prostaglandin synthesis as a mechanism of action for aspirin-like drugs, *Nature New Biol.*, 231, 232, 1979.
50. Oshima, M. et al., Suppression of intestinal polyposis in Apc delta716 knockout mice by inhibition of cyclooxygenase 2 (COX-2), *Cell*, 87, 803, 1996.
51. Takahashi, M. et al., Suppression of azoxymethane-induced aberrant crypt foci in rat colon by nimesulide, a selective inhibitor of cyclooxygenase 2, *J. Cancer Res. Clin. Oncol.*, 122, 219, 1996.
52. Fukutake, M. et al., Suppressive effects of nimesulide, a selective inhibitor of cyclooxygenase-2, on azoxymethane-induced colon carcinogenesis in mice, *Carcinogenesis*, 19, 1939, 1998.
53. Nakatsugi, S. et al., Suppression of intestinal polyp development by nimesulide, a selective cyclooxygenase-2 inhibitor, in Min mice, *Jpn. J. Cancer Res.*, 88, 1117, 1997.
54. Okajima, E. et al., Chemopreventive effects of nimesulide, a selective cyclooxygenase-2 inhibitor, on the development of rat urinary bladder carcinomas initiated by N-butyl-N-(4-hydroxybutyl)nitrosamine., *Cancer Res.*, 58, 3028, 1998.
55. Pentland, A.P. et al., Reduction of UV-induced skin tumors in hairless mice by selective COX-2 inhibition, *Carcinogenesis*, 20, 1939, 1999.
56. Fischer, S.M. et al., Chemopreventive activity of celecoxib, a specific cyclooxygenase-2 inhibitor, and indomethacin against ultraviolet light-induced skin carcinogenesis, *Mol. Carcinog.*, 25, 231, 1999.
57. Kawamori, T. et al., Chemopreventive activity of celecoxib, a specific cyclooxygenase-2 inhibitor, against colon carcinogenesis, *Cancer Res.*, 58, 409, 1998.
58. Hu, P.J. et al., Chemoprevention of gastric cancer by celecoxib in rats, *Gut*, 53, 195, 2004.

59. Lanza-Jacoby, S. et al., The cyclooxygenase-2 inhibitor, celecoxib, prevents the development of mammary tumors in Her-2/neu mice, *Cancer Epidemiol. Biomarkers Prev.*, 12, 1486, 2003.
60. Fenton, C., Keating, G.M., and Wagstaff, A.J., Valdecoxib: A review of its use in the management of osteoarthritis, rheumatoid arthritis, dysmenorrhoea and acute pain, *Drugs*, 64, 1231, 2004.
61. Warner, T.D. and Mitchell, J.A., Cyclooxygenases: new forms, new inhibitors, and lessons from the clinic, *FASEB J.*, 18, 790, 2004.
62. Kivitz, A.J. et al., Reduced incidence of gastroduodenal ulcers associated with lumiracoxib compared with ibuprofen in patients with rheumatoid arthritis, *Aliment. Pharmacol. Ther.*, 19, 1189, 2004.
63. Tiano, H.F. et al., Deficiency of either cyclooxygenase (COX)-1 or COX-2 alters epidermal differentiation and reduces mouse skin tumorigenesis, *Cancer Res.*, 62, 3395, 2002.
64. Appleton, I. et al., Temporal and spatial immunolocalization of cytokines in murine chronic granulomatous tissue. Implications for their role in tissue development and repair processes, *Lab. Invest.*, 69, 405, 1993.
65. Langenbach, R. et al., Prostaglandin synthase 1 gene disruption in mice reduces arachidonic acid-induced inflammation and indomethacin-induced gastric ulceration, *Cell*, 83, 483, 1995.
66. Kitamura, T. et al., Inhibitory effects of mofezolac, a cyclooxygenase-1 selective inhibitor, on intestinal carcinogenesis, *Carcinogenesis*, 23, 1463, 2002.
67. Gupta, R.A. et al., Cyclooxygenase-1 is overexpressed and promotes angiogenic growth factor production in ovarian cancer, *Cancer Res.*, 63, 906, 2003.
68. Grosch, S. et al., COX-2 independent induction of cell cycle arrest and apoptosis in colon cancer cells by the selective COX-2 inhibitor celecoxib, *FASEB J.*, 15, 2742, 2001.
69. Arico, S. et al., Celecoxib induces apoptosis by inhibiting 3-phosphoinositide-dependent protein kinase-1 activity in the human colon cancer HT-29 cell line, *J. Biol. Chem.*, 277, 27613, 2002.
70. Wu, T. et al., The cyclooxygenase-2 inhibitor celecoxib blocks phosphorylation of Akt and induces apoptosis in human cholangiocarcinoma cells, *Mol. Cancer Ther.*, 3, 299, 2004.
71. Kulp, S.K. et al., 3-phosphoinositide-dependent protein kinase-1/Akt signaling represents a major cyclooxygenase-2-independent target for celecoxib in prostate cancer cells, *Cancer Res.*, 64, 1444, 2004.
72. Surh, Y.J., Anti-tumor promoting potential of selected spice ingredients with antioxidative and anti-inflammatory activities: a short review, *Food Chem. Toxicol.*, 40, 1091, 2002.
73. Surh, Y.J., Cancer chemoprevention with dietary phytochemicals, *Nat. Rev. Cancer*, 3, 768, 2003.
74. Surh, Y.J. et al., Molecular mechanisms underlying chemopreventive activities of anti-inflammatory phytochemicals: down-regulation of COX-2 and iNOS through suppression of NF-kappa B activation, *Mutat. Res.*, 480-481, 243, 2001.
75. Subbaramaiah, K. et al., Resveratrol inhibits cyclooxygenase-2 transcription in human mammary epithelial cells, *Ann. N.Y. Acad. Sci.*, 889, 214, 1999.
76. Subbaramaiah, K. et al., Resveratrol inhibits cyclooxygenase-2 transcription and activity in phorbol ester-treated human mammary epithelial cells, *J. Biol. Chem.*, 273, 21875, 1998.

77. Murakami, A. et al., Effects of selected food factors with chemopreventive properties on combined lipopolysaccharide- and interferon-gamma-induced IkappaB degradation in RAW264.7 macrophages, *Cancer Lett.*, 195, 17, 2003.
78. Jang, M. and Pezzuto, J.M., Effects of resveratrol on 12-O-tetradecanoylphorbol-13-acetate-induced oxidative events and gene expression in mouse skin, *Cancer Lett.*, 134, 81, 1998.
79. Martin, A.R. et al., Resveratrol, a polyphenol found in grapes, suppresses oxidative damage and stimulates apoptosis during early colonic inflammation in rats, *Biochem. Pharmacol.*, 67, 1399, 2004.
80. Li, Z.G, et al., Suppression of N-nitrosomethylbenzylamine (NMBA)-induced esophageal tumorigenesis in F344 rats by resveratrol, *Carcinogenesis*, 23, 1531, 2002.
81. Aggarwal, B.B., Kumar, A., and Bharti, A.C., Anticancer potential of curcumin: preclinical and clinical studies, *Anticancer Res.*, 23(1A), 363, 2003.
82. Zhang, F. et al., Curcumin inhibits cyclooxygenase-2 transcription in bile acid- and phorbol ester-treated human gastrointestinal epithelial cells, *Carcinogenesis*, 20, 445, 1999.
83. Goel, A., Boland, C.R., and Chauhan, D.P., Specific inhibition of cyclooxygenase-2 (COX-2) expression by dietary curcumin in HT-29 human colon cancer cells, *Cancer Lett.*, 172, 111, 2001.
84. Plummer, S.M. et al., Clinical development of leukocyte cyclooxygenase 2 activity as a systemic biomarker for cancer chemopreventive agents, *Cancer Epidemiol. Biomarkers Prev.*, 10, 1295, 2001.
85. Nanji, A.A. et al., Curcumin prevents alcohol-induced liver disease in rats by inhibiting the expression of NF-kappa B-dependent genes, *Am. J. Physiol. Gastrointest. Liver Physiol.*, 284, G321, 2003.
86. Shishodia, S. et al., Curcumin (diferuloylmethane) down-regulates cigarette smoke-induced NF-kappaB activation through inhibition of IkappaBalpha kinase in human lung epithelial cells: correlation with suppression of COX-2, MMP-9 and cyclin D1, *Carcinogenesis*, 24, 1269, 2003.
87. Kang, G. et al., Curcumin suppresses lipopolysaccharide-induced cyclooxygenase-2 expression by inhibiting activator protein 1 and nuclear factor kappab bindings in BV2 microglial cells, *J. Pharmacol. Sci.*, 94, 325, 2004.
88. Hong, J. et al., Modulation of arachidonic acid metabolism by curcumin and related {beta}-diketone derivatives: effects on cytosolic phospholipase A2, cyclooxygenases, and 5-lipoxygenase, *Carcinogenesis*, 25, 167, 2004.
89. Chun, K.S. et al., Curcumin inhibits phorbol ester-induced expression of cyclooxygenase-2 in mouse skin through suppression of extracellular signal-regulated kinase activity and NF-kappaB activation, *Carcinogenesis*, 24, 1515, 2003.
90. Singh, J., Hamid, R., and Reddy, B.S., Dietary fat and colon cancer: modulation of cyclooxygenase-2 by types and amount of dietary fat during the postinitiation stage of colon carcinogenesis, *Cancer Res.*, 57, 3465, 1997.
91. Plummer, S.M. et al., Clinical development of leukocyte cyclooxygenase 2 activity as a systemic biomarker for cancer chemopreventive agents, *Cancer Epidemiol. Biomarkers Prev.*, 10, 1295, 2001.
92. Lo, C.J. et al., Fish oil augments macrophage cyclooxygenase II (COX-2) gene expression induced by endotoxin, *J. Surg. Res.*, 86, 103, 1999.
93. Lee, J.Y. et al., Differential modulation of toll-like receptors by fatty acids: preferential inhibition by n-3 polyunsaturated fatty acids, *J. Lipid Res.*, 44, 479, 2003.

94. Bousserouel, S. et al., Different effects of n-6 and n-3 polyunsaturated fatty acids on the activation of rat smooth muscle cells by interleukin-1 betal, *J. Lipid Res.*, 44, 601, 2003.
95. Babcock, T.A. et al., Modulation of lipopolysaccharide-stimulated macrophage tumor necrosis factor-alpha production by omega-3 fatty acid is associated with differential cyclooxygenase-2 protein expression and is independent of interleukin-10, *J. Surg. Res.*, 107, 135, 2002.
96. Boudreau, M.D. et al., Suppression of tumor cell growth both in nude mice and in culture by n-3 polyunsaturated fatty acids: mediation through cyclooxygenase-independent pathways, *Cancer Res.*, 61, 1386, 2001.
97. Cui, Y. et al., Involvement of ERK AND p38 MAP kinase in AAPH-induced COX-2 expression in HaCaT cells, *Chem. Phys. Lipids*, 129, 43, 2004.
98. Kundu, J.K. et al., Inhibition of phorbol ester-induced COX-2 expression by epigallocatechin gallate in mouse skin and cultured human mammary epithelial cells, *J. Nutr.*, 133, 3805S, 2003.
99. Li, Z.G. et al., Inhibitory effects of epigallocatechin-3-gallate on N-nitrosomethylbenzylamine-induced esophageal tumorigenesis in F344 rats, *Int. J. Oncol.*, 21, 1275, 2002.
100. Ahmed, S. et al., Green tea polyphenol epigallocatechin-3-gallate inhibits the IL-1 beta-induced activity and expression of cyclooxygenase-2 and nitric oxide synthase-2 in human chondrocytes, *Free Radic. Biol. Med.*, 33, 1097, 2002.
101. Park, J.W. et al., Involvement of ERK and protein tyrosine phosphatase signaling pathways in EGCG-induced cyclooxygenase-2 expression in Raw 264.7 cells, *Biochem. Biophys. Res. Commun.*, 286, 721, 2001.
102. Murakami, A. et al., Combinatorial effects of nonsteroidal anti-inflammatory drugs and food constituents on production of prostaglandin E2 and tumor necrosis factor-alpha in RAW264.7 murine macrophages, *Biosci. Biotechnol. Biochem.*, 67, 1056, 2003.
103. Heiss, E. et al., Nuclear factor kappa B is a molecular target for sulforaphane-mediated anti-inflammatory mechanisms, *J. Biol. Chem.*, 276, 32008, 2001.
104. Rao, C.V. et al., Enhancement of experimental colon carcinogenesis by dietary 6-phenylhexyl isothiocyanate, *Cancer Res.*, 55, 4311, 1995.
105. Blanco, A. et al., Involvement of tyrosine kinases in the induction of cyclooxygenase-2 in human endothelial cells, *Biochem. J.*, 312 (Pt 2), 419, 1995.
106. Tetsuka, T., Srivastava, S.K., and Morrison, A.R., Tyrosine kinase inhibitors, genistein and herbimycin A, do not block interleukin-1 beta-induced activation of NF-kappa B in rat mesangial cells, *Biochem. Biophys. Res. Commun.*, 218, 808, 1996.
107. Corbett, J.A. et al., Tyrosine kinase inhibitors prevent cytokine-induced expression of iNOS and COX-2 by human islets, *Am. J. Physiol.*, 270(6 Pt 1), C1581, 1996.
108. Liang, Y.C. et al., Suppression of inducible cyclooxygenase and inducible nitric oxide synthase by apigenin and related flavonoids in mouse macrophages, *Carcinogenesis*, 20, 1945, 1999.
109. Lin, C.H. et al., Involvement of protein kinase C-gamma in IL-1beta-induced cyclooxygenase-2 expression in human pulmonary epithelial cells, *Mol. Pharmacol.*, 57, 36, 2000.
110. Mutoh, M. et al., Suppression of cyclooxygenase-2 promoter-dependent transcriptional activity in colon cancer cells by chemopreventive agents with a resorcin-type structure, *Carcinogenesis*, 21, 959, 2000.

111. Chen, C.C. et al., TNF-alpha-induced cyclooxygenase-2 expression in human lung epithelial cells: involvement of the phospholipase C-gamma 2, protein kinase C-alpha, tyrosine kinase, NF-kappa B-inducing kinase, and I-kappa B kinase 1/2 pathway, *J. Immunol.*, 165, 2719, 2000.
112. Ozaki, Y., Kawahara, N., and Harada, M., Anti-inflammatory effect of Zingiber cassumunar Roxb. and its active principles, *Chem. Pharm. Bull. (Tokyo)*, 39, 2353, 1991.
113. Murakami, A. et al., Suppression of dextran sodium sulfate-induced colitis in mice by zerumbone, a subtropical ginger sesquiterpene, and nimesulide: separately and in combination, *Biochem Pharmacol.*, 66, 1253, 2003.
114. Tanaka, T. et al., Chemoprevention of azoxymethane-induced rat aberrant crypt foci by dietary zerumbone isolated from Zingiber zerumbet, *Life Sci.*, 69, 1935, 2001.
115. Murakami, A. et al., Zerumbone, a Southeast Asian ginger sesquiterpene, markedly suppresses free radical generation, proinflammatory protein production, and cancer cell proliferation accompanied by apoptosis: the alpha,beta-unsaturated carbonyl group is a prerequisite, *Carcinogenesis*, 23, 795, 2002.
116. Kirana, C. et al., Antitumor activity of extract of Zingiber aromaticum and its bioactive sesquiterpenoid zerumbone, *Nutr. Cancer*, 45, 218, 2003.
117. Murakami, A. et al., Zerumbone, a sesquiterpene in subtropical ginger, suppresses skin tumor initiation and promotion stages in ICR mice, *Int. J. Cancer*, 110, 481, 2004.
118. Szewczuk, L.M. et al., Resveratrol is a peroxidase-mediated inactivator of COX-1 but not COX-2: a mechanistic approach to the design of COX-1 selective agents, *J. Biol. Chem.*, 279, 22727, 2004.
119. Kawamori, T. et al., Suppression of azoxymethane-induced colonic aberrant crypt foci by a nitric oxide synthase inhibitor, *Cancer Lett.*, 148, 33, 2000.
120. Lim, J.W., Kim, H., and Kim, K.H., NF-kappaB, inducible nitric oxide synthase and apoptosis by Helicobacter pylori infection, *Free Radic. Biol. Med.*, 31, 355, 2001.
121. Schleiffer, R. et al., Nitric oxide synthase inhibition promotes carcinogen-induced preneoplastic changes in the colon of rats, *Nitric Oxide*, 4, 583, 2000.
122. Jover, B. and Mimran, A., Nitric oxide inhibition and renal alterations, *J. Cardiovasc. Pharmacol.*, 38 Suppl 2, S65, 2001.
123. Chen, T. et al., Chemopreventive effects of a selective nitric oxide synthase inhibitor on carcinogen-induced rat esophageal tumorigenesis, *Cancer Res.*, 64, 3714, 2004.
124. Naito, Y. et al., A novel potent inhibitor of inducible nitric oxide inhibitor, ONO-1714, reduces intestinal ischemia-reperfusion injury in rats, *Nitric Oxide*, 10, 170, 2004.
125. Dugo, L. et al., Effects of GW274150, a novel and selective inhibitor of iNOS activity, in acute lung inflammation, *Br. J. Pharmacol.*, 141, 979, 2004.
126. Cuzzocrea, S. et al., Beneficial effects of GW274150, a novel, potent and selective inhibitor of iNOS activity, in a rodent model of collagen-induced arthritis, *Eur. J. Pharmacol.*, 453, 119, 2002.
127. Kankuri, E. et al., Suppression of pro-inflammatory cytokine release by selective inhibition of inducible nitric oxide synthase in mucosal explants from patients with ulcerative colitis, *Scand. J. Gastroenterol.*, 38, 186, 2003.

128. Garvey, E.P. et al., 1400W is a slow, tight binding, and highly selective inhibitor of inducible nitric-oxide synthase in vitro and in vivo, *J. Biol. Chem.*, 272, 4959, 1997.
129. McMillan, K. et al., Allosteric inhibitors of inducible nitric oxide synthase dimerization discovered via combinatorial chemistry, *Proc. Natl. Acad. Sci. U.S.A.*, 97, 1506, 2000.
130. Blasko, E. et al., Mechanistic studies with potent and selective inducible nitric-oxide synthase dimerization inhibitors, *J. Biol. Chem.*, 277, 295, 2002.
131. Tsai, S.H., Lin-Shiau, S.Y., and Lin, J.K., Suppression of nitric oxide synthase and the down-regulation of the activation of NFkappaB in macrophages by resveratrol, *Br. J. Pharmacol.*, 126, 673, 1999.
132. Chan, M.M. et al., Synergy between ethanol and grape polyphenols, quercetin, and resveratrol, in the inhibition of the inducible nitric oxide synthase pathway, *Biochem. Pharmacol.*, 60, 1539, 2000.
133. Matsuda, H. et al., Effects of stilbene constituents from rhubarb on nitric oxide production in lipopolysaccharide-activated macrophages, *Bioorg. Med. Chem. Lett.*, 10, 323, 2000.
134. Imamura, G. et al., Pharmacological preconditioning with resveratrol: an insight with iNOS knockout mice, *Am. J. Physiol. Heart Circ. Physiol.*, 282, 1996, 2002.
135. Chan, M.M. et al., In vivo inhibition of nitric oxide synthase gene expression by curcumin, a cancer preventive natural product with anti-inflammatory properties, *Biochem. Pharmacol.*, 55, 1955, 1998.
136. Onoda, M. and Inano, H., Effect of curcumin on the production of nitric oxide by cultured rat mammary gland, *Nitric Oxide*, 4, 505, 2000.
137. Pan, M.H., Lin-Shiau, S.Y., and Lin, J.K., Comparative studies on the suppression of nitric oxide synthase by curcumin and its hydrogenated metabolites through down-regulation of IkappaB kinase and NFkappaB activation in macrophages, *Biochem. Pharmacol.*, 60, 1665, 2000.
138. Zheng, M. et al., Inhibition of nuclear factor-kappaB and nitric oxide by curcumin induces G2/M cell cycle arrest and apoptosis in human melanoma cells, *Melanoma Res.*, 14, 165, 2004.
139. Khair-El-Din, T. et al., Transcription of the murine iNOS gene is inhibited by docosahexaenoic acid, a major constituent of fetal and neonatal sera as well as fish oils, *J. Exp. Med.*, 183, 1241, 1996.
140. Komatsu, W. et al., Docosahexaenoic acid suppresses nitric oxide production and inducible nitric oxide synthase expression in interferon-gamma plus lipopolysaccharide-stimulated murine macrophages by inhibiting the oxidative stress, *Free Radic. Biol. Med.*, 34, 1006, 2003.
141. Ohata, T. et al., Suppression of nitric oxide production in lipopolysaccharide-stimulated macrophage cells by omega 3 polyunsaturated fatty acids, *Jpn. J. Cancer Res.*, 88, 234, 1997.
142. Narayanan, B.A. et al., Modulation of inducible nitric oxide synthase and related proinflammatory genes by the omega-3 fatty acid docosahexaenoic acid in human colon cancer cells, *Cancer Res.*, 63, 972, 2003.
143. Kielar, M.L. et al., Docosahexaenoic acid ameliorates murine ischemic acute renal failure and prevents increases in mRNA abundance for both TNF-alpha and inducible nitric oxide synthase, *J. Am. Soc. Nephrol.*, 14, 389, 2003.

144. Lin, Y.L. and Lin, J.K., (-)-Epigallocatechin-3-gallate blocks the induction of nitric oxide synthase by down-regulating lipopolysaccharide-induced activity of transcription factor nuclear factor-kappaB, *Mol. Pharmacol.*, 52, 465, 1997.
145. Chan, M.M. et al., Inhibition of inducible nitric oxide synthase gene expression and enzyme activity by epigallocatechin gallate, a natural product from green tea, *Biochem. Pharmacol.*, 54, 1281, 1997.
146. Singh, R. et al., Epigallocatechin-3-gallate inhibits interleukin-1beta-induced expression of nitric oxide synthase and production of nitric oxide in human chondrocytes: suppression of nuclear factor kappaB activation by degradation of the inhibitor of nuclear factor kappaB, *Arthritis Rheum.*, 46, 2079, 2002.
147. Ahmed, S. et al., Green tea polyphenol epigallocatechin-3-gallate inhibits the IL-1 beta-induced activity and expression of cyclooxygenase-2 and nitric oxide synthase-2 in human chondrocytes, *Free Radic. Biol. Med.*, 33, 1097, 2002.
148. Suzuki, M. et al., Protective effects of green tea catechins on cerebral ischemic damage, *Med. Sci. Monit.*, 10, BR166, 2004.
149. Song, E.K., Hur, H., and Han, M.K., Epigallocatechin gallate prevents autoimmune diabetes induced by multiple low doses of streptozotocin in mice, *Arch. Pharm. Res.*, 26, 559, 2003.
150. Lorenz, M. et al., A constituent of green tea, epigallocatechin-3-gallate, activates endothelial nitric oxide synthase by a phosphatidylinositol-3-OH-kinase-, cAMP-dependent protein kinase-, and Akt-dependent pathway and leads to endothelial-dependent vasorelaxation, *J. Biol. Chem.*, 279, 6190, 2004.
151. Ippoushi, K. et al., Effect of naturally occurring organosulfur compounds on nitric oxide production in lipopolysaccharide-activated macrophages, *Life Sci.*, 71, 411, 2002.
152. Chen, Y.H., Dai, H.J., and Chang, H.P., Suppression of inducible nitric oxide production by indole and isothiocyanate derivatives from Brassica plants in stimulated macrophages, *Planta Med.*, 69, 696, 2003.
153. Marczin, N., Papapetropoulos, A., and Catravas, J.D., Tyrosine kinase inhibitors suppress endotoxin- and IL-1 beta-induced NO synthesis in aortic smooth muscle cells, *Am. J. Physiol.*, 265(3 Pt 2), H1014, 1993.
154. Murakami, et al., Synergistic suppression of superoxide and nitric oxide generation from inflammatory cells by combined food factors, *Mutat Res.*, 523, 151, 2003.
155. Vrba, J. et al., Sanguinarine is a potent inhibitor of oxidative burst in DMSO-differentiated HL-60 cells by a non-redox mechanism, *Chem. Biol. Interact.*, 147, 35, 2004.
156. Morre, D.J., Preferential inhibition of the plasma membrane NADH oxidase (NOX) activity by diphenyleneiodonium chloride with NADPH as donor, *Antioxid Redox Signal.*, 4, 207, 2002.
157. Mendes, A.F. et al., Diphenyleneiodonium inhibits NF-kappaB activation and iNOS expression induced by IL-1beta: involvement of reactive oxygen species, *Mediators Inflamm.*, 10, 209, 2001.
158. Dorsam, G. et al., Diphenyleneiodium chloride blocks inflammatory cytokine-induced up-regulation of group IIA phospholipase A(2) in rat mesangial cells, *J. Pharmacol. Exp. Ther.*, 292, 271, 2000.
159. Bandoh, T. et al., Antioxidative potential of fluvastatin via the inhibition of nicotinamide adenine dinucleotide phosphate (NADPH) oxidase activity, *Biol. Pharm. Bull.*, 26, 818, 2003.

160. Odani, K. et al., ML-7 inhibits exocytosis of superoxide-producing intracellular compartments in human neutrophils stimulated with phorbol myristate acetate in a myosin light chain kinase-independent manner, *Histochem. Cell Biol.*, 119, 363, 2003.
161. Wang, J.P. et al., Inhibition of superoxide anion generation by YC-1 in rat neutrophils through cyclic GMP-dependent and -independent mechanisms, *Biochem. Pharmacol.*, 63, 577, 2002.
162. Ohashi, I. et al., Inhibitory effect of a synthetic protease inhibitor (gabexate mesilate) on the respiratory burst oxidase in human neutrophils, *J. Biochem. (Tokyo)*, 118, 1001, 1995.
163. Joseph, G. et al., Inhibition of NADPH oxidase activation by synthetic peptides mapping within the carboxyl-terminal domain of small GTP-binding proteins. Lack of amino acid sequence specificity and importance of polybasic motif, *J. Biol. Chem.*, 269, 29024, 1994.
164. Hart, B.A. and Simons, J.M., Metabolic activation of phenols by stimulated neutrophils: a concept for a selective type of anti-inflammatory drug, *Biotechnol. Ther.*, 3, 119, 1992.
165. Barbieri, S.S. et al., Apocynin prevents cyclooxygenase 2 expression in human monocytes through NADPH oxidase and glutathione redox-dependent mechanisms, *Free Radic. Biol. Med.*, 37, 156, 2004.
166. Orallo, F. et al., The possible implication of trans-resveratrol in the cardioprotective effects of long-term moderate wine consumption, *Mol. Pharmacol.*, 61, 294, 2002.
167. Schneider, S.M. et al., Activity of the leukocyte NADPH oxidase in whole neutrophils and cell-free neutrophil preparations stimulated with long-chain polyunsaturated fatty acids, *Inflammation*, 25, 17, 2001.
168. Wu, G.S. and Rao, N.A., Activation of NADPH oxidase by docosahexaenoic acid hydroperoxide and its inhibition by a novel retinal pigment epithelial protein, *Invest. Ophthalmol. Vis. Sci.*, 40, 831, 1999.
169. Huang, Z.H. et al., N-6 and n-3 polyunsaturated fatty acids stimulate translocation of protein kinase Calpha, -betaI, -betaII and -epsilon and enhance agonist-induced NADPH oxidase in macrophages, *Biochem. J.*, 325 (Pt 2), 553, 1997.
170. Poulos, A. et al., Effect of 22-32 carbon n-3 polyunsaturated fatty acids on superoxide production in human neutrophils: synergism of docosahexaenoic acid with f-met-leu-phe and phorbol ester, *Immunology*, 73, 102, 1991.
171. Nakagawa, T. and Yokozawa, T., Direct scavenging of nitric oxide and superoxide by green tea, *Food Chem. Toxicol.*, 40, 1745, 2002.
172. Miyoshi, N. et al., Benzyl isothiocyanate inhibits excessive superoxide generation in inflammatory leukocytes: implication for prevention against inflammation-related carcinogenesis, *Carcinogenesis*, 25, 567, 2004.
173. Conde, M. et al., Modulation of phorbol ester-induced respiratory burst by vanadate, genistein, and phenylarsine oxide in mouse macrophages, *Free Radic. Biol. Med.*, 18, 343, 1995.
174. Dorseuil, O., Quinn, M.T., and Bokoch, G.M., Dissociation of Rac translocation from p47phox/p67phox movements in human neutrophils by tyrosine kinase inhibitors, *J. Leukoc. Biol.*, 58, 108, 1995.
175. Murakami, A. et al., 1′-Acetoxychavicol acetate, a superoxide anion generation inhibitor, potently inhibits tumor promotion by 12-O-tetradecanoylphorbol-13-acetate in ICR mouse skin, *Oncology*, 53, 386, 1996.

176. Miyake, Y. et al., Identification of coumarins from lemon fruit (Citrus limon) as inhibitors of in vitro tumor promotion and superoxide and nitric oxide generation, *J. Agric. Food Chem.*, 47, 3151, 1999.
177. Nakamura, Y. et al., Suppression of tumor promoter-induced oxidative stress and inflammatory responses in mouse skin by a superoxide generation inhibitor 1′-acetoxychavicol acetate, *Cancer Res.*, 58, 4832, 1998.
178. Murakami, A. et al., Auraptene, a citrus coumarin, inhibits 12-O-tetradecanoylphorbol- 13-acetate-induced tumor promotion in ICR mouse skin, possibly through suppression of superoxide generation in leukocytes, *Jpn. J. Cancer Res.*, 88, 443, 1997.
179. Kim, O.K. et al., Novel nitric oxide and superoxide generation inhibitors, persenone A and B, from avocado fruit, *J. Agric. Food Chem.*, 48, 1557, 2000.
180. Murakami, A. et al., Inhibitory effect of citrus nobiletin on phorbol ester-induced skin inflammation, oxidative stress, and tumor promotion in mice, *Cancer Res.*, 60, 5059, 2000.
181. Murakami, A. et al., Suppressive effects of citrus fruits on free radical generation and nobiletin, an anti-inflammatory polymethoxyflavonoid, *Biofactors*, 12, 187, 2000.
182. Murakami, A. et al., Suppression by citrus auraptene of phorbol ester-and endotoxin-induced inflammatory responses: role of attenuation of leukocyte activation, *Carcinogenesis*, 21, 1843, 2000.
183. Kim, H.W. et al., Screening of edible Japanese plants for suppressive effects on phorbol ester-induced superoxide generation in differentiated HL-60 cells and AS52 cells, *Cancer Lett.*, 176, 7, 2002.
184. Nakamura, Y., Murakami, A., and Ohigashi, H., Search for naturally-occurring antioxidative chemopreventors on the basis of the involvement of leukocyte-derived reactive oxygen species in carcinogenesis, *Asian Pac. J. Cancer Prev.*, 1, 115, 2000.
185. Jiwajinda, S. et al., Suppressive effects of edible Thai plants on superoxide and nitric oxide generation, *Asian Pac. J. Cancer Prev.*, 3, 215, 2002.
186. Adam, O. et al., Anti-inflammatory effects of a low arachidonic acid diet and fish oil in patients with rheumatoid arthritis, *Rheumatol. Int.*, 23, 27, 2003.
187. Tate, G.A. et al., Suppression of monosodium urate crystal-induced acute inflammation by diets enriched with gamma-linolenic acid and eicosapentaenoic acid, *Arthritis Rheum.*, 31, 1543, 1998.
188. Barham, J.B. et al., Addition of eicosapentaenoic acid to gamma-linolenic acid-supplemented diets prevents serum arachidonic acid accumulation in humans, *J. Nutr.*, 130, 1925, 2000.
189. Pischon, T. et al., Habitual dietary intake of n-3 and n-6 fatty acids in relation to inflammatory markers among US men and women, *Circulation*, 108, 155, 2003.
190. Araki, Y. et al., The dietary combination of germinated barley foodstuff plus Clostridium butyricum suppresses the dextran sulfate sodium-induced experimental colitis in rats, *Scand. J. Gastroenterol.*, 35, 1060, 2000.
191. Vega-Lopez, S. et al., Supplementation with omega3 polyunsaturated fatty acids and all-rac alpha-tocopherol alone and in combination failed to exert an anti-inflammatory effect in human volunteers, *Metabolism*, 53, 236, 2004.
192. Chuang, C.H. et al., Vitamin C and E supplements to lansoprazole-amoxicillin-metronidazole triple therapy may reduce the eradication rate of metronidazole-susceptible Helicobacter pylori infection, *Helicobacter*, 7, 310, 2002.

193. Harrison, S.A. et al., Vitamin E and vitamin C treatment improves fibrosis in patients with nonalcoholic steatohepatitis, *Am. J. Gastroenterol.*, 98, 2485, 2003.
194. Bennett, R.T. et al., Suppression of renal inflammation with vitamins A and E in ascending pyelonephritis in rats, *J. Urol.*, 161, 1681, 1999.
195. Ghezzi, P. and Ungheri, D., Synergistic combination of N-acetylcysteine and ribavirin to protect from lethal influenza viral infection in a mouse model, *Int. J. Immunopathol. Pharmacol.*, 17, 99, 2004.
196. Goudev, A. et al., Reduced concentrations of soluble adhesion molecules after antioxidant supplementation in postmenopausal women with high cardiovascular risk profiles — a randomized double-blind study, *Cardiology*, 94, 227, 2000.
197. Hwang, J., Hodis, H.N., and Sevanian, A., Soy and alfalfa phytoestrogen extracts become potent low-density lipoprotein antioxidants in the presence of acerola cherry extract, *J. Agric. Food Chem.*, 49, 308, 2001.
198. Cellini, L. et al., Inhibition of Helicobacter pylori by garlic extract (Allium sativum), *FEMS Immunol Med Microbiol.*, 13, 273, 1996.
199. Rovensky, J. et al., Treatment of experimental adjuvant arthritis with the combination of methotrexate and lyophilized Enterococcus faecium enriched with organic selenium, *Folia Microbiol (Praha)*, 47, 573, 2002.
200. Vinson, J.A. et al., Beneficial effects of a novel IH636 grape seed proanthocyanidin extract and a niacin-bound chromium in a hamster atherosclerosis model, *Mol. Cell Biochem.*, 240, 99, 2002.
201. Klivenyi, P. et al., Additive neuroprotective effects of creatine and cyclooxygenase 2 inhibitors in a transgenic mouse model of amyotrophic lateral sclerosis, *J. Neurochem.*, 88, 576, 2004.
202. Klivenyi, P. et al., Additive neuroprotective effects of creatine and a cyclooxygenase 2 inhibitor against dopamine depletion in the 1-methyl-4-phenyl-1,2,3,6-tetrahydropyridine (MPTP) mouse model of Parkinson's disease, *J. Mol. Neurosci.*, 21, 191, 2003.
203. Swamy, M.V. et al., Modulation of cyclooxygenase-2 activities by the combined action of celecoxib and decosahexaenoic acid: novel strategies for colon cancer prevention and treatment, *Mol. Cancer Ther.*, 3, 215, 2004.
204. Jodoin, J., Demeule, M., and Beliveau, R., Inhibition of the multidrug resistance P-glycoprotein activity by green tea polyphenols, *Biochim. Biophys. Acta.*, 1542, 149, 2002.

15

Food and Food–Drug Synergies: Role in Hypertension and Renal Disease Protection

Manuel T. Velasquez

CONTENTS

15.1 Introduction

Dietary therapy is an integral part of the management of many diseases or clinical disorders. In addition to providing the essential nutrients required for health and survival, the diet is often modified, either quantitatively or qualitatively, or both, for the purpose of correcting nutritional imbalances (deficiencies or excesses) and/or eliminating risk factors that are responsible for or associated with the disease process. However, an even greater possible value for dietary modifications is their potential for synergies that may provide greater benefits in disease prevention and treatment. This chapter presents an overview of the role of dietary factors in hypertension and chronic renal disease and examines the evidence for food and food–drug synergies in the treatment of these two common disorders.

15.2 Hypertension

15.2.1 General Considerations

Hypertension represents one of the most prevalent disorders in industrialized countries and affects about 1 billion people worldwide.[1] Hypertension is also the single most common cause of coronary artery disease, stroke, and chronic renal failure. In addition, it often coexists with other major risk factors, such as obesity, diabetes, and dyslipidemia, which further add to the burden of cardiovascular disease and chronic renal disease. Hypertension is a complex heterogeneous disorder that is thought to result from an interaction between genetic and environmental factors.[2,3] The heterogeneity of hypertension may reflect the multiplicity of factors involved in the regulation of blood pressure (BP). The BP level of a given individual may be viewed as the end result of a complex combination of genetic, physiological, biochemical, and structural factors that interact with each other and adapt to changes in the environment. Among the various environmental factors, diet has long been recognized as playing a substantial role in the pathogenesis of hypertension. Indeed, there is a large body of scientific evidence linking long-term changes in BP and the incidence of hypertension to dietary factors.

15.2.2 Dietary or Food Factors in Hypertension

Of all the dietary factors that have been linked to hypertension, sodium (salt) intake has been the most extensively studied. Experimental studies have shown that high sodium intake can induce hypertension in susceptible animals.[4] Data accumulated from epidemiological, cross-cultural, interventional, and animal studies over the past 50 years indicate that sodium intake is directly related to BP and that lowering sodium intake reduces BP. The largest epidemiological study yet conducted regarding the relation between sodium intake and BP was the International Study of Salt and Blood Pressure or the INTERSALT study.[5] This landmark study, which enrolled over 10,000 men and women 20 to 59 years of age from 52 population samples and 32 countries, convincingly showed that sodium intake (as measured by 24-h urinary sodium excretion) was positively related to BP level, age, and the prevalence of hypertension. Further analyses revealed that an increase of 100 mmol/d of sodium excretion was associated with an increase in systolic BP of 3 to 6 mmHg. Across populations, when individuals aged 25 years were compared with those aged 55 years, there was a 10 mmHg greater rise in systolic BP per 100 mmol/d higher sodium excretion with age. In addition to the INTERSALT study, a recent review[6] of the evidence collected from studies over the last decade about sodium intake–BP relationship concluded that "the evidence continues to demonstrate that higher sodium intake is associated with higher blood pressure levels and other cardiovascular conditions."

Potassium intake has also been implicated in the pathogenesis of hypertension. Population studies have shown that potassium intake is inversely related to BP, particularly among blacks.[7,8] In the INTERSALT study, a lower potassium intake was shown to be associated with higher BP. Potassium depletion has been reported to exacerbate hypertension,[9] even in the absence of changes in sodium intake.[10]

An inverse relationship between calcium intake and BP has been suggested in epidemiological and controlled clinical trials, but this relationship has not been consistently observed in all studies. A meta-analysis pooled from 22 clinical trials using calcium supplements of 0.4 to 2.2 g/d showed a decrease in systolic BP of 0.5 mmHg in normotensive persons and 1.7 mmHg in hypertensive persons.[11] Another meta-analysis of 42 randomized controlled trials using either dietary (dairy) or nondietary calcium supplements showed a reduction in BP of −1.44/0.84 mmHg.[12] Thus, calcium supplementation has only a minimal effect on BP, an effect too small to recommend its use for treating hypertension.

Studies on the relation between magnesium intake and BP have shown inconsistent results. A prospective analysis of a biracial cohort of 7,731 adult participants who were not hypertensive found no association between dietary magnesium intake and incident hypertension.[13] A meta-analysis of 20 randomized clinical trials that included both normotensive and hypertensive individuals showed that magnesium supplementation resulted in only a small overall reduction in BP.[14] However, other controlled clinical trials showed no significant effect of magnesium supplementation on BP.[15,16]

A role for other dietary factors in determining BP changes and the incidence of hypertension is also well documented in large population studies. For example, a prospective study of more than 40,000 women showed that intakes of cereals and meat were directly related to systolic BP, whereas intakes of fruits and vegetables were inversely related to systolic and diastolic pressures.[17] In addition, data from the National Health and Nutrition Examination Survey III (NHANES III), which included over 17,000 adults, showed that systolic BP was positively associated with higher dietary intake of protein and negatively associated with potassium intake.[18]

A more recent prospective cohort study of 1,710 middle-aged men reported a relation of several specific food groups to 7-year blood pressure change.[19] In this study, the average BP increase over the 7-year period was 1.9/0.3 mmHg per year. Beef, veal, lamb, and poultry intakes were noted to be directly related to a greater BP increase, whereas fruit and vegetable intakes were inversely related to BP increase. The systolic BP of men who consumed 14 to 42 cups of vegetables a month (0.5 to 1.5 cups/d) vs. less than 14 cups a month (less than 0.5 cups/d) was estimated to rise 2.8 mmHg less in 7 years (p <.01), whereas the systolic BP of men who consumed 14 to 42 cups of fruit a month versus less than 14 cups a month was estimated to increase 2.2 mmHg less in 7 years. These results suggest that diets higher in fruits and vegetables and lower in animal meats may prevent or delay the development of hypertension and reduce the incidence of overt hypertension.

The evidence for a role of dietary fat in hypertension is mixed. Experimental studies have shown that high fat intake can raise BP or induce hypertension in animals.[20,21] Observational studies in humans also indicate that saturated fat–enriched diets are positively associated with higher BP,[22] whereas diets rich in polyunsaturated fatty acids (PUFA) are negatively associated with BP.[23] However, other studies have found no such associations.[24,25] The source or type of dietary fat appears to have different effects on BP. In laboratory animals, a high saturated fat (lard) or polyunsaturated fat (corn oil) diet induces hypertension.[26] Dietary docosahexaenoic acid (DHA) and PUFA-rich diets with a reduced (n-6)/(n-3) ratio prevent the development of hypertension.[27,28] In a large population-based study of over 4,000 men and women, plasma concentrations of fatty acids associated with dietary saturated fat (16:0, 16:1, and 20:3n-6) were shown to be positively associated with BP, whereas the plasma concentration of polyunsaturated 18:2n-6 or linoleic acid was inversely associated with BP.[29]

Data regarding the role of dietary carbohydrates on BP are limited. Although a high intake of refined sugars can induce hypertension in experimental animals,[30] the role of these types of carbohydrates on BP in humans is uncertain. Contrary to findings in animals, the results of the multiple risk factor intervention trial (MRFIT) have shown that dietary starch, in addition to saturated fat and cholesterol, was positively associated with BP.[23]

15.2.3 Dietary Interventions in the Treatment of Hypertension

The antihypertensive efficacy of dietary sodium restriction is well established.[31] Blood pressure in some individuals is responsive ("salt-sensitive") to variations in sodium intake whereas in others it is not ("salt-resistant"). Such individual differences in salt sensitivity have been attributed to many factors, including age, race, obesity, plasma renin level, sympathetic nervous system activity, insulin resistance, presence of renal failure, and genetic factors. Despite these differences, most data from large randomized controlled trials show that moderate sodium reduction to approximately 100 mmol/d lowers BP by an average of 4.8/2.5 mmHg in hypertensive individuals.[32] The antihypertensive effect of sodium restriction appears to be greater in hypertensives with higher initial BP and in older individuals. In addition, the Trials of Hypertension Prevention (TOHP) study has shown that sodium restriction can prevent progression of high normal BP levels to overt hypertension.[33]

A large number of randomized, controlled trials have reported on the effects of increased potassium intake on BP in normotensive and hypertensive persons. A pooled analysis of 33 trials showed an overall BP reduction of 4.4/2.5 mmHg. Greater BP reductions were observed in hypertensives, blacks, and those consuming high intake of sodium.[34] In addition to its hypotensive effects, increased potassium intake may reduce the risk of stroke.[35]

Despite the reported associations between protein intake and BP, an antihypertensive effect of dietary protein has yet to be confirmed in prospective clinical trials, although there maybe subtle cardiovascular and renal effects unrelated to BP. One randomized controlled trial showed that switching from a typical omnivorous (meat) diet to an ovolactovegetarian diet resulted in a significant fall in systolic BP of about 5 mmHg in patients with mild untreated hypertension.[36] The reduction in BP was not associated with significant changes in urinary sodium or potassium excretion, or body weight. However, it is unclear whether this hypotensive effect is related to the increased fiber intake or a lower protein intake.

The effect of different levels and types of dietary fat on BP has been tested in many clinical trials. In two small trials, a reduction of total fat intake produced small but significant decreases in BP in healthy volunteers and hypertensive subjects.[37,38] Similar results have been observed in earlier studies using low-fat diets with high polyunsaturated to saturated (P/S) ratios.[39] However, one study found no BP effect of low fat diets with different fatty acid compositions.[40] In several randomized trials, fish oil supplementation was found to have a small, dose-dependent hypotensive effect. Two meta-analyses of these trials showed significant antihypertensive effects of 3 to 6 g/d of fish oil, averaging 3.0/1.5 mmHg fall in BP, particularly in hypertensive patients.[41,42] A smaller dose of fish oil, however, had no effect in hypertensive and normotensive persons. DHA appears to have a greater hypotensive effect than eicosapentamoire acid (EPA).[43] In a randomized crossover study, the addition of extra-virgin olive oil rich in monounsaturated fatty acid (MUFA) to a slightly low saturated fat diet lowered BP and reduced the need for antihypertensive medications in hypertensive patients.[44]

Few clinical trials have examined the effect of whole grains on BP. One small study of 43 adult men and women showed that consumption of a hypocaloric diet containing oats for over 6 weeks produced greater decreases in systolic BP than did a hypocaloric diet without oats.[45] In a randomized-controlled trial of 88 hypertensive men and women treated with antihypertensive drugs, consumption of whole oats lowered BP and reduced the need for antihypertensive medications.[46] One smaller study of 36 middle-aged and older men with high-normal to stage I hypertension did not show any significant effect on BP when 14 g/d of dietary fiber in the form of oat was added to their usual diet.[47]

Thus, it appears that clinical intervention trials that have tested certain nutrients or foods individually (namely, calcium, magnesium, plant protein, fat, or whole grains) have shown either a mild or insignificant BP-lowering effect in hypertensive individuals.

15.2.4 Diet Combinations and Food Synergy in the Treatment of Hypertension

There is ample evidence that suggests that a combination of different foods or food groups in a diet can produce additive or synergistic effects on BP reduction. Perhaps, the most compelling evidence of food synergy in BP reduction is provided by the results of the Dietary Approaches to Stop Hypertension (DASH) trial.[48] This was a multicenter randomized trial that compared a diet rich in fruits, vegetables, and low-fat dairy foods with a reduced content of dietary cholesterol, as well as saturated and total fat, and increased contents of potassium, calcium, magnesium, dietary fiber, and protein (DASH diet) to a "control" diet that is typical of dietary intake in the United States. A total of 459 adults participants (with systolic BP of less than 160 mmHg and diastolic BP of 80 to 95 mmHg) were randomly assigned to one of these two diets and were followed for a period of 8 weeks. The amounts of food were titrated to keep body weight constant. After only 2 weeks, the DASH diet lowered BP substantially and significantly, and was highly effective in mild hypertensives with a mean reduction of 11.6/5.3 mmHg. It was also effective in individuals with high normal BP producing a mean reduction of 3.5/2.2 mmHg. Among blacks with hypertension, the DASH diet reduced BP by 13.2/6.1 mmHg. A "fruits and vegetables" diet was included to test the effects of fruits and vegetables alone. This diet produced about half the BP effect of the DASH diet, showing at least that the blood pressure-lowering effect of the DASH diet can be attributed to this food group alone. A second study, the DASH-sodium trial, provides even stronger evidence for food synergy in BP reduction.[49] The DASH-Sodium trial was also a randomized trial that tested the combined effects on BP of the DASH diet and lower sodium intake. In this 16-week trial, 412 adult participants with a BP that ranged between 120 and 159 mmHg systolic and 80 to 95 mmHg diastolic were randomly assigned to either the DASH diet or the "control" diet. In addition, they were randomly given one of three levels of sodium intake: high (150 mmol/d); intermediate (100 mmol/d); or low (50 mmol/d) and the amount of food was titrated so that body weight was kept constant. Reduced sodium intake significantly lowered BP in a stepwise fashion in both the control and the DASH diets. Among participants assigned to the control diet, BP reductions were enhanced at progressively lower sodium intake, and the combined BP-lowering effects of reduced sodium intake and the DASH diet were substantially greater than either alone. Taken together, these two trials have clearly established the independent benefits of the DASH dietary pattern and dietary sodium restriction in the prevention and treatment of hypertension. In light of these findings, the Seventh Report of the Joint National Committee on the Prevention, Detection, and Evaluation, and Treatment of High Blood Pressure (JNC-7) has for the first time included the DASH combination diet as part of the initial nonpharmcologic treatment of hypertension.[50]

A similar dietary approach was used in an earlier smaller controlled trial by Little and co-workers in which a combination of low sodium, low fat, and high fiber diet was compared to the individual components of this diet in 196 hypertensive patients who were already on medications.[51] In this 8-week trial, high fiber diet alone had no significant effects on BP. Low sodium diet produced only a marginal decrease in systolic BP, whereas the low fat diet resulted in a small but significant decrease in seated diastolic BP and weight. The combination of the three diets, however, produced larger and highly significant decreases in both BP and body weight. These findings complement the results of the DASH-Sodium trial and further show that multiple dietary intervention in the form of a low sodium, low fat, high fiber diet, is more effective than any single dietary intervention in lowering BP in hypertensive patients. Such a dietary combination appears to be particularly useful in hypertensive patients on antihypertensive medication.

Other groups of investigators have used different combinations of diets and found similar additive or synergistic BP-lowering effect in hypertensive patients. In a factorial study of parallel design, Burke et al. tested the effects of a combination of protein and soluble fiber in 41 treated hypertensive subjects in whom protein or fiber intake, or both was increased against a background of a standardized diet low in both constituents.[52] At the end of 8-weeks of dietary intervention, the combination of protein and fiber produced significant additive effects on 24-h and awake systolic blood pressure (SBP), with a net reduction in 24-h SBP of 5.9 mmHg that was independent of age, gender, change in body weight, or urinary sodium and potassium. There were no significant interactions between protein and fiber. It should be noted that soy protein rather than animal protein was used in this study. Therefore, it is possible that the observed antihypertensive effect may be partly related to the lower animal meat in the diet. A similar additive effect on ambulatory BP reduction was demonstrated by Bao et al. in a factorial study using a combination of a daily meal of fish rich in n-3 fatty acids and a reduced-fat, energy-restricted diet for 16 weeks in overweight medication-treated hypertensive subjects.[53] In this study, daytime BP fell 6.0/3.0 mmHg with dietary fish alone, 5.5/2.2 mmHg with weight reduction alone, and 13.0/9.3 mmHg with fish and weight loss combined. The hypotensive effects were associated with decreases in heart rate. Given the magnitude of the BP reduction with the combination diet, it was suggested that the need for antihypertensive drugs might have been reduced in these patients.

15.2.5 Food–Drug Synergy in the Treatment of Hypertension

A number of clinical trials have demonstrated additive or synergistic effects on BP reduction with a combination of diet and antihypertensive drug treatment. Uusitupa et al.[54] evaluated the effects of moderate salt restriction alone and in combination with an angiotensin-converting enzyme (ACE) inhibitor cilazapril on office and ambulatory BP in 39 subjects with mild to moderate hypertension and showed additive effects of sodium restriction and ACE inhibition. In this trial, sodium restriction alone reduced office BP by about 7.1/2.8 mmHg and daytime BP 2.8/1.2 mmHg. The addition of cilazapril (2.5 mg/d) to sodium restriction further reduced office BP by 13.2/9.1 mmHg and daytime BP by 5.9/5.3 mmHg. The synergism between the low sodium diet and cilazapril may be related to a reactive increase in angiotensin II induced by sodium restriction, which is blunted by the inhibitory action of cilazapril on angiotensin II production. A study by Howe et al.[55] showed a similar additive antihypertensive effect when a low sodium diet was combined with fish oil in hypertensive patients treated with ACE inhibitors. In this study, four matched groups of 14 hypertensive patients taking either captopril or enalapril were assigned to one of four dietary treatments: low sodium (80 mmol/d) with fish oil (5 g of n-3 fatty acids/d); normal sodium (150 mmol/d) with fish oil; low sodium with olive oil; and normal sodium with olive oil. At the end of the 6-week period of intervention, BP was reduced in all treatment groups. There were no differences in BP reduction between the group taking fish oil and those taking olive oil. However, BP reduction was 4.2 mmHg greater in subjects on a low sodium diet than in subjects taking normal sodium. These data suggest that in hypertensive patients on stable treatment with ACE inhibitors, fish oil or olive oil can lower BP further, and that the hypotensive effect of ACE inhibitors is enhanced by sodium restriction.

A recent randomized trial of 55 hypertensive patients assessed the combined effects of the DASH diet and antihypertensive drug treatment with losartan, an angiotensin II receptor blocker.[56] Patients were randomly assigned to 8 weeks of controlled feeding with either a control diet or the DASH diet. Within each diet arm, losartan (50 mg daily) or a placebo was added for 4 weeks in a double-blind crossover fashion. A significant reduction in systolic ambulatory BP of 5.3 mmHg and a small insignificant change in diastolic BP were noted with the DASH diet alone, whereas no change in ambulatory BP was noted with the control diet. Losartan significantly reduced ambulatory BP by 6.7/1.5 mmHg on the control diet and to greater extent 11.7/6.9 mmHg on the DASH diet. BP reduction was particularly marked in African Americans. This is the first study to show that the DASH diet can enhance the hypotensive effect of a specific class of antihypertensive drug, angiotensin II receptor blocker.

Taken together, the results of prospective randomized trials indicate that certain dietary modifications or combinations of foods can produce additive or synergistic effects on BP reduction. In addition, certain types of diets or foods clearly enhance the efficacy of antihypertensive drugs. However, it is not clear from these studies which specific dietary component(s) in foods is responsible for the hypotensive effects of foods. It is likely that the ability of diets to effectively lower BP may result from the additive contributions of multiple components in foods. Although the mechanisms whereby foods or food constituents lower BP have not been defined in these studies, it is possible that multiple mechanisms or factors are also involved.

15.2.6 Biological Activities of Foods or Food Constituents Related to Protection against Hypertension

In considering the biological actions of foods or food constituents and their contribution to the overall effects on BP, few general comments merit special attention. The control of systemic arterial pressure is highly regulated and involves a complex interplay of multiple mechanisms that act to maintain arterial pressure at a constant level. Any dietary intervention or pharmacological agent that lowers BP by one or more mechanisms is countered by autoregulatory mechanisms that oppose or limit the action of the primary agent. Thus, the failure to detect a BP-lowering effect with any dietary intervention does not necessarily indicate inaction. On the other hand, a full additive or synergistic effect is likely to be seen if some of the foods and food constituents or a combination of foods or nutrients act by different but complementary vasodepressor mechanisms and at the same time inhibit corresponding mechanisms that try to raise BP. The interaction between food intake and BP response is further confounded by the fact that foods contain innumerable compounds or nutrients that may have multiple overlapping or antagonistic mechanisms of action, which make it difficult to disentangle the effect of any one nutrient on BP. Nevertheless, data gathered from mechanistic studies of foods and individual constituents of food and their effects on BP regulation may provide the groundwork for exploring other potential synergies between foods that could be beneficial in the prevention and treatment of hypertension and its complications.

Whole foods and certain constituents of foods have a remarkable variety of biologic activities, some of which may relate to their BP-lowering effects (Table 15.1). The DASH diet, itself, which contains a mixture of fruits, vegetables, and whole grains, has recently been shown to increase antioxidant capacity and lipid-induced oxidative stress (as measured by plasma F2-isoprostanes) in association with a decrease in BP in obese hypertensive

TABLE 15.1

Biological Activities of Foods or Food Components Related to Protection against Hypertension

1. Antioxidant action
2. Increased EDRF or nitric oxide production
3. Vascular smooth muscle relaxation
4. Reduced vascular reactivity to vasopressors
5. Increased arterial compliance
6. Inhibition of thromboxane-induced vasoconstriction

subjects.[57] The Mediterranean diet enriched with olive oil was shown to increase endothelium-dependent vasodilatation in hypercholesterolemic men.[58] A number of bioactive compounds commonly found in fruits, vegetables, and seeds, such as polyphenols, flavonoids, phytoestrogens, carotenoids, and tannins among others are known to have antioxidant activities. In addition, natural dietary polyphenolic compounds have been shown to cause endothelium-dependent vasorelaxation in rat thoracic aorta.[59] Flavonoids have also been shown to increase nitric oxide production[60] or induce vascular smooth muscle relaxation in the aorta.[61] Dietary soy, a rich source of phytoestrogens, has also been shown to reduce vasoconstrictor responses to angiotensin II or phenylephrine.[62] In studies of ovariectomized female spontaneously hypertensive rats (SHR), dietary soy also exerts a vasodepressor effect that appears to be mediated through the autonomic nervous system.[63] Similar vasodilator actions have also been reported for fish oils and individual fatty acids. For example, fish oils dose-dependently inhibit vasoconstriction of forearm resistance vessels in humans subjects[64] and improve arterial compliance in patients with non–insulin-dependent diabetes mellitus.[65] In animal experiments, the hypotensive effect of DHA was associated with enhanced arterial release of ATP.[66] Chronic exposure of cultured endothelial cells to EPA potentiates the release of endothelium-derived relaxing factor (EDRF).[67]

Thus, different types of foods and components in a food have complementary actions on vasomotor function and the endothelium that may partly account for some of the antihypertensive effects of different diets. Some of these vasodepressor actions alone or in combination may also enhance the effects of several antihypertensive drugs, which may explain the synergies between diet and antihypertensive drugs on BP reduction. One interesting study in a genetic animal model revealed that transgenic mice lacking the type 1 angiotensin II [AT1(1A)] receptor exhibited significantly greater decreases in BP when placed on a low-salt diet compared with their wild-type littermates, indicating that deletion of the AT(1A) receptor enhances BP sensitivity to changes in dietary salt intake.[68] This provides a molecular basis for the reported synergistic effect of salt restriction and angiotensin II blockade on BP reduction in hypertensive patients.

15.3 Chronic Kidney Disease (CKD)

15.3.1 General Considerations and Overview of Pathophysiology

CKD has become a major public health problem, and its incidence and prevalence are increasing worldwide with poor outcomes. There is an even greater prevalence of the early stages of CKD when the disease process may still be reversible or modifiable with therapy. Like hypertension, CKD is a major risk factor for the development of CVD. Microalbuminuria, the earliest sign of CKD, is also considered an independent predictor of CVD. Diabetes and hypertension represent the two leading causes of end-stage renal disease and account for the excess morbidity and mortality in patients with CKD.

The pathophysiological basis of CKD is multifactorial and includes a wide variety of disorders or conditions, each of which can cause progressive loss of renal function and nephron mass that culminates in end-stage renal disease (ESRD) (Figure 15.1). Often when renal function falls below a certain level, CKD progresses unrelentingly to ESRD, even when the original disease that initiated the renal injury is no longer active. The factors or mechanisms involved in the development and progression of CKD are complex. Several factors, including hyperglycemia, hypertension, hyperlipidemia, immunologic factors, genetic diseases, as well as diet and other environmental factors may initiate renal injury through various mechanisms that alter intrarenal hemodynamics, modulate cell growth and extracellular matrix (ECM) production, and induce inflammation and fibrogenesis. Increased glomerular capillary pressure or glomerular hypertension is considered the major stimulus that may initiate or perpetuate progressive renal injury in a variety of conditions, including diabetes, reduced renal mass, immune disorders, and aging. Glomerular cell proliferation and mesangial ECM accumulation are fundamental structural abnormalities in both human and experimental models of renal disease. A central pathological feature common to all forms of CKD is inflammation consisting of mononuclear cell infiltration in the renal interstitium. In addition, structural alterations in the tubules, such as tubular cell hypertrophy, and renal vascular abnormalities, including endothelial proliferation and smooth muscle hypertrophy, also occur in association with the glomerular and interstitial lesions. These structural changes are thought to be key events in the early stages of evolution of CKD and ultimately converge on common pathways that lead to progressive glomerular scarring, tubular atrophy, and interstitial fibrosis.

Several mediators, including activation of vasoactive peptides, growth factors, and cytokines; release of reactive oxygen species (ROS); and modulation of gene transcription have been suggested to play a role in renal disease progression. The vasoactive peptide angiotensin II is considered to be a central mediator of glomerular hemodynamic and nonhemodynamic changes associated with progressive renal damage. Angiotensin II also activates several growth factors, such as platelet-derived growth factor, trans-

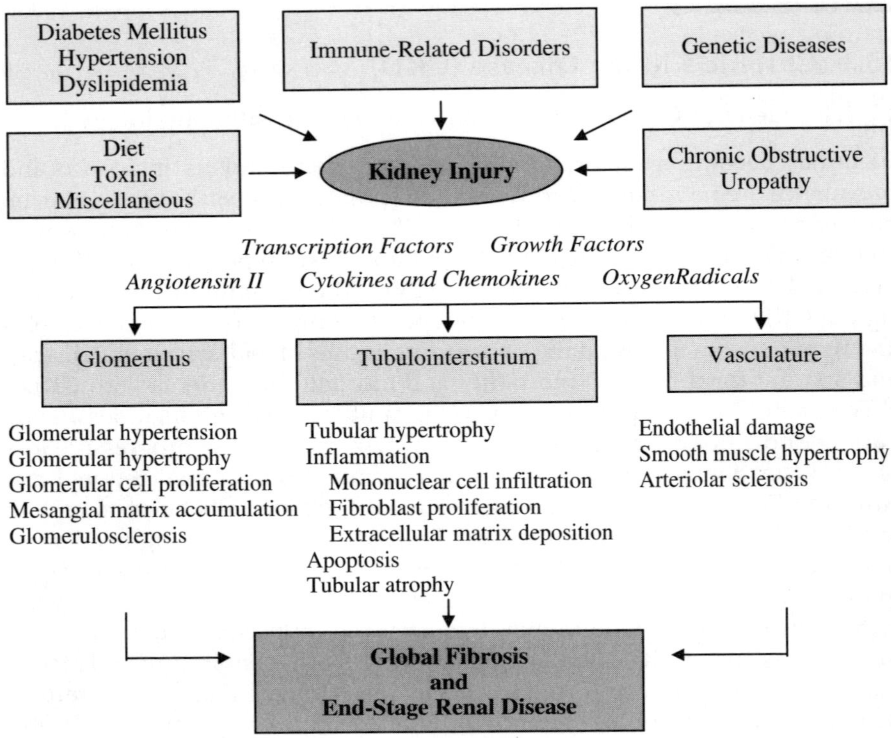

FIGURE 15.1
Pathophysiology of Chronic Kidney Disease.

forming growth factor-beta (TGF-β), and several adhesion molecules and chemoattractants, each of which are known to be involved in renal disease progression. Modulators of gene transcription, namely nuclear factor-kappa B (NF-κB) and activator protein-1 (AP-1), and ROS have emerged as important mediators of renal injury associated with inflammation and oxidative stress. In addition, local release of various cytokines stimulates fibroblast proliferation and matrix synthesis. The relative contribution of these mediators may vary depending upon the nature of the inciting stimulus, the underlying renal damage, and the stage of the evolution of CKD.

15.3.2 Dietary Factors in CKD

The role of various dietary factors in the progression of CKD has been investigated extensively in both animals and humans and described in detail in several reviews.[69–72]

Dietary salt is well documented to have detrimental effects on the kidney.[73] High sodium intake induces myocardial and renal fibrosis in normotensive as well as in hypertensive rats.[74] Epidemiological and interventional studies in humans also indicate that high salt intake increases the risk of cardiovascular and renal diseases, independently of other risk factors.[72] These effects of salt have been traditionally ascribed to the increased BP associated with high salt intake. However, recent evidence suggests dietary salt has direct effects on the kidney, independent of its ability to raise blood pressure.[75] For example, high salt intake has been shown to increase the production of TGF-β1 in aortic endothelium and kidney cortex of Sprague Dawley rats, an immediate and persistent effect that occurred without changes in systemic arterial pressure.[76] In studies of patients with type 2 diabetes, a high salt diet increased the fractional clearances of albumin and IgG, independent of the changes in BP.[77] In a recent study of 839 patients with essential hypertension, urinary sodium excretion was positively correlated with proteinuria, independently of gender, age, body mass index, and systolic BP.[78]

It has long been recognized that a high protein diet has deleterious effects on the kidney. In several animal models, high protein intake aggravates renal injury and accelerates the progression of CKD, whereas low protein intake produces the opposite effects.[69,70] In short term studies of humans, protein loading increases glomerular filtration rate (GFR) in normal volunteers,[79] as well as in diabetics[80] and in patients with chronic renal insufficiency.[81]

Experimental studies have demonstrated that dietary lipids can cause renal damage and increase progression of CKD.[82–85] In rats with experimental renal disease, high-fat and high-cholesterol diet induced or aggravated not only glomerular injury but also tubulointerstitial damage and inflammation, effects attributed to increased oxidant stress.[82,83] High dietary fat also was shown to increase renal cyst progression in a genetic rodent model of polycystic kidney disease[84] and induce severe glomerulosclerosis in hamsters.[85] A detrimental renal effect of a high intake of refined carbohydrates has also been demonstrated in experimental animals. Feeding high fructose or sucrose in rats has been shown to increase proteinuria and glomerular mesangial lesions and glomerulosclerosis in several rodent models.[86–88]

Collectively, these studies provide convincing evidence for the independent role of various dietary factors in the initiation and progression of CKD. High intakes of sodium, animal protein, saturated fat, or refined carbohydrates, all appear to induce or exacerbate renal damage in several experimental models of CKD. Given the multifactorial nature of CKD, each of these diets may produce synergistic renal deleterious effects with other pathogenic factors, such as diabetes, hypertension, immune disorders, and genetic factors and further accelerate renal disease progression, common in many forms of CKD.

15.3.3 Dietary Modifications in the Treatment of CKD

To date, there are no randomized clinical trials that have evaluated the long-term effects of sodium restriction on the progression of CKD in humans. In experimental studies, dietary salt restriction was shown to reduce proteinuria and prevent glomerular hypertrophy and sclerosis in subtotally nephrectomized rats with established renal disease.[89] In a short-term clinical trial, sodium restriction also reduced albuminuria in type 2 diabetic patients with normal blood pressure.[90] However, in view of the proven benefits of low sodium diet in hypertension and the strong evidence of increased risk of renal damage and cardiovascular disease associated with high sodium intake, dietary sodium restriction is generally accepted as an important preventive and therapeutic strategy in patients with CKD, particularly hypertensive or diabetic patients. Moreover, it is a common observation that patients with CKD often present with increased body fluid and sodium retention and, as a consequence, their BP is difficult to control without dietary salt restriction.

The effect of restriction of dietary protein intake in the progression of CKD has been studied in many clinical trials.[70] Most studies suggest that low protein diets have beneficial effects on CKD progression, although some studies do not show a clear benefit. The Modification of Diet in Renal Disease (MDRD) study the largest clinical trial to date on dietary protein restriction and CKD progression, failed to show a benefit in slowing the rate of decline in GFR with lower protein intakes.[91] However, a subsequent analysis showed a significant effect of the low protein diet in slowing progression, which was most evident in those patients with the highest rate of decline in GFR.[92] Additional evidence for a beneficial effect of dietary protein restriction on the progression of CKD is provided by the results of other randomized, controlled trials conducted in patients with diabetic and nondiabetic renal disease. A meta-analysis of these trials (including the MDRD trial) showed that dietary protein restriction was effective in delaying renal disease progression and that the overall risk of renal failure or death was reduced with low protein diet, as compared with nonrestricted protein intake.[93]

Evidence has emerged that changing the source or type of dietary protein may have a beneficial effect on renal function and renal disease.[94,95] In several animal models of CKD, consumption of soybean and soy-based food products has been shown to limit or reduce proteinuria and renal pathological damage, effects that are not attributable to changes in the level of protein or caloric intake.[94–97] In addition to soybeans, other plant seeds, particularly flaxseed, have also been shown to have similar protective effects on the kidney in animals with various forms of CKD.[98–101] In studies of humans with various types of CKD, soy protein also appears to moderate proteinuria and preserve renal function.[102–104] A similar beneficial renal effect has also been reported with dietary flaxseed supplementation in patients with lupus nephritis.[105] However, most of these clinical studies are limited by the relatively short duration of the dietary interventions and the inclusion of a small number of patients. Larger prospective randomized trials are needed to confirm whether soy protein or flaxseed provide long-term benefits in patients with CKD.

Experimental and clinical studies have also shown a beneficial effect of dietary fatty acids on the progression of CKD.[106] Dietary fatty acid or fish oil supplementation has been shown to reduce proteinuria and minimize glomerular and tubulointerstitial damage in several animal models with various types of renal disease, such as salt-loaded stroke-prone spontaneously hypertensive rats,[107] obese Zucker rats,[108] and murine models of lupus nephritis.[109] In a multicenter, placebo-controlled, randomized trial, fish oil supplementation significantly reduced renal disease progression in patients with IgA nephropathy, particularly those with moderately advanced disease.[110]

13.3.4 Food Synergy in the Treatment of CKD

Despite the numerous reports of a beneficial effect of different diets or foods on CKD, there have been only a few studies that have tested a combination of diet or foods for possible synergistic effects on renal disease reduction. In a recently well conducted randomized trial, Facchini and Saylor[111] evaluated the effect of a carbohydrate-restricted, low-iron-available, polyphenol-enriched (CR-LIPE) diet in 191 patients with type 2 diabetes with reduced renal function and proteinuria. In this study, patients were randomized to either a CR-LIPE diet consisting of a reduced carbohydrate (50% less from the previous level of intake) but enriched with iron-poor white meats (poultry and fish) and other proteins (dairy, eggs, and soy) or a standard protein-restricted (0.8 g/kg) diet, isocaloric for ideal body weight maintenance. Over a mean follow-up of 3.9 years, doubling of serum creatinine was significantly less (21%) in patients on CR-LIPE than in control patients on the standard diet (39%). Similarly, renal replacement therapy and mortality occurred less (20%) in CR-LIPE patients than in control patients (39%). Thus, the CR-LIPE combination diet was 40 to 50% more effective than standard protein restriction in delaying the rate of renal function loss and reducing all-cause mortality in diabetic patients with nephropathy. These effects were independent of gender, BP, hemoglobin A_{1c}, and other predictors of progression, and were more apparent in individuals with initially high serum creatinine levels.

Robinson et al.[112] evaluated the effects of two types of fish oil diet containing different mixtures of fatty acids in the (NZB × NZW) F_1 mouse, a murine model for human systemic lupus erythematosus. This mouse strain develops progressive autoimmune renal disease usually at about 5 months of age and fatally succumbs to renal failure at 6 to 12 months of age. Mice were each provided with a diet containing ethyl esters of two purified n-3 fatty acids, eicosapentaenoic acid (EPA-E) and docosahexaenoic acid (DHA-E), a refined fish oil triglycerides (FO), which contained 55% n-3 fatty acids, or beef tallow (BT), which contained no n-3 fatty acids. Diets were given before the onset of overt renal disease at age 22 weeks, and continued thereafter for 14 weeks. Diets containing 10% FO, 10% EPA-E, or 6 or 10% DHA-E attenuated the severity of renal disease compared with the BT diet, whereas diets containing either 3 or 6% EPA-E or 3% DHA-E were less effective. Moreover, the two diets containing 3:1 mixtures of EPA-E and DHA-E alleviated the renal disease to a greater extent than expected for either of these fatty acids given singly, indicating that the renal protective effects of fish oil was related to the synergistic effects of at least two n-3 fatty acids.

Using the same animal model, Jolly et al.[113] studied the long-term effects of combining a fish oil diet with food restriction in a factorial design. In this study, female (NZB $\times$ NZW) F_1 mice were assigned to four different types of diet: 5 g/100 g corn oil, *ad libitum* consumption (CO/AL); 5 g/100 g corn oil, 40% food restricted (CO/FR); 5 g/100 g fish oil + 0.5 g/100 g corn oil, *ad libitum* consumption (FO/AL); and 5 g/100 g fish oil + 0.5 g/100 g corn oil 40% food restricted (FO/FR). In two of the four dietary groups, e.g., FO/AL and FO/FR, fish oil enriched with n-3 fatty acids was substituted for corn oil. However, a smaller amount of corn oil (0.5/100 g of diet) was added to these two fish oil diets as a source of linoleic acid to prevent essential fatty acid deficiency. All diets contained essentially similar amounts of casein, dextrose, cornstarch, oil, cellulose, minerals, and vitamin mixtures. Animals were provided each diet and studied beginning at 5 months of age until mice were sacrificed at 8 months of age. Mice fed the FO/AL diet had an extended life span of 345 days compared to mice fed the CO/AL diet that had an average life span of 242 days. Furthermore, life span was extended maximally to 645 days in mice fed the FO/FR compared with mice fed the CO/FR diet that had a life span of 494 days. The combination of dietary FO and FR was far more effective than either treatment individually in prolonging their survival. Additionally, mice fed both CO/FR and FO/FR had less pronounced renal pathological lesions, as well as suppressed renal cytokine levels (interferon g, interleukins-10 and 12, and tumor necrosis factor-alpha [TNF-α]) and lower NF-κB levels. The suppression of cytokine levels appears to be more pronounced in mice fed FO/FR. Overall, these data suggest that FO/FR is much more effective at inhibiting inflammatory disease in mice with autoimmune renal disease and that the renal protective effect appears to be related to suppression of transcription factor NF-κB and inflammatory cytokines.

15.3.5 Food–Drug Synergy in the Treatment of CKD

Several studies in humans and animals have documented additive or synergistic effects of a combination of diet and drugs in the treatment of CKD. Houlihan et al.[114] examined the effects of dietary sodium restriction (80 to 85 mmol/d) on the efficacy of angiotensin II receptor blocker losartan in 20 hypertensive subjects with type 2 diabetes mellitus and urinary albumin excretion. In this study, the subjects were randomized to losartan (50 mg/d) or placebo. Drug therapy was given in two 4-week phases separated by a washout period. In the last 2 weeks of each phase, patients were then randomly assigned to low- or regular sodium diets. In the placebo group, there were no significant changes in 24-h ambulatory blood pressure (ABP) and urinary albumin to creatinine ratio (ACR) between regular and low-sodium diet. However, in the losartan group, a low-salt diet compared with a normal sodium diet further lowered ABP by about 9.7/5.5 mmHg and substantially reduced ACR by about 29%, indicating additive effects of the combination of low sodium diet and losartan in lowering both BP and proteinuria.

Along similar lines, Ganesvoort et al.[115] evaluated the effects of single treatment with enalapril (10 mg once daily), low-protein diet (LPD, 50% reduction in protein intake), and the combination of both in 14 patients with nondiabetic renal disease with overt proteinuria. Baseline measurements were performed while patients were on a normal protein diet (NPD). In one group (group A), the effects of a LPD were first examined. Thereafter, the effects of addition of ACE inhibitor to LPD were investigated. In the second group (group B), the combination therapy was reversed, that is, first the effects of ACE inhibitor were studied, thereafter, the effects of addition of LPD to ACE inhibitor were investigated. Each treatment lasted for 2 months. LPD reduced proteinuria by 17% in patients without ACE inhibitor treatment (group A) and similarly by 19% in patients with ACE inhibitor treatment (group B). However, the ACE inhibitor reduced proteinuria by 32% during the NPD (group B) and similarly by 43% during the LPD (group A). A similar additive antiproteinuric effect of protein restriction and enalapril has also been observed by Hutchison et al.[116] in studies of rats with passive Heymann nephritis.

Additionally, a study by Peters et al.[117] further showed a greater benefit on renal disease reduction when a low protein diet was combined with both an ACE inhibitor and an angiotensin II receptor blocker in a rat model of experimental glomerulonephritis. In this study, a single treatment with the ACE inhibitor enalapril, angiotensin II receptor blocker losartan, or low protein diet significantly reduced glomerular TGF-β production by about 45% in these animals. However, when these two drugs were combined with a low-protein diet, a greater reduction in pathological TGF- expression was observed with of a total of 65% reduction for enalapril and 60% for losartan. The reduction in TGF-β expression was associated with decreased proteinuria, glomerular matrix accumulation, and overproduction of fibronectin and PAI-1. Since maximal pharmacological doses of enalapril and losartan were used in this study, which presumably induced complete angiotensin II blockade, it was suggested that the additive effects of dietary protein restriction might be related to mechanisms other than inhibition of the renin–angiotensin system.

15.3.6 Biological Actions of Foods or Food Constituents Related to Renal Disease Protection

There are several other physiological or biological actions of foods or food constituents that may relate to their protective effects on the kidney (Table 15.2). These have been reviewed in detail in several publications.[70,95,118–120] Several constituents in foods, notably, flavonoids in fruits and vegetables,

TABLE 15.2

Biological Activities of Foods or Food Components Related to Protection of the Kidney

1. Reduction of intraglomerular pressure
2. Inhibition of mesangial cell growth and proliferation
3. Inhibition of protein tyrosine kinases and DNA topoisomerases I and II
4. Suppression of angiogenesis
5. Modulation of TGF-β and other growth factors
6. Inhibition of cytokine-mediated activation of transcription factors
7. Inhibition of platelet activating factor and platelet aggregation
8. Modulation of immune function

phytoestrogens in soybeans and flaxseed, and fatty acids in fish oils, all have been reported to have antioxidative, antiproliferative, and antiinflammatory activities that may explain their protective effects in various types of CKD. In particular, the biological actions of isoflavones in soybeans and lignans in flaxseed have been well characterized both *in vitro* and *in vivo*. These include inhibition of cell growth and proliferation via estrogen-mediated mechanisms or nonestrogen-mediated pathways through inhibition of protein tyrosine kinases and DNA topoisomerases I and II, modulation of growth factors involved in ECM synthesis and fibrogenesis, inhibition of cytokine-induced activation of transcription factors, inhibition of angiogenesis, suppression of platelet activating factor and platelet aggregation, and immunomodulatory activity.

Similarly, dietary fatty acids have a broad spectrum of biological actions, many of which also affect cell proliferation, inflammation, and immune function. Fish oil has been shown to inhibit mesangial cell proliferation *in vitro* and *in vivo*.[121] Dietary fatty acids also inhibit neutrophil and monocyte chemotaxis, and reduce leukocyte inflammatory potential and leukotriene production. Among the fatty acids, the n-3 fatty acids (particularly EPA and DHA from fish oil) appear to have the greatest antiinflammatory and immunomodulatory activities, with n-6 fatty acids being intermediate, followed by monounsaturated fatty acids (-linolenic acid). Other reported properties of n-3 FA include modulation of endothelial activation, reduction of vascular adhesion molecules, and inhibition of platelet and mesangial production of thromboxane A_2, a powerful vasoconstrictor and inducer of platelet activation. EPA was recently shown to suppress TNF-α production and expression induced by lipopolysaccharide in human monocytes, an effect that was associated with inhibition of NF-κB activation.[122] A novel action of EPA is inhibition of detachment-induced apoptosis or "anoikis" in endothelial cells, an action that may preserve vascular integrity against oxidative stress.[123]

In summary, several different diets and food constituents appear to have favorable biological actions on kidney function and structure that may explain some of their protective effects in various types of CKD. One or more components in foods may have a beneficial effect singly, additively, or synergistically with other active components.

15.4 Diet and Food Safety Issues

Current dietary guidelines recommend moderate salt restriction of about 6 g/d (2.4 g or 110 mmol of sodium/d) for both prevention and treatment of hypertension. Such moderate reduction has been shown to be generally safe, easily achieved, and free from adverse effects. However, an educational effort is often required to successfully maintain long-term compliance to salt restriction and avoid potential adverse reactions. There have been reports of increased total and low-density cholesterol levels, plasma renin, plasma catecholamines, and insulin resistance in some trials of sodium restriction, but these effects occur only in the acute setting when sodium intake is severely reduced.[122–126] Severe sodium depletion resulting in profound hypotension may occasionally occur, particularly in elderly individuals and patients with impaired renal function in whom the renal ability to conserve sodium in response to sodium restriction is reduced.

High intakes of complex carbohydrates may have unfavorable effects on glucose and lipid metabolism. Diets with high glycemic index may worsen postprandial hyperglycemia and glucose control, particularly in subjects with impaired glucose tolerance or diabetes. Therefore, foods with low glycemic index are preferred in such individuals.

Even though soybeans and soy-based foods have been consumed by humans for decades, questions have been raised regarding their safety. Because of their structural similarity to endogenous estrogens, soy isoflavones may have estrogenlike activities that may have a negative impact on reproductive organs, endocrine function, cancer, and other aspects of human health. However, there are no long-term studies that consumption of large amounts of soy isoflavones in the diet produce deleterious effects in humans.[127]

There are some reports suggesting that fish oils or PUFAs may have adverse effects on lipid metabolism, glucose control, and hemostasis.[128] These include increased *in vivo* lipid peroxidation, worsening of glycemic control in diabetic subjects, and increased bleeding diathesis. Such effects, however, have been observed with very high intakes of fish oils or PUFAs, doses that are much larger than those currently recommended for general human consumption.

Although there are reported associations between protein intake and BP in populations, there is no conclusive evidence that high protein diets cause adverse effects in hypertensive individuals. However, caution is advised regarding diets high in animal meat in individuals with underlying CKD, since such diet may have detrimental effects on renal function.

Concerns have been raised regarding the nutritional safety of protein-restricted diets in patients with chronic renal failure with the argument that such diets may cause a negative nitrogen protein balance and increase the risk of malnutrition.[129] However, the results from the MDRD study indicate that the low protein regimens were not associated with any signs of malnutrition or higher rates of mortality.[130] In addition, a review of the evidence from several controlled clinical trials in CKD patients have shown the adequacy of low protein diets (0.6 g/kg/d) or supplemented very low protein diets (0.3 g/kg/d) in maintaining nutrition.[131] Thus, protein-restricted diets, rather than causing malnutrition, tend to prevent it, provided that the diet contains sufficient amounts of calories and essential amino acids.

One of the most serious adverse effects of both diet and drug therapy in CKD is hyperkalemia. This side effect is likely to be encountered in patients with advanced renal failure in whom potassium excretion is impaired. The potential for hyperkalemia may be increased in such patients who are eating potassium-rich foods or are treated with ACE inhibitors or angiotensin II-receptor blockers, since these agents can further reduce potassium excretion as a result of their inhibitory effects on aldosterone secretion. However, this complication can be avoided in the clinical setting with appropriate dietary education and close monitoring of the serum potassium level and renal function.

15.5 Conclusions

In conclusion, a large body of evidence indicates that diet plays an important role in the pathogenesis of both hypertension and CKD. Diet or foods in a diet assume an even greater significance in the treatment of these two common disorders in that certain dietary modifications or specific food combinations can produce additive or synergistic effects on both BP reduction and renal disease protection. In addition, certain diets or specific foods alone or in combination also enhance the hypotensive and renal protective effects of antihypertensive drugs, and thus provide additional benefits in the treatment of hypertension and CKD. Dietary sodium restriction and diets rich in fruits and vegetables, low in saturated and total fat, and high in PUFAs (fish oil) appear to have beneficial effects on BP and renal disease reduction. However, it remains unclear which specific dietary components in foods or diet are responsible for their beneficial effects on BP and the kidney. Several potential mechanisms whereby foods or their constituents may lower BP and protect the kidney have been discussed and include a wide spectrum of physiological and biological activities that favorably affect the endothelium, vasomotor function, as well as kidney function and structure. Synergism between foods may stem from the additive effects of several components that have different but complementary mechanisms of actions on BP reduction and renal protection, which may account for their effectiveness in controlling hypertension and slowing disease progression in various types of CKD. It is possible that there may be other food synergies yet to be discovered that may be useful for both hypertension and CKD. More research is needed to explore other innovative food and food–drug combinations for potential synergies in the treatment of hypertension and CKD.

References

1. World Health Report, Reducing risks, promoting healthy life,: World Health Organization, Geneva, Switzerland, 2002. http://www.who.int/whr/2002.
2. Yamori, Y. et al., Gene-environment interaction in hypertension, stroke and atherosclerosis in experimental models and supportive findings from a world-wide cross-sectional epidemiological survey: a WHO-cardiac study, *Clin. Exp. Pharmacol. Physiol. Suppl.*, 20, 43, 1992.
3. Pauzova, S., Tremblay, J., and Hamet, P., Gene-environment interactions in hypertension, *Curr. Hypertens. Rep.*, 1, 42, 1999.
4. Tobian, L., Lessons from animal models that relate to human hypertension, *Hypertension*, 17(Suppl. I), I-52, 1991.
5. Intersalt Cooperative Research Group. Intersalt: an international study of electrolyte excretion and blood pressure: results for 24-hour urinary sodium and potassium excretion, *Br. Med. J.*, 297, 319, 1988.
6. Chobanian, A.V. et al., National Heart, Lung, and Blood Institute Workshop on Sodium and Blood Pressure: a critical review of current scientific evidence, *Hypertension*, 35, 858, 2000.
7. He, J. and Whelton, P.K., What is the role of dietary sodium and potassium in hypertension target organ injury, *Am. J. Med. Sci.*, 317, 152, 1999.
8. Morris, R.C., Jr. et al., Normotensive salt sensitivity. Effects of race and dietary potassium, *Hypertension*, 33, 18, 1999.
9. Khrisna, G.G. and Kapoor, S.C., Potassium depletion exacerbates essential hypertension, *Ann. Intern. Med.*, 157, 77, 1991.
10. Coruzzi, P. et al., Potassium depletion and salt sensitivity in essential hypertension, *J. Clin. Endocrinol. Metab.* 86, 2857, 2001.
11. Allender, P.S. et al., Dietary calcium and blood pressure: a meta-analysis of randomized clinical trials, *Ann. Intern. Med.*, 124, 825, 1996.
12. Griffith, L.E. et al., The influence of dietary and nondietary calcium supplementation on blood pressure, *Am. J. Hypertens.* 12, 84, 1999.
13. Peacock, J.M. et al., Relationship of serum and dietary magnesium to incident hypertension: Atherosclerosis Risk in Communities (ARIC) Study, *Ann. Epidemiol.* 9, 159, 1999.
14. Jee, S.H. et al., The effect of magnesium supplementation on blood pressure: a meta-analysis of randomized clinical trials, *Am. J. Hypertens.* 15, 691, 2002.
15. Yamamoto, M.E. et al., Lack of blood pressure effect with calcium and magnesium supplementation in adults with high-normal blood pressure: results from Phase I of the Trials of Hypertension Prevention (TOHP), *Ann. Epidemiol.* 5, 96, 1995.
16. Sacks, F.M. et al., Effect on blood pressure of potassium, calcium and magnesium in women with low habitual intake, *Hypertension*, 31, 131, 1998.
17. Ascherio, A. et al., Prospective study of nutritional factors, blood pressure, and hypertension among US women, *Hypertension*, 27, 1065, 1996.

18. Hajjar, I.M. et al., Impact of diet on blood pressure and age-related changes in blood pressure in the US population, *Arch. Int. Med.*, 161, 589, 2001.
19. Miura, K. et al., Relation of vegetable, fruit, and meat intake to 7-year blood pressure change in middle-aged men: The Chicago Western Electric Study, *Am. J. Epidemiol.* 159, 572, 2004.
20. Langley-Evans, S.C. et al., Influence of dietary fats upon systolic blood pressure in rats, *Int. J. Food Sci. Nutr.*, 47, 417, 1996.
21. Wilde, D.W. et al., High-fat diet elevates blood pressure and cerebrovascular muscle Ca^{2+} current, *Hypertension*, 35, 832, 2000.
22. Salonen, J.T. et al., Blood pressure, dietary fats, and antioxidants, *Am. J. Clin. Nutr.*, 48, 1226, 1988.
23. Stamler, J. et al., Relationship to blood pressure of combinations of dietary macronutrients: findings of the Multiple Risk Factor Intervention Trial (MRFIT), *Circulation*, 94, 2417, 1996.
24. Ascherio, A. et al., A prospective study of nutritional factors and hypertension among US men, *Circulation*, 86, 1475, 1992.
25. Witteman, J.C. et al., A prospective study of nutritional factors and hypertension among US women, *Circulation* 80, 1320, 1989.
26. Kaufman, L.N., Peterson, M.M., and Smith, S.M., Hypertensive effect of polyunsaturated fat, *Metabolism*, 43, 1, 1994.
27. Kimura, S., et al., Dietary docosahexaenoic acid (22:6n-3) prevents the development of hypertension in SHRSP, *Clin. Exp. Pharmacol. Physiol.* 22 (Suppl. 1), S306, 1995.
28. de Wilde M.C., et al., Dietary fatty acids alter blood pressure, behavior and brain membrane composition of hypertensive rats, *Brain Res.*, 988, 9, 2003.
29. Grimsgaard, S. et al., Plasma saturated and linoleic fatty acids are independently associated with blood pressure, *Hypertension*, 34, 478, 1999.
30. Preuss, H.G. et al., Sugar-induced blood pressure elevations over the life span of three substrains of Wistar rats, *Am. J. Clin. Nutr.* 17, 36, 1998.
31. Weinberger, M.H. et al., Dietary sodium restriction as adjunctive treatment of hypertension, *JAMA*, 259, 2561, 1988.
32. Cutler, J.A., Follmann, D., and Allender, P.S., Randomized trials of sodium restriction: an overview, *Am. J. Clin. Nutr.*, 64(Suppl), 643S, 1997.
33. Trials of Hypertension Prevention Collaborative Research Group: The effects of nonpharmacologic interventions on blood pressure of persons with high normal levels: Results of the Trials of Hypertension Prevention, Phase I, *JAMA*, 267, 1213, 1992.
34. Whelton, P.K. et al., Effects of oral potassium on blood pressure: meta-analysis of randomized controlled clinical trials, *JAMA*, 277, 1624, 1997.
35. Bazzano, L.A. et al., Dietary potassium intake and risk of stroke in US men and women. National Health and Nutrition Examination Survey I Epidemiologic Follow-up Study, *Stroke*, 32, 1473, 2001.
36. Margetts, B.M. et al., Vegetarian diet in mild hypertension: a randomized controlled trial, *Br. Med. J.*, 293, 1468, 1986.
37. Rantala, M. et al., Apolipoprotein E phenotype and diet-induced alteration of blood pressure, *Am. J. Clin. Nutr.*, 65, 543, 1997.
38. Straznicky, N.E. et al., Hypotensive effect of low-fat, high-carbohydrate diet can be independent of changes in plasma insulin concentrations, *Hypertension*, 34, 580, 1999.

39. Iacono, J.M., Dougherty, R.M., and Puska, P., Dietary fat and blood pressure in humans, *Klin. Wochenschr.*, 68(Suppl.) 20, 23, 1990.
40. Aro, A. et al., Lack of effect on blood pressure by low fat diets with different fatty acid compositions, *J. Hum. Hypertens.*, 12, 383, 1998.
41. Morris, M.C., Sacks, F., and Rosner, B., Does fish oil lower blood pressure? A meta-analysis of controlled trials, *Circulation*, 88, 523, 1993.
42. Appel, L.J. et al., Does supplementation of diet with "fish oil" reduce blood pressure? A meta-analysis of controlled clinical trials, *Arch. Intern. Med.*, 153, 1429, 1993.
43. Mori, T.A. et al., Differential effects of eicosapentaenoic acid docosahexaenoic acid on vascular reactivity of the forearm circulation in hyperlipidemic, overweight men, *Circulation*, 102, 1264, 2000.
44. Ferrara, L.A. et al., Olive oil and reduced need for antihypertensive medications, *Arch. Intern. Med.*, 160, 837, 2000.
45. Saltzman, E. et al., An oat-containing hypocaloric diet reduces systolic blood pressure and improves lipid profile beyond effects of weight loss in men and women, *J. Nutr.*, 131, 1465, 2001.
46. Pins, J.J. et al., Do whole-grain oat cereals reduce the need for antihypertensive medications and improve blood pressure control, *J. Fam. Pract.*, 51, 353, 2002.
47. Davy, B.M. et al., Oat consumption does not affect resting casual and ambulatory 24-h arterial blood pressure in men with high-normal blood pressure to stage I hypertension, *J. Nutr.*, 132, 394, 2002.
48. Appel, L.J. et al., A clinical trial of the effects of dietary patterns on blood pressure, *N. Engl. J. Med.*, 336, 1117, 1997.
49. Sacks, F.M. et al., Effects on blood pressure of reduced dietary sodium and the dietary approaches to stop hypertension (DASH) diet, *N. Engl. J. Med.*, 344, 3, 2001.
50. Chobanian, A.V. et al., The Seventh Report of the Joint National Committee on Prevention, Detection, Evaluation, and Treatment of High Blood Pressure: the JNC 7 report, *JAMA*, 289, 2560, 2003.
51. Little, P. et al., A controlled trial of a low sodium, low fat, high fibre diet in treated hypertensive patients: the efficacy of multiple dietary intervention, *Postgrad. Med. J.*, 66, 1990.
52. Burke, V. et al., Dietary protein and soluble fiber reduce ambulatory blood pressure in treated hypertensives, *Hypertension*, 38, 821, 2001.
53. Bao, D.Q. et al., Effects of dietary fish and weight reduction on ambulatory blood pressure in overweight hypertensives, *Hypertension*, 32, 710, 1998.
54. Uusitupa, M. et al., Effects of moderate salt restriction alone and in combination with cilazapril on office and ambulatory blood pressure, *J. Hum. Hypertens.*, 10, 319, 1996.
55. Howe, P.R. et al., Effect of sodium restriction and fish oil supplementation on BP and thrombotic risk factors in patients treated with ACE inhibitors, *J. Hum. Hypertens.*, 8, 43, 1994.
56. Conlin, P.R. et al., The DASH diet enhances the blood pressure response to losartan in hypertensive patients, *Am. J. Hypertens.*, 16, 337, 2003.
57. Lopes, H.F et al., DASH diet lowers blood pressure and lipid-induced oxidative stress in obesity, *Hypertension*, 41, 422, 2003.
58. Fuentes, F. et al., Mediterranean and low-fat diets improve endothelial function in hypercholesterolemic men, *Ann. Intern. Med.*, 134, 1115, 2001.

59. Andriambeloson, E. et al., Natural dietary polyphenolic compounds cause endothelium-dependent vasorelaxation in rat thoracic aorta, *J. Nutr.* 128, 2324, 1998.
60. Benito, S. et al., A flavonoid-rich diet increases nitric oxide production in rat aorta, *Br. J. Pharmacol.* 135, 910, 2002.
61. Ajay, M., Gilani, A.U., and Mustafa, M.R., Effects of flavonoids on vascular smooth muscle of the isolated rat thoracic aorta, *Life Sci.* 74, 603, 2003.
62. Martin, D.S. et al., Pressor responsiveness to angiotensin in soy-fed spontaneously hypertensive rats, *Can. J. Physiol. Pharmacol.*, 80, 1180, 2002.
63. Martin, D.S. et al., Dietary soy exerts an antihypertensive effect in spontaneously hypertensive female rats, *Am. J. Physiol.Regul. Integr. Comp. Physiol.*, 281, R553, 2001.
64. Chin, J.P.F. et al., Fish oils dose-dependently inhibit vasoconstriction of forearm resistance vessels in humans, *Hypertension*, 21, 22, 1993.
65. McVeigh, G.E. et al., Fish oil improves arterial compliance in non-insulin dependent diabetes mellitus, *Arterioscler. Thromb.*, 14, 1425, 1994.
66. Hashimoto, M. et al., The hypotensive effect of docosahexaenoic acid is associated with enhanced release of ATP from the caudal artery of aged rats, *J. Nutr.*, 129, 70, 1999.
67. Boulanger, C et al., Chronic exposure of cultured endothelial cells to eicosapentaenoic acid potentiates the release of endothelium-derived relaxing factor(s), *Br. J. Pharmacol.*, 99, 176, 1990.
68. Mangrum, A.J., Gomez, R.A., and Norwood, V.F., Effects of AT1(1A) receptor deletion on blood pressure and sodium excretion during altered dietary salt intake, *Am. J. Physiol. Renal Physiol.*, 283, F447, 2002.
69. Brenner, B.M., Meyer, T.W., and Hostetter, T.H., Dietary protein intake and the progressive nature of kidney disease: the role of hemodynamically mediated glomerular injury in the pathogenesis of progressive glomerular sclerosis of aging, renal ablation, and intrinsic renal disease, *N. Engl. J. Med.*, 307, 652, 1982.
70. Klahr, S., Buerkert. J., and Purkerson, M.L., Role of dietary factors in the progression of chronic renal disease, *Kidney Int.*, 24, 579, 1983.
71. Schreiner, G.F. and Klahr, S., Diet and kidney disease: the role of dietary fatty acids, *Proc. Soc. Exp. Biol. Med.*, 197, 1, 1991.
72. Boero, R., Pignataro, A., and Quarello, F., Salt intake and kidney disease, *J. Nephrol.*, 15, 225, 2002.
73. de Wardener, H.E. and MacGregor, G.A., Harmful effects of dietary salt in addition to hypertension, *J. Hum. Hypertens.*, 16, 213, 2002.
74. Yu, H.C.M. et al., Salt induces myocardial and renal fibrosis in normotensive and hypertensive rats, *Circulation*, 98, 2621, 1998.
75. Sanders, P.W., Salt intake, endothelial cell signaling, and progression of kidney disease, *Hypertension*, 43, 142, 2004.
76. Ying, W-Z. and Sanders, P.W., Dietary salt modulates renal production of transforming growth factor-β in rats, *Am. J. Physiol.*, 274 (4 Pt 2), F635, 1998.
77. Yoshioka, K. et al., Glomerular charge and size selectivity assessed by changes in salt intake in type 2 diabetic patients. *Diabetes Care*, 21, 482, 1998.
78. Du Cailar G., Ribstein, G., and Mimran, A., Dietary sodium and target organ damage in essential hypertension, *Am. J. Hypertens.*, 14, 68S, 2002.
79. Kontessis, P. et al., Renal, metabolic, and hormonal responses to ingestion of animal and vegetable proteins, *Kidney Int.*, 38, 136, 1990.

80. Lopes de Faria, J.B. et al., Renal functional response to protein loading in type 1 (insulin-dependent) diabetic patients on normal or high salt intake, *Nephron*, 76, 411, 1997.
81. Bilo, H.J. et al., Effects of chronic and acute protein administration on renal function in patients with chronic renal insufficiency, *Nephron*, 53, 181, 1989.
82. Eddy, A.A., Interstitial inflammation and fibrosis in rats with diet-induced hypercholesterolemia, *Kidney Int.*, 50, 1139, 1996.
83. Scheuer, H., et al., Oxidant stress in hyperlipidemia-induced renal damage, *Am. J. Physiol. Renal Physiol.*, 278, F633, 2000.
84. Jayapalan, S. et al., High dietary fat intake increases renal cyst disease progression in Han:SPRD-cy rats, *J. Nutr.*, 130, 2356, 2000.
85. Popov, D., Simionescu, M., and Shepherd, P.R., Saturated-fat diet induces moderate diabetes and severe glomerulosclerosis in hamsters, *Diabetologia*, 46, 1408, 2003.
86. Velasquez, M.T. et al., Effect of carbohydrate intake on kidney function and structure in SHR/N-cp rats, *Diabetes*, 38, 679, 1989.
87. Zaoui, P. et al., High fructose-fed rats: a model of glomerulosclerosis involving the renin-angiotensin system and renal gelatinases, *Ann. N.Y. Acad. Sci.*, 878, 716, 1995.
88. Manitius, J., Baines, A.D., and Roszkiewicz, A., The effect of high fructose intake on renal morphology and renal function in rats, *J. Physiol. Pharmacol.*, 46, 179, 1995.
89. Dworkin, L.D. et al., Salt restriction inhibits renal growth and stabilizes injury in rats with established renal disease, *J. Am. Soc. Nephrol.*, 7, 437, 1996.
90. Imanishi, M. et al., Sodium sensitivity related to albuminuria appearing before hypertension in type 2 diabetic patients, *Diabetes Care*, 24, 111, 2001.
91. Klahr, S. et al., The effects of dietary protein restriction and blood pressure control on the progression of chronic renal disease: Modification of Diet in Renal Disease Study Group, *N. Engl. J. Med.*, 330, 877, 1994.
92. Levey, A.S. et al., Effects of dietary protein restriction on the progression of moderate renal disease in the Modification of Diet in Renal Disease Study, *J. Am. Soc. Nephrol.*, 7, 2616, 1996.
93. Pedrini, M.T. et al., The effects of dietary protein restriction on the progression of diabetic and non-diabetic renal disease: a meta-analysis, *Ann. Intern. Med.*, 124, 627, 1996.
94. Williams A.J., Baker, F., and Walls, J., Effect of varying quantity and quality of dietary protein intake in experimental renal disease in rats, *Nephron*, 46, 83, 1987.
95. Velasquez, M.T. and Bhathena, S.J., Dietary phytoestrogens: a possible role in renal disease protection, *Am. J. Kidney Dis.*, 37, 1056, 2001.
96. Ogborn, M.R. et al., Soy protein modification of rat polycystic kidney disease, *Am. J. Physiol.*, 274(3Pt2), F541, 1998.
97. Maddox, D.A. et al., Protective effects of a soy diet in preventing obesity-linked renal disease, *Kidney Int.*, 61, 96, 2002.
98. Ingram A.J. et al., Effects of flaxseed and flax oil diets in a rat-5/6 renal ablation model, *Am. J. Kidney Dis.*, 25, 320, 1995.
99. Ogborn, M.R. H, et al., Flaxseed ameliorates interstitial nephritis in rat polycystic kidney disease, *Kidney Int.*, 55, 417, 1999.

100. Velasquez, M.T. et al., Dietary flaxseed meal reduces proteinuria and ameliorates nephropathy in an animal model of type 2 diabetes mellitus, *Kidney Int.*, 64, 2100, 2003.
101. Hall, A.V. et al.: Abrogation of MRL/*lpr* lupus nephritis by dietary flaxseed, *Am. J. Kidney Dis.*, 22, 326, 1993.
102. Jibani M.M. et al., Predominantly vegetarian diet in patients with incipient and early clinical diabetic nephropathy: effects on albumin excretion rate and nutritional status, *Diabet. Med.*, 8, 949, 1991.
103. D'Amico G. et al.: Effect of vegetarian soy diet on hyperlipidaemia in nephrotic syndrome, *Lancet*, 339, 1131, 1992.
104. Soroka N. et al., Comparison of a vegetable-based (soya) and an animal-based low-protein diet in predialysis chronic renal failure patients, *Nephron*, 79(2), 173, 1998.
105. Clark, W.F. et al., Flaxseed in lupus nephritis: a two-year nonplacebo-controlled crossover study, *J. Am. Coll. Nutr.*, 20, 143, 2001.
106. Lefkowith, J.B. and Klahr, S., Polyunsaturated fatty acids and renal disease, *Proc. Soc. Exp. Biol. Med.*, 213, 13, 1996.
107. Kasiske, B.L. et al., Impact of dietary fatty acid supplementation on renal injury in obese Zucker rats, *Kidney Int.*, 39, 1125, 1991.
108. Hobbs, L.M., Rayner, T.E., and Howe, P.R., Dietary fish oil prevents the development of renal damage in salt-loaded stroke-prone spontaneously hypertensive rats, *Clin. Exp. Pharmacol. Physiol.*, 23, 508, 1996.
109. Clark, W.F. and Parbtani, A., ω-3 fatty acid supplementation in clinical and experimental lupus nephritis, *Am. J. Kidney Dis.*, 23, 664, 1994.
110. Donadio, J.V., Jr. et al., A controlled trial of fish oil in IgA nephropathy, *N. Engl. J. Med.*, 331, 1194, 1994.
111. Facchini, F.S. and Saylor, K.L., A low-iron-available, polyphenol-enriched, carbohydrate-restricted diet to slow progression of diabetic nephropathy, *Diabetes*, 52, 1204, 2003.
112. Robinson, D.R. et al., Suppression of autoimmune disease by dietary n-3 fatty acids, *J. Lipid. Res.*, 34, 1435, 1993.
113. Jolly, C.A. et al., Life span is prolonged in food-restricted autoimmune-prone (NZB × NZW) F1 mice fed a diet enriched with (n-3) fatty acids, *J. Nutr.*, 131, 2753, 2001.
114. Houlihan, C.A. et al., A low-sodium diet potentiates the effects of losartan in type 2 diabetes, *Diabetes, Care* 25, 663, 2002.
115. Gansevoort, R.T., de Zeeuw, D., and de Jong, P.E.,Additive antiproteinuric effect of ACE inhibition and a low-protein diet in human renal disease, *Nephrol. Dial. Trasplant.*, 10, 497, 1995.
116. Hutchison, F.N. et al., Differing actions of dietary protein and enalapril on renal function and proteinuria, *Am. J. Physiol.*, 258, F126, 1990.
117. Peters, H., Border, W.A., and Noble, N.A., Angiotensin II blockade and low-protein diet produce additive therapeutic effects in experimental glomerulonephritis, *Kidney Int.*, 57, 1493, 2000.
118. Nijveldt, R.J. et al., Flavonoids: a review of probable mechanisms of action and potential applications, *Am. J. Clin. Nutr.*, 74, 418, 2001.
119. Setchell, K.D., Phytoestrogens: the biochemistry, physiology, and implications for human health of isoflavones, *Am. J. Clin. Nutr.*, 68 (Suppl 6), 1333S, 1998.
120. Simopolous, A.P., ω-3 fatty acids in inflammation and autoimmune diseases, *J. Am. Coll. Nutr.*, 21, 495, 2002.

121. Grande, J.P. et al., Suppressive effects of fish oil on mesangial cell proliferation in vitro and in vivo, *Kidney Int.*, 57, 1027, 2000.
122. Zhao, Y., et al., Eicosapentaenoic acid prevents LPS-induced TNF-alpha expression by preventing NF-kappa B activation, *J. Am. Coll. Nutr.*, 23, 71, 2004.
123. Suzuki, T. et al., Eicosapentaenoic acid protects endothelial cells against anoikis through restoration of cFLIP, *Hypertension*, 42, 342, 2003.
124. Egan, B.M. and Stepniakowski, K.D., Adverse effects of short-term very-low-salt diets in subjects with risk-factor clustering, *Am. J. Clin. Nutr.*, 65(Suppl), 671S, 1997.
125. Graudal, N., Galloe, A., and Garred, P., Effects of sodium restriction on blood pressure, renin, aldosterone, catecholamines, cholesterols, and triglyceride, *JAMA*, 279, 1383, 1998.
126. Gomi, T. et al., Strict dietary sodium reduction worsens insulin sensitivity by increasing sympathetic nervous activity in patients with primary hypertension, *Am. J. Hypertens.*, 11, 1048, 1998.
127. Setchell, K.D.R., Soy isoflavones — Benefits and risks from nature's selective estrogen receptor modulators, *J. Am. Coll. Nutr.*, 20, 354S, 2001.
128. Eritsland, J., Safety considerations of polyunsaturated fatty acids, *Am. J. Clin. Nutr.*, 71, 197, 2000.
129. Walser M. et al.: Should protein intake be restricted in predialysis patients, *Kidney Int.*, 55, 771, 1999.
130. Kopple, J.D. et al., Effect of dietary restriction on nutritional status in the Modification of Diet in Renal Disease study, *Kidney Int.*, 52, 778, 1997.
131. Aparicio, M., Chauveau, P., and Combe C., Are supplemented low protein diets nutritionally safe? *Am. J. Kidney Dis.*, 37(Suppl 2), S71, 2001.

16

Milk Proteins in Food–Food and Food–Drug Synergy on Feeding Behavior, Energy Balance, and Body Weight Regulation

Alfred Aziz and G. Harvey Anderson

CONTENTS

16.1 Introduction

Obesity is a metabolic disorder of energy balance that has reached the proportions of an epidemic worldwide, and that has a complex etiology involving both genetic and environmental factors.[1] However, genetic components cannot solely account for the rapid increase in the incidence of obesity that has occurred in the last two or three decades because gene shifts do not occur this rapidly.[2] Therefore, environmental factors are primary factors in the imbalance between energy intake and energy expenditure that leads to body weight gain. Strategies to treat obesity have relied primarily on either dietary or drug interventions, and neither has proven to be satisfactory. However, for the future, emerging knowledge of how food components interact to trigger satiety or interact with drug strategies to prevent or treat obesity provide optimism for addressing this challenge.

All macronutrients provide energy when metabolized and can therefore contribute to the energy imbalance that results in obesity. However, macronutrients are different in their ability to suppress food intake. Protein is more satiating than carbohydrate, which in turn is more satiating than fat.[3] Studies in both animals and humans have confirmed that protein suppresses food intake the most among the three macronutrients.[4,5] This high satiating power of protein might be a contributor to the success claimed by certain diets, such as Atkins and Protein Power, in achieving and maintaining weight loss.[6,7]

Not only is there variation among macronutrients in their ability to suppress food intake, but within a macronutrient class the source is a determinant as well. For example, in humans, polyunsaturated fats have been reported to suppress food intake more than monounsaturated and saturated fats,[8] although the evidence is not conclusive.[9] Among carbohydrates, glucose-containing drinks suppress food intake consumed 1 hr. or hour later more than drinks containing sucrose and fructose.[10,11] Protein source is also a factor determining the magnitude of food intake suppression in humans. Whey protein suppresses food intake more than soy or egg albumen.[12]

In recent years, it has been established that the digestion of certain proteins gives rise to bioactive peptides (BAP) that possess many physiological functions, such as the regulation of food intake.[3] Of particular interest to the problem of obesity are those BAP that have appetite suppressive and ponderostatic properties. BAP that affect food intake regulation through satiety hormone receptors have been found in milk proteins and soy.[13,14] Peptides exhibiting opioid-like activity in the periphery lead to the inhibition of eating.[13,14] Similarly, the digestion of casein, *in vivo* or *in vitro*, during cheese processing yields a 160 amino acid peptide, caseinomacropeptide (CMP), which is a potent secretagogue of the satiety hormone cholecystokinin (CCK).[15,16] Milk proteins also contain angiotensin converting enzyme (ACE) inhibitory peptides,[17] shown to be antiadipogenic.[18] Thus the presence of BAP in proteins provides the possibility of developing functional foods that, alone or in combination with other food components or drugs, will have antiobesity benefits.

In addition, the recent advances in molecular techniques and their application in the fields of genetics, endocrinology, and neuroendocrinology have widened the horizons for the development of pharmacological agents to treat metabolic diseases. The discovery of genes causing obesity, their expression products (peptide hormones), and the biological actions of these hormones offer a plethora of opportunities for development of drugs that manipulate the system of energy regulation. For example, much research is focusing on hormone agonists or antagonists that trigger on or off the receptor signal transduction pathway leading to a biological response that suppresses food intake and/or increases energy expenditure.

The purpose of this chapter is to discuss food–food synergy and food–drug synergy in the regulation of body weight. The food–food synergy or food–drug synergy is defined as the ability of the combination of foods or the combination of food constituents with drugs to elicit a greater effect on the physiological system investigated than the foods, food components, or drugs alone. The concept is illustrated based primarily on the interaction on food intake and energy balance regulatory systems between components of dairy products, particularly milk proteins and calcium.[18] The combination of milk proteins and other dairy constituents exerts a synergistic effect on markers of energy homeostasis (food–food synergy). With respect to food–drug synergy, there is a synergistic effect between milk proteins and the glucagon-like peptide-1 (GLP-1) receptor agonist, exendin-4 (Ex-4), on food intake.[19,20]This and other possible food–drug synergies are discussed.

16.2 The Regulation of Food Intake and Energy Balance

To understand the basis of interactions among food components and intake regulation, a review of the physiological mechanisms regulating food intake and energy balance is required.

An understanding of the physiological and molecular mechanisms regulating food intake and energy homeostasis has increased markedly in the past decade. A model for the regulation of food intake and energy homeostasis has emerged.[21] This model proposes that both long-term and short-term food intake are distinct but overlap in matching energy intake with requirements. Long term food intake and energy balance are regulated by humoral signals circulating in proportion to adipose mass, namely leptin and insulin, which alter the expression of orexigenic (neuropeptide Y [NPY], agouti related protein [AgRO], orexins A and B [ORX], and melanin concentrating hormone [MCH]) and anorexigenic (proopiomelanocortin/x-melanocyte stimulating hormone [POMC/MSH], cocaine–amphetamine related transcript [CART], corticotropin releasing hormone [CRH], thyrotropin releasing hormone [TRH]) neuropeptides in discrete hypothalamic nuclei, and which modulate the activity of the sympathetic nervous system, which is involved in energy expenditure. These adiposity signals exert effects in the central nervous system (CNS) that are slow in onset and offset (e.g., hours to days), but which are sustained over long intervals. Short-term food intake, or meal size, is regulated by fast-acting satiety signals arising from the gastrointestinal tract, mainly gut hormones (e.g., CCK, GLP-1, and peptide YY [PYY]), and from the metabolism of nutrients (e.g., glucose, fatty acids, and amino acids), and are relayed to the brain stem. It is also proposed that the overall energy status (adiposity signals) dictates the responsiveness to these short-term satiety signals through neuronal pathways connecting the hypothalamus and the brain stem.[21]

Integration of the short- and long-term signals for the control of food intake is supported by neuroanatomical and behavioral research. Neuronal connections have been identified between the brain stem and the hypothalamus, particularly between the paraventricular nucleus (PVN) and the nucleus of the tract solitarius (NTS).[22] Thus the sensitivity of the NTS neurons to satiety signals could be influenced by neuronal input from the PVN.[21] Furthermore, leptin and melanocortin receptor-4 receptors are expressed in the NTS,[23,24] making it the target of circulating leptin and neurons releasing α-MSH and AgRP. The NTS is also the only brain center other than the arcuate nucleus to express the POMC gene,[25] further implicating the NTS in the processing of information relating to long-term regulation of food intake. The concept of integration of short- and long-term signals for the control of food intake is supported by the specific example that insulin enhances the satiating effect of CCK.[26–29]

16.2.1 The Role of Gut Hormones in Regulating Short-Term Food Intake

Gut hormones play a very important role in initiating the satiety response to food ingestion because they are released into the circulation upon the ingestion of macronutrients, and their actions are exerted in CNS areas involved in the regulation of feeding behavior. Gut hormones, with the exception of ghrelin, suppress food intake. CCK is the most documented gut hormone with respect to its effect on satiety. However, other gut hormones implicated in the satiety response to a meal include GLP-1,[30] gastrin-releasing peptide (GRP), glucose-dependent insulinotropic polypeptide–gastric inhibitory polypeptide (GIP), PYY, galanin, and enterostatin.

16.2.2 Macronutrients and Gut Hormones

Gut hormones are secreted upon ingestion of food, but the ability of different types and sources of macronutrients to stimulate their release has received little attention. However, to illustrate that this occurs, this section focuses on the effect of macronutrients, particularly protein, on the secretion of CCK and GLP-1 and on the production from dietary proteins of BAP that possess opioid-like activity in the gut.

16.2.2.1 CCK

Protein (casein) stimulates CCK release more than carbohydrate (glucose) and fat (a soybean emulsion) in the rat.[31] Also, the type and form of dietary proteins and their susceptibility to protease action determines the degree of CCK release.[32–34] The CCK-releasing peptide, secreted by the stomach, is susceptible to degradation by peptidases upon entry into the duodenum. The presence of food proteins, and peptides arising from their digestion, has a sparing effect on the CCK-releasing peptide, which allows more of it to act on the I cells of the small intestine to stimulate CCK release.[35,36]

16.2.2.2 GLP-1

All macronutrients stimulate GLP-1 release, but the role of protein is less clear than that of carbohydrate and fat. Carbohydrates that utilize the sodium–glucose transporter (SGLT), such as glucose, galactose, and sucrose, but not fructose and lactose, stimulate GLP-1 release.[37,38] Ingestion of fermentable fiber increases proglucagon (PG) gene expression (GLP-1 is a post-translational cleavage product of proglucagon protein) in rat ileum through mechanisms involving the production of short-chain fatty acids (SCFA),[39,40] that act from the systemic side of the L-cell.[41]

GLP-1 release upon fat ingestion depends on both the chain length and the degree of saturation of fatty acids.[42] *In vitro* stimulation of the L cells is specific to monounsaturated fatty acids (MUFA) with $C \geq 16$ and a free carboxyl group. Consistent with this observation, a diet containing olive oil, rich in MUFA, resulted in higher plasma GLP-1 concentrations in rats than a diet containing only coconut oil, rich in saturated fatty acids (SAFA).[43] Similar observations were reported in humans consuming a MUFA-rich vs. a SAFA-rich diet.[44]

In humans, proteins or amino acids have been reported to have no effect on or to increase plasma GLP-1 concentrations.[45–51] In rats, protein hydrolysates, unlike protein and amino acids, stimulated GLP-1 secretion *in vitro* and *in vivo*, and increased PG expression in cultured cell lines.[48]

16.2.2.3 Opioids

Opioid signaling appears to be involved in protein-, but not carbohydrate- or fat-induced satiety. In rats, inhibition of eating elicited by intact casein or soy protein can be blocked by naloxone methiodide, an opioid receptor antagonist that does not enter the brain from the circulation.[13,14] Similarly, the effect of casein or soy hydrolysates on food intake was partially reversed by naloxone at a dose that does not increase food intake by itself.[14] The duration and the strength of the interaction between the opioid receptors and the preloads depended on the type and form of the proteins. The strongest interaction occurred with intact casein and its hydrolysate, suggesting higher opioid activity in casein than in soy, whereas the most prolonged interaction occurred with intact soy protein and its hydrolysate, suggesting that the release of opioid peptides from soy is slow.

The foregoing illustrates that macronutrients differ in their ability to stimulate the release of satiety hormones from the gut and that within a macronutrient class, the source is also a factor. This leads to the hypothesis that food–food synergies, such as those that would arise from combining the sources of macronutrients that have the strongest releasing properties, could maximize the release of gut peptides, and hence the suppression of food intake. For example, combining milk proteins with monomeric carbohydrates utilizing the SGLT transporter, monounsaturated fat, and fermentable fiber might maximize gut peptide secretion and have a synergistic effect on satiety, leading to a more rapid meal termination and prolonged intermeal interval. This hypothesis has not yet been tested.

16.3 Food–Food Synergy on Energy Intake, Subjective Appetite, and Body Weight Regulation: The Role of Dairy Components

Although the effects of macronutrients, individual foods, and their constituents on energy intake, subjective measures of appetite, and body weight have been extensively documented, the data on the effect of any combination of these on such parameters are limited. However, the potential of such combinations can be illustrated by interactions among dairy food constituents on parameters related to energy homeostasis.

The consumption of dairy products is inversely associated with body weight, in particular body fat in both children[52,53] and adults.[54–58] Several components of dairy might account for this antiobesity effect, including calcium, proteins, and peptides derived from their digestion, branched-chain amino acids (BCAA), conjugated linoleic acid (CLA), and medium-chain triglycerides (MCT). Evidence for a synergistic effect among the different components of dairy arises from the observations that consumption of dairy products results in antiobesity effects that are greater than that due to the consumption of calcium supplements alone.[18]

16.3.1 Milk Proteins and Their Components

The interest in milk proteins as participants in the adiporegulatory functions of dairy arises from the observations that they play a role in the regulation of food intake, energy homeostasis, and metabolism. Particularly, milk proteins exert a suppressive effect on food intake, possess encrypted BAP, which with physiological and endocrine functions, and contain large amounts of BCAA, which modulate protein synthesis in skeletal muscles.

16.3.1.1 Milk Proteins and Food Intake

There are two major proteins in milk: micellar casein, which makes up approximately 80% of milk proteins, and the soluble whey proteins that account for the remaining 20%. The differences in the physical properties of casein and whey also account for the differences in their physiological effects, including their effect on food intake. In one study, *ad libitum* intake of a buffet meal was significantly lower 90 min after the consumption of a preload containing 48 g of whey than after a preload containing the same amount of casein.[59] In a recent study by Moore,[60] subjects ate less of an *ad libitum* pizza meal 90 min after preloads of complete milk proteins. Casein and whey suppressed intake of a pizza meal more than a water preload, but there were no significant differences in energy intake among the protein treatments. However, when the pizza intake was measured 150 min after the consumption of the preloads, casein suppressed food intake more than whey, whereas complete milk proteins had an intermediate effect. The discrepancy between the results of Hall et al.[59] and Moore[60] might arise from methodological differences. In the former, half of the energy in the preloads was derived from carbohydrate and fat, whereas in the latter the preloads were given as pure protein sources. Furthermore, the whey protein in Hall's study might have contained up to 20% CMP, a peptide believed to have a strong satiating power, whereas the whey protein isolate used by Moore contained less than 5% CMP.

The effects of casein and whey on food intake are consistent with their categorization a "slow" and a "fast" protein, respectively.[61] Whey is a fast protein that, along with caseinomacropeptide and other small peptides derived from casein digestion, remains soluble in the acidic medium of the stomach and is emptied at a relatively rapid rate from the stomach. On the other hand, the remainder of the casein fraction precipitates and empties slowly from the stomach. The changes in plasma amino acid profiles after the consumption of whey and casein reflect their rate of digestion and absorption. Whey ingestion leads to a fast but short and transient increase in plasma amino acid concentrations, whereas casein results in a prolonged plateau with no defined peak that can be sustained for more than 7 hrs. or hours.[61,62]

The differences between whey and casein in the suppression of food intake does not, however, associate with plasma amino acid concentrations after their ingestion,[60] corroborating previous findings in rats.[63] Thus satiety signals arising from the gut are more likely to provide an explanation for the differential effects of casein and whey on food intake. Furthermore, the observations that the antiobesity effects of dairy products were evident at constant protein intakes[18] suggest that the contribution of the protein component of dairy might be mediated through other mechanisms. Specifically, the antiobesity effect of the milk proteins might be attributed to ACE inhibitor peptides and to their high content of BCAA.

16.3.1.2 Antiobesity Effect of ACE Inhibitory Peptides

The hydrolysis of milk proteins gives rise to a number of BAP that exert several physiological functions. Among these BAP, peptides that exhibit ACE inhibitory activity might act synergistically with calcium to modulate adipocyte lipid metabolism. ACE is an enzyme that hydrolyzes the vasodilatory bradykinin and angiotensin I to vasoconstrictive inactive fragments and angiotensin II, respectively.[17] Angiotensin II also up-regulates fatty acid synthase in adipose tissue and thus is lipogenic.[64] In concordance with this, ACE inhibition in mice and subjects with high blood pressure cause a small weight reduction.[18] Furthermore, a whey-derived ACE inhibitor enhanced the antiobesity effects of dietary calcium in transgenic agouti mice placed on a diet with a moderate energy deficit.[18]

Other ACE inhibitory peptides are encrypted in milk proteins and released upon their digestion *in vitro* and *in vivo*.[17] They are collectively referred to as casokinins and lactokinins, depending on the protein fraction they are derived from. However, in order to exert physiological effects, these peptides must resist enzymatic degradation pre- and post-absorption. In this regard, some casokinins and lactokinins have been found to exert hypotensive effects in rats.[17] Thus it is possible that different ACE inhibitory peptides derived from milk proteins interfere with lipid metabolism in the adipose tissue. However, when a lactokinin was given with calcium, the combination neither reduced body weight and body fat, nor maintained skeletal muscle mass to the same extent as milk or whey, suggesting that other BAP and/or constituents of proteins in whey and milk could also have antiobesity functions.[18] Among BAP, those with opioid antagonist activity[65] could exert adiporegulatory effects through reduction of postprandial insulin rise.[66] Another possible candidate for the antiobesity effect of milk proteins are the BCAA, which account for an average of 21% of total amino acids in milk proteins.[60]

16.3.1.3 The Role of BCAA in Energy Partitioning

Amino acids, including the BCAA, have many metabolic roles beyond their use for protein synthesis, and their involvement in these metabolic processes is proportional to their dietary intake. It has been hypothesized that BCAA exert antiobesity effects through shifting dietary energy from adipose tissue to skeletal muscle.[67] Among the BCAA, leucine is involved in many metabolic pathways related to energy production in the skeletal muscle, transamination reactions, glycemic control, and of particular interest to the antiobesity properties of dairy, protein synthesis in skeletal muscle.[67]

The rate of protein synthesis in the skeletal muscle is dependent on the intracellular concentrations of leucine.[67] Thus, leucine supplementation stimulates muscle protein synthesis even during catabolic periods such as energy restriction and exercise.[68,69] It has been proposed that this mechanism explains the sparing effect of muscle mass during periods of weight loss by a diet rich in dairy products.

The mechanisms of leucine-mediated regulation of protein synthesis in skeletal muscles involve downstream components of the insulin signaling pathway. Specifically, leucine stimulates the kinase activity of the mammalian target of rapamycine (mTOR) that controls the translational process of muscle protein synthesis through phosphorylation of different proteins.[67] Therefore, stimulation of muscle protein synthesis by BCAA, especially by leucine, might draw on triglyceride stores in adipose tissue to provide the energy required to sustain protein synthesis.

16.3.2 Adiposity Regulation by Dietary Calcium

Calcium, independent of other dairy components, has an antiobesity effect. However, when consumed in dairy products, its effects are potentiated, illustrating food component synergy.

16.3.2.1 Observational Studies

An antiobesity effect of dietary calcium has been suggested by observational and epidemiological studies and by experimental studies in animals and humans. The association between dietary calcium and body weight and fat mass was reported in the 1980s during an investigation of the antihypertensive effect of dairy products in obese African-American men.[54] The daily consumption of calcium (1000 mg) for 1 year resulted in a decrease of fat mass by almost 5 kg. An inverse association between dietary calcium intake and body weight was also reported in the first National Health and Nutrition Examination Survey (NHANES I) database.[70] An explanation for the effect of dietary calcium on body weight has been offered by the observation of increased fat oxidation with high calcium intake, suggesting that calcium modulates energy partitioning.[71]

16.3.2.2 Animal Studies

The report that increased calcium intake reduced both body weight and weight gain in lean and fatty Zucker rats[72] prompted investigations into the role of calcium and dairy products in energy homesostasis. For this aim, transgenic mice expressing in adipose tissue the *agouti* gene, which exhibit diet-induced, adult-onset obesity, have been used.[64] The rapid weight and fat gain, increased lipogenesis, and reduced lipolysis that are induced by a high fat, high sucrose, low calcium diet (0.4%) were substantially inhibited by a high calcium diet (1.2%) fed at identical *ad libitum* and moderately restricted energy intake.[18] Furthermore, these effects were enhanced when the source of calcium was nonfat dry milk compared with calcium carbonate.[54]

Energy partitioning resulting in reduction of body fat and sparing of muscle mass due to calcium consumption has also been shown. After weight loss on a high calcium–low energy diet, aP2-agouti transgenic mice were given *ad libitum* access to a diet low in calcium, high in calcium, or high in dairy.[73] The high calcium diets, and more so the high dairy diet, limited the weight and fat regain, prevented the suppression of lipolysis and fat oxidation, and increased skeletal muscle fat oxidation, suggesting that components of dairy other than calcium are involved in regulating energy balance and substrate oxidation.

16.3.2.3 Human Studies

As in animal studies, calcium supplementation alone appears to benefit weight control, but there is clearly a synergy between calcium and other components of dairy products. Initial experimental studies of the effect of adding calcium to the diet were aimed at improving markers of bone metabolism, but retrospective analyses of the data showed that increasing calcium intake by 300 to 1,000 mg/d was associated with a 3 to 10 kg reduction in body weight.[74,75] However, in more recent clinical trials, increasing dietary calcium intake in the form of supplements has not been found to be as effective as increased intake through dairy products. In one study,[76] 32 subjects were placed on energy-restricted diets differing in their calcium content and source for 24 weeks. Subjects receiving the high calcium treatments lost more weight, total fat, and trunk fat than subjects receiving the low calcium–dairy treatment. However, subjects receiving their calcium from dairy sources lost even more weight, total fat, and trunk fat than subjects supplemented with calcium carbonate. Furthermore, an improvement in markers of glycemic control and blood pressure, with no change in lipid parameters, was observed with the high dairy treatment. Similarly, a moderately energy-restricted diet supplemented with three servings of yogurt for 12 weeks resulted in a reduction of 31% in the loss of lean body mass loss compared with the control group.[77] This improved body composition upon dairy consumption has been also reported in subjects who maintained their regular energy intake and did not lose weight,[78] suggesting that dairy consumption also causes a redistribution of dietary energy from adipose to muscle tissue, leading to a net fat mass loss.

16.3.2.4 Mechanisms of Adiposity Regulation by Calcium

The effect of dietary calcium on weight loss, and particularly fat loss, has been attributed to the modulation of intracellular calcium concentrations $[Ca^{2+}]i$ in adipocytes. Consistent with this, increased $[Ca^{2+}]i$ in adipocytes of the obese agouti mutant mice account for their obese phenotype.[79,80] Under conditions of low dietary calcium intake, the calcitrophic hormones parathyroid hormone and 1,25-dihydroxyvitamin D (1,25 $(OH)_2D_3$) increase $[Ca^{2+}]i$, and thus account for the shifts in adipose tissue metabolism.[18] $[Ca^{2+}]i$ modulates lipid metabolism in adipose tissue by decreasing and increasing the expression and/or the activity of lipogenic and lipolytic enzymes, respectively.[64] Increases in $[Ca^{2+}]i$ up-regulate the expression and activity of fatty acid synthase,[81–83] and inhibit lipolysis through direct activation of phosphodiesterase 3B, which decreases cAMP and the subsequent activity of hormone sensitive lipase.[83,84]

Insulin appears to be necessary for the full expression of the $[Ca^{2+}]i$-mediated, agouti-induced obesity. Two lines of evidence support this theory. First, hyperplasia of the agouti-expressing B-cell and hyperinsulinemia precede the development of obesity in the agouti mutant mice.[85] Second, in transgenic mice expressing agouti in the adipose tissue, obesity develops only upon administration of either exogenous insulin or a high sucrose diet that leads to hyperinsulinemia.[86,87]

Accumulating evidence indicates that 1,25 $(OH)_2D_3$ induces lipogenesis and inhibits lipolysis and apoptosis in adipose tissue through both genomic and nongenomic vitamin D receptors.[88,89] Part of the genomic-mediated actions of 1,25 $(OH)_2D_3$ on lipid metabolism has been attributed to a decrease in the expression of uncoupling protein 2 (UCP2), a mitochondrial proton leak that is also involved in fatty acid transport and oxidation.[90]

Although higher calcium intakes are associated with less obesity, its role is clearly enhanced by other components of dairy. In particular, milk proteins (through BAP and BCAA), MCT, and CLA affect energy homeostasis.

16.3.3 Milk Fat and the Regulation of Food Intake, Body Weight, and Adiposity

In addition to protein and calcium, the fat content of dairy products, particularly MCT and CLA, might have antiobesity roles.

16.3.3.1 The Role of MCT

MCT, containing 6- to 12-carbon fatty acids, are metabolized differently from the long-chain triglycerides (LCT). The former are directly absorbed into the portal system and rapidly oxidized by the liver, whereas the latter are packaged into chylomicrons, enter the lymphatic circulation, and are substantially taken up by adipocytes for storage.[91] The rapid oxidation of MCT has been hypothesized to exert antiobesity effects through increasing energy expenditure, decreasing fat storage, and eliciting a faster satiety response than LCT.

MCT increase energy expenditure, measured as thermogenesis, compared with LCT in both animals and humans, in a dose-dependent manner.[92,93] The increase in energy expenditure is attributed to both a higher thermic effect of food upon consumption of MCT compared with LCT and a greater fat oxidation.[92,94] It is unclear though whether MCT sustains the increase in energy expenditure in the long term. Few studies have investigated the effect of MCT compared to LCT on energy expenditure for periods greater than 1 week. One of these showed that there were no differences in energy expenditure after 2 weeks of treatment, suggesting that the effect of MCT might be transient.[95] Another study showed that body weight and subcutaneous fat decreased more after a 4-week treatment with MCT than with LCT.[96] These reductions were associated with greater energy expenditure and fat oxidation. Interestingly, the effects of MCT were stronger in subjects with lower initial body weight, suggesting that MCT might be more useful in preventing weight gain than in promoting weight loss.

In addition to affecting energy expenditure, many animal and human studies have reported enhanced satiety and low food intake, with or without a decrease in body weight after MCT, compared with LCT ingestion.[92] Reduced food intake was associated with increases in β-hydroxybutyrate concentrations[97] and gut peptide release. CCK concentrations are increased in plasma after feeding MCT in rats,[98,99] but not in humans.[100,101] In contrast, the plasma concentrations of the satiety hormone PYY were higher after LCT ingestion.[102] Other gut hormones, such as GLP-1, may be involved in the satiety response to MCT. GLP-1 secretion depends on the chain length and degree of saturation of the fatty acid, but this has been based on studies of fatty acids of chain length between 14 and 18 carbons.[42] Furthermore, GLP-1 synthesis and secretion are enhanced by ingestion of fermentable fiber and systemic infusion of short-chain fatty acids,[39–41] suggesting that MCT ingestion could lead to an increase in plasma GLP-1 concentrations.

It has been proposed that the increase in energy expenditure, satiety, and the reduction in food intake upon consumption of MCT would translate into a decrease in body weight and fat mass. Although most animal studies report lower body weight and smaller fat cells, similar effects are not consistently observed in humans.[92,96] These discrepancies might be due to the amount of MCT in the diet or to gender differences in the effect of MCT, which is more potent in males than in females.[96]

16.3.3.2 The Role of CLA

The antiobesity effects of dairy products could also be contributed to by CLA. Dairy products are rich in CLA, a group of positional and geometric isomers of linoleic acid,[103,104] which has been shown in some studies to reduce subjective appetite,[105] body weight, and fat deposition.[103,104]

CLA ingestion affects an array of proteins controlling energy expenditure and lipid metabolism in the adipose tissue.[103] It increases energy expenditure through up-regulation of UCP2 expression in adipose tissue, and reduces lipid storage by down-regulating the expression of transcription factors involved in adipocyte proliferation and differentiation as well as the expression of lipogenic enzymes, such as lipoprotein lipase. Furthermore, CLA increases fat oxidation through up-regulation of carnitine palmitoyltransferase activity, which stimulates β-oxidation.[103] These actions appear to be isomer specific, such that the commercially available *trans*-10, *cis*-12 isomer is more potent at exhibiting these effects than the naturally occurring *cis*-9, *trans*-11,[103] leaving uncertain the contribution of CLA to the antiobesity effects of dairy products.

16.4 Food–Drug Synergy, Food Intake, and Body Weight

For achieving and maintaining weight loss, combining two different intervention regimens has potentially more benefit than using either approach alone. For example, combining a hypocaloric diet with increased physical activity is more successful in reducing body weight than physical activity alone.[106] However, the potential for a synergy between a pharmacological agent and a food on food intake and weight loss has received little attention.

16.4.1 Pharmacological Treatment of Obesity

Pharmacological intervention for the treatment of obesity is often necessary when alternative treatments have failed in producing and maintaining weight loss in obese individuals with BMI > 27 kg/m^2 and/or exhibiting comorbidities, such as type 2 diabetes, dyslipidemias, and hypertension.[107] Moderate weight reduction is associated with a disproportionate decrease in obesity-related morbidities.[108,109] Unfortunately, when food intake is voluntarily reduced, counterregulatory neuroendocrine responses limit weight loss by increasing appetite and decreasing energy expenditure.[110] Thus, the use of pharmacological agents might help induce weight loss and maintain it.

Antiobesity drugs available at present can be classified into two main categories: (1) intestinal fat absorption inhibitors and (2) agents that modulate neurotransmitter physiology in the brain.[111] The Food and Drug Administration has approved the long-term use of orlistat and sibutramine, and the short-term use (up to 3 months) of phentermine for the treatment of obesity. Orlistat (Xenical, Hoffman-LaRoche, Nutley, NJ), which inhibits pancreatic and gastrointestinal lipases, reduces the absorption of dietary fat by approximately 30%. Sibutramine inhibits serotonin and catecholamine reuptake in brain neurons, whereas phentermine is a noradrenergic agent.[112] However, many more drugs are currently undergoing preclinical and clinical trials for the management of body weight in obesity. Some of these drugs were originally developed to treat other pathological conditions, such as amyotrophic lateral sclerosis (ciliary neurotrophic factor), epilepsy (topiramate and zonisamide), depression (bupropion), and diabetes (metformin).[112] Moreover, the recent discovery of gut–brain peptides and the understanding of their mechanisms of actions in the hypothalamus and other brain areas involved in the regulation of food intake and energy expenditure has opened the path for the development of new classes of antiobesity drugs. The effects on food intake, appetite, energy expenditure, and weight loss of peptide receptor agonists and antagonists, and modulators of their intracellular signal transduction pathways are being investigated.[112] Examples include agonists of the melanocortin-3 and -4 receptors (to which x-MSH is an endogenous ligand), GLP-1 receptors (exendin-4), and CCK-A receptors, antagonists for the NPY Y2 (PYY is an endogenous antagonist of NPY Y2 receptor), and Y5 receptors (to which NPY is the endogenous ligand), MCH and endocannabinoid receptors, as well as inhibitors of protein tyrosine phosphatase 1B, which negatively regulates insulin and leptin signaling pathways.[112]

Because macronutrients can stimulate the synthesis and release of these gut–brain peptides and/or neurotransmitters and because the actions of these peptides and/or neurotransmitters overlap in feeding centers of the brain, it can be hypothesized that the combination of macronutrients and peptide-related drugs could have a synergistic effect on food intake, appetite suppression, and body weight reduction. The benefits of food–drug combination would extend beyond synergistically reducing food intake and body weight because the doses of the drug could be reduced, thus minimizing adverse side effects associated with their use.

16.4.2 Food–Drug Synergies: Examples

In the following, four examples of food–drug synergies are proposed. These include (1) dairy protein and exendin-4; (2) high-protein or high carbohydrate diets and sibutramine and/or phentermine; (3) high-protein diets and leptin: and (4) fermentable fiber and orlistat.

16.4.2.1 Dairy Protein, Exendin-4, and Food Intake

Ex-4, a 39 amino acid peptide isolated from lizard (*Heloderma*) venom, shares 53% sequence homology with the mammalian GLP-1.[113] Ex-4 has a high affinity for and acts as a potent agonist to the GLP-1R.[113,114] The greater potency of Ex-4 over GLP-1 is attributed mainly to its longer half-life in circulation, due to its resistance to the action of the enzyme dipeptidyl peptidase IV (DPP-IV)[115] and neutral endopeptidases,[116] which are responsible for the rapid degradation of GLP-1 *in vivo*.

Synthetic Ex-4 (Exenatide, Amylin Pharmaceuticals, Inc., San Diego, CA) has been primarily targeted at the treatment of hyperglycemia in type 2 diabetes,[117] but its strong anorectic effects allow it to be a promising tool for the treatment of hyperphagia and obesity. In fact, Ex-4 has been shown to reduce both food intake[4,19,20,118,119] and body weight[120] in different animal models.

Protein ingestion has been recently shown to have a synergistic effect with Ex-4 in reducing food intake in rats. Investigation of the combined effect of protein and Ex-4 on feeding behavior was stimulated by the interest in elucidating the role of GLP-1 receptors in protein-induced suppression of food intake.[19,20] In these studies, fasted rats were treated with an i.p. injection of Ex-4 (0.5 μg/rat) 5 min prior to the administration of whey and casein preloads by gavage. Food was introduced 30 min after the administration of the preloads, and food intake was measured every hour for the first 3 h during the dark cycle and then at the end of the feeding period. Both Ex-4 alone and protein preloads alone suppressed food intake, but rats ate less at any time of measurement when they received the combination treatment than when they received each treatment alone, indicating a synergistic effect between Ex-4 and the protein on food intake. For example, during the first hour of feeding, rats ate 6.3, 4.1, 4.8, and 3.6 g after control, whey alone, Ex-4 alone, and the combined treatment Ex-4 and whey, respectively (Figure 16.1A). Similarly, at the end of feeding cycle, rats ate less after receiving the combined treatment than after receiving each treatment alone (Figure 16.1B). These results indicated that the activation of the GLP-1 receptors is involved in protein-induced suppression of food intake and suggested that GLP-1 might be involved in the satiety response to protein ingestion. Furthermore, Ex-4 combination with either protein hydrolysates or amino acids suppressed food intake more than each of the treatments alone, suggesting that both amino acids and peptides derived from the digestion of whey and casein induce suppression of food intake in part through the GLP-1 receptors.[20]

Although these results suggest that a combination of a high-protein diet with a low dose of Ex-4 might benefit weight loss in humans, the combination also led to hyperglycemia in rats.[19] At the present time, the origin of this hyperglycemia is unknown, but it also serves to illustrate that food–drug synergies occur. Further studies are needed to characterize the mechanisms underlying these synergies.

16.4.2.2 High-Protein or High-Carbohydrate Diets and Sibutramine or Phentermine

Because the synthesis of serotonin and the catecholamines is under control of precursor amino acids, tryptophan (Trp) and tyrosine (Tyr), respectively,[121] a synergistic effect between macronutrient composition of the diet and sibutramine or phentermine on food intake and body weight is likely to

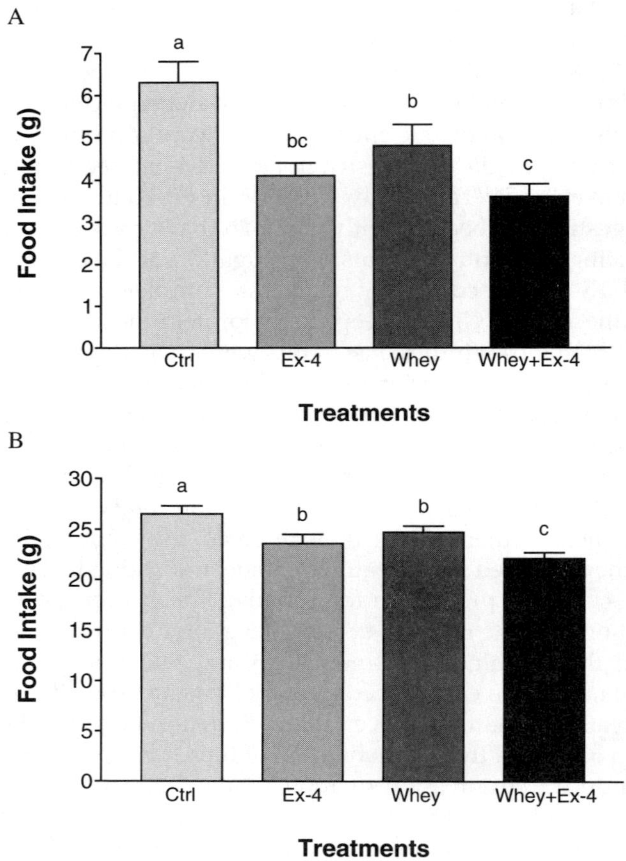

FIGURE 16.1
Effect of coadministering whey and Ex-4 on food intake by rats during (A) 0 to 1 h and (B) 0 to 14 h. N=16 rats, whey = 1 g/2.5 ml; Ex-4 = 0.5 μg/rat. Treatment with different letters are significantly different by one-way ANOVA ($p < .05$) followed by *post-hoc* Duncan's multiple range test. Adapted from Aziz, A. and Anderson, G.H., *J. Nutr.*, 132, 990, 2002.

occur. Sibutramine inhibits the reuptake of serotonin and catecholamines, whereas phentermine stimulates the release of norepinephrine.[112]

The availability of Trp to the brain is subject to dietary influences, and because Trp hydroxylase is not saturated at normal brain Trp concentrations, these fluctuations partly determine serotonin synthesis.[122] Carbohydrate intake increases serotonin concentrations by increasing Trp uptake by the brain as a result of the action of insulin. Insulin suppresses the release of free fatty acids from adipose tissue, thus allowing more Trp binding to albumin, and lowers the concentrations of the other large neutral amino acids (LNAA), especially the BCAA, by increasing their uptake by peripheral tissues. Thus, Trp is given a competitive advantage for uptake by the common carrier system at the blood–brain barrier.

Both synthesis and turnover of the catecholamines are affected by Tyr availability.[121] Pharmacological doses of the precursor amino acids Tyr and Phe suppress food intake in rats.[123,124] Brain Tyr concentrations increase after single meals of both carbohydrate and protein, with protein having the greatest effect.[125]

Thus altering the macronutrient composition of the diet could enhance the effect of sibutramine or phentermine on food intake and body weight. A calorie-restricted diet high in either carbohydrate or protein has the potential to enhance the antiobesity effects of sibutramine by increasing serotonin or norepinephrine synthesis, respectively. On the other hand, high protein diets would be predicted to be more effective than high carbohydrate diets in potentiating the effect of phentermine.

16.4.2.3 High-Protein Diets and Leptin

The effects of high-protein diets on food intake, body weight, and adiposity might be enhanced also by a low-dose leptin treatment. The use of leptin for the treatment of obesity has proved disappointing,[126] mainly because leptin concentrations are elevated in obesity.[127] The inefficacy of high leptin concentrations and leptin treatment in reducing food intake and body weight is attributed to the development of leptin resistance in the obese state.[128] Weight loss per se results in reductions in leptin concentrations that are accompanied by reductions in energy expenditure, thus limiting further weight loss and even reversing it.[110] However, administration of a low dose of leptin brings back the hormonal and metabolic milieu to the state prior to weight loss, thus helping maintain reduced body weight.[129] Therefore, coupling low-dose leptin treatment with a high protein diet, perhaps one high in dairy, can be hypothesized to reduce food intake and appetite, lower body weight and adipose mass, and preserve muscle mass more than either treatment can achieve alone.

16.4.2.4 Fermentable Fiber and Orlistat

A possible synergy on reduction of food intake and body weight might be achieved by combining orlistat treatment with a diet high in fermentable fiber. Generally, dietary fiber might help regulate food intake and energy balance through their physical and chemical properties that enhance satiety signals and improve metabolic control.[130] In particular, fermentable fiber has been shown to increase the synthesis of GLP-1 through a mechanism possibly involving SCFA.[39–41] Recently, administration of 120 mg orlistat to type 2 diabetic subjects resulted in significantly higher postprandial GLP-1 concentrations compared with a placebo.[131] This effect is thought to be due to decreased fat absorption and subsequent increased fat contact with GLP-1-secreting L-cells in the distal intestines. Thus, a diet rich in fermentable fiber can enhance the effect of orlistat on GLP-1 secretion by increasing the synthesis of GLP-1 intestinal L-cells, leading to enhanced satiety and possibly greater weight loss.

Although the concomitant use of energy-restricted diets and drugs to reduce body weight has been widely used, specific food–drug synergy based on the recent advances in the understanding of food intake and energy balance regulation is a new concept warranting testing. However, the examples provided are sufficient to encourage exploration, and it can be anticipated that many other interactions would emerge as new drugs are developed.

16.5 Safety Issues

The use of drugs to treat obesity, and any other condition, is associated with potential adverse effects. The history of the pharmacological treatment of obesity provides many examples of adverse effects of drugs on physiological systems.[112] In one instance, the combination of the serotonergic agent fenfluramine and the catecholaminergic agent phentermine was probably the most effective pharmacological treatment of obesity, resulting in 15 to 20 % reduction in body weight after 28 weeks.[132] However, the use of this combination was discontinued when it was found that fenfluramine and its active enantiomer dexfenfluramine had adverse effects on the cardiovascular physiology, and that they were exacerbated by the concomitant use of phentermine.[133] Such limitations illustrates the failure of the use of antiobesity drugs.

Although the safety of the three drugs approved so far for the treatment of obesity (sibutramine, phentermine, and orlistat) has been evaluated, adverse side effects have been reported upon their use. Sibutramine and phentermine treatments result in a dose-dependent increase in blood pressure and heart rate that are associated with increased activity of sympathetic nervous system.[112] Other side effects include dry mouth, constipation, and insomnia.[112] The adverse effects of the lipase inhibitor, or listat are gastrointestinal related. They include steatorrhea, increased frequency of evacuation episodes, and flatulence. Furthermore, orlistat use decreases the absorption of the fat-soluble vitamins, a problem that can be corrected by taking these vitamins in supplement forms before meals.[112] The possible food–drug synergies described earlier might alleviate the adverse side effects associated with these drugs and other drugs undergoing clinical trials by reducing the therapeutic dose required.

16.6 Conclusions

The unique role of proteins, in particular milk proteins, in the regulation of food intake and energy balance has been used in the discussion to provide a framework for proposing dietary strategies aimed at managing body weight through food–food and food–drug combinations. The synergistic effects between milk proteins and other components of dairy stress the importance of the consumption of whole foods or food–food combinations, rather than isolated food components, and provide a rationale for the development of functional foods containing an ideal mixture of these components that will optimize their beneficial health effects. Furthermore, we proposed that high-protein diets, especially dairy-rich diets, and high fiber diets could serve as useful adjunct therapy to pharmacological treatment of obesity, reducing the possibility of adverse reactions to the drug alone by reducing the dose required and yet enhancing its benefits in reducing or maintaining body weight.

References

1. Speakman, J.R., Obesity: the integrated roles of environment and genetics, *J. Nutr.*, 134 (8 Suppl), 2090S, 2004.
2. Widdowson, P.S., Obesity in diabetes and the impact of leptin, *Diab. Rev. Int.*, 6, 2, 1997.
3. Anderson, G.H. and Moore S.E., Dietary proteins in the regulation of food intake and body weight in humans, *J. Nutr.*, 134, 974, 2004.
4. Peters, C.T. et al., A glucagon-like peptide-1 receptor agonist and an antagonist modify macronutrient selection by rats, *J. Nutr.*, 131, 2164, 2001.
5. Anderson, G.H., Regulation of food intake, in *Modern Nutrition in Health and Disease*, Shils, M.E., Olson, J.A., and Shike, M., Eds., Lea & Febiger, Philadelphia, 1994, chap. 35.
6. Foster, G.D. et al., A randomized trial of a low-carbohydrate diet for obesity, *N. Engl. J. Med.*, 348, 2082, 2003.
7. Samaha, F.F. et al., A low-carbohydrate as compared with a low-fat diet in severe obesity, *N. Engl. J. Med.*, 348, 2074, 2003.
8. Lawton, C.L. et al., The degree of saturation of fatty acids influences post-ingestive satiety, *Br. J. Nutr.*, 83, 473, 2000.
9. Alfenas, R.C. and Mattes, R.D., Effect of fat sources on satiety, *Obes. Res.*, 11, 183, 2003.
10. Anderson, G.H. et al., Inverse association between the effect of carbohydrates on blood glucose and subsequent short-term food intake in young men, *Am. J. Clin. Nutr.*, 76, 1023, 2002.
11. Anderson, G.H. and Woodend, D., Consumption of sugars and the regulation of short-term satiety and food intake, *Am. J. Clin. Nutr.*, 78, 843S, 2003.
12. Anderson, G.H. et al., Protein source, quantity and time of consumption as factors in determining the effect of protein on short-term food intake in young men, *J. Nutr.*, 134, 3011, 2004.
13. Froetschel, M.A. et al., Opioid and cholecystokinin antagonists alleviate gastric inhibition of food intake by premeal loads of casein in meal-fed rats, *J. Nutr.*, 131, 3270, 2001.
14. Pupovac, J. and Anderson, G.H., Dietary peptides induce satiety via cholecystokinin-A and peripheral opioid receptors in rats, *J. Nutr.*, 132, 2775, 2002.

15. Corring, T., Beaufrere, B., and Maubois, J.L., Release of cholecystokinin in humans after ingestion of glycomacropeptide (GMP), in *International Whey Conference,* Rosemont, IL, 1997.
16. Pedersen, N.L. et al., Caseinomacropeptide specifically stimulates exocrine pancreatic secretion in the anesthetized rat, *Peptides,* 21, 1527, 2000.
17. FitzGerald, R.J., Murray, B.A., and Walsh, D.J., Hypotensive peptides from milk proteins, *J. Nutr.*, 134, 980S, 2004.
18. Zemel, M.B., Role of calcium and dairy products in energy partitioning and weight management, *Am. J. Clin. Nutr.*, 79, 907S, 2004.
19. Aziz, A. and Anderson, G.H., Exendin-4, a GLP-1 receptor agonist, modulates the effect of macronutrients on food intake by rats, *J. Nutr.*, 132, 990, 2002.
20. Aziz, A. and Anderson, G.H., Exendin-4, a GLP-1 receptor agonist, interacts with proteins and their products of digestion to suppress food intake in rats, *J. Nutr.*, 133, 2326, 2003.
21. Schwartz, M.W. et al., Central nervous system control of food intake, *Nature*, 404, 661, 2000.
22. Ter Horst, G.J. et al., Ascending projections from the solitary tract nucleus to the hypothalamus. A Phaseolus vulgaris lectin tracing study in the rat, *Neuroscience*, 31, 785, 1989.
23. Mountjoy, K.G. et al., Localization of the melanocortin-4 receptor (MC4-R) in neuroendocrine and autonomic control circuits in the brain, *Mol. Endocrinol.*, 8, 1298, 1994.
24. Mercer, J.G., Moar, K.M., and Hoggard, N., Localization of leptin receptor (Ob-R) messenger ribonucleic acid in the rodent hindbrain, *Endocrinology*, 139, 29, 1998.
25. Bronstein, D.M. et al., Evidence that beta-endorphin is synthesized in cells in the nucleus tractus solitarius: detection of POMC mRNA, *Brain. Res.*, 587, 269, 1992.
26. Figlewicz, D.P. et al., Intracisternal insulin alters sensitivity to CCK-induced meal suppression in baboons, *Am. J. Physiol.*, 250, R856, 1986.
27. Barrachina, M.D. et al., Synergistic interaction between leptin and cholecystokinin to reduce short-term food intake in lean mice, *Proc. Natl. Acad. Sci. U.S.A.*, 94, 10455, 1997.
28. Emond, M. et al., Central leptin modulates behavioral and neural responsivity to CCK, *Am. J. Physiol.*, 276, R1545, 1999.
29. Matson, C.A. and Ritter, R.C., Long-term CCK-leptin synergy suggests a role for CCK in the regulation of body weight, *Am. J. Physiol.*, 276, R1038, 1999.
30. Woods, S.C., Gastrointestinal satiety signals I. An overview of gastrointestinal signals that influence food intake, *Am. J. Physiol.*, 286, G7, 2004.
31. Douglas, B.R. et al., The influence of different nutrients on plasma cholecystokinin levels in the rat, *Experientia*, 44, 21, 1988.
32. Liddle, R.A. et al., Proteins but not amino acids, carbohydrates, or fats stimulate cholecystokinin secretion in the rat, *Am. J. Physiol.*, 251, G243, 1986.
33. Miyasaka, K. et al., Feedback regulation by trypsin: evidence for intraluminal CCK-releasing peptide, *Am. J. Physiol.*, 257, G175, 1989.
34. Herzig, K.H. et al., Diazepam binding inhibitor is a potent cholecystokinin-releasing peptide in the intestine, *Proc. Natl. Acad. Sci. USA*, 93, 7927, 1996.
35. Cuber, J.C. et al., Luminal CCK-releasing factors in the isolated vascularly perfused rat duodenojejunum, *Am. J. Physiol.*, 259, G191, 1990.

36. Sharara, A.I. et al., Evidence for indirect dietary regulation of cholecystokinin release in rats, *Am. J. Physiol.*, 265, G107, 1993.
37. Sasaki, H. et al., GLP-1 secretion coupled with Na/glucose transporter from the isolated perfused canine ileum, *Digestion* 54, 365, 1993.
38. Ritzel, U. et al., Release of glucagon-like peptide-1 (GLP-1) by carbohydrates in the perfused rat ileum, *Acta. Diabetol.*, 34, 18, 1997.
39. Reimer, R.A. and McBurney, M.I., Dietary fiber modulates intestinal proglucagon messenger ribonucleic acid and postprandial secretion of glucagon-like peptide-1 and insulin in rats, *Endocrinology*, 137, 3948, 1996.
40. Reimer, R.A. et al., A physiological level of rhubarb fiber increases proglucagon gene expression and modulates intestinal glucose uptake in rats, *J. Nutr.*, 127, 1923, 1997.
41. Tappenden, K.A. et al., Short-chain fatty acids increase proglucagon and ornithine decarboxylase messenger RNAs after intestinal resection in rats, *J. Parenter. Enteral. Nutr.*, 20, 357, 1996.
42. Rocca, A.S. and Brubaker, P.L., Stereospecific effects of fatty acids on proglucagon-derived peptide secretion in fetal rat intestinal cultures, *Endocrinology*, 136, 5593, 1995.
43. Rocca, A.S. et al., monounsaturated fatty acid diets improve glycemic tolerance through increased secretion of glucagon-like peptide-1, *Endocrinology*, 142, 1148, 2001.
44. Beysen, C. et al., Interaction between specific fatty acids, GLP-1 and insulin secretion in humans, *Diabetologia*, 45, 1533, 2002.
45. Morgan, L. et al., GLP-1 secretion in response to nutrients in man, *Digestion*, 54, 374, 1993.
46. Layer, P. et al., Ileal release of glucagon-like peptide-1 (GLP-1). Association with inhibition of gastric acid secretion in humans, *Dig. Dis. Sci.*, 40, 1074, 1995.
47. Plaisancie, P. et al., Luminal glucagon-like peptide-1(7-36) amide-releasing factors in the isolated vascularly perfused rat colon, *J. Endocrinol.*, 145, 521, 1995.
48. Cordier-Bussat, M. et al., Peptones stimulate both the secretion of the incretin hormone glucagon-like peptide 1 and the transcription of the proglucagon gene, *Diabetes*, 47, 1038, 1998.
49. Kreymann, B. et al., Glucagon-like peptide-1 7-36: a physiological incretin in man, *Lancet*, 2, 1300, 1987.
50. Elliott, R.M. et al., Glucagon-like peptide-1 (7-36) amide and glucose-dependent insulinotropic polypeptide secretion in response to nutrient ingestion in man: acute post-prandial and 24-h secretion patterns, *J. Endocrinol.*, 138, 159, 1993.
51. Herrmann, C. et al., Glucagon-like peptide-1 and glucose-dependent insulin-releasing polypeptide plasma levels in response to nutrients, *Digestion*, 56, 117, 1995.
52. Carruth, B.R. and Skinner, J.D., The role of dietary calcium and other nutrients in moderating body fat in preschool children, *Int. J. Obes. Relat. Metab. Disord.*, 25, 559, 2001.
53. Skinner, J.D. et al., Longitudinal calcium intake is negatively related to children's body fat indexes, *J. Am. Diet. Assoc.*, 103, 1626, 2003.
54. Zemel, M.B. et al., Regulation of adiposity by dietary calcium, *FASEB J.*, 14, 1132, 2000.
55. Pereira, M.A. et al., Dairy consumption, obesity, and the insulin resistance syndrome in young adults: the CARDIA Study, *JAMA*, 287, 2081, 2002.

56. Albertson, A.M. et al., Ready-to-eat cereal consumption: its relationship with BMI and nutrient intake of children aged 4 to 12 years, *J. Am. Diet. Assoc.*, 103, 1613, 2003.
57. Jacqmain, M. et al., Calcium intake, body composition, and lipoprotein-lipid concentrations in adults, *Am. J. Clin. Nutr.*, 77, 1448, 2003.
58. Phillips, S.M. et al., Dairy food consumption and body weight and fatness studied longitudinally over the adolescent period, *Int. J. Obes. Relat. Metab. Disord.*, 27, 1106, 2003.
59. Hall, W.L. et al., Casein and whey exert different effects on plasma amino acid profiles, gastrointestinal hormone secretion and appetite, *Br. J. Nutr.*, 89, 239, 2003.
60. Moore, S.E., The effects of milk proteins on the regulation of short-term food intake and appetite in young men, M.Sc. thesis, University of Toronto, Toronto, 2004.
61. Boirie, Y. et al., Slow and fast dietary proteins differently modulate postprandial protein accretion, *Proc. Natl. Acad. Sci. USA*, 94, 14930, 1997.
62. Dangin, M. et al., The digestion rate of protein is an independent regulating factor of postprandial protein retention, *Am. J. Physiol.*, 280, E340, 2001.
63. Anderson, G.H. et al., Dissociation between plasma and brain amino acid profiles and short-term food intake in the rat, *Am. J. Physiol.*, 266, R1675, 1994.
64. Zemel, M.B., Role of dietary calcium and dairy products in modulating adiposity, *Lipids*, 38, 139, 2003.
65. Meisel, H., Biochemical properties of regulatory peptides derived from milk proteins, *Biopolymers*, 43, 119, 1997.
66. Froetschel, M.A., Bioactive peptides in digesta that regulate gastrointestinal function and intake, *J. Anim. Sci.*, 74, 2500, 1996.
67. Layman, D.K. and Baum, J.I., Dietary protein impact on glycemic control during weight loss, *J. Nutr.*, 134, 968S, 2004.
68. Gautsch, T.A. et al., Availability of eIF4E regulates skeletal muscle protein synthesis during recovery from exercise, *Am. J. Physiol.*, 274, C406, 1998.
69. Anthony, J.C. et al., Leucine stimulates translation initiation in skeletal muscle of postabsorptive rats via a rapamycin-sensitive pathway, *J. Nutr.*, 130, 2413, 2000.
70. McCarron, D.A., Calcium and magnesium nutrition in human hypertension, *Ann. Intern. Med.*, 98, 800, 1983.
71. Melanson, E.L. et al., Relation between calcium intake and fat oxidation in adult humans, *Int. J. Obes. Relat. Metab. Disord.*, 27, 196, 2003.
72. Bursey, R.D., Sharkey, T., and Miller, G.D, High calcium intake lowers weight in lean and fatty Zucker rats, *FASEB J.*, 3, A265(abstr), 1989.
73. Sun, X. and Zemel., M.B., Calcium and dairy inhibition of weight and fat regain during ad libitum feeding following energy restriction in aP2-agouti transgenic mice, *FASEB J.*, 17, A746(abstr), 2003.
74. Davies, K.M. et al., Calcium intake and body weight, *J. Clin. Endocrinol. Metab.*, 85, 4635, 2000.
75. Heaney, R.P., Davies, K.M., and Barger-Lux, M.J., Calcium and weight: clinical studies, *J. Am. Coll. Nutr.*, 21, 152S, 2002.
76. Zemel, M.B. et al., Calcium and dairy acceleration of weight and fat loss during energy restriction in obese adults, *Obes. Res.*, 12, 582, 2004.
77. Zemel M.B. et al., Dairy (yogurt) augments fat loss and reduces central adiposity during energy restriction in obese subjects, *FASEB J.*, 17, A1088(abstr), 2003.

78. Zemel M.B. et al., Interaction between calcium, dairy and dietary macronutrients in modulating body composition in obese mice, *FASEB J.*, 16, A369(abstr), 2002.
79. Zemel, M.B. et al., Agouti regulation of intracellular calcium: role in the insulin resistance of viable yellow mice, *Proc. Natl. Acad. Sci. USA*, 92, 4733, 1995.
80. Kim, J.H. et al., The effects of calcium channel blockade on agouti-induced obesity, *FASEB. J.*, 10, 1646, 1996.
81. Claycombe, K.J. et al., Transcriptional regulation of the adipocyte fatty acid synthase gene by agouti: interaction with insulin, *Physiol. Genomics*, 3, 157, 2000.
82. Xue, B.Z. and Zemel, M.B., Relationship between human adipose tissue agouti and fatty acid synthase (FAS), *J. Nutr.*, 130, 2478, 2000.
83. Xue, B.Z. et al., The agouti gene product inhibits lipolysis in human adipocytes via a Ca^{2+}-dependent mechanism, *FASEB J.*, 12,. 1391, 1998.
84. Xue, B.Z. et al., Mechanism of intracellular calcium ($Ca^{2+}i$) inhibition of lipolysis in human adipocytes, *FASEB J.*, 15, 2527, 2001.
85. Xue, B.Z. et al., The agouti gene product stimulates pancreatic beta-cell Ca^{2+} signaling and insulin release, *Physiol. Genomics*, 1, 11, 1999.
86. Mynatt, R.L. et al., Combined effects of insulin treatment and adipose tissue-specific agouti expression on the development of obesity, *Proc. Natl. Acad. Sci. USA*, 94, 919, 1997.
87. Zemel, M.B., Mynatt, R.L., and Dibling, D., Synergism between diet-induced hyperinsulinemia and adipocyte-specific agouti expression, *FASEB J.*, 13, A733 (abstr), 1999.
88. Shi, H. et al., 1 alpha,25-Dihydroxyvitamin D_3 modulates human adipocyte metabolism via nongenomic action, *FASEB J.*, 15, 2751, 2001.
89. Ye, W.Z. et al., Vitamin D receptor gene polymorphisms are associated with obesity in type 2 diabetic subjects with early age of onset, *Eur. J. Endocrinol.*, 145, 181, 2001.
90. Shi, H. et al., 1 alpha,25-dihydroxyvitamin D_3 inhibits uncoupling protein 2 expression in human adipocytes, *FASEB J.*, 16, 1808, 2002.
91. Babayan, V.K., Medium chain triglycerides and structured lipids, *Lipids*, 22, 417, 1987.
92. St-Onge, M.P. and Jones, P.J., Physiological effects of medium-chain triglycerides: potential agents in the prevention of obesity, *J. Nutr.*, 132, 329, 2002.
93. Dulloo, A.G. et al., Twenty-four-hour energy expenditure and urinary catecholamines of humans consuming low-to-moderate amounts of medium-chain triglycerides: a dose-response study in a human respiratory chamber, *Eur. J. Clin. Nutr.*, 50, 152, 1996.
94. Hill, J.O. et al., Thermogenesis in humans during overfeeding with medium-chain triglycerides, *Metabolism*, 38, 641, 1989.
95. White, M.D., Papamandjaris, A.A., and Jones, P.J., Enhanced postprandial energy expenditure with medium-chain fatty acid feeding is attenuated after 14 d in premenopausal women, *Am. J. Clin. Nutr.*, 69, 883, 1999.
96. St-Onge, M.P. and Jones, P.J., Greater rise in fat oxidation with medium-chain triglyceride consumption relative to long-chain triglyceride is associated with lower initial body weight and greater loss of subcutaneous adipose tissue, *Int. J. Obes. Relat. Metab. Disord.*, 27,1565, 2003.
97. Bray, G.A., Lee, M., and Bray, T.L., Weight gain of rats fed medium-chain triglycerides is less than rats fed long-chain triglycerides, *Int. J. Obes.*, 4, 27, 1980.

98. Furuse, M. et al., Feeding behavior in rats fed diets containing medium chain triglyceride, *Physiol. Behav.*, 52, 815, 1992.
99. Bellissimo, N. and Anderson, G.H., Cholecystokinin-A receptors are involved in food intake suppression in rats after intake of all fats and carbohydrates tested, *J. Nutr.*, 133, 2319, 2003.
100. McLaughlin, J. et al., Fatty acid chain length determines cholecystokinin secretion and effect on human gastric motility, *Gastroenterology*, 116, 46, 1999.
101. Barbera, R. et al., Sensations induced by medium and long chain triglycerides: role of gastric tone and hormone, *Gut*, 46(1), 32, 2000.
102. Maas, M.I., et al., Release of peptide YY and inhibition of gastric acid secretion by long-chain and medium-chain triglycerides but not by sucrose polyester in men, *Eur. J. Clin. Invest.*, 28, 123, 1998.
103. Wang, Y. and Jones, P.J., Dietary conjugated linoleic acid and body composition, *Am. J. Clin. Nutr.*, 79, 1153S, 2004.
104. Wang, Y. and Jones, P.J., Conjugated linoleic acid and obesity control: efficacy and mechanisms, *Int. J. Obes. Relat. Metab. Disord.*, 28, 941, 2004.
105. Kamphuis, M.M. et al., Effect of conjugated linoleic acid supplementation after weight loss on appetite and food intake in overweight subjects, *Eur. J. Clin. Nutr.*, 57, 1268, 2003.
106. Miller, Y.D. and Dunstan, D.W., The effectiveness of physical activity interventions for the treatment of overweight and obesity and type 2 diabetes, *J. Sci. Med. Sport.*, 7, 52, 2004.
107. Executive summary of the clinical guidelines on the identification, evaluation, and treatment of overweight and obesity in adults, Expert Panel on the Identification, Evaluation, and Treatment of Overweight and Obesity in Adults, *Arch. Int. Med.*, 158, 1855, 1998.
108. Goldstein, D.J., Beneficial effects of modest weight loss, *Int. J. Obes. Relat. Metabol. Disord.*, 16, 397, 1992.
109. Blackburn, G., Effect of degree of weight loss on health benefits, *Obes. Res.*, 3, 2112S, 1995.
110. Chan, J.L. et al., The role of falling leptin levels in the neuroendocrine and metabolic adaptation to short-term starvation in healthy men, *J. Clin. Invest.*, 111, 1409, 2003.
111. Padwal, R., Li, S.K., and Lau, D.C.W., Long-term pharmacotherapy for overweight and obesity: a systematic review and meta-analysis of randomized controlled trials, *Int. J. Obes. Relat. Metabol. Disord.*, 27, 1437, 2003.
112. Korner, J. and Aronne, L.J., Pharmacological approaches to weight reduction: therapeutic targets, *J. Clin. Endocr. Metabol.*, 89, 2616, 2004.
113. Goke, R. et al., Exendin-4 is a high potency agonist and truncated exendin-(9-39)-amide an antagonist at the glucagon-like peptide 1-(7-36)-amide receptor of insulin-secreting beta-cells, *J. Biol. Chem.*, 268, 19650, 1993.
114. Thorens, B. et al., Cloning and functional expression of the human islet GLP-1 receptor. Demonstration that exendin-4 is an agonist and exendin-(9-39) an antagonist of the receptor, *Diabetes*, 42, 1678, 1993.
115. Drucker, D.J., Glucagon-like peptides, *Diabetes*, 47, 159, 1998.
116. Doyle, M.E. et al., The importance of the nine-amino acid C-terminal sequence of exendin-4 for binding to the GLP-1 receptor and for biological activity, *Regul Pept.*, 114, 153, 2003.

117. Kolterman, O. G. et al., Synthetic exendin-4 (exenatide) significantly reduces postprandial and fasting plasma glucose in subjects with type 2 diabetes, *J. Clin. Endocrinol. Metab.*, 88, 3082, 2003.
118. Rodriquez de Fonseca, F. et al., Peripheral versus central effects of glucagon-like peptide-1 receptor agonists on satiety and body weight loss in Zucker obese rats, *Metabolism*, 49, 709, 2000.
119. Young, A.A. et al., Glucose-lowering and insulin-sensitizing actions of exendin-4: studies in obese diabetic (ob/ob, db/db) mice, diabetic fatty Zucker rats, and diabetic rhesus monkeys (Macaca mulatta), *Diabetes*, 48, 1026, 1999.
120. Szayna, M. et al., Exendin-4 decelerates food intake, weight gain, and fat deposition in Zucker rats, *Endocrinology*, 141, 1936, 2000.
121. Wurtman, R.J., Hefti, F., and Melamed, E., Precursor control of neurotransmitter synthesis, *Pharmacol. Rev.*, 32, 315, 1980.
122. Anderson, G. H., Diet, neurotransmitters and brain function, *Br. Med. Bull.*, 3795, 1981.
123. Morris, P. et al., Food intake and selection after peripheral tryptophan, *Physiol. Behav.*, 40, 155, 1987.
124. Bialik, R. J et al., Route of delivery of phenylalanine influences its effect on short-term food intake in adult male rats, *J. Nutr.*, 119, 1519, 1989.
125. Glanville, N. T. and Anderson, G. H., The effect of insulin deficiency, dietary protein intake, and plasma amino acid concentrations on brain amino acid levels in rats, *Can. J. Physiol. Pharmacol.*, 63, 487, 1985.
126. Heymsfield, S.B. et al., Recombinant leptin for weight loss in obese and lean adults: a randomized, controlled, dose-escalation trial, *JAMA*, 282, 1568, 1999.
127. Smith, S.R., The endocrinology of obesity, *Endocrinol. Metabol. Clin. North Am.*, 25, 921, 1996.
128. El-Haschimi, K. et al., Two defects contribute to hypothalamic leptin resistance in mice with diet-induced obesity, *J. Clin. Invest.*, 105, 1827, 2000.
129. Rosenbaum, M. et al., Low dose leptin administration reverses effects of sustained weight-reduction on energy expenditure and circulating concentrations of thyroid hormones, *J. Clin. Endocrinol. Metab.*, 87, 2391, 2002.
130. Burton-Freeman, B., Dietary fiber and energy regulation, *J. Nutr.*, 130, 272S, 2000.
131. Damci, T. et al., Orlistat augments postprandial increases in glucagon-like peptide 1 in obese type 2 diabetic patients, *Diabetes Care*, 27, 1077, 2004.
132. Weintraub, M., Long-term weight control: the National Heart, Lung, and Blood Institute funded multimodal intervention study, *Clin. Pharmacol. Ther.*, 51, 581, 1992.
133. Connolly, H.M. et al., Valvular heart disease associated with fenfluramine-phentermine. *N. Engl. J. Med.*, 337, 581, 1997.

Section VI

Ergogenics

17

Caffeine, Creatine, and Food–Drug Synergy: Ergogenics and Applications to Human Health

Terry E. Graham and Lesley L. Moisey

CONTENTS

17.1 Introduction

Caffeine and creatine are two of the most commonly employed ergogenic aids. For example, Kanayama et al.[1] surveyed clients of five gymnasiums in the United States. Of the men, 47% reported having used creatine and 26% had used ephedrine; comparable responses for the women were 7 and 13%, respectively. A brief review by Rawson and Clarkson[2] stated that 17 to 74% of various athletic groups use creatine supplementation, often for periods of many months. Melia et al.[3] surveyed over 1600 Canadian school children (11 to 18 years of age), and 27% reported having used caffeine for the specific purpose of enhancing sport performance within a 12-month period. The popularity of these compounds is likely attributable to a number of factors: they are well researched and publicized, they have been proven to have benefits to some athletes in some situations, they are perceived by the public to be safe and most likely are safe, they are not currently regulated by sport federations, and they are readily available.

Both caffeine and creatine are common elements of the diets of many North Americans, and it is difficult to establish whether they are nutrients, natural health products, nutraceuticals, and/or drugs. As with many supplements and natural health products, possible food and/or drug synergies have not been extensively investigated. Many researchers have proposed that these compounds operate via simple, straightforward mechanisms; however they are complex and likely have multiple actions. In addition, both have applications beyond athletic performance, including applications to human health. While they are very different in their structure and influence human physiology in very different ways, there is evidence that there may be interactions between caffeine and creatine.

This chapter considers caffeine in the greatest detail because there is a far greater body of knowledge concerning this compound. Each substance is reviewed first as an ergogenic aid, followed by examination for food and/or drug synergies that could influence its actions and/or metabolism, and then consideration of human health issues. Potential safety issues are included in the discussion of each substance throughout this review.

17.2 Caffeine

17.2.1 The Compound and Its Mode of Action

Caffeine (trimethylxanthine) is one of a number of methylxanthines that share similar physiological and pharmacological properties. There are three dimethylxanthines: theophylline, theobromine, and paraxanthine. Caffeine (Table 17.1) and the first two dimethylxanthines occur in a variety of food

TABLE 17.1
Caffeine Content of Various Beverages, Foods, and Medicinals

Product	Serving Size	Caffeine (mg)
Coffee		
Brewed	8 oz	135
Roasted and ground, percolated	8 oz	118
Roasted and ground, drip	8 oz	179
Roasted and ground, decaffeinated	8 oz	3
Instant	8 oz	106
Instant, decaffeinated	8 oz	5
Coffee Specialties		
Tim Horton's coffee	8 oz	85
Starbucks coffee	8 oz	250
Starbucks espresso coffee	1 oz	35
Tea		
Tea, average blend	8 oz	43
Tea, green	8 oz	30
Tea, leaf or bag	8 oz	50
Chocolate Beverages		
Chocolate milk	8 oz	8
Hot-cocoa mix, 1 envelope	8 oz	5
Chocolate Cake and Cookies		
Chocolate cake	80 g	6
Chocolate cookies	15 g	1
Chocolate chip Cookies	20 g	4
Chocolate brownies	42 g	10
Chocolate Candy		
Fudge	25 g	11
Chocolate bar, Hershey's	1.5 oz	10
Chocolate bar, Hershey's Dark	1.5 oz	31
Baking Chocolate		
Baker's, unsweetened	1 oz	25
Baker's, German sweet	1 oz	8
Baker's, semisweet	1 oz	13
Frozen Desserts		
Jello Pudding Pops	47 g	2
Starbucks Frappucino bar	2.5 oz	15
Ice Cream		
Haagen-Dazs coffee ice cream	8 oz	58
Haagen-Dazs, coffee fudge ice, low fat	1 cup	30
Health choice cappuccino, chocolate chunk	1 cup	8
Starbucks coffee ice cream	1 cup	40

TABLE 17.1 (Continued)

Caffeine Content of Various Beverages, Foods, and Medicinals

Product	Serving Size	Caffeine (mg)
Yogurt		
Ben & Jerry's No fat coffee fudge	8 oz	85
Haagen-Dazs coffee frozen, fat free	1 cup	40
Dannon coffee yogurt	8 oz	45
Dannon light cappuccino yogurt	8 oz	<1
Colas		
Canada Dry cola	12 oz	30
Canada Dry cola, diet	12 oz	1
Coca Cola	12 oz	46
Coca Cola, diet	12 oz	46
Jolt	12 oz	100
Pepsi	12 oz	38
Caffeinated Waters		
Aqua Blast	16.9 oz (500 ml)	90
Aqua Java	16.9 oz (500 ml)	50
Java Water	16.9 oz (500 ml)	125
Krank 20	16.9 oz (500 ml)	100
Water Joe	16.9 oz (500 ml)	60
Energy Drinks		
AMP	8 oz	77
Arizona Rx Power	8 oz	30
Arizona Energy	8 oz	30
Battery	8 oz	76
Blue Ox	8 oz	76
Jones Soda Energy	8 oz	43
Jones Soda WhoopAss	8 oz	50
Red Bull	8 oz	80
Sobe Energy Rush	8 oz	79
Sobe No Fear	8 oz	158
Over the Counter Medications		
No Doz Vivarin, maximum strength	1 tablet	100
No Doz Vivarin, regular strength	1 tablet	100
Anacin	1 tablet	33
Excedrin	1 tablet	65
Midol	1 tablet	33
Vanquish	1 tablet	33
Cold Remedies		
Coryban-D	1 tablet	30
Triaminicin	1 tablet	30
Diuretics	1 tablet	100

Source: Modified from Harland, B.F., *Nutrition*, 16, 522, 2000.

products. Paraxanthine does not occur in any plant source, but, in humans, it is the dominant dimethylxanthine produced by the liver from caffeine. The half-life of caffeine is 4 to 6 h and although the plasma concentration of caffeine can increase to approximately 40 μM following ingestion of large amounts of coffee (i.e., two to three large mugs of coffee), more commonly concentrations range from 5 to 20 μM. The levels of the dimethylxanthines are much lower, although paraxathine can reach 5 to 8 μM. The structure of these xanthines is similar to that of adenosine, and they can bind to and antagonize adenosine receptors. The resulting effects are the same regardless of which xanthine is binding to the receptor, and for simplicity we will only refer to caffeine, although both theophylline and paraxathine are more potent antagonists than caffeine. There are several forms of adenosine receptors (A_1, A_{2A}, A_{2B}, and A_3), and all but the A_3 receptor are antagonized by the xanthines at physiological concentrations of 5 to 20 μM.[4] This antagonism requires significant tonic activation of the receptors by adenosine. Antagonism of A_1 receptors could result in inhibition of either G_i input onto adenyl cyclase or $G_{\beta,\gamma}$. The latter are subunits of the heterotrimeric G protein that can have actions separate from the G_α subunit that mediates inhibition of adenylate cyclase. The $G_{\beta,\gamma}$ subunit affects calcium release, potassium channels, and voltage-sensitive calcium channels.[4] Antagonism of A_2 receptors would remove the G_s stimulatory effect on adenyl cyclase.

Adenosine receptors are ubiquitous, occurring throughout the nervous system, and in the vascular endothelium, heart, liver, adipose tissues, and muscle.[5–8] Thus the actions that result from caffeine are dependent on which type of receptors it blocks and in which tissue the receptors are located. Furthermore, within the central nervous system, A_1 receptors are dominant in the hippocampus, cortex, and cerebellum while A_{2a} receptors are concentrated in the dopamine-rich, GABA-ergic region. The sympathetic nervous system is stimulated when the central nervous system is exposed to caffeine. There are a number of reports that caffeine increases circulating levels of epinephrine,[9–13] and we have reported an increase in norepinephrine "spill-over" from the leg of humans both at rest and in exercise. This raises the possibility that some of the actions of caffeine are secondary to this sympathetic stimulation.

Caffeine can also have intracellular actions that may be independent of adenosine receptors. It can act as a phosphodiesterase inhibitor and stimulates calcium-release channels. However, these actions require pharmacological or lethal concentrations (500 to 5000 μM) of caffeine, and Daly and Fredholm[4] stated that the methylxanthines are only weak phosphodiesterase inhibitors even at these high concentrations.

17.2.2 Sources of Caffeine

Caffeine is the world's most frequently consumed drug and is found naturally occurring in more than 60 different plant species.[14] Caffeine, theophyl-

TABLE 17.2

Global Coffee Consumption in 2001 per Continent

Region	2001 Consumption (kg/person/year)	% Difference from the World Average
World	1.1	—
Europe	3.9	+254.5
European Union	5.1	+363.6
North and Central America	3.4	+209.1
North America developed	4.1	+272.7
Central America	2.0	+81.8
Oceania	2.2	+100.0
South America	1.7	+54.5
Africa	0.6	45.5
Asia	0.3	72.7

Source: Food and Agricultural Organization, Coffee food balance sheet, Rome, 2001.

line, and theobromine are most commonly found in the *Coffee arabica, Thea sinensis, Theobroma cocoa,* and *Cola nitida* plants from which coffee, tea, chocolate, and kola, respectively, are derived.[15] While caffeine is commonly identified with coffee beans in the North American society, plants such as guarana actually have a greater concentration of caffeine than do coffee beans, and new foods and beverages are appearing that contain "guarana extract" without listing caffeine as an ingredient.

It is currently estimated that 80% of adult Americans consume caffeine-containing products every day,[16] and it is likely that caffeine consumption patterns are similar in Canada. The primary sources of caffeine in our diet are coffee, tea, and soft drinks,[17] but there has also been an increase in the production of a number of novelty foods and beverages that contain caffeine, including water, chewing gum, and alcoholic beverages. Table 17.1 provides a comprehensive list of the caffeine content found in common North American beverages, foods, and medicinals. In 2001, according to the Food Balance Sheets established by the Food and Agricultural Organization of the United Nations, global coffee production was 7,203,000 metric tons[18] and is second only to oil as a world trade commodity. Countries of the European Union are the highest consumers of coffee in the world while the developed North American countries also consume a high amount in comparison to the rest of the world (Table 17.2). It has been suggested that coffee consumption is responsible for 54% of all caffeine consumption in the world,[19] and in North America, coffee is the predominant source of caffeine in the diet.[20]

Estimating average caffeine consumption in populations and groups of specific interest has proven to be an elusive task because caffeine concentration often varies in products because of a number of factors, some of which include nonstandardized serving sizes, processing methods, and caffeine source. In assessing food and beverage consumption in Canada and the United States, it is apparent that there has been a trend toward increasing coffee, tea, and soft drink consumption (Table 17.3). Between 1993 and 2003,

TABLE 17.3

Per Capita Annual Beverage and Cocoa Consumption, Canada and the United States: 1993-2003

	1993	1994	1995	1996	1997	1998	1999	2000	2001	2002	2003
Canada											
Coffee[a] (kg)	4.38	4.86	4.34	4.64	4.49	4.53	4.57	4.64	4.96	4.48	4.07
Coffee[b] (L)	81.76	88.13	84.95	86.54	83.22	84.73	87.92	89.70	89.76	90.52	N/A
Tea[c] (kg)	0.78	0.71	0.65	0.62	0.72	0.80	0.87	0.89	0.93	0.91	1.16
Tea[b] (L)	54.03	49.31	44.88	43.35	50.29	55.38	60.47	61.68	64.64	63.24	N/A
Cocoa[d] (kg)	1.80	1.28	1.10	1.40	1.39	1.38	1.39	1.40	1.38	1.40	1.42
Soft drinks[b] (L)	102.8	108.9	109.5	110.7	112.6	117.3	117.0	113.1	113.6	112.4	N/A
United States											
Coffee[a] (kg)	4.09	3.68	3.59	3.95	4.14	4.23	4.45	4.68	4.27	N/A	N/A
Tea[b] (kg)	0.40	0.40	0.38	0.37	0.35	0.40	0.40	0.38	0.40	N/A	N/A
Cocoa[c] (kg)	2.41	2.18	2.05	2.36	2.27	2.45	2.55	2.68	2.55	N/A	N/A
Soft drinks (Lr)	184.0	183.2	179.4	176.4	177.2	181.3	188.1	186.2	N/A	N/A	N/A

[a] Green bean equivalent.
[b] Disappearance adjusted for retail, household, cooking and plate loss.
[c] Dry leaf equivalent.
[d] Bean equivalent.

Source: Food and Agricultural Organization, Coffee food balance sheet, Rome, 2001; Statistics Canada, Food consumption in Canada (part I and part II, 2002), 32-229-XIB, 2003.

coffee consumption by the average Canadian increased from almost 82 to just over 90 L/year.[21]

In North American adults, it is estimated that 60 to 75% of total caffeine intake comes from coffee where as 15 to 30% is derived from tea.[22] In contrast, the primary sources of caffeine in North American children are soft drinks and chocolate.[22] A recent study conducted in southern Ontario estimated the average caffeine intake in adults ages 30 to 75 years to be between 288 and 426 mg/d,[23] which is equivalent to 4.1 to 6.1 mg caffeine per kilogram body weight in a 70-kg individual. Clearly, caffeine is a widely consumed drug in our society and a typical part of the average consumer diet. As will be illustrated in the following section, caffeine is a potent ergogenic aid when ingested in a dose of 3 to 6 mg per kilogram body weight and this dose has also been associated with insulin resistance (Section 17.2.6). However, the wide range of food products containing caffeine presents many opportunities for food–caffeine interactions.

17.2.3 Caffeine as an Ergogenic Aid

Ergogenic aids can act by facilitating work capacity and/or power output. The former is a major component of endurance and the latter is critical in performance that requires completing a task as quickly as possible. It is redundant to provide yet another review of caffeine's effect on work capacity. There have been a number of such reviews by this author[24–27] and others.[28–31] The vast majority of the studies of the last 15 years have shown that caffeine has a great impact on work capacity (Figure 17.1). That is, one can produce the same power output for a longer period of time after consuming caffeine, and the enhancement can be as much as 10 to 20 min in efforts that cause fatigue in 1 to 2 h[13,32] and as little as a few seconds in efforts lasting 1 to 10 min.[33,34] While this does not directly relate to many athletic events where the goal is to reach a finish line quickly, it would be very useful as a training tool to increase training volume. Often scientists have elected to study caffeine and work in this manner because it is easier to quantify the nature of the exercise using traditional laboratory equipment, and for those who are interested in metabolic regulation, this design provides a steady state.

Early studies of performance often used field trials,[33,35–37] which can be subject to environmental changes and make it very difficult to make detailed measures other than performance time. Contemporary advances in exercise equipment have facilitated studies in which power output can be altered in a very controlled manner. This has allowed investigators to design simulated races and time trials.[38–42] Again the general consensus is that caffeine enhances performance. The mechanisms of action for the ergogenic properties of caffeine remain elusive and without this information it is difficult to address synergies with foods and drugs. Most ergogenic aids, including creatine (see Section 17.3), have a specific effect (i.e., increased reaction time, expanded blood volume, or increased muscle strength) that gives an advan-

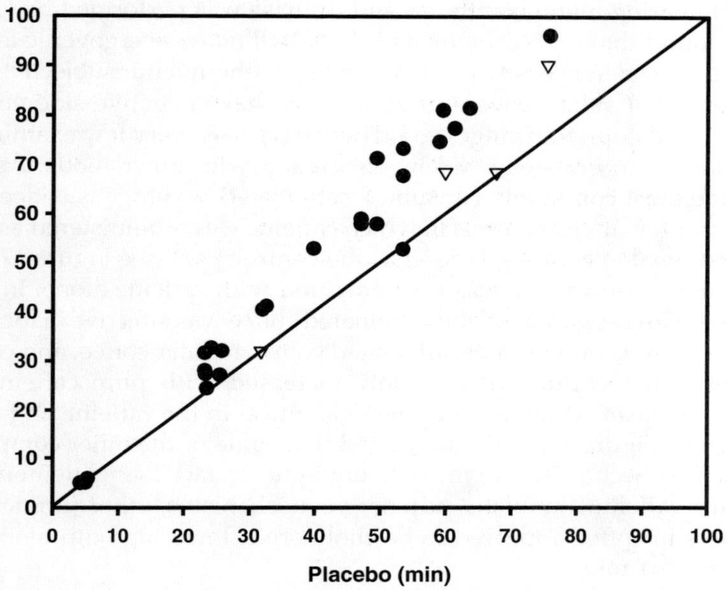

FIGURE 17.1
A summary of data from examinations of caffeine or coffee ingestion and exercise duration. The data plotted are mean data from a number of investigations[11,13,34,43–46,50,56,145–151] that had subjects either ingest placebo or decaffeinated coffee on one occasion and caffeine (circles) or caffeinated coffee (triangles) on the other occasion before exercising to exhaustion. The line is the line of identity. Thus any point above the line indicates that caffeine or caffeinated coffee increased endurance.

tage to a narrow range of activities. One of the interesting aspects of these examinations is that caffeine has a positive effect on exercise that lasts as little as 1 min and as long as 2 h, and enhances both aerobic and muscle strength endurance. There is little doubt that the physiological limitations of these various activities are quite different and yet they are influenced by caffeine. This suggests that there are multiple actions of caffeine.

17.2.4 Caffeine–Food Interactions and Ergogenics

There are many possible caffeine–food interactions. We are not aware of any studies that have examined exercise responses and the interactions of caffeine with specific foods or nutrients. As noted above, dimethylxanthines can be consumed rather than caffeine, or caffeine could be ingested as a component of coffee, tea, soft drinks, sport drinks, etc. While there have been a few investigations using these modes of administration prior to or during exercise, in almost every case the studies have not included a comparison with pure caffeine ingestion.

The vast majority of the studies in this area have administered caffeine in its pure form. Rarely have other methylxanthines been tested, and the only study comparing methylxanthines and exercise was performed by Greer et al.[43] We found that both caffeine and theophylline were ergogenic and that there was no difference between compounds, although our subjective observation was that subjects were more likely to have negative side effects of nausea after theophylline ingestion. There have been very few examinations of caffeine as an ergogenic aid in association with other foods. As noted above, the most commonly consumed caffeinated beverage is coffee. There have been a few investigations in which caffeine was administered as coffee, and decaffeinated coffee was used as the control[40,44–46] (see Figure 17.1), but this administration mode was not compared with caffeine alone. In all but one of these investigations,[45] the caffeinated coffee was effective in increasing endurance. We[11] compared decaffeinated coffee, regular coffee, and caffeine, and found that endurance was only increased with pure caffeine even though the plasma caffeine levels were identical in the caffeine and regular coffee trials (Figure 17.1). We suggested that some of the other components of coffee (see Section 17.2.6) must be ergolytic. In fact Tse[47,48] demonstrated that while caffeine stimulates adrenergic mechanisms, other (unidentified) substances in coffee appeared to be cholinergic, lowering both blood pressure and heart rate.

Sport drinks are commonly ingested prior to and during exercise. We are aware of only three studies that have carefully examined the ingestion of caffeine in solutions of carbohydrates and electrolytes.[39,49,50] Two of these demonstrated that caffeine combined with carbohydrates[50] and electrolytes[39] was superior to noncaffeinated drinks. Similarly, Cox et al.[38] examined cola that was either decaffeinated or caffeinated in a simulated cycle time trial and found the caffeinated cola to be ergogenic. These studies consisted of a series of experiments in which they compared ingestion of cola beverages with and without caffeine incorporated to caffeine ingestion with and without carbohydrates. They concluded that the caffeinated cola ingestion was effective, and this was mainly due to the caffeine and not the carbohydrate. While more studies are required, our tentative conclusion is that coffee is less effective than pure caffeine as an ergogenic aid, and that caffeinated beverages that also contain electrolytes and carbohydrates in concentrations similar to sport drinks are more effective than pure caffeine.

There have been concerns that the diuretic effects of caffeine could interfere with its ergogenic potential. The caffeine-induced diuresis takes several hours to develop, and if exercise takes place within this period, there does not appear to be an effect on sweat rate, plasma volume, electrolyte shifts, or urine production.[37,39,49,51–53] Both Armstrong[54] and Maughan and Griffin[55] have reviewed this topic and concluded that ingestion of caffeinated beverages resulted in the same urine production as the consumption of water, and there was no evidence of fluid-electrolyte imbalance.

The science of caffeine–food interactions is in its infancy. While the data are limited, it appears that caffeine and theophylline have similar ergogenic properties. Furthermore, caffeine in the form of coffee may be an inferior mode of consumption, while there is a synergy among caffeine and carbohydrates and electrolytes in fluid form. The interaction of caffeine and creatine is discussed in Section 17.3.6.

17.2.5 Caffeine–Drug Interactions and Ergogenics

It is uncertain whether characteristics such as caffeine consumption habits and the person's sex affect the ergogenic responses. While traditionally scientists have the subjects withdraw from all caffeine sources for 24 to 48 h prior to testing, we[56] have shown that the ergogenic effects are present and are not different following 0, 2, or 4 d of withdrawal from caffeine. In addition, Bell et al.[57] reported that caffeine administered to habitual caffeine users and nonusers resulted in similar ergogenic effects. Thus, it appears that neither the acute nor the chronic caffeine habits of the person are critical factors.

We are not aware of any study that has directly compared the ergogenic responses of men and women to caffeine. Studies that have examined female subjects[42] have demonstrated a caffeine-induced ergogenic response. There are reports[58,59] that women and men may not have the same capacity for metabolizing caffeine. However, McLean and Graham[60] performed a detailed comparison between fit young adult men and women (not using oral contraceptives), and they had very similar caffeine pharmacokinetics. Furthermore, neither menstrual cycle position, exercise, nor dehydration influenced the pharmacokinetics for the women. In contrast, women who are experiencing high levels of steroid hormones (oral contraceptive users or pregnant women) do have a decreased caffeine catabolism.[61] This would result in higher plasma caffeine levels and a longer half-life. These implications suggest that a lower dose of caffeine would be effective in these particular populations of women, but there is no reason to suspect that the ergogenic effects of caffeine would be altered. We are unaware of any study that has examined the possible interaction of oral contraceptives on the ergogenic effects of caffeine. To our knowledge, the only drug that has been examined in combination with caffeine for putative ergogenic purposes is ephedrine. If caffeine is acting via stimulation of the sympathetic nervous system, coingesting it with a sympathomimetic could be synergetic. The Canadian military has investigated the possible synergy of caffeine and ephedrine as an ergogenic aid. Bell and colleagues[62] reported that neither caffeine nor ephedrine were ergogenic when taken before performing intense exercise, but the combination resulted in increased time to fatigue. While this suggests that the two compounds are synergistic, it is surprising that they failed to find that caffeine alone was ergogenic. Subsequently, they came to a similar conclusion when subjects performed a 10-km run.[63] Once again, the results had a high degree of variability.

Recently, Shekelle et al.[64] conducted a meta-analysis of the impact of ephedrine on athletic performance. They remarked that very few studies had been conducted, mainly performed by Bell and colleagues.[62] This review also identified that several of the investigations only compared the combination of caffeine and ephedrine to placebo and did not include treatments with each drug separately. The studies do illustrate that the combination of caffeine and ephedrine is ergogenic, but it is uncertain whether the combination of caffeine and ephedrine has a greater ergogenic effect than caffeine alone. While sympathomimetics such as ephedrine (a nonselective adrenergic agonist) and related compounds are banned in most sports, they are frequently combined with caffeine in medications and supplements (often as ephedra) for weight loss (see Section 17.2.7). We are not aware of studies that have examined ephedra and caffeine under exercise conditions.

17.2.6 Caffeine, Foods, and Health and Safety Issues: Insulin Resistance

There is a wide range of health-related topics where caffeine could be discussed. It is possible that caffeine could affect nutrient assimilation. Recently, Johnston et al.[65] observed that caffeinated coffee altered the normal responses of gut incretins to a mixed meal. These hormones are potent stimuli to pancreatic beta cell stimulation and may play a role in satiety.[66] These findings need to be explored further.

Given that the theme of this text is food–drug synergy and safety, we use caffeine, coffee, and insulin actions as the example of food synergies. In a subsequent section dealing with drug interactions, we address the synergy between caffeine and ephedrine or ephedra, particularly with respect to weight loss. As noted previously, caffeine can antagonize adenosine receptors. Adenosine is known to facilitate the action of insulin on glucose uptake by adipocytes.[67,68] In contrast, when caffeine is ingested prior to performing exercise, there is no impact on either plasma insulin concentration or muscle glucose uptake during the exercise.[69] However, in this situation, insulin concentration is low in the resting subject, and it then declines even further during exercise. The subject's active muscles are able to take up glucose independent of insulin. In this circumstance, even if caffeine interfered with the actions of insulin, the impairment would be difficult to detect. Thus we resolved to examine the potential interaction of caffeine and insulin when insulin secretion is stimulated. In the initial study[70] we had lean, young, adult males ingest caffeine and 1 h later, consume 75 g of carbohydrates, i.e., an oral glucose tolerance test. During the subsequent 2 h, the plasma insulin concentration was 60% higher in the caffeine trial and despite this enhancement in insulin availability, blood glucose was 24% greater in the caffeine trial. We have subsequently observed a similar caffeine-induced insulin resistance (20 to 25% lower than placebo) in obese, young men both before and after a 12-week nutrition-exercise intervention that resulted in an 8% weight loss and a 60% increase in insulin sensitivity.[71] In addition, Lane et al.[72] found that caffeine ingestion prior to consuming a liquid meal (containing 75 g of carbohydrates) resulted in a 21 and 48% greater blood glucose and insulin response, respectively, in individuals with type 2 diabetes. Similarly, we[73] have studied middle-aged males with type 2 diabetes; they responded to caffeine by a modest increase in insulin and a large, prolonged accumulation

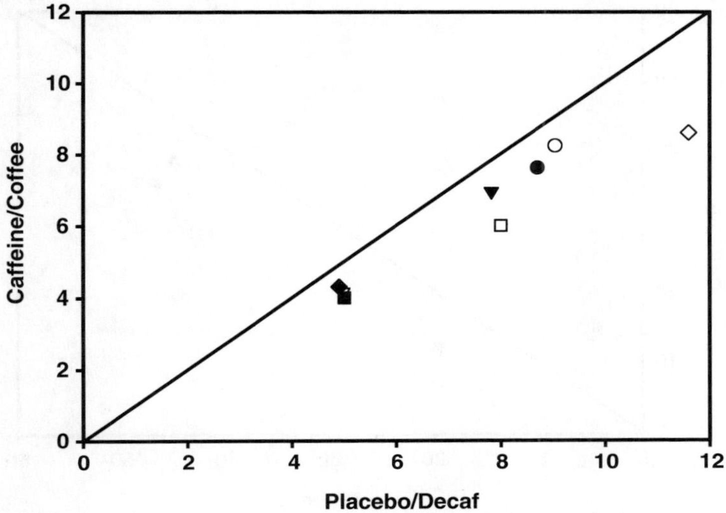

FIGURE 17.2
A summary of data from five studies of caffeine or caffeinated coffee ingestion on the insulin sensitivity index. The data are the mean data from Battram (unpublished: lean subjects with caffeine [open circle] or coffee [closed circle]), Chown[152] (lean men, closed triangle; obese men, open triangle), Petrie[71] (obese men, before [closed square] and after [open square] weight loss), Robinson et al.[73] (type 2 diabetics [closed diamond] and Thong and Graham[80] (lean, fit men [open diamond]. In each study the male subjects ingested either placebo or decaffeined coffee on one occasion and caffeine or caffeinated coffee on the other occasion. One hour later the subject ingested 75 g of glucose in liquid form. As in Figure 17.1, the line is the line of identity and any point that is below the line represents a situation in which the insulin sensitivity index was reduced by caffeine or caffeinated coffee. Insulin sensitivity index was calculated by the method of Matsuda and DeFronzo.[74]

of glucose in the circulation that lasted several hours. From these data one can estimate insulin sensitivity by calculating the "insulin sensitivity index."[74] Figure 17.2 summarizes the results from these investigations and others from our laboratory.

We[75,76] and others[77,78] have employed hyperinsulinemic clamps rather than an oral glucose tolerance test. In every study (Figure 17.3), methylxanthine administration resulted in decreased insulin sensitivity. De Galan et al.[77] have shown that this occurs in individuals with type 1 diabetes, and they also demonstrated that theophylline elicits insulin resistance similar to caffeine. There can be little doubt that acute administration of caffeine impedes the action of insulin. However, the insulin clamp method does not identify which tissues have reduced their glucose uptake.

Recently, Pencek et al.[79] have demonstrated that infusion of caffeine into the portal vein of conscious dogs results in an increase in net hepatic glucose uptake. In a hyperinsulinemic–euglycemic clamp, insulin sensitivity is based on the rate of glucose infusion that is necessary to maintain a constant blood glucose level. If caffeine increased hepatic glucose uptake, then there must

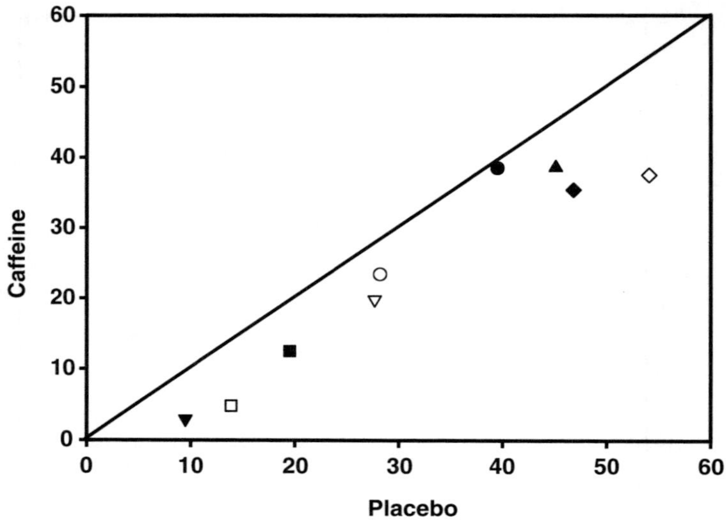

FIGURE 17.3
A summary data from four studies employing hyperinsulinemic clamps with or without caffeine or theophylline. The figure and data (glucose infusion rates [μmol/kg·min]) are organized as in Figure 17.2. The data are mean data from studies by De Galan et al.[77] (theophylline and type 1 diabetics at 5.0, 3.5, and 2.5 m*M* glucose [open triangles, closed squares, and open squares, respectively] and controls at the same glucose concentrations [closed circles, open circles, and closed triangles, respectively]), as well as euglycemia by Greer et al.[75] (lean, healthy men, closed diamond), Thong et al.[76] (lean, healthy men, open diamond), and Keijzers et al.[78] (healthy men, closed triangle).

be a greater impairment of glucose uptake by other tissues in order for whole-body disposal to be depressed. Thong et al.[76] examined leg metabolism using direct Fick techniques during the insulin clamp and observed that leg-muscle glucose uptake was suppressed by approximately 50%. Given that muscle composes about 35 to 40% of the body, presumably the effect on muscle more than balances the opposite influence of caffeine in the liver. We had anticipated that caffeine was inhibiting insulin's ability to promote glucose disposal in muscle by inhibiting the postreceptor signaling events of the hormone. However, analysis of muscle biopsies for a number of insulin signaling proteins failed to show any impact of caffeine. Keijzers et al.[78] have speculated that the mechanism of action is via the sympathetic nervous system, and subsequently Thong and Graham[80] reported that administration of the beta adrenergic antagonist propranolol abolished the influence of caffeine ingestion on glucose and insulin during an oral glucose tolerance test. Thus the stimulatory effect of caffeine on the sympathetic nervous system appears to be an important factor.

Given these recent studies, one would anticipate that coffee would be a detrimental dietary factor for anyone who is glucose intolerant or diabetic. However, there have been a number of recent epidemiological studies that have concluded exactly the opposite. They have reported that heavy, habitual

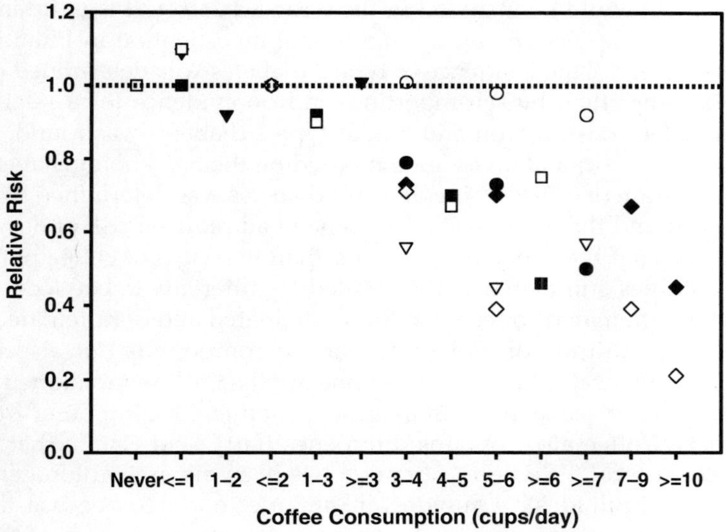

FIGURE 17.4
A summary of data from six investigations of relative risk (RR) of type 2 diabetes and coffee consumption. The horizontal dotted line is a RR of 1.0. The data are from van Dam and Feskens[81] (closed circles), Reunanen et al.[87] (open circles), Saremi et al.,[88] Knowler et al.[90] (closed triangles), Rosengren et al. [83] (open triangles, female subjects), Salazar-Martinez et al.[82] (closed squares, men and open squares, women), and Tuomilehto et al.[84] (closed diamonds, men, and open diamonds, women). The *x*-axis in nonlinear and is based on categories defined by each of the studies represented.

coffee consumption (greater than five to seven cups of coffee per day) may be protective against the development of type 2 diabetes.[81–86] When data from the epidemiological studies assessing the relative risk of type 2 diabetes according to coffee consumption are pooled, there appears to be a positive relationship between increased coffee consumption and decreased risk of developing type 2 diabetes (Figure 17.4). Despite the general consensus of these investigations, some studies have not replicated these findings and have shown no association between coffee intake and onset of type 2 diabetes.[87,88] We are aware of 11 studies that had population sample sizes ranging from 1,361 to 126,210 individuals. In the majority of these studies, individuals were stratified into various groupings of coffee consumption (ranging from never or less than 1 cup of coffee per day to greater than 10 cups per day) based on compiled dietary or food frequency questionnaires. During the follow-up period of the investigations, the number of new cases of type 2 diabetes among study participants was tracked and subsequent statistical analyses were used to determine whether a potential association between habitual coffee consumption and incidence of type 2 diabetes existed.

A significant weakness of six of these investigations is that the incidence of type 2 diabetes was either self-reported[81,82,87] or identified through record linkage.[83–85] Approximately 35% of cases of type 2 diabetes are unreported,[89] and thus they would be included in the wrong data set. It is of interest that in an original, population-based longitudinal investigation in Pima Indians by Saremi et al.,[88,90] the incidence of type 2 diabetes was determined directly by OGTT rather than by self-reporting, and no evidence for a relationship between coffee consumption and risk of type 2 diabetes was found. In contrast, in a cross-sectional investigation based on the Stockholm Diabetes Prevention Program ($n = 7949$),[86] incidence of diabetes was determined by OGTT, and it was found that both men and women had reduced risk of developing type 2 diabetes if they consumed greater than five cups of coffee per day.

Of the studies summarized, three failed to differentiate between caffeinated and decaffeinated coffee.[81,83,84] Both caffeinated and decaffeinated coffee consist of a multitude of biologically active compounds but also possess substantial chemical differences from one another.[14,15] As mentioned in Section 17.2.4, Tse[47,48] isolated an unidentified, cholinergic compound from coffee extracts. Coffee also contains diterpenes (fatty acid esters) that elevate plasma cholesterol.[91] Recently, attention has been given to chlorogenic acid and lactones (quinides).[4] Quinides are unique to coffee because they are formed during the roasting of the bean and they are not found in other caffeinated foods. Quinides have a variety of actions including antagonizing the mu opiod receptor. Of particular interest to the present discussion, the quinides have been reported to inhibit the adenosine transporter. This would result in an accumulation of interstitial adenosine, and this would in turn act contrary to caffeine on adenosine receptors. Shearer et al.[92] recently reported that chronic administration of quinides to rats increased insulin sensitivity. In contrast to caffeine, these compounds did not affect muscle because skeletal muscle glucose uptake was not enhanced, and she speculated that the quinides stimulated hepatic glucose uptake. There are many compounds in coffee that could have biological effects. Some of these may be specific to coffee and are not present in other caffeinated foods or beverages. Thus one must be very careful at applying findings in a general fashion. One example of this is the increasing usage of guarana extract in products. This may well add caffeine to the product, and it may be adding other active ingredients as well.

The marked contrast between the acute, negative effects of caffeine ingestion on insulin sensitivity and the observation that habitual coffee ingestion is associated with decreased risk for type 2 diabetes presents two possibilities. Caffeine in coffee may not be effective and/or chronic consumption of caffeinated coffee may result in the habituation to caffeine, allowing the effects of other biologically active compounds such as quinides to remain unchallenged by the actions of caffeine. Presently we do not know if humans habituate to either the effects of caffeine or to the effects of compounds such as the quinides. If the former occurs, it is rapidly reversed. Most of the subjects in the studies described above have regularly consumed caffeinated coffee for years. In the experiments, they must withdraw from all caffeine for 48 h prior to testing and they are quite responsive to caffeine.

Although, collectively, these investigations have reported significant associations and are based on data compiled from large sample sizes with an average follow-up of approximately 13.5 years, there are factors that warrant cautious interpretation of these studies. Brown et al.[23] assessed total caffeine intake of adults in Ontario, Canada, and placed the subjects into quartiles. While regular coffee was the most common source of caffeine intake, they found that coffee intake severely underestimated the total intake, and if used alone, it resulted in serious misclassification. For example, of 93 subjects in the quartile of total caffeine intake of 116 to 230 mg/d, only 2% were correctly classified by coffee intake, while 48% were incorrectly placed in the 1 to 115 mg/d quartile, and 49% were in the nonuser quartile! In studies such as those reviewed in this section, those subjects who consume five or more cups of coffee a day are also heavy caffeine consumers. However, the findings of Brown et al.[23] strongly suggest that some of the subjects consuming less coffee could also have heavy caffeine consumption as well. The authors then created a hypothetical case-control distribution to provide odds ratio estimates for both threshold and dose-response associations between caffeine intake and the hypothetical disease. A hypothetical 10-fold increase in risk was completely obscured when only coffee intake was employed rather than total caffeine intake. They concluded that the tendency to equate coffee and caffeine exposure is not accurate and can produce misleading conclusions regarding caffeine.

Whether coffee consumption is protective against type 2 diabetes and what mechanism accounts for the potentially protective effect of coffee are questions that remain to be elucidated. Clearly, coffee is a complex food, and there are many compounds that could promote or oppose the actions of caffeine. Compounds such as the quinides and diterpenes are specific to coffee because they are formed when the bean is roasted. Not only must one be cautious of generally applying the effects of caffeine to coffee, but it is also very important not to extrapolate the studies of coffee ingestion to consumption of tea or other foods containing caffeine.

Caffeine and coffee were selected as the example for this topic because of the large body of literature concerning this subject. It is clear that one cannot safely apply findings from studies of caffeine ingestion to coffee. Two recent studies suggest that this is also true for other substances. Choi et al.[93] provided growing rats with caffeinated cola for 28 weeks. Compared to pair-fed control animals, the treated rats gained less weight and had a greater sensitivity to insulin. In contrast, Brand-Miller et al.[94] compared the glycemic and insulinemic responses of a wide range of products with or without chocolate (cocoa powder). The glycemic responses were not affected by the chocolate, but the insulinemic responses were on average 28% greater, implying that some aspects of the chocolate created an insulin resistance. The results of these two studies suggest the contrast between coffee and caffeine is not unique and that the metabolic responses to chocolate-flavored foods and colas are also unique.

17.2.7 Caffeine and Health and Safety Issues: Weight Loss Supplements

Caffeine has been studied as a potential aid in promoting weight loss. When it is administered acutely, there is a very modest increase in resting metabolic rate and in dietary-induced thermogenesis.[95–99] The effect was found to be small, there was no evidence for increased fat oxidation (i.e. decrease in respiratory exchange ratio), and chronic ingestion of caffeine with diet intervention[100] was found to be no more effective than diet intervention alone. Thus, investigators explored the putative synergistic effects of combining caffeine administration with the sympathomimetic, ephedrine.[96,100] Various studies[101–104] have demonstrated that the combination of caffeine and ephedrine taken acutely is effective in increasing whole-body metabolic rate in humans. Chronic ingestion of these drugs has been shown to result in a greater weight loss[64,104] than placebo treatments, but the possible side effects and risks have made the supplement controversial.

Ephedrine is found in its organic form in a Chinese herb, ma huang, or Chinese ephedra (*Ephedra sinica*). The active ingredients of this herb consist of ephedrine and related alkaloids (mostly ephedrine, pseudoephedrine, methylephedrine, norephedrine, and norpseudoephedrine).[105,106] As noted earlier, caffeine is found in many plants, including coffee, tea, cocoa, guarana, and kola nut. Thus, natural health products can be constructed to include caffeine and symphathomimetics, and many companies have marketed such supplements claiming to promote weight loss.

There are very few long-term trials of caffeine and ephedrine mixtures. The primary investigation was a double-blind placebo-controlled study by Astrup et al.[100] in which 180 obese patients were treated by diet and ephedrine, caffeine, a combination of the two drugs, or placebo 3 times a day for 24 weeks. The group receiving the combination supplement lost a significantly greater amount of weight than the other three groups. Dietary restriction was not individualized, and even intake was not frequently monitored.[100,107]

Caffeine and drug synergy was further examined with respect to aspirin (ASA) (often referred to as "the stack").[108,109] Daly et al.[96] investigated ASA in combination with ephedrine and caffeine on the basis that the ASA could enhance the sympathetic response by inhibiting prostaglandins that inhibit norepinephrine.[110] Another 8-week, double-blind placebo-controlled trial completed by Daly et al.[96] compared an ephedrine (75 to 150 mg), caffeine (150 mg), and ASA (330 mg) mixture to a placebo in 24 obese subjects with no restrictions on energy intake. There was a significantly greater weight loss within the treatment group vs. placebo. Although this investigation did not compare the combination of caffeine and ephedrine with and without ASA, it appears that it is the basis for many natural health products that include ASA.

Subsequent placebo-controlled, double-blind trials with obese subjects using caffeine and ephedrine or ephedra treatments have consistently found the supplement to result in greater weight loss.[104,111,112] It is important to note that dietary and exercise controls were minimal, and in one study, they concluded that dietary restriction was not accurate because of a significant amount of underreporting.[111] As noted below, the most common and prolonged side effect of caffeine and ephedrine is suppression of appetite. Astrup et al. estimated that 80% of fat lost was due to the anorectic effect of the compound and about 20% was due to the thermogenic effect of the combination.[113] A number of investigations have examined ingestion of caffeine and ephedrine for potential side effects. Studies[102,114,115] examining the acute effects have generally focused on the cardiovascular impact of these drugs. Generally, a single dose elevates both systolic and diastolic blood pressure and heart rate. For example, Astrup et al.[100] reported a 5 to 7 beat/min increase in heart rate and an 8 to 10 mmHg increase in systolic blood pressure over 3 h with different drug doses while diastolic blood pressure decreased. Long-term trials consistently show that subjective side effects are present (usually consisting of insomnia, palpitations, nausea, tremor, and headache) but often are described as transient and disappear within 2 to 4 weeks.[100,111,112,116] No significant changes in blood pressure were found in chronic studies,[107,111,117–119] and Greenway[104] also noted that there was no influence on serum lipids.

Haller and Benowitz[120] performed an independent review of approximately 140 adverse event reports submitted to the U.S. Food and Drug Administration between June 1, 1997, and March 31, 1999, to determine risk to the consumer. Of these reports, 43 cases were considered to be definitely or probably related to ephedra alkaloids, 44 cases were considered to be possibly related to ephedra alkaloids, and the remaining cases were either unrelated or it was impossible to establish causation. They concluded that ephedra alkaloids could be potentially fatal for some individuals. Recently, Chen et al.[121] reported five cases where patients suffered myocardial infarctions while using ephedra-containing products, and they concluded that ephedrine predisposes patients to ischemic and hemorrhagic strokes. However, Kalman[122] reanalyzed his previous work[123] in which overweight subjects consumed ephedra and caffeine for 2 weeks. Reanalysis confirmed the original conclusion that there were no statistically significant differences between treatment and placebo groups within specific event types, but the former did have more overall adverse effects. The most common were dry mouth, increased activity, and upper respiratory tract infections, all of which occurred in 20% of subjects. There were no serious adverse effects, and they observed no differences in echocardiograms, electrocardiograms, and blood pressure. Shekelle et al.[64] also conducted a meta-analysis of published reports on ephedra and ephedrine and weight loss. After screening 530 articles, they examined 52 controlled studies and 65 case reports. There were no reports of serious adverse effects among the 1,706 subjects in the 52 controlled studies, and they concluded that caffeine was synergistic with ephedrine or ephedra and resulted in a greater weight loss of 0.8 to 1.0 kg/month compared to placebo. They also estimated that there was a 2.2 to 3.6 greater risk of psychiatric, autonomic, or gastrointestinal symptoms and heart palpitations. In the case studies, the adverse events included 5 deaths, 5 myocardial infarctions, 11 cerebrovascular accidents, 4 seizures, and 8 psychiatric cases. In contrast, Greenway[104] reviewed the safety and efficacy of caffeine and ephedrine use in weight loss. He concluded that caffeine and ephedrine do act synergistically to promote weight loss, that they are as effective as diethylpropion, and superior to dexfenfluramine in inducing weight loss. Greenway concluded that the randomized, double-blind placebo-controlled trials have shown that the side effects of the drugs are mild and transient, and the cause–effect relationships in the case study reports of adverse effects are unclear. He pointed out that the number of case reports of adverse events is very small relative to the billions of caffeine–ephedrine doses consumed per year and that the weight loss benefits to the obese person outweigh the risks. These studies have not been controlled for subject characteristics and include a wide range of ages and body composition among both men and women. There could be a subset of people who are more susceptible to cardiovascular complications and side effects.

Currently there are very few pharmaceutical or herbal combinations available for weight loss. In some cases the side effects of pharmaceuticals are too severe to make them effective products. For example, fenfluramine has been associated with valvular heart disease,[124] and there are limited options for anorectic drugs due to the negative dependence effects seen with certain addictive amphetamines.[117]

17.3 Creatine

17.3.1 The Mode of Action

The work by Hultman and Greenhaff in the early 1990's has resulted in a great deal of scientific interest in creatine supplementation. Creatine exists in the body both in the free (Cr) and phosphorylated (CrP) form. The latter, phosphocreatine, is vital in tissues as an "energy buffer." Cr and CrP are found in tissues that can experience intense energy demands (skeletal and cardiac muscle, retina, brain, spermatozoa, etc.). These tissues contain both ATP and CrP, and when ATP is hydrolyzed to produce ADP and energy, CrP reacts with the ADP to reform ATP. The resulting Cr is rephosphorylated when the mitochondria produce more ATP. The Cr–CrP reaction is also important in transferring the ATP formed inside the mitochondria to the cytosol. The formation of Cr consumes hydrogen ions, and thus it can act as a buffer to the acidosis generated by glycolysis. In skeletal muscle, brief, intense contractions rely heavily on this ATP–CrP pathway. During these contractions the ATP to ADP ratio remains remarkably constant while the CrP to Cr ratio declines markedly.

17.3.2 Creatine Production and Metabolism

Creatine monohydrate is a very commonly used supplement in sports, taken for the purpose of increasing muscle mass and strength. Muscle contains about 95% of the body's creatine, but it cannot synthesize the compound. Creatine is a nonessential nutrient that is obtained primarily from meat and fish, and it is absorbed almost completely intact in the intestine. It can also be synthesized by the liver and, to a modest degree, by the pancreas and kidneys, from the amino acids arginine, glycine, and methionine. In humans, the kidney begins the synthesis by forming ornithine and guanidinoacetate from arginine and glycine. Guanidinoacetate is then transported to the liver where it is methylated to creatine using methionine.

Slow twitch, or type I, muscle fibers have 5 to 15% lower levels of Cr stores,[118,125,126] reflecting the role of type II fibers in bolistic activity. Type I fibers have been reported to take up Cr to a greater degree during supplementation.[118,125] The muscle and other tissues are able to take up creatine from the circulation using a membrane-based transporter. The transporter is saturable and is sodium- and chloride-dependent, and is susceptible to both hormonal and dietary regulation. Both insulin and catecholamines stimulate the transporter, but it appears that the most important regulator is plasma Cr.[125] The latter also down-regulates the production of guanidinoacetate in the kidney, resulting in decreased endogenous production of Cr. Cr has a long half-life in muscle (about 2% of the body's Cr is excreted per day), and it is converted nonenzymatically to creatinine and lost in the urine.

17.3.3 Creatine as an Ergogenic Aid

While meat and fish are relatively rich in Cr, it is not possible to consume enough to increase the body's Cr stores above normal levels. The normal intake is about 1 g/d and the body normally synthesizes 1 g/d. On the other hand, ingestion of creatine monohydrate results in a rapid, 15 to 20-fold increase in plasma Cr.[118,125,126] During the first few days of supplement ingestion, the body retains most of the additional Cr, and there is a reduction in urine production due to the osmotic load. Subsequently, up to 90% of the Cr is excreted unaltered in the urine. Thus the common supplement ingestion procedure is typically to consume 20 g/d for 5 d and then to decrease this to a "maintenance dose" (2 to 5 g/d). The consensus statement of the American College of Sports Medicine[126] is that this initial large supplementation is not necessary and that a steady intake of 3 g/d will result in a similar enhancement, although over a longer period of time (i.e., 30 d vs. 4 to 6 d). Even this more modest intake is impossible via the normal diet. Meat has only 4 to 5 g/kg and some of this is destroyed during cooking. If Cr supplementation is stopped, the muscle Cr stores slowly return to normal over many weeks (decreasing by about 2 g/d).

There is considerable variability in the impact of creatine loading on muscle stores. Since the major dietary sources of Cr are meat and fish, there is speculation that vegetarians may have the greatest responses. There are anecdotal reports that those with lower initial muscle total Cr concentrations (Cr + CrP) increase to a greater extent. However, Branch[127] performed a meta-analysis of 100 studies and concluded that there was no association between the initial muscle concentration and the percent increase in Cr content with supplementation. It appears the upper limit for muscle total Cr is about 160 mmol/kg dry weight, and Branch[127] concluded that the average increase with supplementation was 18%.

Exercise prior to Cr ingestion appears to enhance muscle uptake,[125,126] and this is specific for the exercised muscles. This means that a local factor is involved, but it is well known that total muscle Cr is not changed by acute exercise. Insulin is thought to regulate the Cr transporter, and exercised muscle is insulin sensitive with regard to GLUT 4. It may be that a similar response is induced in the Cr transporter.

When a person begins to "Cr load," there is a rapid weight gain (1 to 3 kg) that occurs within a few (5 to 7 d) days.[118,119,126,127] This has been attributed to the reduction in urine output as described previously. There are a number of reports of a slow gradual weight gain with maintenance supplementation, but there are very few long term studies.[118,125–127] There have been hundreds of studies of Cr loading and exercise performance or capacity. In contrast to the investigations of caffeine, the findings have been somewhat inconsistent. This may, in part, be due to the nature of the exercise. It is very technically difficult to show significant changes in activity that only lasts a few seconds. The general consensus from a number of reviews[118,125,127] and roundtable discussions of experts[2,126] is that Cr loading is ergogenic for short, intense exercise, particularly if the activity is repeated. The major process that appears to be enhanced is the speed at which CrP can be restored after intense contractions. There is no evidence that Cr loading enhances maximal isometric strength, maximal rate of force production, or aerobic activity. Nevertheless, the findings of the various studies are inconsistent. This has been attributed[118,119,125,128] to faulty experimental protocols, interindividual variability of degree of change in muscle Cr stores, coupled with a lack of documentation of the muscle Cr concentration, small sample size, lack of crossover experimental designs, and poor dietary controls (including meat and caffeine intake).

Generally Cr supplementation coupled with resistance or strength training is positive in increasing body mass and lean mass, most likely because of greater training capacity. This increase in body weight may be helpful in some sports but detrimental in others. The most common side effect is the rapid weight gain of several kilograms early in the supplementation. This can have a negative impact on athletic performance and has been attributed to increased body water.[119,125] Other side effects that have been considered include gastrointestinal distress, cramps, and heat intolerance, but most reviews[118,126,127] conclude that weight gain is the only documented side effect of supplementation in healthy adults. There have been no long term studies even though some athletic populations are thought to use the supplement for months, if not years. The fact that it is widely used and there are very few reports of problems suggests that the side effects are minimal.

There are concerns that supplementation should not be used by people who have kidney dysfunction or pathologies. In chronic kidney disease where the glomerular filtration rate is compromised, circulating creatinine levels and oxidative stress can greatly increase. This can result in the formation of toxic creatinine degradation products in a variety of tissues and in the gut by intestinal bacteria. These products can aggravate the kidney disorder.[125]

17.3.4 Mechanism of Action

At a simplistic level, the mechanism of action is fairly obvious: an enhancement of muscle Cr, and especially CrP, should facilitate the buffering of the critical ATP stores during intense contractions and also facilitate the restoration of high energy stores to homeostasis following contractions. One naively tends to associate ATP use in muscle only with contraction mechanisms, but it is also critical for relaxation, and the rate at which the cell relaxes is important to performance. Hespel et al.[118] point out that the sarcoplasmic reticulum (SR) Ca^{2+}-ATPase is very sensitive to the ATP to ADP ratio and tightly coupled to Cr kinase. This ATPase uses up to 40 to 50% of the ATP during contractions, and Van Leemputte et al.[129] found that Cr supplementation shortens the relaxation time of human muscle. As noted earlier, slow twitch or type I fibers have lower levels of Cr stores and take up Cr to a greater degree during supplementation.[118,125] McGuire et al.[130] found that rodent slow twitch muscle (soleus) responded to Cr supplementation with an approximate 10% faster relaxation time following an isometric twitch and fatigue resistance was enhanced. In contrast, the fast twitch muscle (extensor digitorum longus) was not affected.

Increasing muscle Cr stores should facilitate the performance of repeated bouts of intense activity. This would facilitate anaerobic training, which, in turn could produce the observed effects of Cr supplementation. However, the actions of this nutrient may well be more complex. There is evidence that Cr supplementation can directly facilitate muscle protein synthesis when the muscle undergoes resistance exercise. Hespel et al.[131] examined Cr supplementation in subjects who had one leg immobilized for 2 weeks and then rehabilitated for 10 weeks. Supplementation did not influence the muscle atrophy during immobilization (10% decrease in cross-sectional area) or the loss of thigh power (25%), but during rehabilitation, the limb increased in volume more rapidly and had a greater capacity to produce force even though the training workload was the same as in those receiving placebo. Supplementation did not alter plasma growth hormone, testosterone, or cortisol. However, training in combination with supplementation resulted in expression of myogenic transcription factor MRF4 and prevented an increase in myogenin protein expression. This suggests that there can be effects isolated to those muscles specifically exercised. And this is compatible with the earlier report that previously exercised muscle is more receptive to the uptake of Cr.

While Cr supplementation did not alter muscle atrophy during the immobilization,[132] it did prevent a 20% immobilization-induced decline in GLUT 4 content that occurred in the placebo group. During 10 weeks of rehabilitation, the muscle content of GLUT 4 was facilitated by 40% while in the control group GLUT 4 was only restored to the preimmobilization concentration. This could be important in the interaction of Cr and carbohydrate ingestion (see Section 17.3.5).

On the basis of findings from studies with animal models using supraphysiological doses of Cr, there has been speculation that Cr supplementation would result in a decrease in skeletal muscle Cr transporter. However, Tarnopolsky et al.[133] examined this in detail and found no evidence for such an effect. They found no change in mRNA for the transporter in the muscle of young adults after 8 to 9 d of supplementation and no change in the transporter protein concentration after 2 months of supplementation and resistance training. This is obviously an area that requires far more investigation.

17.3.5 Creatine–Food Interactions and Ergogenics

The coingestion of Cr with large amounts of simple carbohydrates (up to 100 g of carbohydrate per 5 g of Cr) has been shown to enhance muscle uptake, most likely as a result of the increased insulin that, in turn, may stimulate the Cr transporter.[2,125,126] It is not clear whether this only hastens the normal process of increasing the muscle Cr concentration or whether the tissue actually stores more Cr. In addition, it is not known if this enhances the ergogenic effects of Cr supplementation nor is it established if repeated coingestion is beneficial in the long term.

This interaction with insulin and carbohydrates presents the possibility that Cr supplementation and expansion of the muscle Cr pool could be linked to glycogen. Op't et al.[134] found that when rats were supplemented with Cr for 5 d, total muscle Cr increased predominantly in the soleus (slow twitch) muscle, and there was a 40% increase in muscle glycogen as well. However, there were no changes in circulating insulin concentration or in muscle glucose transport rate, muscle GLUT 4 content, or glycogen synthase activity. As noted above, this same group found that Cr supplementation had a positive impact on muscle GLUT 4 in humans during rehabilitation following immobilization, but in that investigation there was no consistent impact on muscle glycogen. It is not known why the findings are not consistent between studies. One must note that not only was the species studied and protocol different, but also that the human muscle that was analyzed would be a mixture of fiber types.

17.3.6 Creatine–Drug Interactions and Ergogenics

An aspect that clearly is central to this review is a possible interaction between caffeine and creatine. Intuitively, one would not expect an interaction because caffeine is commonly identified with ergogenic effects in prolonged, aerobic exercise while Cr is associated with ergogenic effects for brief, intense aerobic contractions. On the other hand, both are ergogenic and there is evidence that they may both affect aspects of excitation–contraction coupling. Thus, if there is an interaction, one might expect it to be synergistic. Surprisingly, Hespel and coworkers[118,135] reported the exact opposite findings. They had subjects ingest placebo or Cr for 6 days while a third group consumed the same Cr supplementation but on the last 3 days they also ingested caffeine. The subjects completed intense, "anaerobic" exercise tests about 20 h after the last dietary treatment. The ingestion of caffeine did not affect Cr incorporation into the muscle because the two Cr treatments both increased total muscle Cr by 4 to 6%. The Cr group improved their knee extensor torque output by 10 to 23%, while there was no improvement in the group that also ingested caffeine with the Cr. This finding is even more remarkable when one realizes that assessment was performed 20 h after the last caffeine ingestion. The half-life of caffeine is 4 to 6 h, thus there would be very little caffeine remaining in the circulation.

These findings were examined further[136] using a similar nutritional supplementation regime in a randomized crossover design protocol. They also included a trial with 3 d of caffeine supplementation without Cr ingestion as well as one where the only caffeine ingested was a single, acute dose (5 mg/kg) 1 h prior to testing. The exercise testing employed electric stimulation of the quadriceps and detailed assessments of the contractions. Cr supplementation shortened the muscle relaxation time by approximately 5% while 3 d of caffeine ingested lengthened it by 10%. Daly and Fredholm[4] report that A_1 receptors in neurons activate potassium channels and inhibit calcium channels. If the A_1 receptor functions in a similar fashion in skeletal muscle, then antagonism could lead to a lengthening of the relaxation time. However, it is surprising that an acute dose of caffeine had no effect on relaxation time and yet the 3-d treatment was effective even though the circulating level of caffeine would be very low at the time of testing! Short-term ingestion of caffeine negated the effects of Cr supplementation on relaxation time (performance was not measured) even though there would be little caffeine in the circulation during the time of testing. This suggests that some of the actions of the supplements require prolonged exposure and are long lasting, perhaps acting at the level of gene expression. As noted above, this same research group has reported evidence that Cr supplementation may alter gene expression. We are not aware of any comparable evidence for caffeine, but this does raise the intriguing question: Does repeated ingestion of caffeine alter gene expression in muscle?

Doherty et al.[137] had subjects ingest Cr for 6 d and then complete a treadmill running test that lasted approximately 3 to 4 min. Prior to one test, the subjects ingested 5 mg/kg of caffeine. Caffeine resulted in a 10% increase in endurance, while Cr supplementation had no effect. These results may seem contrary to the findings that caffeine interferes with the effects of Cr supplementation. However, one would not expect Cr supplementation to have an ergogenic effect in this exercise situation. Similarly, Hespel et al.[136] did not find an interaction between supplements when caffeine was only ingested acutely.

Unfortunately, this intriguing paradox does not appear to have been investigated further, and many questions remain unanswered and the mechanisms remain to be established. In addition, it remains unknown if coffee consumption has the same effect as caffeine. If this were the case, this could confound many long-term Cr supplementation studies that have not controlled for caffeine and coffee ingestion. The American College of Sport Medicine[126] suggested that coffee ingestion does not interfere with the ergogenic effects of Cr, but did not provide any references. However, as discussed in Section 17.2.6, one must not transpose findings from studies using caffeine to complex beverages such as coffee.

17.3.7 Creatine and Health

Bioenergetic dysfunction can be a factor in apoptosis that is associated with neurodegenerative and neuromuscular diseases as well as that in normal aging. The conclusions of various reviews on the topic of Cr supplementation and the muscle mass of the elderly are very inconsistent. There is some suggestion that Cr stores decline with age and that following exercise, the resynthesis of CrP is slower. Wyss and Kaddurah-Daouk[125] concluded that supplementation of Cr was not only effective in middle-aged individuals, but also that the ergogenic benefits increased with age. Brose et al.[138] completed a detailed study with men and women over 65 years old and, unlike many studies in this area, theirs employed direct measures of body composition and muscle biopsies. Cr supplementation combined with resistance exercise over 14 weeks improved muscle Cr concentration by 27% and resulted in a greater increase in fat free mass, body weight, and a greater improvement in strength of various muscle groups. The training resulted in hypertrophy of type I fibers, but there was no difference between supplementation and placebo. However, Eijnde et al.[139] conducted a thorough study in which men and women aged 55 to 75 years received Cr supplementation for up to 1 year while undergoing an exercise program that involved a combination of aerobic and strength training. There was no impact of the supplement on the training responses. However, muscle Cr was only modestly elevated and surprisingly, there was no improvement in maximal isometric strength over the year in either group. The responses of such groups may be dependent on the quality of the subjects and the nature of the training program.

Tarnopolsky et al.[133] found that 4 months of Cr supplementation and resistance training did not influence skeletal muscle Cr transporter content.

In both of these studies,[133,138] the elderly had normal initial levels of total CR and this increased substantially during supplementation. Their work showed no sign of the muscle of subjects who were more than 65 years of age having an unusual response to Cr supplementation.

Tarnopolsky and Parise[140] reported that CrP as well as ATP concentrations are lower in the muscles of patients with several neuromuscular diseases. Tarnopolsky et al.[141] also found that such patients also had lower concentrations of Cr transporter protein in their muscles, while generally they had normal levels of mitochondrial Cr kinase. This implies that the reduced Cr in their muscles was directly related to the transporter. Benefits of Cr supplementation are speculated for a variety of disease states. Tarnopolsky and Beal[142] reviewed this topic, and they concluded that there was substantial evidence from studies of animal models that Cr supplementation can provide neuroprotective effects and that clinical studies with patients are promising. Cr supplementation increases brain as well as muscle total Cr concentration, and this may protect against neuronal degeneration and chemically mediated neurotoxicity, in part by attenuating the accumulation of markers of oxidative stress. The one area where fairly extensive work has been conducted is in neuromuscular diseases that are characterized by low muscle Cr concentrations, and muscle atrophy and weakness such as inflammatory myopathy, mitochondrial cytopathy, and muscular dystrophy. Tarnopolsky and coworkers have contributed significantly to this area. They[140] found that Cr supplementation increased the muscle strength of patients with neuromuscular disorders or mitochondrial cytopathologies. Subsequently, they have recently reported[143] that boys with Duchanne muscular dystrophy responded positively to 4 months of Cr supplementation. They increased handgrip strength and fat free mass and had a reduction in urinary N-telopeptides, a marker of bone breakdown. Conversely, they[144] found no effect of a similar supplementation in adults with myotonic dystrophy type 1. In this group of patients, magnetic resonance spectroscopy demonstrated that the supplement did not alter intramuscular total Cr. No effect could be expected if the treatment was not able to increase the Cr store.

17.4 Conclusions

Caffeine and Cr are two of the most common and most effective ergogenic aids. Caffeine may have interactions with a variety of compounds, some of which appear to be found in beverages such as coffee, thus limiting the ability to generalize the findings of caffeine to caffeinated foods and beverages. Caffeine is synergistic with ephedrine and ephedra in weight loss supplements and possibly also as an ergogenic aid. However, the potential for cardiovascular complications implies that the use of this combination should be restricted and supervised by medical personnel.

There is a great deal of evidence that Cr supplementation is effective in enhancing the ability of muscle to produce repeated bouts of intense exercise. There is also evidence that muscle hypertrophy can occur. There is no consensus regarding whether this is due to the facilitation of the volume resistance training or to direct actions on gene expression. Unfortunately the vast majority of studies have been descriptive. There is evidence that the initial level of muscle Cr is a deciding factor in the effectiveness of Cr supplementation. The most exciting applications of Cr supplementation are in situations where the muscle mass is compromised because of atrophy, sarcopenia, or neuromuscular disorders. The only food or drug interaction that was identified is the paradox that caffeine ingestion for several days may inhibit the effectiveness of Cr.

Both caffeine and Cr are examples of nutritional supplements that are effective and also illustrate that the actions of these compounds are diverse and complicated. There are subsets of the population that may have different responses to the supplements and situations when there are interactions with other foods or drugs. These interactions may result in altered responses to the supplement and one should not think of the compounds as simple nutrients that have only one action on the body.

Acknowledgment

The work by the authors was supported by the Natural Science and Engineering Research Council of Canada (NSERC), and L. Moisey held an NSERC industrial scholarship sponsored by Gatorade.

References

1. Kanayama, G. et al., Over-the-counter drug use in gymnasiums: an underrecognized substance abuse problem? *Psychother. Psychosom.*, 70, 137, 2001.
2. Rawson, E.S., and Clark, P.M., Scientifically debatable: is creatine worth its weight? *Sports Science Exchange*, 16, 1, 2003.
3. Melia, P., Pipe, A., and Greenberg,L., The use of anabolic-androgenic steroids by Canadian students, *Clin. J. Sports Med.*, 6, 9, 1996.
4. Daly, J.W. and Fredholm, B.B., Mechanisms of action of caffeine on the nervous system, in *Coffee, Tea, Chocolate And The Brain*, Nehlig, A., Ed., CRC Press, Boca Raton, FL, 2004, chap.1.
5. Reppert, S.M. et al., Molecular cloning and characterization of a rat A1-adenosine receptor that is widely expressed in brain and spinal cord, *Mol. Endocrinol.*, 5, 1037, 1991.
6. Dixon, A.K. et al., Tissue distribution of adenosine receptor mRNAs in the rat, *Br. J. Pharmacol.*, 118, 1461, 1996.

7. Hohimer, A.R. et al., Effect of exercise on uterine blood flow in the pregnant pygmy goat, *Am. J. Physiol. 246,* H207, 1984.
8. Fredholm, B.B. et al., Actions of caffeine in the brain with special reference to factors that contribute to its widespread use, *Pharmacol. Rev.,* 51, 83, 1999.
9. Robertson, D. et al., Tolerance to the humoral and hemodynamic effects of caffeine in man, *J. Clin. Invest.,* 67, 1111, 1981.
10. Benowitz, N.L. et al., Sympathomimetic effects of paraxanthine and caffeine in humans, *Clin. Pharmacol.,* 58, 684, 1995.
11. Graham, T.E., Hibbert, E., and Sathasivam, P., The metabolic and exercise endurance effects of coffee and caffeine ingestion, *J. Appl. Physiol.,* 85, 883, 1998.
12. Van Soeren, M.H. et al., Caffeine metabolism and epinephrine responses during exercise in users and nonusers, *J. Appl. Physiol.,* 75, 805, 1993.
13. Graham, T.E. and Spriet, L.L., Metabolic, catecholamine, and exercise performance responses to various doses of caffeine, *J. Appl. Physiol.,* 78, 867, 1995.
14. Spiller, A.M., The coffee plant and its processing, in *Caffeine,* Spiller, G.A., Ed., CRC Press, Boca Raton, FL, 1998, chap. 5.
15. Spiller, A.M., The chemical components of coffee, in *Caffeine,* Spiller, G.A., Ed., CRC Press, Boca Raton, FL, 1998, chap. 6.
16. Harland, B.F., Caffeine and nutrition, *Nutrition,* 16, 522, 2000.
17. Lundsberg, L.S., Caffeine consumption, in *Caffeine,* Spiller, G.A., Ed., CRC Press, Boca Raton, FL, 1998, chap. 9.
18. Food and Agricultural Organization, Coffee food balance sheet, Rome, 2001. Source: FAOSTAT statistical databases.
19. Gilbert, R.M., Caffeine consumption, in *The Methylxanthine Beverages and Foods: Chemistry, Consumption, and Health Effects*, Spiller, G.A., Ed., Alan R. Liss, Inc., New York, 1984, chap.9.
20. Nawrot, P. et al., Effects of caffeine on human health, *Food Addit. Contam.,* 20, 1, 2003.
21. Statistics Canada, Food consumption in Canada (part I and part II, 2002), 32-229-XIB, Minister of Industry, Ottawa, 2003.
22. D'Amicis, A. and Viani, R., The consumption of coffee, in *Caffeine, Coffee, and Health*, Garattini, S., Ed., Raven Press, New York, 1993, chap.1.
23. Brown, J. et al., Misclassification of exposure: coffee as a surrogate for caffeine intake, *Am.J. Epidemiol.,* 153, 815, 2001.
24. Graham, T.E., The possible actions of methylxanthines on various tissues, in *The Clinical Pharmacology of Sport and Exercise,* Reilly, T. and Orme, M., Eds., Elsvier Science B. V., Amsterdam, 1997, p. 257.chap no???
25. Graham, T.E., Caffeine and exercise: metabolism, endurance and performance, *Sports Med.,* 31, 785, 2001.
26. Thong, F.S. and Graham, T.E., The putative roles of adenosine in insulin- and exercise-mediated regulation of glucose transport and glycogen metabolism in skeletal muscle, *Can. J. Appl. Physiol.,* 27, 152, 2002.
27. Graham, T.E., Caffeine, coffee and ephedrine: impact on exercise performance and metabolism, *Can. J. Appl. Physiol.,* 26 Suppl, S103, 2001.
28. Tarnopolsky, M.A., Caffeine and endurance performance, *Sports Med.,* 18, 109, 1994.
29. Nehlig, A. and Debry, G., Caffeine and sports activity: a review, *Int. J. Sports Med.,* 15, 215, 1994.
30. Conlee, R.K., Amphetamine, caffeine, and cocaine, in *Ergogenics — Enhancement of Performance in Exercise and Sport*, Lamb, D.R. and Williams, M.H., Eds., Wm. C. Brown, Ann Arbor, MI, 1991, chap.8.

31. Spriet, L.L., Caffeine and performance, *Int. J. Sport Nutr.*, 5, S84, 2000.
32. Graham, T.E. and Spriet, L.L., Performance and metabolic responses to a high caffeine dose during prolonged exercise, *J. Appl. Physiol.*, 71, 2292, 1991.
33. Collomp, K. et al., Benefits of caffeine ingestion on sprint performance in trained and untrained swimmers, *Eur. J. Appl. Physiol.*, 64, 377, 1992.
34. Jackman, M. et al., Metabolic, catecholamine, and endurance responses to caffeine during intense exercise, *J. Appl. Physiol.*, 81, 1658, 1996.
35. Cohen, B.S. et al., Effects of caffeine ingestion on endurance racing in heat and humidity, *Eur. J. Appl. Physiol.*, 73, 358, 1996.
36. Berglund, B. and Hemmingsson, P., Effects of caffeine ingestion on exercise performance at low and high altitudes in cross-country skiing, *Int. J. Sports Med.*, 3, 234, 1982.
37. MacIntosh, B.R. and Wright, B.M., Caffeine ingestion and performance of a 1500 meter swim, *Can. J. Appl. Physiol.*, 20, 168, 1995.
38. Cox, G.R. et al., Effect of different protocols of caffeine intake on metabolism and endurance performance, *J. Appl. Physiol.*, 93, 990, 2002.
39. Kovacs, E.M.R., Stegen, J.H.C.H., and Brouns, F., Effect of caffeinated drinks on substrate metabolism, caffeine excretion, and performance, *J. Appl. Physiol.*, 85, 709, 1998.
40. Wiles, J.D. et al., Effect of caffeinated coffee on running speed, respiratory factors, blood lactate and perceived exertion during 1500-m treadmill running, *Br. J. Sp. Med.*, 26, 116, 1992.
41. Bruce, C.R. et al., Enhancement of 2000-m rowing performance after caffeine ingestion, *Med. Sci. Sports Exerc.*, 32, 1958, 2000.
42. Anderson, M.E. et al., Improved 2000- meter rowing performance in competitive oarswomen after caffeine ingestion, *Int. J. Sport Nutr. Exerc. Metab.*, 10, 464, 2000.
43. Greer, F., Friars, D., and Graham, T.E., Comparison of caffeine and theophylline ingestion: exercise metabolism and endurance, *J. Appl. Physiol.*, 89, 1837, 2000.
44. Costill, D.L., Dalsky, G.P., and Fink, W.J., Effects of caffeine ingestion on metabolism and exercise performance, *Med. Sci. Sports*, 10, 155, 1978.
45. Butts, N.K. and Crowell, D., Effect of caffeine ingestion on cardiorespiratory endurance in men and women, *Res. Q. Exerc. Sport*, 56, 301, 1985.
46. Trice, I. and Haymes, E.M., Effects of caffeine ingestion on exercise-induced changes during high-intensity, intermittent exercise, *Int. J. Sport Nutr.*, 5, 37, 1995.
47. Tse, S.Y.H., Coffee contains cholinomimetic compound distinct from caffeine. 1: purification and chromatographic analysis, *J. Pharmaceut. Sci.*, 80, 665, 1991.
48. Tse, S.Y.H., Cholinomimetic compound distinct from caffeine contained in coffee. II: Muscarinic actions, *J. Pharm. Sci.*, 81, 449, 1992.
49. Wemple, R.D., Lamb, D.R., and McKeever, K.H., Caffeine vs caffeine-free sports drinks: effects on urine production at rest and during prolonged exercise, *Int. J. Sports Med.*, 18, 40, 1997.
50. Sasaki, H. et al., Effect of sucrose and caffeine ingestion on performance of prolonged strenuous running, *Int. J. Sports Med.*, 8, 261, 1987.
51. Wells, C.L. et al., Physiological responses to a 20-mile run under three fluid replacement treatments, *Med. Sci. Sports Exerc.*, 17, 364, 1985.
52. Falk, B. et al., Effects of caffeine ingestion on body fluid balance and thermoregulation during exercise, *Can. J. Physiol. Pharmacol.*, 68, 889, 1990.

53. Engels, H.-J. and Haymes, E.M., Effects of caffeine ingestion on metabolic responses to prolonged walking in sedentary males, *Int. J. Sport Nutr.*, 2, 386, 1992.
54. Armstrong, L.E., Caffeine, body fluid-electrolyte balance, and exercise performance, *Int. J. Sport Nutr. Exerc. Metab.*, 12, 189, 2002.
55. Maughan, R.J., and Griffin, J., Caffeine ingestion and fluid balance: a review, *J. Hum. Nutr. Dietet.*, 16, 411, 2003.
56. Van Soeren, M.H. and Graham, T.E., Effect of caffeine on metabolism, exercise endurance, and catecholamine responses after withdrawal, *J. Appl. Physiol.*, 85, 1501, 1998.
57. Bell, D.G. and McLellan, T.M., Exercise endurance 1, 3, and 6 h after caffeine ingestion in caffeine users and nonusers, *J. Appl. Physiol.*, 93, 1227, 2002.
58. Lane, J.D. et al., Menstrual cycle effects on caffeine elimination in the human female, *Eur. J. Clin. Pharmacol.*, 43, 543, 1992.
59. Collomp, K. et al., Effects of moderate exercise on the pharmacokinetics of caffeine, *Eur. J. Clin. Pharmacol.*, 40, 279, 1991.
60. McLean, C. and Graham, T.E., Effects of menstrual cycle position, exercise and thermal stress on caffeine pharmacokinetics in eumenorrheic women, *J. Appl. Physiol.* 93, 1471, 2001.
61. Arnaud, M.J., Metabolism of caffeine and other components of coffee, in *Caffeine, Coffee, and Health*, Garattini, S., Ed., Raven Press, New York, 1993, chap.3.
62. Bell, D.G., Jacobs, I., and Zamecnik, J., Effects of caffeine, ephedrine and their combination on time to exhaustion during high-intensity exercise, *Eur. J. Appl. Physiol.*, 77, 427, 1998.
63. Bell, D.G., McLellan, T.M., and Sabiston, C.M., Effect of caffeine and ephedrine on 10 km run performance, *Med. Sci. Sports. Exerc.*, 34, 344, 2002.
64. Shekelle, P.G. et al., Efficacy and safety of ephedra and ephedrine for weight loss and athletic performance: a meta-analysis, *JAMA*, 289, 1537, 2003.
65. Johnston, K.L., Clifford, M.N., and Morgan, L.M., Coffee acutely modifies gastrointestinal hormone secretion and glucose tolerance in humans: glycemic effects of chlorogenic acid and caffeine, *Am. J. Clin. Nutr.*, 78, 728, 2003.
66. Wynne, K., Stanley, S., and Bloom, S., The gut and regulation of body weight, *J. Clin. Endocrinol. Metab.*, 89, 2576, 2004.
67. Steinfelder, H.J. and Petho-Schramm, S., Methylxanthines inhibit glucose transport in rat adipocytes by two independent mechanisms, *Biochem. Pharmacol.*, 40, 1154, 1990.
68. Palmer, T.M., Taberner, P.V., and Houslay, M.D., Alterations in G-protein expression, Gi function and stimulatory receptor-mediated regulation of adipocyte adenylyl cyclase in a model of insulin-resistant diabetes with obesity, *Cell. Signal.*, 4, 365, 1992.
69. Graham, T.E. et al., Caffeine ingestion does not alter carbohydrate or fat metabolism in human skeletal muscle during exercise. *J. Physiol.*, 529, 837, 2000.
70. Graham, T.E. et al., Caffeine ingestion elevates plasma insulin response in humans during an oral glucose tolerance test, *Can.J. Physiol. Pharmacol.*, 79, 559, 2001.
71. Petrie, H.J. et al., Caffeine ingestion increases the insulin response to an oral-glucose-tolerance test in obese men before and after weight loss, *Am. J. Clin. Nutr.*, 80, 22, 2004.
72. Lane, J.D. et al., Caffeine impairs glucose metabolism in type 2 diabetes, *Diabetes Care*, 27, 2047, 2004.

73. Robinson, L.E. et al., Caffeine ingestion before an oral glucose tolerance test impairs blood glucose management in men with type 2 diabetes, *J. Nutr.*, 134, 2528, 2004.
74. Matsuda, M. and DeFronzo, R.A., Insulin sensitivity indices obtained from oral glucose tolerance testing: comparison with the euglycemic insulin clamp, *Diabetes Care*, 22, 1462, 1999.
75. Greer, F. et al., Caffeine ingestion decreases glucose disposal during a hyperinsulinemic euglycemic clamp in sedentary humans, *Diabetes*, 50, 2349, 2001.
76. Thong, F.S.L. et al., Caffeine-induced impairment of insulin action but not insulin signaling in human skeletal muscle is reduced by exercise, *Diabetes*, 51, 583, 2001.
77. de Galan, B.E. et al., Theophylline improves hypoglycemia unawareness in type 1 diabetes, *Diabetes*, 51, 790, 2002.
78. Keijzers, G.B. et al., Caffeine can decrease insulin sensitivity in humans, *Diabetes Care*, 25, 364, 2002.
79. Pencek, R.R. et al., Portal vein caffeine infusion enhances net hepatic glucose uptake during a glucose load in conscious dogs, *J. Nutr.*, 134, 3042, 2004.
80. Thong, F.S. and Graham, T.E., Caffeine-induced impairment of glucose tolerance is abolished by beta-adrenergic receptor blockade in humans, *J. Appl. Physiol.*, 92, 2347, 2002.
81. van Dam, R.M. and Feskens, E.J., Coffee consumption and risk of type 2 diabetes mellitus, *Lancet*, 360, 1477, 2002.
82. Salazar-Martinez, E. et al., Coffee consumption and risk for type 2 diabetes mellitus, *Ann. Intern. Med.*, 140, 1, 2004.
83. Rosengren, A. et al., Coffee and incidence of diabetes in Swedish women: a prospective 18-year follow-up study, *J. Intern. Med.*, 255, 89, 2004.
84. Tuomilehto, J. et al., Coffee consumption and risk of type 2 diabetes mellitus among middle-aged Finnish men and women, *JAMA*, 291, 1213, 2004.
85. Carlsson, S. et al., Coffee consumption and risk of type 2 diabetes in Finnish twins, *Int. J. Epidemiol.*, 33, 616, 2004.
86. Agardh, E.E. et al., Coffee consumption, type 2 diabetes and impaired glucose tolerance in Swedish men and women, *J. Intern. Med.*, 255, 645, 2004.
87. Reunanen, A., Heliovaara, M., and Aho, K., Coffee consumption and risk of type 2 diabetes mellitus, *Lancet*, 361, 702, 2003.
88. Saremi, A., Tulloch-Reid, M., and Knowler, W.C., Coffee consumption and the incidence of type 2 diabetes, *Diabetes Care*, 26, 2211, 2003.
89. Harris, M.I. et al., Prevalence of diabetes, impaired fasting glucose, and impaired glucose tolerance in U.S. adults. The Third National Health and Nutrition Examination Survey, 1988–1994. *Diabetes Care*, 21, 518, 1998.
90. Knowler, W.C. et al., Diabetes mellitus in the Pima Indians: incidence, risk factors and pathogenesis, *Diabetes Metab. Rev.*, 6, 1, 1990.
91. Urgert, R. and Katan, M.B., The cholesterol-raising factor from coffee beans, in *Annual Review of Nutrition*, McCormick, D.B., Bier, D.M. and Goodridge, A.G. Eds., Annual Reviews Inc., Palo Alto, California, 1997,p. 305.
92. Shearer, J. et al., Quinides of roasted coffee enhance insulin action in conscious rats, *J. Nutr.*, 133, 3529, 2003.
93. Choi, S.B., Park, C.H., and Park, S., Effect of cola intake on insulin resistance in moderate fat-fed weaning male rats, *J. Nutr. Biochem.*, 13, 727, 2002.
94. Brand-Miller, J. et al., Cocoa powder increases postprandial insulinemia in lean young adults, *J. Nutr.*, 133, 3149, 2003.

95. Acheson, K.J. et al., Caffeine and coffee: their influence on metabolic rate and substrate utilization in normal weight and obese individuals, *Am. J. Clin. Nutr.*, 33, 989, 1980.
96. Daly, P.A. et al., Ephedrine, caffeine and aspirin: safety and efficacy for treatment of human obesity, *Int. J. Obesity*, 17, S73, 1993.
97. Dulloo, A.G. et al., Normal caffeine consumption: influence on thermogenesis and daily energy expenditure in lean and post-obese human volunteers, *Am. J. Clin. Nutr.*, 49, 44, 1989.
98. Astrup, A. et al., Caffeine: a double-blind, placebo-controlled study of its thermogenic, metabolic, and cardiovascular effects in healthy volunteers, *Am. J. Clin. Nutr.*, 51, 759, 1990.
99. Bracco, D. et al., Effects of caffeine on energy metabolism, heart rate, and methylxanthine metabolism in lean and obese women, *Am. J. Physiol*, 32, E671, 1995.
100. Astrup, A. et al., The effect and safety of an ephedrine/caffeine compound compared to ephedrine, caffeine and placebo in obese subjects on an energy restricted diet, A double blind trial, *Int. J. Obes.*, 16, 269, 1992.
101. Vallerand, A.L., Jacobs, I., and Kavanagh, M.F., Mechanism of enhanced cold tolerance by an epindrine-caffeine mixture in humans, *J. Appl. Physiol.*, 67, 438, 1989.
102. Astrup, A. et al., Thermogenic synergism between ephedrine and caffeine in healthy volunteers: a double-blind, placebo-controlled study, *Metabolism*, 40, 323, 1991.
103. Horton, T.J. and Geissler, C.A., Aspirin potentiates the effects of ephedrine on the thermogenic response to a meal in obese but not in lean women, *Int. J. Obes.*, 15, 359, 2000.
104. Greenway, F.L., The safety and efficacy of pharmaceutical and herbal caffeine and ephedrine use as a weight loss agent, *Obes. Rev.*, 2, 199, 2001.
105. White, L.M. et al., Pharmacokinetics and cardiovascular effects of ma-huang (Ephedra sinica) in normotensive adults, *J. Clin. Pharmacol.*, 37, 116, 1997.
106. Gurley, B.J. et al., Ephedrine pharmacokinetics after the ingestion of nutritional supplements containing Ephedra sinica (ma huang), *Ther. Drug Monit.*, 20, 439, 1998.
107. Breum, L. et al., Comparison of an ephedrine/caffeine combination and dexfenfluramine in the treatment of obesity, A double-blind multi-centre trial in general practice, *Int. J. Obes. Relat. Metab. Disord.*, 18, 99, 1994.
108. Dulloo, A.G. and Miller, D.S., Aspirin as a promoter of ephedrine-induced thermogenesis: potential use in the treatment of obesity, *Am. J. Clin. Nutr.*, 45, 564, 1987.
109. Dulloo, A.G. and Miller, D.S., Ephedrine, caffeine and aspirin: "over-the-counter" drugs that interact to stimulate thermogenesis in the obese, *Nutrition.*, 5, 7, 1989.
110. Dulloo, A.G., Ephedrine, xanthines and prostaglandin-inhibitors: actions and interactions in the stimulation of thermogenesis, *Int. J. Obes. Relat. Metab. Disord.*, 17 Suppl 1, S35, 1993.
111. Molnar, D. et al., Safety and efficacy of treatment with an ephedrine/caffeine mixture. The first double blind placebo controlled pilot study in adolescents, *Int. J. Obes.*, 24, 1573, 2000.
112. Boozer, C.N. et al., An herbal supplement containing ma huang-guarana for weight loss: a randomized, double-blind trial, *Int. J. Obes.*, 25, 316, 2001.

113. Astrup, A. et al., The effect of ephedrine/caffeine mixture on energy expenditure and body composition in obese women, *Metabolism.*, 41, 686, 1992.
114. Horton, T.J. and Geissler, C.A., Post-prandial thermogenesis with ephedrine, caffeine and aspirin in lean, pre-disposed obese and obese women, *Int. J. Obes. Relat. Metab. Disord.*, 20, 91, 1996.
115. Troiano, R.P. et al., The relationship between body weight and mortality: a quantitative analysis of combined information from existing studies, *Int. J. Obes. Relat. Metab. Disord.*, 20, 63, 1996.
116. Norregaard, J. et al., The effect of ephedrine plus caffeine on smoking cessation and postcessation weight gain, *Clin. Pharmacol. Ther.*, 60, 679, 1996.
117. Bray, G.A., A concise review on the therapeutics of obesity, *Nutrition.*, 16, 953, 2000.
118. Hespel,P. et al., Creatine supplementation: exploring the role of the creatine kinase/phosphocreatine system in human muscle, *Can. J. Appl. Physiol.*, 26 Suppl, S79, 2001.
119. Lemon, P.W., Dietary creatine supplementation and exercise performance: why inconsistent results? *Can. J. Appl. Physiol.*, 27, 663, 2002.
120. Haller, C.A. and Benowitz, N.L., Adverse cardiovascular and central nervous system events associated with dietary supplements containing ephedra alkaloids, *N. Engl. J. Med.*, 343, 1833, 2000.
121. Chen, C. et al., Ischemic stroke after using over the counter products containing ephedra, *J. Neurol. Sci.*, 217, 55, 2004.
122. Kalman, D.S., An acute clinical trial evaluating the cardiovascular effects of an herbal ephedra-caffeine weight loss product in healthy overweight adults, *Int. J. Obes. Relat. Metab. Disord.*, 28, 1355, 2004.
123. Kalman, D. et al., An acute clinical trial evaluating the cardiovascular effects of an herbal ephedra-caffeine weight loss product in healthy overweight adults, *Int. J. Obes. Relat. Metab. Disord.*, 26, 1363, 2002.
124. Gardin, J.M. et al., Valvular abnormalities and cardiovascular status following exposure to dexfenfluramine or phentermine/fenfluramine, *JAMA*, 283, 1703, 2000.
125. Wyss, M. and Kaddurah-Daouk, R., Creatine and creatine metabolism, *Physiol. Rev.*, 80, 1107, 2000.
126. Terjung, R.L. et al., The physiological and health effects of oral creatine supplementation. *Med. Sci. Sports Exerc.*, 32, 706, 2000.
127. Branch, J.D., Effect of creatine supplementation on body composition and performance: a meta-analysis, *Int. J. Sport Nutr. Exerc. Metab.*, 13, 198, 2003.
128. Gibala, M.J., Nutritional supplementation and resistance exercise: what is the evidence for enhanced skeletal muscle hypertrophy? *Can. J. Appl. Physiol.* 25, 524, 2000.
129. Van Leemputte,M., Vandenberghe, K., and Hespel, P., Shortening of muscle relaxation time after creatine loading, *J. Appl. Physiol.*, 83, 840, 1999.
130. McGuire, M., Bradford, A., and MacDermott, M., The effects of dietary creatine supplements on the contractile properties of rat soleus and extensor digitorum longus muscles, *Exp. Physiol.*, 86, 185, 2001.
131. Hespel, P. et al., Oral creatine supplementation facilitates the rehabilitation of disuse atrophy and alters the expression of muscle myogenic factors in humans, *J. Physiol.*, 536, 625, 2001.
132. Op't, E.B. et al., Effect of oral creatine supplementation on human muscle GLUT4 protein content after immobilization, *Diabetes*, 50, 18, 2001.

133. Tarnopolsky, M. et al., Acute and moderate-term creatine monohydrate supplementation does not affect creatine transporter mRNA or protein content in either young or elderly humans, *Mol. Cell Biochem.*, 244, 159, 2003.
134. Op't, E.B. et al., Effect of creatine supplementation on creatine and glycogen content in rat skeletal muscle, *Acta. Physiol. Scand.*, 171, 169, 2001.
135. Vandenberghe, K. et al., Caffeine counteracts the ergogenic action of muscle creatine loading, *J. Appl. Physiol.*, 80, 452, 1996.
136. Hespel, P., Op't, E.B., and Van Leemputte, M., Opposite actions of caffeine and creatine on muscle relaxation time in humans, *J. Appl. Physiol.*, 92, 513, 2002.
137. Doherty, M. et al., Caffeine is ergogenic after supplementation of oral creatine monohydrate, *Med. Sci. Sports Exerc.*, 34, 1785, 2002.
138. Brose, A., Parise, G., and Tarnopolsky, M.A., Creatine supplementation enhances isometric strength and body composition improvements following strength exercise training in older adults, *J. Gerontol. A Biol. Sci. Med. Sci.*, 58, 11, 2003.
139. Eijnde, B.O. et al., Effects of creatine supplementation and exercise training on fitness in men 55–75 yr old, *J. Appl. Physiol.*, 95, 818, 2003.
140. Tarnopolsky, M.A. and Parise, G., Direct measurement of high-energy phosphate compounds in patients with neuromuscular disease, *Muscle Nerve*, 22, 1228, 1999.
141. Tarnopolsky, M.A. et al., Creatine transporter and mitochondrial creatine kinase protein content in myopathies, *Muscle Nerve*, 24, 682, 2001.
142. Tarnopolsky, M.A. and Beal, M.F., Potential for creatine and other therapies targeting cellular energy dysfunction in neurological disorders, *Ann. Neurol.*, 49, 561, 2001.
143. Tarnopolsky, M.A. et al., Creatine monohydrate enhances strength and body composition in Duchenne muscular dystrophy, *Neurology*, 62, 1771, 2004.
144. Tarnopolsky, M. et al., Creatine monohydrate supplementation does not increase muscle strength, lean body mass, or muscle phosphocreatine in patients with myotonic dystrophy type 1, *Muscle Nerve*, 29, 51, 2004.
145. Cadarette, B.S. et al., Effects of varied dosages of caffeine on endurance exercise to fatigue, in *Biochemistry of Exercise. International Series of Sport Sciences*, Knuttgen, H.G., Vogel, J.A., and Poortmans, J., Eds., Human Kinetics, Champaign, IL, 1982, p. 871.
146. Pasman, W.J. et al., The effect of different dosages of caffeine on endurance performance time, *Int. J. Sports Med.*, 16, 225, 1995.
147. Bell, D.G. and McLellan, T.M., Exercise endurance 1, 3, and 6 h after caffeine ingestion in caffeine users and nonusers, *J. Appl. Physiol.*, 93, 1227, 2002.
148. Perkins, R. and Williams, M.H., Effect of caffeine upon maximal muscular endurance of females, *Med. Sci. Sports.*, 7, 221, 1975.
149. Collomp, K. et al., Influence de la prise aigue ou chronique de cafeine sur la performance et les catecholamines au cours d'un exercice maximal, *C.R. Soc. Biol.*, 184, 87, 1990.
150. Mohr, T. et al., Caffeine ingestion and metabolic responses of tetraplegic humans during electrical cycling, *J. Appl. Physiol.*, 85, 979, 1998.
151. Spriet, L.L. et al. Caffeine ingestion and muscle metabolism during prolonged exercise in humans, *Am. J. Physiol.* 262, E891, 1992.
152. Chown, S. Caffeine increases the insulin/glucose response to an OGTT in obese, resting males, *Can. J. Appl. Physiol.* 26, S249, 2001.

Section VII

Experimental Designs

18

Designing Experiments for Food–Drug Synergy: Health Aspects

Lyn M. Steffen

CONTENTS

18.1 Introduction

The prevalence of food–drug synergy that occurs in the hospital or at home is unknown. However, with over 80% of the U.S. adult population consuming at least one prescription drug, herb, supplement, or over-the-counter drug during the previous week, and 50% consuming at least one prescription drug per week,[1] the concern is raised about the increasing potential occurrence of adverse food–drug synergy. In this chapter, "food–drug synergy" refers to the interaction of a food (or food components) and a specific drug (or drugs) conferring a greater health benefit or adverse reaction than either the food (or food component) or drug alone. However, other chapters in this book expand this definition to include additive effects of multiple foods, or foods and drugs, to result in a health benefit; or the ability of a food or drug to attenuate an adverse effect of a food or drug. The majority of these interactions are pharmacokinetic interactions, such that a single food or beverage or combination of foods may change the absorption, bioavailability, or metabolism of a drug resulting in its decreased effectiveness or enhanced absorption, which may or may not be desirable. Furthermore, individual characteristics, such as age, gender, weight, and health status, may also change the action of a consumed food and/or drug. Thus, in addition to the individual characteristics, a significant adverse or beneficial health outcome may potentially occur when a food or beverage and drug are consumed together.

18.1.1 An Emerging Problem of Adverse Effects of Food Intake on Drug Action

The bioavailability and safety of many drugs may be tested in the fasted or fed state of mostly healthy adults. The test meal recommended by the FDA is one that is high in calories and total fat,[2] but does not include typical foods that U.S. adults consume today, such as ready-to-eat, fortified breakfast cereals, fortified orange juice, or grapefruit juice. Because many individuals in the U.S. population are focused on prevention and consuming a healthy diet, many fortified foods and nutrient-modified foods have been developed and are in today's marketplace. Some of these foods are fortified with calcium, iron, and zinc — ions shown to interact with drug metabolism.[3] Other foods in the marketplace or meal patterns of individuals that may influence drug metabolism vary in composition of nutrients and food compounds, thereby increasing the possibility of food–drug interactions. Even though physicians and pharmacists counsel their patients or clients regarding food and beverage effects on a specific drug, information is not available about the effect of most foods and beverages on drug action or health effects. Well-designed studies are needed to elucidate the potentially adverse or beneficial effect of food–drug synergy that may be associated with coadministration of various foods or beverages with prescription or over-the-counter drugs. The purpose of this report is to describe factors for consideration in designing experiments that elucidate food–drug synergy and potential challenges that may arise.

18.2 Diet and Food Factors

The mechanisms by which most foods or nutrients interact with a drug are chelation, adsorption, change in gastric pH, change in urinary pH (influencing renal clearance), and decreased absorption. The results of these food–drug synergies range from insignificant to major health consequences. Singh,[4] Schmidt and Dahhoff, [5] Fleischer et al.,[6] and Harris et al.[7] provide excellent reviews of food–drug synergy studies conducted in both adults and children. Several examples of food–drug interactions studies are shown by medical condition in Table 18.1.

18.2.1 Food and Drug Administration (FDA) Requirements

Hundreds of new drugs are being developed each year. To determine whether a drug is to be consumed in the fed or fasting state, food effect studies are conducted for new drug products during its development period to assess the influence of food intake on drug absorption, metabolism, and bioavailability.[2] The FDA recommends testing the effectiveness of a drug concomitantly with intake of a high-fat meal, about 58% of calories from fat that includes eggs fried in butter, buttered toast, sausage, and whole milk. No other dietary pattern is required for testing drugs with food intake, despite the national average intake of fat being about 35% of calories from fat. No requirement for testing food–drug interactions is mandated for other foods in the marketplace, such as grapefruit juice or calcium-fortified orange juice, that are likely to interact with many drugs.[2] Although, the agency sponsoring the drug may choose to conduct additional studies to better understand the relation between food and drug intake, more studies are needed to systematically investigate food–drug synergy.

18.2.2 Composition of Foods and Meals

The nutrient composition or food compound composition of a food may influence the action of a drug. With prevention being a focus in health care, the food industry has responded with many new "functional" food products on the market — foods rich in vitamins, minerals, protein, soy, or other food compounds. Examples of these foods include calcium fortified juice, bread, and milk; nutrition bars, drinks, breakfast cereal, and other foods fortified with 100% of the U.S. dietary reference intake (DRI) of vitamins and minerals in men and women. Additionally, with the increasing prevalence of over-

TABLE 18.1

Studies Exploring Food–Drug Interactions

Ref.	Food	Drug	Study Design	Population	Health Effect of the Interaction
Drugs for Cardiovascular Disease					
Suvarna	Cranberry juice	Warfarin	Case study	Male CVD patient	Flavonoid inhibition of cytochrome P450 activity resulting in change of INR > 50; patient died from GI and pericardial hemorrhage
Cambria-Kelly	Soy milk	Warfarin	Case study	70 year old male CVD patient	Decreases the effect of warfarin absorption or metabolism resulting in subtherapeutic INR values
Bovill	Vitamin K foods (0.5–1.06 mg)	Warfarin	Clinical trials and prospective studies	Non-hospitalized, free-living patient population	Vitamin K foods (0.5 mg of vitamin K_1) act as a coagulant to decrease the effect of warfarin
Koytchev	Standard test meal vs.	Diprafenone	Experimental study	15 healthy males, 20–25 years	Drug absorption is influenced (blockage of the gut enzymes permits a larger amount of the drug to reach the liver) resulting in a 50% increase in the bioavailability of drug after eating food.
Bailey, Dresser	Grapefruit juice, segments, and extract	Felodipine	Randomized, 4-way crossover study design	12 healthy men and women aged 18–40 years	With food intake there is an inhibition of presystemic drug metabolism mediated by CYP3A4. Grapefruit juice and whole fruit increased drug bioavailability by 3-fold that may produce drug toxicity

Parker	Grapefruit juice	Digoxin	Open-label, unblinded crossover study	7 healthy men and women	
Drugs for Weight Loss					
Heck	Olestra potato chips	Orlistat	Case study	16-year old African American girl	Abdominal pain, fatty, oily stools
Drugs for Immunosuppression					
Zimmerman	High-fat meal	Sirolimus (rapamycin)	Randomized 2-way crossover study design	23 healthy men and women aged 19–43 years	Reduced rate of absorption resulting in increased bioavailability of the drug
Carver	Testing 5 meals of same volume and 680 kcal: high-calorie protein, fat, and carbohydrate liquid meals, non-caloric viscous meal, and control meal	Indinavir (600 mg) with 100 ml water	Randomized 4-way crossover study design	7 male HIV-infected patients mean age 41 years who had adequate organ function at baseline	The protein meal elevated the gastric pH, therefore, reducing the absorption of the drug resulting in treatment failure
Drugs for Type 2 Diabetes					
Delrat	Fasted or fed state	Gliclazide modifed release	Randomized, 2-way cross-over study design	16 healthy men and women mean age 26 years old	There was no difference in bioavailability of drug between the fasted or fed state
Antibiotic Drugs					
Wallace	Orange juice and calcium-fortified orange juice	Levofloxacin	Randomized 3-way crossover study design	16 healthy men and women, mean age 38 years old	Calcium-fortified orange juice decreased bioavailability of drug resulting in treatment failure and potential promotion of antibiotic resistance

TABLE 18.1 (Continued)

Studies Exploring Food–Drug Interactions

Ref.	Food	Drug	Study Design	Population	Health Effect of the Interaction
Neuhofel	Calcium-fortified orange juice, orange juice, and water	Ciprofloxacin	Randomized, 3-way cross-over study design	15 healthy men and women, aged 18+ years old	Calcium-fortified orange juice decreased bioavailability of drug resulting in treatment failure and potential promotion of antibiotic resistance
Gastrointestinal Drugs					
Offman	Red wine, grapefruit juice	Cisapride	Randomized 3-way cross-over study design	12 healthy men, 19–41 years old	Inhibition of intestinal cytochrome p450 3A4 activity resulted in increased bioavailability for both red wine and grapefruit juice; this interaction may produce prolongation of the QTc interval.
Neurological Drugs					
Simon	Foods high in protein (comparison of low protein meal vs. high protein meal)	LevoDOPA	Experimental study	20 advanced Parkinson patients (10 years duration)	High protein diet impairs the clinical effect of the drug

weight and obese individuals in the U.S. population, there is also an increasing number of popular weight loss diets in the marketplace that instruct how to manipulate the nutrient composition of the diet by increasing or decreasing fat, carbohydrate, and/or protein, or limit food intake to a few foods for weight loss. Meanwhile, adverse health effects may result from concomitant intake of a drug with high levels of a particular nutrient or food. Examples of studies designed to test the effectiveness of drugs with food intake are shown in Table 18.1. This table summarizes several studies by medical condition, the study design, study population, test drug, treatment diet, food or beverage, and health effect.[8–20]

18.2.3 Macronutrients

The bioavailability of many drugs is increased when consumed with a high fat diet;[4,5] but this is not always the case. The bioavailability of pravastatin was decreased by 31% with concurrent intake of a high fat meal.[21] Fat intake slows down gastric emptying; therefore, it is likely that bioavailability of most drugs will be enhanced when coadministered with meals that are high in fat.[22] The clinical outcome of such synergy may result in toxic levels of the drug in the blood. A meal high in dietary protein may also enhance the absorption of a drug.[20]

18.2.4 Fiber

The fiber content of a meal influences drug absorption, such as lower absorption of both lovastatin and digoxin with high fiber intake.[23,24] Thyroxin absorption is also reduced with high intake of wheat bran. Lower absorption of any drug influences its effectiveness and, therefore, may result in treatment failure. However, fiber intake may also relieve discomfort from constipation when taking opioids, such as morphine.

18.2.5 Fat Substitutes

With the increasing prevalence of obesity, the food industry has manufactured food products, such as fat substitutes, that provide fewer calories and thus facilitate lower energy intake in consumers. In the case study of a female diagnosed with type 2 diabetes, coadministration of the fat substitute Olestra and the oral agent orlistat resulted in serious GI distress.[10] It is important to understand the effect of concomitant food and drug intake on the health of the patient.

18.2.6 Fortified Foods

Some fortified foods contain vitamins and minerals at doses as high as in supplements. Examples of fortified foods include orange juice and bread fortified with calcium and breakfast cereal fortified with multiple vitamins and minerals. It is possible for these foods to interact with several drugs commonly prescribed for hypertension, high cholesterol, diabetes, infections, or other medical conditions, and thereby result in treatment failure of the drug. The antibiotic fluoroquinolone, which has been around since the 1980s, is known to interact with multivalent ions, such as calcium, magnesium, aluminum, iron, and zinc.[25] Therefore, patients are warned to consume these drugs with foods and beverages other than those containing these multivalent minerals. However, it is becoming increasingly difficult to know which foods and beverages are high in nutrients that may have synergistic effects with certain drugs. Most of these synergy studies are not conducted using calcium-fortified food products but are instead extrapolated from milk or yogurt studies.[3,25]

18.2.7 Fruit Juice and Flavonoids

Several hundred studies have been conducted to determine the effectiveness of many different drugs when taken with grapefruit juice on the associated clinical health effects.[26] Grapefruit juice interacts with more than 25 medications by inhibiting cytochrome P4503A4 (CYP450)-mediated drug metabolism[27–29] as well as modulating transporter activity, such as P-glycoprotein.[4,26,30,31] A single glass of grapefruit juice taken with or even 24 h prior to consumption of certain drugs can produce a clinically relevant event, including increased frequency of hemodynamic-related adverse events.[26] Recovery from this food–drug interaction takes about 3 d after a single exposure to grapefruit juice.[32] Time course is another factor to consider regarding the interaction of a food and drug. It is important to note that the whole fruit also causes the same adverse clinical health effects as the juice.[33]

Different fruit juices and their constituents interact with drugs, such as fexofenadine and cyclosporine, by altering the activity of transporters such as P-glycoprotein and reducing the drug bioavailability. Grapefruit, orange, and apple juices all markedly lowered plasma fexofenadine concentrations compared with a similar amount of water intake. Seville orange juice enhanced felodipine bioavailability, although regular orange juice did not; this interaction may be due to the food compound content, bergamottin and naringin, of Seville oranges.[34] Cranberry juice, which contains flavonoids, is known to inhibit cytochrome P450 enzymes.[35]

The calcium channel blocker felodipine was first shown to be synergistic with grapefruit juice in 1989.[36] The several classes of drugs exhibiting synergy with grapefruit juice include calcium channel antagonist CNS modulators, HMG-CoA reductase inhibitors, and several other agents. Clinical health effects involving the calcium channel agonists, agents that manage hypertension and angina pectoris, are increased heart rate and orthostatic hypotension.[37,38] Clinical effects resulting from the synergy between cyclosporine, an immunosuppressive agent, and grapefruit juice may include nephrotoxicity, hypertension, and cerebral toxicity.[26] Increased bioavailability of cizapride, a prokinetic agent used for GI disorders, occurs with concomitant consumption of grapefruit juice. High plasma concentrations of cizapride have resulted in serious cardiac adverse effects, such as tachycardia, palpitations, QT prolongation, and torsade de pointes.[39] Eight case studies reported the interaction between cranberry juice, which contains flavonoids, and warfarin intake that resulted in bleeding or death.[8]

18.2.8 Caffeine

Caffeine is found in food and beverages, including coffee, tea, soft drinks, and chocolate. Food and beverages containing caffeine should be avoided while taking bronchodilators, such as aminophylline and theophylline, because both the bronchodilator and caffeine stimulate the central nervous system.

18.2.9 Alcohol

The synergy between alcohol and many drugs can be very dangerous because the combination of the drug and alcohol may cause drowsiness and slowed reactions. Many physicians and pharmacists discourage the use of alcohol while taking any medication.

18.2.10 Probiotics

Probiotics or live bacteria, such as lactobacillus and bifidobacterium, are added to foods for prevention and treatment of diarrhea. In a study investigating combined antibiotic and probiotic use in pediatric diarrhea patients, the use of *Saccharomyces boulardii* decreased the diarrhea rate from 32.3 to 11.4% (p <.05).[40] Additionally, probiotic lactobacillus GG supplementation beneficially affects *Helicobacter pylori* therapy-related side effects and overall treatment tolerance.[41] In seven clinical trials, probiotics were added to a therapeutic regimen of antibiotics, resulting in an increased cure rate in two studies and reduced side effects in four.[42]

18.2.11 Other Dietary Factors

Other dietary factors that may influence food–drug synergy are amount or volume of food or beverage consumed,[4] timing of consumption of the meal or beverage intake relative to drug consumption,[32] texture of the meal (viscous or fiber vs. liquid),[4] and intake of herbs and vitamin supplements.[43,44] Consistent nutrient composition of meals for patients consuming theophylline for asthma, especially children, is important for maintaining therapeutic blood levels of the drug.

TABLE 18.2

Factors to Consider in Designing Food–Drug Interaction Studies

Study Component	Factor
Hypothesis	What do you want to know?
Experimental design	Crossover design Parallel-arm design
Study population Inclusion and exclusion criteria	Individual characteristics: Health status: healthy or patients with a specific condition Age: children, young adult, middle-aged, elderly Gender Pregnancy
Drug exposure	Formulation Dose Timing and duration of administration
Randomized groups	Treatment: Dietary factor-of-interest Control: Standard FDA diet or other
Dietary factor-of-interest	Macronutrients, meal effects, fiber effects Vitamin or mineral fortified food effects Volume effects (amount of food, beverage) Timing of administration of food Beverages: dairy products, alcohol, caffeinated beverages, fortified juice
Other factors	There are many other factors. These are examples: Physiological status Body composition Hydration status Consuming other multiple drugs
Measurable outcome-of-interest	Drug or health effects
Statistical issues	Sample size and power Variability, reliability Effect size Dropout rate and compliance

18.3 Experimental Design

In addition to an excellent research team, the key components in designing controlled experiments are: (1) a testable study hypothesis and (2) a study design compatible with testing the hypothesis, including study participants (healthy volunteers or patients), test drug (dose and formulation), test meal or single food or beverage, an appropriate outcome variable (significant clinical event), a study protocol, and a plan for data management, quality control, and analysis (Table 18.2 presents these study components). For more detailed information about study design, the reader is directed to textbooks about designing clinical experiments.[45–47]

18.3.1 Study Hypothesis

What is your research question? The research question is based upon a set of study objectives. The following questions may facilitate the planning stages of the study:

- What do you want to know?
- What impact does the food–drug interaction have on health?
- What clinically relevant event do you expect?
- How does a particular meal pattern or individual food or beverage influence the action of a particular drug?
- Does it last several hours, if there is a food effect?
- Does the clinical outcome differ between drug formulations? The study question may then be restated as a study hypothesis that takes into account the drug and food to be tested, the study design, and the study population.

18.3.2 Study Design

The next step for the research team, which should include a statistician as one of the team members, is to select an appropriate study design. Common experimental study designs used to study the effects of food on the action of a drug include randomized crossover and parallel-arm designs. In a randomized crossover design, the participant is assigned to all treatment diets in a randomized order. In a parallel-arm design, the participant is randomly assigned to receive only one diet treatment, such that different groups of participants receive different test diets. The major difference between the two study designs is the lower variability demonstrated using the crossover design compared with the parallel-arm design. The test diet groups will be compared using the within-person difference in the crossover study design, while the between-person difference will be compared in the parallel-arm design. The major advantage for the crossover design is the smaller sample size necessary to detect a minimal detectable difference between treatment groups compared with the other design.

18.3.3 Study Population

Who will be in the study? Characteristics of individuals influence drug action and need to be taken into account when designing a study to elucidate food–drug interactions. Additionally, food choices differ given the characteristics of the population, such as age, gender, and health status, for example. The majority of published studies testing food effects of drug actions include healthy, young adults as the study participants, although some published studies reported particular drugs tested in patients for whom the drug was intended.[4]

The study population should be suitable to achieve the study objectives. The following questions may facilitate identification of the study population. What segment of the population is taking this drug? Is the drug usually prescribed to children, middle-aged, or elderly adults? Who will be included and excluded in this clinical study? To answer the study question, it is important to define the study population using specific criteria to exclude and include certain potential study participants. Given the drug of interest, common inclusion criteria are age (within a certain age range), gender (either male or female or both), nutritional or health status (normal weight, obese, or both, etc.), or certain disease state (healthy, hypertension, cystic fibrosis, etc.). Common exclusion criteria include outside the specified age range, pregnancy, certain medical conditions or disease states, nutritional status, and allergies to foods or drugs as examples. Safety of the study population in conducting these studies is always a concern. The following are factors to consider in identifying the study population:

18.3.3.1 Age

18.3.3.1.1 The Elderly

On a given day, an average of 6.5 medications (including OTCs) are consumed by individuals over 70 years of age.[1] More than 30% of all prescription drugs and 40% of over-the-counter (OTC) drugs are consumed by individuals over the age of 65 years.[1]

With increasing age, individuals become more sensitive to medications, which may result in more adverse side effects. Aging is also associated with many physical and physiological changes in the body. Chronic diseases, for which single or multiple drug therapies are prescribed, are more common in the elderly. Additionally, the elderly are at risk of excessive use or misuse of medications, for which there are many reasons.[48,49] Physiological changes that occur with aging include gastrointestinal tract changes that may affect drug absorption, including an increase in the pH of the stomach; decreased splanchnic blood flow; and decreased intestinal motility. Body composition changes with aging include decreased lean mass, decreased body water, and increased fat stores. These body changes may contribute to a reduced volume of distribution of drug, an increased retention of fat-soluble drugs in the fat stores, and greater availability of free drug to diffuse to receptor sites. Metabolism of drugs may be slower in the elderly because of aging or declines in nutritional status or liver function. Because glomerular filtration rates decline with age, certain drugs may be eliminated slowly in the elderly.

There is a great need to study the elderly because they (1) are at high risk of chronic disease, (2) purchase about one-third of the prescribed drugs in the United States, and (3) are at high risk for adverse health effects of food–drug interactions. The challenge in studying this population is that many are taking multiple drugs, some have poor nutritional status, and all have many physiological changes taking place.

18.3.3.1.2 Children

Children's responses to drugs are different than those of adults because of their differences in physiology and metabolism.[50] Studies of the effect of drugs in children should be determined in children rather than extrapolating from adult studies. Children are able to tolerate larger doses of drug than adults, perhaps because of greater clearance by the liver and/or kidney. Disease affects the disposition of drugs in both adults and children. For example, drug clearance is greater in children with cystic fibrosis than in healthy children.[51] Therefore, a higher dose of drug is necessary in children with cystic fibrosis. Additionally, several studies suggest that children are more responsive to food effects than adults.[52]

18.3.3.1.3 Pregnancy

Few studies have published results of drugs tested in pregnant women. In a study conducted among over 150,000 women who delivered a baby between 1996 and 2000, 64% were prescribed medications other than the prenatal vitamins during their pregnancy. Of these, almost 40% were prescribed a drug for which safety during pregnancy was not established.[53] Clearly, more research is needed to establish drug safety during pregnancy as well as to determine the potential for food–drug synergy in a population taking prenatal vitamins.

18.3.3.2 Gender

Women take more medications (prescription or nonprescription drugs, vitamins, and supplements) than men: 94% of women and 91% of men 65 years and over reported taking at least 1 medication in the past week, 57% of women and 44% of men took 5 or more, and 12% of both men and women took 10 or more during the previous week.[1] The overlap in use of prescription and nonprescription drugs, herbals, and/or supplements, in addition to consumption of foods and beverages, may potentially result in a clinically adverse interaction.

18.3.3.3 Physiological Status

Consider the physiological status of the individual. Poor nutritional status may lead to drug toxicity because of a decreased ability to metabolize drugs. Dehydration may significantly decrease the distribution volume of a drug because of decreases in the size of the aqueous compartment. This may also reduce glomerular filtration rate. Body composition may influence the dosing of the drug. There is a need to determine whether drug dosing (multiple doses or duration of doses) alters the volume of distribution of the drug given the weight of the patient.

18.3.4 Drug Considerations

Over 200 new drugs have come on the market in the past 2 years. More than likely, however, very few have been tested for the effects of food–drug synergy. In designing food–drug synergy studies, the following issues concerning the drug should be taken into consideration: formulation of the drug, dose size, and duration and timing of coadministration.

18.3.4.1 Drug Formulation

Meals may have a different effect on a drug depending on its formulation, such as the conventional or controlled-release drugs. Different preparations or formulations of a drug may differ in their bioavailability when consumed with meals vs. fasting. For example, the bioavailability of Theo-24, an ultra-long-acting theophylline is increased with a high-fat vs. low-fat meal.[49] In contrast, no difference was demonstrated in pharmacokinetic properties between a controlled release and immediate release formulation of isradipine under fasted or fed conditions.[54]

18.3.4.2 Drug Dose

One factor often overlooked in food–effect studies is the drug dose. Singh reports a number of studies showing that multiple dosage is less affected by food intake compared with single doses.[4] However, this area needs further research, especially with so many new drugs being available in recent years.

18.3.4.3 Timing and Duration of Coadministration

The timing of the meal or administration of the drug may influence the rate of drug availability for some drugs, but not all. Grapefruit juice does not need to be ingested with the drug to produce an adverse effect.[26] Even 12 h after consuming the juice, the bioavailability of lovastatin was two times greater compared with levels without grapefruit juice intake. Other drugs are not affected by food or beverage intake.[4,16,55]

18.4 Conclusions

There is a tremendous need to conduct studies to determine whether the combination of a particular drug and a food or beverage result in an adverse or beneficial health effect. Food effects commonly occur with nutrient dense foods, fortified and functional foods, fruit juices, and alcohol. In addition to selection of the treatment food or beverage and test drug, the experimental design should also take into consideration the population for which the drug was intended: children, pregnant women, adult or elderly women and men, or patients with the intended health condition. Other factors to consider in designing studies are the drug formulation, dosing, and timing and duration of the drug effect. More studies are needed to systematically investigate the synergy between food and drugs. Continued failure of a drug treatment will prolong an illness or infection; however, continued failure may also result in discontinuation of an otherwise appropriate drug for medical management. Finally, the results of these studies should provide more labeling information for better patient care. With many new foods in the marketplace, especially fruit juices, fortified foods, and functional foods and beverages, physicians and pharmacists should educate their patients or clients about the adverse or beneficial health effects of certain food and drug combinations.

References

1. Kaufman, D.W. et al., Recent patterns of medication use in the ambulatory adults population of the U.S.: The Slone Survey, *JAMA*, 287, 337, 2002.
2. Guidance for Industry: Food-effect bioavailability and fed bioequivalence studies. Accessed on August 7, 2004: http://www.fda.gov/cder/guidance/index.htm.
3. Wallace, A.W. and Amsden, G.W., Is it really OK to take this with food? Old interactions with a new twist, *J. Clin. Pharmacol.*, 42, 437, 2002.
4. Singh, B., Effects of food on clinical pharmacokinetics, *Clin. Pharmacokinet.*, 37, 213, 1999.
5. Schmidt, L.E. and Dahhoff, K., Food-drug interactions, *Drugs, 62, 1481,* 2002.
6. Fleisher, D. et al., Drug, meal and formulation interactions influencing drug absorption after oral administration: clinical implications, *Clin. Pharmacokinet.*, 36, 233, 1999.
7. Harris, R.Z., Jang, G.R., and Tsunoda, S., Dietary effects on drug metabolism and transport, *Clin. Pharmacokinet., 42, 1071,* 2001.
8. Suvarna, R., Pirmohamed, M., and Henderson, L., Possible interaction between warfarin and cranberry juice, *Br. Med. J., 327, 1454,* 2003.
9. Cambria-Kiely, J.A., Effect of soy milk on warfarin efficacy, *Ann. Pharmacother.*, 36, 1893, 2002.
10. Heck, A.M. et al., Additive gastrointestinal effects with concomitant use of Olestra and Orlistat, *Ann. Pharmacother.*, 36, 1003, 2002.
11. Franco, V. et al., Role of dietary vitamin K intake in chronic oral anticoagulation: prospective evidence from observational and randomized protocols, *Am. J. Med.*, 16, 651, 2004.
12. Koytchev, R. et al., Influence of food on the bioavailability and some pharmacokinetic parameters of diprafenone — novel antiarrhythmic agent, *Eur. J. Clin. Pharmacol.*, 50, 315, 1996.
13. Bailey, D.G. et al., Grapefruit-felodipine interaction: effect of unprocessed fruit and probable active ingredients, *Clin. Pharmocol. Ther.*, 68, 468, 2000.
14. Zimmerman, J.J. et al., The effect of a high-fat meal on the oral bioavailability of the immunosuppressant sirolimus (Rapamycin), *J. Clin. Pharmacol.*, 39, 1155, 1999.

15. Carver, P.L. et al., Meal composition effect on the oral bioavailability of Indinavir in HIV-infected patients, *Pharm. Res.*, 16, 718, 1999.
16. Delrat, P., Paraire, M., and Jochemsen, R., Complete bioavailability and lack of food-effect on pharmacokinetics of gliclazide 30 mg modified release in healthy volunteers, *Biopharm. Drug Dispos.*, 23, 151, 2002.
17. Wallace, A.W., Victory, J.M., and Amsden, G.W., Lack of bioequivalence when levofloxacin and calcium-fortified orange juice are coadministered to healthy volunteers, *J. Clin. Pharmacol.*, 43, 539, 2003.
18. Neuhofel, A.L. et al., Lack of bioequivalence of ciprofloxacin when administered with calcium-fortified orange juice: a new twist on an old interaction, *J. Clin. Pharmacol.*, 42, 461, 2002.
19. Offman, E.M. et al., Red wine-cisapride interaction: comparison with grapefruit juice, *Clin. Pharmacol. Ther.*, 70, 17, 2001.
20. Simon, N. et al., The effects of a normal protein diet on levodopa plasma kinetics in advanced Parkinson's disease, *Parkinsonism Related Disorders*, 10, 137, 2004.
21. Pan, H.Y. et al., Effect of food on pravastatin pharmacokinetics and pharmacodynamics, *Int. J. Clin. Pharmacol. Ther. Toxicol.*, 31, 291, 1993.
22. Ingwersen, S.H., Mant, T.G., and Larsen, J.J., Food intake increases the relative oral bioavailability of vanoxerine, *Br. J. Clin. Pharmacol.*, 35, 308, 1993.
23. Richter, W.O., Jacob, B.G., and Schwatdt, P., Interaction between fiber and lovastatin, [letter], *Lancet*, 338, 706, 1991.
24. Huupponen, R., Seppala, P., and Iisalo, E., Effect of guar gum, a fiber preparation, on digoxin and penicillin absorption in man, *Eur. J. Clin. Pharmacol.*, 26, 279, 1984.
25. Neuhofel, A.L. et al., Lack of bioequivalence of ciprofloxacin when administered with calcium-fortified orange juice: a new twist on an old interaction, *J. Clin. Pharmacol.*, 42, 461, 2002.
26. Dahan, A. and Altman, H., Food-drug interaction: grapefruit juice augments drug bioavailability – mechanism, extent and relevance, *Eur. J. Clin. Nutr.*, 58, 1, 2004.
27. Lown, K.S. et al., Grapefruit juice increased felodipine oral availability in humans by decreasing intestinal CYP3A protein expression, *J. Clin. Invest.*, 99, 2545, 1997.
28. Bailey, D.G., Malcolm, J.M.O., and Spence, J.D., Grapefruit juice–drug interactions. *Br. J. Clin. Pharmocol.*, 46, 101, 1998.
29. Dresser, G.K., Spence, J.D., and Bailey, D.G., Pharmacokinetic-pharmacodynamic consequences and clinical relevance of cytochrome P450 3A4 inhibition, *Clin. Pharmacokinet.*, 38, 41, 2000.
30. Dresser, G.K. et al., Fruit juices inhibit organic anion transporting polypeptide-mediated drug uptake to decrease the oral availability of fexofenadine, *Clin. Pharmacol. Ther.*, 71, 11, 2002.
31. Dresser, G.K. and Bailey, D.G., The effects of fruit juices on drug disposition: a new model for drug interactions, *Eur. J. Clin. Invest.*, 33, 10, 2003.
32. Greenblatt, D.J. et al., Time course of recovery of cytochrome P4503A function after single doses of grapefruit juice, *Clin. Pahrmacol. Ther.*, 74, 121, 2003.
33. Bailey, D.G. et al., Grapefruit-felodipine interaction: effect of unprocessed fruit and probable active ingredients, *Clin. Pharmocol. Ther.*, 68, 468, 2000.

34. Malhotra, S. et al., Seville orange juice-felodipine interaction: comparison with dilute grapefruit juice and involvement of furocoumarins, *Clin. Pharmacol. Ther.*, 69, 14, 2001.
35. Hodek, P., Trefil, P., and Stiborova, M., Flavonoids-potent and versatile biologically active compounds interacting with cytochromes P450, *Chem. Biol. Interact.*, 139, 1, 2002.
36. Bailey, D.G. et al., Ethanol enhances the hemodynamic effects of felodipine, *Clin. Invest. Med.*, 12, 357, 1989.
37. Bailey, D.G. et al., Interaction of citrus juices with felodipine and nifedipine, *Lancet*, 337, 268, 1991.
38. Lundahl, J.U. et al., The interaction effect of grapefruit juice is maximal after the first glass, *Eur. J. Clin. Pharmacol.*, 54, 75, 1998.
39. Michalets, E.L. and Williams, C.R., Drug interactions with cisapride: clinical implications, *Clin. Pharmacokinet.*, 39, 49, 2000.
40. Erdeve O., Tiras U., and Dallar Y. The probiotic effect of Saccharomyces boulardii in a pediatric age group, *J. Tropical Ped.*, 50, 234, 2004.
41. Armuzzi A. et al, Effect of lactobacillus GG supplementation on antibiotic-associated gastrointestinal side effects during Helicobacter pylori eradication therapy: a pilot study, *Digestion.* 63, 1, 2001.
42. Hamilton-Miller JMT. The role of probiotics in the treatment and prevention of Helibacter pylori infection, *Int J Antimicrob. Agents.*, 22, 360, 2003.
43. Sorensen, J.M., Herb–drug, food–drug, nutrient–drug, and drug–drug interactions: mechanisms involved and their medical implications, *J. Altern. Complem. Med.*, 3, 293, 2002.
44. Morimoto, T., Effect of St. John's wort on the pharmacokinetics of theophylline in healthy volunteers, *J. Clin. Pharmacol.*, 44, 95, 2004.
45. Dennis, B.H. et al., *Well-Controlled Diet Studies in Humans: A Practical Guide to Design and Management*, American Dietetic Association, Chicago, 1997.
46. Hulley, S.B. et al., *Designing Clinical Research,* 2nd edition,. Williams & Wilkins, Baltimore, 2001.
47. Campbell, D. and Stanley, J., *Experimental and Quasi-Experimental Designs*, Rand McNally, Chicago, 1963.
48. McCabe, B.J., Prevention of food-drug interactions with special emphasis on older adults, *Curr. Opin. Clin. Nutr. Metab. Care,* 7, 21, 2004.
49. Utermohlen, V., Diet, nutrition, and drug interactions, in Shils, M.E., Olson, J.A., and Shike, M., *Modern Nutrition in Health and Disease,* 9th edition, Lea & Febiger, Philadelphia, 1998.
50. Crom, W.R., Pharmakokinetics in the child, *Environ. Health Perspec.*, 102, 111, 1994.
51. Prandota, J., Drug disposition in cystic fibrosis: progress in understanding pathophysiology and pharmacokinetics, *Pediatr. Infect. Dis. J.*, 6, 1111, 1987.
52. Dupuis, L.L. et al., Influence of food on the bioavailability of oral methotrexate in children, *J. Rheumatol.*, 22, 1570, 1995.
53. Andrade, S.E. et al., Prescription drug use in pregnancy, *Am. J. Obstet. Gynecol.*, 191, 398, 2004.
54. Holmes, D.G. and Kutz, K., Bioequivalence of a slow-release and a non-retard formulation of isradipine, *Am J. Hypertens.*, 6 Suppl, 70, 1993.
55. Welty D.F. et al., The temporal effect of food on tacrine bioavailability, *J Clin Pharmacol.* 34, 985, 1994.

19

Designing Experiments for Food–Drug Synergy: Safety Aspects

V.J. Feron, J.P. Groten, R.J.J. Hermus, D. Jonker, I. Meijerman, G.J. Mulder, F. Salmon, and E.D. Schoen

CONTENTS

19.1 Introduction

Food is essential to life, and optimized nutrition (functional foods) contributes to health and well-being. However, optimized foods also need to be safe according to the criteria defined in current food regulations, though in many cases, new concepts and new procedures will need to be developed and validated to assess functional food safety.[1–3]

The development of potent and effective drugs continues to be associated with concern regarding drug safety. The administration of a bioactive compound to humans is always accompanied by some element of risk that cannot be entirely avoided by extensive preclinical animal toxicity studies and the most rigorous and exhaustive clinical trials of a new drug in humans (phase I, II, and III studies) before it is introduced into the therapeutic market.[4] Therefore, after the drug has come onto the market (phase IV), studies are carried out under the normal conditions of use specified in the so-called Drug Master File.[3]

The safety evaluation of combined exposures to different foods or food components and drugs should focus on those combinations that have been shown or are expected to prevent or to reduce disease to an extent greater than that known for exposure to the separate substances. In a strict sense, detection of antagonism leading to lowered or less severe toxicity of a combination of chemicals is beyond the scope of hazard identification and risk assessment. However, because of its potential importance for the application of combinations of foods and drugs, antagonism should be considered in designing experiments. Particularly, in the case of anticancer drugs, reduction of side effects by nutrients or nonnutritive bioactive dietary components is of great health significance.

A variety of systems and designs to study the toxicity of combined chemical exposures (or chemical mixtures) as well as methods to analyze the data obtained are available.[5–25] Making the right choice is crucial for a successful study yielding interpretable results and allowing scientifically sound conclusions.[26]

After a short discussion on what foods and drugs have in common, definitions and basic concepts in mixture toxicology as well as types of possible toxicological interactions are briefly described. Major test systems and study designs are dealt with in some detail, including their strengths and limitations and taking into account that foods are complex chemical mixtures themselves. For hazard identification of combinations of foods, food components, and drugs, studies in experimental animals are still almost unavoidable. Possibilities will be discussed as to how far *in vitro* and *in silico* methods can or should be used. Using two examples, the choice of the test system and the use of the selected study design are illustrated.

19.2 What Foods and Drugs Have in Common

To better understand the toxicological implications of combined exposures to foods, food components, and drugs, a short section is devoted to what foods (nutrients) and drugs have in common.

A balanced mixture of nutrients (a balanced diet) is a prerequisite for human health, and, in fact is the preeminent "drug" of life. Both nutrients and drugs are bioactive, body-oriented chemicals. Unlike food-oriented additives and other (regulated) nonnutritive food components (e.g., residues of pesticides, disinfectants or solvents), nutrients have small margins of safety (margins between the recommended and the toxic doses).[27] Therefore, nutrients (essential to life) are also the food chemicals of greatest health concern.[20,27,28] Dietary imbalance may easily result in nutritional deficiencies but also in exceeding the (small) margin of safety of certain nutrients.

The toxicity of drugs is evaluated along the whole process of drug development and weighed against expected effectiveness. Studies to detect and identify severe toxic effects are performed in the early phase of the development whereas acceptable side effects within the therapeutic window are determined in patients at later stages. However, side effects are nowadays less well tolerated by patient populations. Occasionally, severe toxicity (side effects) has to be accepted, for instance in the case of anticancer and anti-HIV drugs. Clearly, for many drugs the margins of safety are small and sometimes absent. Because both nutrients and drugs are bioactive chemicals with often small or no margins of safety, they are priority chemicals with respect to possible adverse effects and health risks of combined exposures. It is not only toxicologically plausible, but it has also been demonstrated experimentally that the risk of adverse effects due to combined exposures increases with decreasing size of the margin of safety of the individual chemicals.[25,29–35] Moreover, from these studies it appeared that combined exposure to chemicals at (minimum) toxic effect levels of the individual compounds may lead to all kinds of (unexpected) adverse effects or absence of expected adverse effects due to additive actions or synergistic or antagonistic interactions.

From a toxicological point of view, foods are complex chemical mixtures, and in addition to nutrients, many commonly consumed foods contain non-nutritive bioactive compounds that may positively or negatively affect health. Seen as separate chemicals, these bioactive constituents are toxicologically similar to drugs. However, as present in foods, they are part of a complex chemical mixture and as such their biological activity (e.g., their toxicity) might be influenced by the food matrix.

In brief, aspects such as bioactivity, body orientation, essence for health, small margins of safety, and influence of the food matrix should be taken into account when designing experiments for hazard identification of combined exposures to foods, food components, and drugs.

19.3 Terminology and Basic Concepts in Mixture Toxicology

This section briefly describes a number of key definitions and basic concepts considered relevant for proper understanding of research on mixtures or combinations of chemicals.

19.3.1 Terminology

- A *mixture* of chemicals is characterized by simultaneity of exposure to the constituents as a result of their joint occurrence.[36,37]
- A *simple mixture* is defined as a mixture that consists of a relatively small number of chemicals, say 10 or less, the composition of which is qualitatively and quantitatively fully known (e.g., a cocktail of pesticides).[25,37–39]
- A *complex mixture* is defined as a mixture that consists of tens, hundreds, or thousands of chemicals, the composition of which is qualitatively and/or quantitatively not fully known (e.g., diesel exhaust, drinking water, food).[25,37,38]
- In a *(specified) combination* of chemicals, all chemicals are known, regardless of whether they occur as a mixture. The exposures to the individual chemicals may be sequential, or partly or completely overlapping and may involve different sources, routes, duration, and times.[36]
- *Combined or joint action* is defined as any outcome of exposure to multiple chemicals, regardless of source or of spatial or temporal proximity.[25,37,40]
- *Aggregate exposure* and *aggregate risk assessment* consider exposure and risk accumulated over time and across sources, environmental pathways, or exposure routes for a single chemical.[25,37,40]
- *Cumulative risk* is the combined risks from aggregate exposures to multiple chemicals, and *cumulative risk assessment* is the analysis and characterization of the combined health risk from multiple chemicals.[25,37,40]

19.3.2 Basic Concepts

To study and characterize the toxicity of simple mixtures one can make use of empirical and mechanistic models. In the last decade, empirical models have played a dominant role in identifying health and safety characteristics of chemical mixtures. "Empirical" means that only information on doses or concentrations and effects is available in addition to quantitative-dose and concentration-response relationships.[18] Empirical models are based on the work of pioneers in mixture toxicology, half a century ago, who defined three types of actions for combinations of chemicals that are still widely used today: independent (or dissimilar) joint action, similar joint action, and interaction.[41,42]

19.3.2.1 Independent (Dissimilar) Joint Action

Independent (dissimilar) joint action is also referred to as *simple independent action*[43] or *response addition*.[44,45] This type of joint action is noninteractive, i.e., the chemicals in the mixture do not affect the toxicity of one another. In other words, the chemicals are assumed to behave independently of one another so that the body's response to the first chemical is the same whether or not the second chemical is present. The modes of action and possibly the nature and site of the toxic effect differ among the chemicals in the mixture. The toxicity of the mixture can be predicted (calculated) from the dose-response curves of the individual chemicals. Response is expressed as the probability that an effect appears (viz., the likelihood of an individual or a proportion of a population showing an effect). The response to a mixture depends not only on the dose, but also on the correlation of the tolerances, which can vary between –1 and +1. In case the individual most sensitive to chemical 1 is also most sensitive to chemical 2, the susceptibilities (tolerances) are considered to show complete, positive correlation ($r = +1$). In this case, the response to the mixture of chemicals 1 and 2 would be equal to that attributed to the most toxic chemical. In contrast, if the correlation of tolerances would be completely negative ($r = -1$; the individual most sensitive to chemical 1 is least sensitive to chemical 2), the response to the mixture would be equal to the sum of the responses of the individual chemicals. If there is no correlation of tolerances ($r = 0$), then the chemicals are assumed to produce toxicity independently, and the mixture response is calculated by the standard formula for statistical independence:

$$P_{mix}(d_1,d_2) = P_1(d_1) + P_2(d_2)\ [P_1(d_1) * P_2(d_2)]$$

where $P_1(d_1)$, $P_2(d_2)$ and $P_{mix}(d_1,d_2)$ are the probabilities that an effect is induced by chemical 1 at dose d_1, chemical 2 at dose d_2, and their mixture, respectively. An important characteristic of response addition is that a chemical does not contribute to the mixture response when it is present at a level below its individual effect threshold.[25]

19.3.2.2 Similar Joint Action

Similar joint action[41,42] is also referred to as *simple similar action*,[43] *dose addition*,[44,45] or *concentration addition*.[46] Like independent joint action, similar joint action is noninteractive. The chemicals produce similar but independent effects, so that one chemical can be substituted at a constant proportion for the other. Under the narrow definition of dose addition,* the chemicals are assumed to behave similarly in terms of mode of action and primary physiological processes (uptake, metabolism, distribution, elimination), and to have similarly shaped (parallel) dose-response curves and complete positive correlation of individual susceptibilities. The chemicals differ only in their potencies. In practice, since information on the mode of action and toxicokinetics is often lacking, the requirement of toxicological similarity is usually relaxed to that of similarity of target organs.[45] The toxicity of the mixture can be calculated using summation of the doses of the individual chemicals after adjustment for the differences in potencies. The adding of doses implies that the summed dose can be high enough to induce a toxic effect even when the dose of each individual chemical is at a level below its individual effect threshold.

It should be realized that the preceding theoretical distinction between dose and response addition generally does not hold so strictly in whole organisms because of the complexity and interdependence of their physiological systems. When a mixture contains many chemicals, it is unlikely that the mode of toxic action is the same for all chemicals and the application of full dose addition would overestimate the toxicity of the mixture. On the other hand, it is also unlikely that all chemicals in such a mixture have completely different modes of action. It is more reasonable to assume an intermediate form of noninteractive joint action.[25,37]

19.3.2.3 Interaction

Interaction, in a broad sense, is defined as one chemical influencing the biological action of the other.[46] Operationally, interaction can be defined as the type of joint action showing a mixture response which deviates from that expected on the basis of (dose or response) addition. Interactive joint actions can be less than additive (e.g., antagonistic, inhibitory, infra- or subadditive) or greater than additive (e.g., synergistic, potentiating, supraadditive). Terms such as antagonism or synergism indicate in which direction a response to a mixture differs from what is expected under the assumption of additivity. However, they provide no information about the mechanisms or quantitative aspects of interactions.

Often, three types of mechanisms for underlying interactions are distinguished: direct chemical–chemical, toxicokinetic, and toxicodynamic mechanisms.[37]

* Broader definitions allow for nonlinear or nonparallel curves, imperfect correlation of tolerances, or different modes (not sites) of primary action.[11,46,47]

In direct *chemical–chemical interactions*, one chemical directly interacts with another, causing a chemical change in one or more of the compounds. In many cases, this mechanism results in decreased toxicity (less than additive effect) and is one of the common principles of antidotal treatment. A well-known example of chemical–chemical interactions leading to greater than additive effects is the formation of carcinogenic nitrosoamines in the stomach through the reaction of noncarcinogenic nitrite (from drinking water or food) with amines (e.g., from fish protein).

Toxicokinetic interactions involve alterations in metabolism (biotransformation) or disposition of a chemical. Interactions during absorption, distribution, metabolism, and excretion are often distinguished. Essentially, toxicokinetic interactions alter the amount of the toxic agents reaching the cellular target sites without qualitatively affecting the toxicant–receptor site interaction. With respect to their toxicological consequences, interactions in the process of metabolism (enzyme induction or inhibition) are considered most relevant. However, the impact of alterations in absorption, distribution, or excretion is not to be neglected and can have life threatening consequences even at low doses, e.g., in case of impaired renal function.[48,49]

Toxicodynamic interactions affect a tissue's response or susceptibility to toxic injury. They include, for example, immunomodulation, alterations in protective factors (depletion or induction), and changes in tissue repair or hemodynamics.[45] Alternatively, toxicodynamic interactions are described as interactions occurring at or among cellular receptor sites. Interactions at the same receptor site resulting in antagonism have been termed "receptor antagonism" (e.g., the antagonistic effect of oxygen on carbon monoxide). Interactions resulting from different chemicals acting on different receptor sites and causing opposite effects have been termed "functional antagonism" (e.g., opposing effects of histamine and noradrenaline on vasodilatation and blood pressure).[50]

Drug–drug interactions have been reported in the past[47,51] and are presently being reported with increasing frequency in the medical and pharmaceutical literature, thus emphasizing the necessity of determining which of those interactions require attention in the clinical setting. It is imperative that health care practitioners be given tools to focus on the most important drug interactions in order to improve clinical outcomes and patients' well-being. Moreover, in several reviews on chemicals of occupational or environmental concern, examples of interactions have been documented.[47,52,53]

19.4 Test Systems and Study Designs

Given the diversity of scenarios for exposure to mixtures or combinations of chemicals and the wide variety of questions to be addressed in the safety evaluation of such exposures, it is not surprising that there is no "one size fits all" design and method of data analysis for studying the toxicity of mixtures or combined exposures.[14]

Moreover, a number of test systems ranging in principle from studies in volunteers to computer simulations are available. An important issue in toxicology is the suitability of the data obtained with experimental animals for human risk assessment. Because it is not possible to use humans in long-term toxicological studies, the use of animals will continue to be necessary. However, the data obtained in animal studies can be better extrapolated to the exposure situation in humans by utilizing bridging studies with *in vitro* models combined with computational approaches. There are also several types of modeling approaches (empirical or mechanistic). Empirical models are used to collect quantitative information on dose-response relationships while the use of mechanistic models is based on information on biological mechanisms at the target site or organ, allowing dose-response relationships to be described as physico(bio)chemical equations (e.g., competitive agonism, Michaelis-Menten kinetics) for receptor interactions or substrate–enzyme kinetics.

To make the right choice regarding test system, study design and methods of data analysis is a prerequisite, if not a *conditio sine qua non,* for successfully studying a certain aspect of the safety of combined exposures to foods, food components, and drugs. The choice should be made by a team of experienced experts consisting of a nutritionist, pharmacist, mixture toxicologist, and a toxicology-oriented biostatistician. The following factors determine to a large extent the choice to be made:

- Number of constituents (two or more than two individual components or a food which itself is a complex chemical mixture);
- Number of dose levels to be tested (dose levels of the combination and/or the individual components; need or desirability to establish dose-effect and dose-response curves);
- Extent to which the toxicity of the combination of chemicals has to be characterized (the relative contribution of the constituents to the toxicity of the combination as well as the mechanism underlying potential joint or interactive effects);
- Desirability of detecting potential antagonistic effects (clear adverse effect levels have to be included);
- Type and amount of toxicological information on the individual components already available (target organs, critical effects, mechanisms underlying the toxic effects, observed-adverse-effect levels and no-observed-adverse-effect levels (NOAEL) of the individual components; data on adverse effects of the individual components in humans);
- History of (safe) use in humans;
- Anticipated exposure scenarios;

- Available resources (budget, personnel, facilities) and time frame (these practicalities may dictate a less than optimal design).

19.4.1 Test Systems

19.4.1.1 In Vivo Systems

Studies in experimental animals and human volunteers are indispensable for the safety evaluation of combined exposures to foods, food components, and drugs. For ethical reasons, studies in volunteers can only be carried out if careful evaluation of all available data leads to the conclusion (to be drawn by an independent ethical committee) that no unacceptable risk is being run. The end points should be "short term" and indicative of reversible disturbances of physiology rather than of cell, tissue, or organ damage.

Pharmaco- or toxicodynamic interaction may be caused by a large variety of mechanisms. When similar mechanisms and/or effects are found in animals and in humans, then animal studies can be used to characterize the potential interaction.[54] Toxicokinetic studies will usually pick up interactions at the absorption, distribution, metabolism, excretion (ADME) level and thus, will contribute to more confident interspecies extrapolation. However, differences in drug metabolism pathways between species may make interactions at the ADME level species specific.

To avoid unacceptable risks in volunteers, toxicity testing in animals usually has to precede safety studies in humans. However, for reasons of animal welfare and ethics, the number of studies in experimental animals as well as the number of animals used should be as small as possible, which means that any study in animals should be carefully planned, well designed, and conducted in conformity with the principles of good laboratory practice. In this respect it is very helpful that for a wide variety of validated standard animal toxicity tests international guidelines developed by the Organisation for Economic Cooperation and Development are available.[55] Obviously, when selecting an animal model, its suitability for predicting effects in humans should be considered.

19.4.1.2 In Vitro Systems

Apart from mutagenicity assays, the greatest use of *in vitro* methods is for elucidating metabolism and the mechanisms underlying toxic effects or responses to xenobiotics, including food components and drugs.[56,57] In terms of mechanistic understanding, interactions between compounds may occur in the kinetic or the dynamic phase. The most obvious cases for interactions in the kinetic phase are enzyme induction or inhibition because metabolism is an important determinant of toxicity. Compounds that influence the amount of biotransformation enzymes can have large effects on the action of other chemicals. Drug–drug interactions mediated by the drug metabolizing enzyme cytochrome P450 are rather common and can lead to serious clinical effects.[58] Indeed, clearance pathways by cytochrome P450 enzymes of the liver and gut have proven especially vulnerable given that many of the drug interactions that result in large (greater than 50%) changes in exposure do so through inhibition or induction of cytochrome P450 in the liver. It should, however, be kept in mind that this is not the only mechanism responsible for drug–drug interactions with clinically serious consequences, and that every possible clearance pathway for a substrate (such as active renal secretion, drug degradation in the gut, biliary excretion, and secretion based on cellular transport mechanisms) may be altered by an interacting compound. Therefore, a practical approach to defining *in vitro* the interaction potential of drugs is based on a mechanistic evaluation in three steps: (1) identification of the major enzymes involved in the clearance of the drug, (2) evaluation of the inhibitory potential of the drug toward metabolizing enzymes, and (3) evaluation of the induction potential of the drug toward metabolic systems.

Because of major (qualitative and quantitative) differences between human and animal metabolizing enzymes, the most useful *in vitro* systems have been developed from human liver.[59] Liver microsomes, hepatocytes, liver slices, and cell lines expressing individual human metabolizing enzymes are commonly used in the early phases of drug development to determine the interaction potential of a drug candidate. A guidance document for industry from the U.S. Food and Drug Administration[60] describes techniques and approaches to study *in vitro* metabolism-based interactions, *in vitro–in vivo* correlations, the timing of such studies, and the labeling of drug products based on such data.

Of special interest to food and drug toxicologists are systems using pieces of intestine and intestinal cells, for instance, to study interactions at the absorption level among (micro) nutrients, other food components, and drugs. A validated model very suitable for studying such interactions is the multicompartimental dynamic computer-controlled *in vitro* gastrointestinal model simulating the conditions of the stomach and the small and large intestines, including peristaltic movements, water absorption, and absorption of fermentation products.[61–63] It consists of a gastric–small-intestinal part and a large-intestinal part that can operate independently of one another but can also be connected to each other. A limitation of the model is the absence of intestinal epithelium, implying that there are no physiological interactions with enterocytes and no intestinal xenobiotic enzyme activities. This means that the model cannot simulate the response of the body to the bioaccessible chemicals in the "gastrointestinal content." However, the model can be combined with intestinal segments in transport chambers or with a Caco-2 system (colon cancer cells differentiated to a monolayer of epithelial cells), which makes it possible to predict type of transport and absorption rate *in vivo*.[64,65] This *in vitro* gastrointestinal model has been shown to be a powerful screening tool in food and drug research, reducing the number of experimental animal studies substantially.[66–69]

19.4.1.3 Physiologically Based Pharmacokinetic Modeling and in Silico Systems

Early screening systems, like *in vitro* preparations of human microsomes can give an indication if a pharmacokinetic interaction between a new and an existing drug is possible. However, it is difficult to interpret the relevance of such an *in vitro* interaction for the clinical situation. Therefore, recently a physiologically based pharmacokinetic (PBBK) approach has been introduced to integrate human pharmacokinetics of both substrate and inhibitor (e.g., an old and new drug) with *in vitro* inhibition constants. The model contains a detailed gastrointestinal tract submodel to predict portal blood concentrations from an oral dose and, for the time being, uses a two-compartment model for the distribution within the body. Drug-specific parameters are chosen such that they can all be obtained from *in vitro* data. The following *in vitro* parameters are needed: intestinal absorption in Caco-2 system, intrinsic liver clearance, and tissue–blood or tissue–plasma partition coefficients. Interaction between substrate and inhibition in the liver is described by inhibition constant K_i. The model was tested with a substrate and an inhibitor of CYP3A4 by simulating the effect of an oral dose of 200 mg ketoconazole on 6 mg midazolam. Because CYP3A4 is also active in the small intestine, metabolism and inhibition of the gastrointestinal tract were added to these model compartments. The model was validated by comparing the plasma kinetics of the two compounds individually with literature data and then used to predict the interaction between the two compounds (C_{max}, area under the curve). Predictions were compared with experimental inhibition data, showing a pronounced ameliorative effect of ketoconazole on the clearance of midazolam.[70]

PBPK models have been used in mixture toxicology mainly for two purposes:

1. To estimate the internal dose (in the target tissue) of the individual components that results from external exposure to a mixture or combination of chemicals. PBPK models for simple mixtures have been developed and successfully applied,[71–73] and occasionally, very sophisticated models have been used to deal with complex mixtures.[74–76]
2. To investigate interactions in the toxicokinetic phase.

In the past decade, considerable knowledge on the mechanistic background of specific interactions has been acquired, especially on interactions caused by inhibition or induction of different P450 isoenzymes.[77] Methods that describe binary interactions have been successfully used for health risk assessment of mixtures of organic compounds.[78] Several PBPK models that offer the possibility of incorporating interference between compounds in the same metabolic pathway have been described.[79–81] Using a model for competitive inhibition of metabolism between all compounds, Haddad et al.[80] and Krishnan et al.[82] described an approach that involves the development

ing an unbalanced diet and nutritional deficiencies. In such a situation it might be worthwhile to consider the use of the so-called "top-*n*" or "pseudo top *n*" approach. These approaches have been suggested for the safety evaluation of complex chemical mixtures such as welding fumes, workplace atmospheres, and indeed also foods.[18,36,87] The top *n* approach begins with the identification of the *n*, say four or five or eight, most risky (not the most toxic!) chemicals in a complex mixture. The pseudo top *n* approach starts off with identifying the *n* most risky classes of chemicals followed by identification of a representative chemical or pseudochemical for each class, using the lumping technique. The selected pseudo top *n* chemicals are either representative chemicals of each class or pseudochemicals representing a fictitious average of a certain class. The lumping technique is based on grouping chemicals with relevant similarities, such as the same target organ and/or similar mode of action.[74] The pseudo top *n* approach is suggested for complex mixtures that consist of many, widely varying chemicals with no obvious ranking of individual constituents according to potential health risk, and thus, seems to be particularly suitable for foods. Identification of the top *n* or pseudo top *n* might not be easy because of lack of relevant data. However, for commonly used foods, available data on chemical composition, intake levels, and toxicity might help a team of experienced nutritionists and food toxicologists in establishing these priority chemicals or classes of them. Once the top *n* or pseudo top *n* chemicals have been identified, they will be approached as a simple, defined mixture, assuming that hazard and potential risk of the mixture of the top *n* or pseudo top *n* chemicals represent the hazard and risk of the entire mixture. A very similar approach is successfully being used in the United States to identify the priority substances (the top *n* substances) that are released from hazardous waste sites and that pose the greatest risk to human health.[88–90]

19.4.2.2 Component-Based Studies

Compared with whole-combination studies, a more specific and more informative approach is to study the combined toxicity of the components and to compare the results with the toxicity of the individual components. To be able to ascribe the adverse effect of the combination to dose addition (similar joint action) or effect or response addition (dissimilar joint action) or to synergistic (or antagonistic) interaction or to combinations of these, dose-effect or dose-response curves for each of the individual components are needed.[20] For component-based studies, several experimental designs are available, and the choice mainly depends on the number of components and the complexity of the combination.[18]

19.4.2.2.1 Isobolographic Method

The isobolographic method is the classical approach to determine whether two chemicals interact[19,22,47,91–93] An isobologram is a graphical representation of the joint effect of two chemicals in which the doses of chemicals 1 and 2 are given on the *x*- and *y*-axis, respectively, and the experimentally determined dose combinations of 1 and 2, which all cause the same effect (e.g., 50% mortality), are plotted and connected by a line: the isoeffect line or isobole (or contour of constant response). This experimentally determined line is then compared with the theoretical isoeffect line based on the assumption of additivity. Correspondence of the two lines indicates additivity, and differences between these lines indicate departure from additivity. Isoboles below the line of additivity indicate synergism (in the presence of chemical 1, less of chemical 2 is required to generate the response predicted in case of additivity); those above it indicate antagonism. The isobolographic method requires a large number of data points (extensive studies) that are not fully exploited. Another disadvantage is that there is no easy statistical basis for conclusions to be drawn. Also, because of its graphical nature and use of perpendicular axes, isobolograms are unsuitable for combinations of more than three chemicals. For a detailed description of the basic principles of the method, including a discussion about its strengths and limitations, the reader is referred to Cassee et al.[20] More complex versions of the isobolographic method are available, such as the construction of an additivity envelope[94] or the use of a system of parallel coordinate axes representing hyperdimensional figures plus a polynomial model to characterize interaction effects.[6]

19.4.2.2.2 Interaction-Index Method

The interaction-index method proposed by Berenbaum[95,96] is related to the isobolographic method (both use isoeffective doses) but does not require plotting of the isobologram and can be used for mixtures or combinations of any number of chemicals. Under Berenbaum's definition of additivity, noninteractive combinations satisfy the equation:

$$d_1/D_1 + d_2/D_2 + \ldots + d_i/D_i = 1;$$

D_1, D_2, … D_i are doses of the individual chemicals 1, 2, … *i* that produce some specified effect when given alone, and d_1, d_2, …d_i are their doses in a combination that produces the same effect. The sum of the fractions on the left side of the equation is termed the interaction index, which is less than 1 for synergy, 1 for zero interaction (additivity), and greater than 1 for antagonism. These criteria are independent of the type of effect under consideration, the shapes of the dose-response curves, or the homogeneity of the target population, and do not require any assumptions about mechanisms of action of the chemicals. The interaction index covers combinations of an active chemical with a chemical that does not affect the endpoint of interest (for the inactive chemical D_i may be assumed to be infinite so that d_i/D_i is zero).

As with the isobolographic method, a problem of the interaction index method is the statistical analysis; it is not immediately clear how different

To analyze the data obtained from combination studies using (fractional) factorial designs, effect–response surface analysis is particularly suitable. This widely used method permits the use of readily available statistical methods, and thus accounts for variability in the experimental data.[92,98] Clear descriptions of the effect–response surface method are presented by Cassee et al.[20] and Tallarida.[22] For further details of this methodology, including discussions on dose dependency of interactions and statistical analysis of the data, the reader is referred to Sühnel,[17] Greco et al.,[12] and Groten et al.[18]

19.4.2.2.4 Departure from Additivity

Instead of modeling the concentration–response relationship for a mixture of chemicals to detect departures from additivity, Berenbaum[99] and Gennings[13,100] have proposed methods based on the concentration-response relationships of each individual chemical. In this "additivity approach" the concentration-response relationships of the individual chemicals are used to calculate the expected response for a given combination, under the assumption of additivity. Then the predicted response is compared with the response for that combination observed experimentally. For a mixture of k chemicals, the number of groups required would be $(m * k) + 1$ (m levels of k chemicals + the combination), which is much less than the m^k groups required for a complete factorial design. A disadvantage of this additivity approach is that it can only show whether the effect of the whole mixture deviates from additivity; it is unable to identify the chemicals that cause interaction. Steps 1 and 2 of the study on mycotoxins by Tajima et al.[23] described above in some detail (see Sections 19.4.2.1.1 and 19.4.2.2.3) may serve as an example of testing for "departure from additivity," using the dose-response relationships of the individual mycotoxins to calculate the expected response for a certain combination, under the assumption of additivity.

19.4.2.2.5 General Approaches in Drug Development

Early *in vitro* and *in vivo* pharmacological and toxicological investigations enhance the quality and efficiency of drug development, in some cases fully addressing a question of interest, in others providing information to guide further studies. The early elucidation of metabolism, for example, permits *in vitro* investigation of drug interaction potential that in turn provides information useful in guiding the clinical program. Metabolism data can also provide information on the relevance of the preclinical toxicology program and allows the early identification of drugs that are likely to have a large interindividual pharmacokinetic variability due to the involvement of polymorphic enzymes. An integrated approach that considers interaction potential at all stages of drug development is most useful and should include (1) preclinical *in vitro* studies to determine which interaction studies should be conducted *in vivo*, (2) early phase *in vivo* studies to assess the most potential interaction suggested by the *in vitro* data, and (3) late-phase population pharmacokinetic studies to expand the range of interactions studied, including unexpected ones, and to examine pharmacodynamic interactions such as synergisms. These steps address the goals of risk assessment (determination of whether an important interaction is present), risk management (adjustment in drug dosing in the presence of an interacting component), and risk communication (provision of labeling statement on how to manage the risk). In terms of risk management, the magnitude of the interaction may be so great or the effect of the interacting component may be so pervasive that special actions might be required, e.g., one drug may be removed from the market, or labeling may state that the drug and the interacting component should not be given concurrently.

19.5 Examples

Two examples are described to illustrate the way in which a study can be designed that contributes to establishing "safe" dose levels for combinations of foods, food components, and drugs. The two combinations chosen are (1) soy and tamoxifen and (2) grape seed extract (GSE) and doxorubicin (DOX). It was assumed that all four substances possess anticancer activity and that both combinations have been shown to be more effective than the separate substances. To optimize clinical application of these combinations, information about their toxicity is crucial. There is a substantial body of data on the toxicity of soy and soy isoflavones,[101–105] tamoxifen,[106–109]and DOX,[110] but toxicity data on GSE[111] and on the combinations mentioned are scarce or nonexistent.[112,113]

The first example concerns a standard 4-week toxicity study in rats comparing the toxicity of combinations of soy and tamoxifen with that of the individual substances. Review of the available toxicological information on both substances led to the conclusion that at present such a study is most suitable as a first step of a testing strategy, ultimately resulting in establishing optimal dose levels of tamoxifen for patients on soy-based diets.* The second example deals with *in vitro* studies addressing the biotransformation, toxicokinetics, and the possible cytotoxicity of combinations of DOX and GSE. This *in vitro* study might be a first step toward understanding the mechanism of toxicity of the combined toxicity of these compounds. To translate such *in vitro* findings into dosage regimes or therapeutic advice, *in vivo* studies as well as clinical trials are necessary.

* For the sake of these examples, it was assumed that this is a justifiable conclusion. However, in reality experts currently involved in studies on health and safety aspects of combined exposures to soy and tamoxifen may reach a different conclusion.

PXR, indicating the possibility of interaction with DOX. Further studies, therefore, are warranted.

Besides biotransformation by CYPs, phase II conjugation reactions can also play a substantial role in the metabolic conversion of a drug. Intact liver systems, such as isolated human hepatocytes and subcellular liver fractions, but also suitable cell lines, can be used to study the effect of GSE on phase II enzyme activity and the availability of necessary cofactors, like glutathione.[115] Gluthatione S-transferase (GST) is especially of interest because increased expression of GSTπ, an isoenzyme of GST, has been associated with resistance of cancer cells to DOX.[119] Because DOX is supposed to be cardiotoxic through the formation of an oxidative semiquinone metabolite, and myocardial cells contain low concentrations of catalase, superoxide dismutase, and glutathione peroxidase, it would also be necessary to test the effect of GSE on these enzymes.

19.5.2.3 **Drug Transport**

Inhibition or induction of drug transporters such as P-glycoprotein (MDR1) and Multidrug Resistance Protein 2 (MRP2) can influence oral bioavailability and elimination by the liver, possibly affecting efficacy and toxicity of drugs. The effect of GSE on DOX transport can be studied by several *in vitro* systems, using several concentrations of GSE and DOX: (1) transport assays in which apical–basal transport through cultured monolayers of cells (CaCo-2, HCT-8, T8, and MDCK) is measured, (2) drug accumulation and efflux assays where the accumulation of a drug or substrate is measured within cells, (3) ATPase assay where the activity of a transporter is measured indirectly by measuring the ATP-ase activity, and (4) labeling and binding assays.[120]

19.5.2.4 **Pharmacodynamics**

DOX disrupts the uncoiling of DNA by topoisomerase II, intercalates between DNA strands, and causes DNA lesions. Therefore, the replication of rapidly dividing tumor cells will be inhibited preferentially.[110] DOX can also stimulate Fas-receptor mediated apoptosis. The possibility that GSE interferes with the capability of DOX to inhibit tumor growth and induce apoptosis can be determined by exposing a representative tumor cell panel to several, clinically relevant concentrations of DOX and GSE. Cell growth and apoptosis can then be measured by specific, commercially available assays. The same approach can be used to study possible cytotoxic effects of the combination of DOX and GSE on nontumor cells, for instance, Berse cells and human liver cells.

19.5.2.5 **Clinical Toxicology**

Potential genotoxicity and carcinogenicity of DOX could change when DOX and GSE are combined. However, genotoxicity and carcinogenicity studies are not required for phase I clinical trials in cancer patients. Depending on the results of the *in vitro* studies with DOX and GSE, an appropriate physiologically based computer model can be built to extrapolate the DOX–GSE interaction to the pharmacokinetic or pharmacodynamic relationship *in vivo*. The advantage of an *in silico* approach at this stage would be the possibility of simulating various patient populations by introducing a Monte-Carlo analysis of various relevant parameters, such as metabolic capacity, that might be highly variable between individuals. To translate the *in vitro* findings about possible interactions between DOX and GSE into a dosage adjustment or therapeutic advice, both *in vivo* studies and clinical trials based on the outcome of the *in vitro* studies are necessary.

19.6 Conclusions

In addition to knowledge about test systems, study designs and methods of data analysis, knowledge of the basic concepts of combination (mixture) toxicology is crucial for designing relevant, scientifically sound studies regarding the safety evaluation of combined exposures to foods, food components, and drugs. Therefore, the best guarantee for a successful study is the formation of a team of experienced experts (for instance, a nutritionist, pharmacist, mixture toxicologist, and biostatistician) that discusses and finally defines the study to be performed or the testing strategy to be followed.

For many drugs side effects are unavoidable, so prevention or reduction of such effects may be achieved through simultaneous or sequential exposure to (functional) foods or food chemicals. Clearly, studies aimed at evaluating the safety of combinations of food, food components, and drugs should be designed in a way that also allows for the detection of antagonistic effects.

For ethical, economic, and practical reasons, studies in experimental animals should be carried out only when alternatives are not available or are expected to produce inadequate information. This is generally true for toxicity studies but is of particular relevance for combination toxicity studies because in these latter studies the number of test groups will increase exponentially with increasing numbers of chemicals and dose levels, leading to unjustifiably large numbers of animals and an unmanageable study size, and thus, ultimately to impracticable studies. This problem can partly be solved by using fractionated factorial designs, keeping the number of animals reasonably low, and the number of test groups manageable.[87] Another part of the solution seems to be further development of *in vitro* systems in combination with computational approaches (*in silico* methods) and small-scale mechanistic studies in human volunteers.[83,121] Obviously, for the safety evaluation of combined exposures to foods and drugs, a testing strategy should be developed based on a step-by-step and question-and-answer approach, focusing on the right study at the right moment. This seems to be an efficient,

37. Jonker, D. et al., Safety evaluation of chemical mixtures and combinations of chemical and non-chemical stressors, *Rev. Environ. Health,* 19, 83, 2004.
38. Feron, V.J. et al., Toxicology of chemical mixtures: challenges for today and the future, *Toxicology,* 105, 415, 1995.
39. Feron, V.J., Groten, J.P., and Bladeren, P.J. van, Exposure of humans to complex chemical mixtures: hazard identification and risk assessment, *Arch. Toxicol.,* Suppl. 20, 363, 1998.
40. United States Environmental Protection Agency, Framework for cumulative risk assessment, EPA/600/P-02/001F, 01 Jan 2003, United States Environmental Protection Agency, Office of Research and Development, National Center for Environmental Assessment, Washington, D.C., 2003.
41. Bliss, C.I., The toxicity of poisons applied jointly, *Ann. Appl. Biol.,* 26, 585, 1939.
42. Plackett, R.L. and Hewlett, P.S., Quantal responses to mixtures of poisons, *J. Roy. Statist. Soc., Series B,* 14, 143, 1952.
43. Finney, D.J., *Probit Analysis,* Cambridge University Press, Cambridge, 1971.
44. United States Environmental Protection Agency, Guidelines for the health risk assessment of chemical mixtures, *Fed. Regis.,* 51 (185) 34014–34025, 1986.
45. United States Environmental Protection Agency, Supplementary Guidance for Conducting Health Risk Assessment of Chemical Mixtures, EPA/630/R-00/002, United States Environmental Protection Agency, Washington, D.C., 2000.
46. Kodell, R.L. and Pounds, J.G., Assessing the toxicity of mixtures of chemicals, in *Statistics in Toxicology,* Krewski, D. and Franklin, C., Eds., Gordon and Breach, New York, 1991, p. 559.
47. Calabrese, E.J., *Multiple Chemical Interactions,* Lewis Publishers, Inc., Chelsea, 1991.
48. Brown, B.A. et al., Clarithromycin-associated digoxin toxicity in the elderly, *Clin. Infect. Dis.,* 24, 92, 1997.
49. Wakasugi, H. et al., Effect of clarithromycin on renal excretion of digoxin: interaction with P-glycoprotein, *Clin. Pharmacol. Ther.,* 64, 123, 1998.
50. Mumtaz, M.M. and Hertzberg, R.C., The status of interactions data in risk assessment of chemical mixtures, in *Hazard Assessment of Chemicals,* Vol. 8, Saxena, J., Ed., Taylor and Francis, Washington, D.C., 1993, p. 47.
51. Aarons, L., Kinetics and drug-drug interactions, in *International Encyclopedia of Pharmacology and Therapeutics*, Section 122, Phamacokinetics: Theory and Methodology, Rowland, M. and Tucker, G.T., Eds., Pergamon Press, Oxford, 1986, p. 163.
52. Vouk, V.B. et al., *Methods for Assessing the Effects of Mixtures of Chemicals*, Scope 30, SGOMSEC 3, John Wiley & Sons, Chichester, 1987.
53. World Health Organisation, Health Effects of Combined Exposures in the Work Environment, WHO Technical Report Series no. 662, World Health Organisation, Geneva, 1981.
54. Note for Guidance on the Investigation of Drug Interaction, Committee for Proprietary Medicinal Products, CPMP/EWP/560/95; http://www.emea.eu.int, access date: 21 April 2005.
55. Feron, V.J., Introduction to adverse effects of food and nutrition, in *Food Safety and Toxicity,* Vries, J. de, Ed., CRC Press, Boca Raton, FL, 1997, chap. 8.
56. Spielmann, H., and Goldberg, A. M., In vitro methods, in *Toxicology,* Marquardt, H., Schäfer, S.G., McCLellan, R.O., and Welsch, F., Eds., Academic Press, San Diego, 1999, chap. 49.

57. Spielmann, H., In-vitro-Methoden, in *Lehrbuch der Toxikologie,* Marquardt, H., and Schäfer, S., Eds., Wissenschaftliche Verlaggesellschaft mbH, Stuttgart, 2004, chap. 48.
58. Ishigam, M. et al., Inhibition of in vitro metabolism of simvastatin by itraconazole in humans and prediction of in vivo drug-drug interactions, *Pharm. Res.,*18, 622, 2001.
59. Wrighton S.A., Ring B.J., and Vanden Branden M., The use of *in vitro* metabolism techniques in the planning and interpretation of drug safety studies, *Toxicol. Path.,* 23, 199, 1995.
60. Food and Drug Administration, Drug Metabolism/Drug Interactions in the Drug Development Process: Studies *in Vitro,* Food and Drug Administration, http://www.fda.gov/cder, 1997, access date: 20 April 2005.
61. Minekus, M. et al., A multicompartimental dynamic computer-controlled model simulating the stomach and small intestine, *ATLA,* 23, 197, 1995.
62. Minekus, M., Development and validation of a dynamic model of the gastrointestinal tract, PhD thesis, Utrecht University, Utrecht, 1998.
63. Minekus, M. et al., A computer-controlled system to simulate the conditions of the large intestine with peristaltic mixing, water absorption and absorption of fermentation products, *Appl. Microbiol. Biotech.,* 53, 108, 1999.
64. Duizer, E. et al., Effects of cadmium chloride on the paracellular barrier function of intestinal epithelial cell lines, *Toxicol. Appl. Pharmacol.,* 155, 117, 1999.
65. Barthe, L., Woodley, J., Houin, G., Gastrointestinal absorption of drugs: methods and studies, *Fund. Clin. Pharmacol.,* 13, 154, 1999.
66. Krul, C. et al., Application of a dynamic *in vitro* gastrointestinal tract model to study the availability of food mutagens, using heterocyclic aromatic amines as model compounds, *Food Chem. Toxicol.,* 38, 783, 2000.
67. Venema, K. et al., TNO's in vitro large intestinal model: an excellent screening tool for functional food and pharmaceutical research, *Nutrition,* 24, 558, 2000.
68. Krul, C.A.M. et al., Metabolism of sinigrin (2-propenyl glucosinolate) by the human colonic microflora in a dynamic *in vitro* large-intestinal model, *Carcinogenesis,* 23, 1009, 2002.
69. Krul, C.A.M. et al., Intragastric formation and modulation of N-nitrosodimethylamine in a dynamic in vitro gastrointestinal model under human phsiological conditions, *Food Chem. Toxicol.,* 42, 51, 2004.
70. Freidig, A.P. et al., Evaluation of in vitro drug-drug interaction data using PBPK models, *Drug Metabolism Rev.,* 35, 22, 2003.
71. Yang, R.S.H. et al., The application of physiologically based pharmacokinetic/pharmacodynamic (BPK/PD) modeling for exploring risk assessment approaches of chemical mixtures, *Toxicol.Lett.,* 79, 193, 1995.
72. Simmons, J.E., Application of physiologically based pharmacokinetic modeling to combination toxicology, *Food Chem. Toxicol.,* 34, 1067, 1996.
73. Tardif, R. et al., Physiologically based pharmacokinetic modeling of a ternary mixture of alkyl benzenes in rats and humans, *Toxicol. Appl. Pharmacol.,* 144, 120, 1997.
74. Verhaar, H.J.M. et al., A proposed approach to study the toxicology of complex mixtures of petroleum products: the integrated use of QSAR, lumping analysis and PBPK/PD modeling, *Environ. Health Perspect.,* 105, 179, 1997.
75. El-Masri, H.A. et al., Applications of computational toxicology methods at the Agency for Toxic Substances and Disease Registry, *Int. J. Hyg. Environ. Health,* 205, 63, 2002.

113. Jones, J.L. et al., Genistein inhibits tamoxifen effects on cell proliferation and cell cycle arrest in T47D breast cancer cells, *Am. Surg.*, 68, 575, 2002.
114. Sharma, G. et al., Synergistic anti-cancer effects of grape seed extract and conventional cytotoxic agent doxorubicin against human breast carcinoma cells, *Breast Cancer Res. Treat.*, 85, 1, 2004.
115. Brandon, E.F. et al., An update on in vitro test methods in human hepatic drug biotransformation research: pros and cons, *Toxicol. Appl. Pharmacol.*, 189, 233, 2003.
116. Synold, T.W., Dussault, I., and Forman, B.M., The orphan nuclear receptor SXR coordinately regulates drug metabolism and efflux, *Nat. Med.*, 7, 584, 2001.
117. Willson, T.M. and Kliewer, S.A., PXR, CAR and drug metabolism, *Nat. Rev. Drug Discov.*, 1, 1259, 2002.
118. Raucy, J. L., Regulation of CYP3A4 expression in human hepatocytes by pharmaceuticals and natural products, *Drug Metab. Dispos.*, 31, 533, 2003.
119. Goto, S. et al., Doxorubicin-induced DNA intercalation and scavenging by nuclear glutathione S-ransferaseπ *FASEB J.*, 15, 2702, 2001.
120. Varma, M.V. et al., P-glycoprotein inhibitors and their screening: a perspective from bioavailability enhancement, *Pharmacol. Res.*, 48, 347, 2003.
121. Suk, W.A., Olden, K., and Yang, R.S.H., Chemical mixtures research: significance and future perspectives, *Environ. Health Persp.*, 110 (Suppl. 6), 891, 2002.

Index

D

E

M

N

O

U

V

W